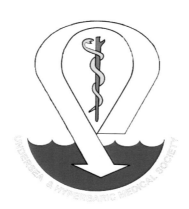

UNDERSEA AND HYPERBARIC MEDICAL SOCIETY

Hyperbaric Oxygen Therapy
INDICATIONS

14TH EDITION

Richard E. Moon MD
Chair and Editor

Undersea and Hyperbaric Medical Society
631 US Highway 1, Suite 307
North Palm Beach, FL 33408
USA

Copyright © 2019 Undersea and Hyperbaric Medical Society

ISBN: 978-1-947239-16-6

Library of Congress Catalog Number: 2019940027

Published by: Best Publishing Company
631 U.S. Highway 1, Suite 307
North Palm Beach, Florida 33408

Printed and bound in the United States of America

Table of Contents

Preface

The application of air under pressure (hyperbaric air) dates back to 1667, when Nathaniel Henshaw proposed a hypo-hyperbaric room pressurized and depressurized with an organ bellows.[1] In the nineteenth century, Simpson wrote a treatise on the use of compressed air for certain respiratory diseases.[2] The medicinal uses of oxygen were first reported by Beddoes in 1794,[3] while the first article describing adjunctive uses of hyperbaric oxygen therapy (HBO_2) was written by Fontaine in 1879,[4] who constructed a mobile operating room which could be pressurized. He observed that pressurized patients were not as cyanotic after the use of nitrous oxide during induction of anesthesia as compared to patients anesthetized at atmospheric pressure. In addition, he noted that hernias were much easier to reduce. Also around that time, the work of Paul Bert[5] and J. Lorrain-Smith[6] showed that oxygen under pressure had potentially deleterious consequences on the human body with side effects that included central nervous system and pulmonary toxicity. The efforts of Churchill-Davidson and Boerema in the 1950s and 1960s spurred the modern scientific use of clinical hyperbaric medicine.

In 1967, the Undersea Medical Society was founded by six United States Naval diving and submarine medical officers with the explicit goal of promoting diving and undersea medicine. In short order, this society expanded to include those interested in clinical hyperbaric medicine. In recognition of the dual interest by members in both diving and clinical applications of compression therapy, the society was renamed The Undersea and Hyperbaric Medical Society in 1986. It remains the leading not for profit organization dedicated to reporting scientifically and medically efficacious and relevant information pertaining to hyperbaric and undersea medicine.

In 1972, an ad hoc Medicare committee was formed to evaluate the efficacy of hyperbaric oxygen therapy for specified medical conditions. The focus was to determine if this treatment modality showed therapeutic benefit and merited insurance coverage. The growth of the body of scientific evidence that had developed over the preceding years supported this endeavor and recognition for the field. In 1976, the Hyperbaric Oxygen Therapy Committee became a standing committee of what was then the UMS. The first Hyperbaric Oxygen Committee Report was published in 1977 and served as guidance for practitioners and scientists interested in HBO_2. The report is usually published every three to five years and was last published in 2014. Additionally, this document continues to be used by the Centers for Medicare and Medicaid Services and other third party insurance carriers in determining payment.

The report, currently in its 14th edition, has grown in size and depth to reflect the evolution of the literature. To date, the committee recognizes 14 indications for which scientific and clinical evidence supports the use of HBO_2.

The Undersea and Hyperbaric Medical Society continues to maintain its reputation for its expertise on hyperbaric therapy. With leading experts authoring chapters in their respective fields, this publication continues to provide the most current and up to date guidance and support for scientists and practitioners of hyperbaric oxygen therapy.

Richard E. Moon MD
Editor, UHMS Committee Chair

References

1. Henshaw N. Aero-Chalinos or a register for the air for the better preservation of health and cure of diseases, after a new method. London. 1677.
2. Simpson A. Compressed Air as a Therapeutic Agent in the Treatment of Consumption, Asthma, Chronic Bronchitis and Other Diseases. Edinburgh: Sutherland and Knox; 1857.
3. Beddoes T, Watt J. Considerations of the Medicinal Use of Factitious Airs, and on the Manner of Obtaining Them in Large Quantities, First Edition, part II. Bristol: Bulgin and Rossier; 1794.
4. Fontaine JA. Emploi chirurgical de l'air comprime. Union Med. 1879;28:445.
5. Bert P. Barometric Pressure [Hitchcock MS, Hitchcock FA, translation]. Bethesda, MD: Undersea Medical Society; 1978. P. 579.
6. Lorrain-Smith J. The pathological effects due to increase of oxygen tension in the air breathed. J Physiol. 1899; 24:19-35.

Members of the Hyperbaric Oxygen Therapy Committee

Richard Moon MD (Chair)

Dirk Bakker MD
Robert Barnes MD
Michael Bennett MD
Enrico Camporesi MD
Paul Cianci MD
James Clark MD
William Dodson, MD
John Feldmeier DO
Laurie Gesell MD
Neil B. Hampson MD
Brett Hart MD
Enoch Huang MD
Irving Jacoby MD
Robert Marx DDS
Heather Murphy-Lavoie MD
Richard Roller MD
Ben Slade MD
Michael Strauss MD
Stephen Thom MD, PhD
Keith Van Meter MD
Lindell Weaver MD
Wilbur T. Workman MS

I. Background

The Undersea and Hyperbaric Medical Society (UHMS) is an international scientific organization which was founded in 1967 to foster exchange of data on the physiology and medicine of commercial and military diving. Over the intervening years, the interests of the Society have enlarged to include clinical hyperbaric oxygen therapy. The society has grown to over 2,000 members and has established the largest repository of diving and hyperbaric research collected in one place. Clinical information, an extensive bibliographic database of thousands of scientific papers, as well as books, and technical reports which represent the results of over 100 years of research by military and university laboratories around the world are contained in the UHMS Schilling Library, holdings are now part of the Duke University Library, Durham, NC. The results of ongoing research and clinical aspects of undersea and hyperbaric medicine are reported annually at scientific meetings and in *Undersea and Hyperbaric Medicine* published bi-monthly. Previously the society supported two journals, *Undersea Biomedical Research* and the *Journal of Hyperbaric Medicine*. These two journals were merged in 1993 into *Undersea and Hyperbaric Medicine*.

UHMS headquarters is located at:

631 US Highway 1, Suite 307
North Palm Beach, FL 33408
Phone: 561-776-6110 / 1-877-533-UHMS (8467)
FAX: 919-490-5149
Email: uhms@uhms.org
Internet: www.uhms.org

II. Hyperbaric Oxygen: Definition

The UHMS defines hyperbaric oxygen (HBO_2) as an intervention in which an individual breathes near 100% oxygen intermittently while inside a hyperbaric chamber that is pressurized to greater than sea level pressure (1 atmosphere absolute [ATA]). For clinical purposes, the pressure must equal or exceed 1.4 ATA while breathing near 100% oxygen. The United States Pharmacopoeia (USP) and Compressed Gas Association (CGA) Grade A specify medical grade oxygen to be not less than 99.0% by volume, and the National Fire Protection Association (NFPA) specifies USP medical grade oxygen.

In certain circumstances hyperbaric oxygen therapy represents the primary treatment modality while in others it is an adjunct to surgical or pharmacologic interventions.

The NFPA classifies chambers according to occupancy for the purposes of establishing minimum construction and operation requirements.[1]

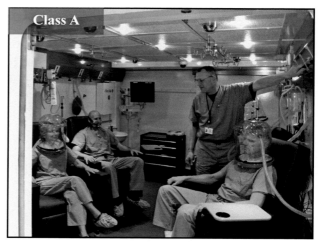

Figure 1. Multiplace Chamber

Photograph courtesy of Lindell Weaver MD, of Intermountain Medical Center, Murray, Utah. Fink DL8 multiplace chamber, Fink Engineering, Melbourne, Australia.

1. Class A – Human, multiple occupancy

2. Class B – Human, single occupancy

3. Class C – Animal, no human occupancy

Clinical treatments can be carried out in either a Class A (multi) or B (mono) chamber system. In a Class B system, the entire chamber is pressurized with near 100% oxygen, and the patient breathes the ambient chamber oxygen directly. A Class A system holds two or more people (patients, observers, and/or support personnel); the chamber is pressurized with compressed air while the patients breathe near 100% oxygen via masks, head hoods, or endotracheal tubes. It is important to note that Class B systems can and are pressurized with compressed air while the patients breathe near 100% oxygen via masks, head hoods, or endotracheal tubes.

According to the UHMS definition and the determination of The Centers for Medicare and Medicaid Services (CMS) and other third-party carriers, breathing medical grade near-100% oxygen at 1 atmosphere of pressure or exposing isolated parts of the body to 100% oxygen does not constitute HBO_2 therapy. The patient must receive the oxygen by inhalation within a pressurized chamber. Current information indicates that pressurization should be to 1.4 ATA or higher.

The literature of HBO_2 treatment began to appear during the 1930s as navies and universities around the world began studies in oxygen breathing at elevated pressures as a way to more safely decompress divers and to treat decompression sickness and arterial gas embolism. During the 1960s, HBO_2 was incorporated in standard treatment tables of the U.S. Navy. Extensive research on oxygen toxicity was undertaken to establish safe limits, overall safety, and medical and physiologic aspects of the compressed gas environment. These efforts led to a vast body of literature which underpins modern HBO_2 therapy.

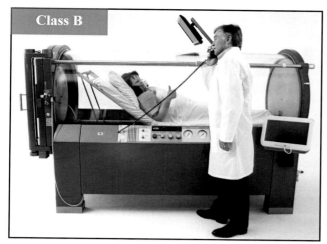

Figure 2. Monoplace Chamber
Photograph courtesy of Sechrist Industries.

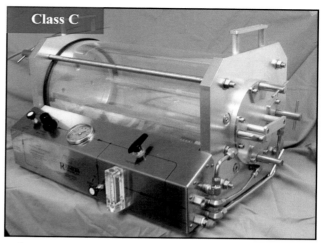

Figure 3. Animal Chamber
Photograph courtesy of Reimers Systems.

In 1976, recognizing the need for meticulous scrutiny of emerging clinical applications of HBO_2, the Executive Committee of the UHMS established the Hyperbaric Oxygen Therapy Committee. The Committee was charged with the responsibility of continuously reviewing research and clinical data and rendering recommendations regarding clinical efficacy and safety of HBO_2. To achieve this goal, the multispecialty committee is comprised of practitioners and scientific investigators in the fields of internal medicine, infectious diseases, pharmacology, emergency medicine, general surgery, orthopedic surgery, trauma surgery, thoracic surgery, otolaryngology, oral and maxillofacial surgery, anesthesiology, pulmonology, critical care, radiation oncology and aerospace medicine.

Since 1976, the Committee has met annually to review research and clinical data. From the 28 indications for which third-party reimbursement was recommended in the 1976 and 1979 reports, the number of recognized indications has been refined to 14 in the current report. These indications are those for which in vitro and in vivo pre-clinical research data as well as extensive positive clinical experience and study have become convincing.

Evidence considered by the Committee includes sound physiologic rationale; in vivo or in vitro studies that demonstrate effectiveness; controlled animal studies, prospective controlled clinical studies; and extensive clinical experience from multiple, recognized hyperbaric medicine centers.

The Committee requires that experimental and clinical evidence submitted for the efficacy of HBO_2 treatment for a disorder be at least as convincing as that for any other currently accepted treatment modality for that disorder. Studies in progress will continue to clarify mechanisms of action, optimal oxygen dosage, duration of exposure times, frequency of treatments, and patient selection criteria. The Committee recommends third party reimbursement of HBO_2 therapy for the disorders included in the accepted conditions category. Currently, most insurance carriers have established HBO_2 reimbursement policies.

The Committee also reviews cost effectiveness and has established guidelines for each entity. Results show that, in addition to its clinical efficacy, HBO_2 therapy yields direct cost savings by successfully resolving a high percentage of difficult and expensive disorders, thereby minimizing prolonged hospitalization. However, the Committee recommends that each individual hyperbaric facility, whether monoplace or multiplace, establish its own charges consistent with the actual local costs of providing such service.

III. Utilization Review for Hyperbaric Oxygen Therapy

A utilization review section is presented for each recognized HBO_2 indication. It is recommended that utilization review be obtained if the number of HBO_2 treatments is to exceed the recommended number of treatments for that indication. Such review should involve discussion of the clinical case with another qualified hyperbaric medicine physician from an outside institution. If that individual agrees that additional HBO_2 therapy is warranted, treatment may exceed the usually prescribed number of treatments.

IV. Acceptance (Addition) of New Indications for Hyperbaric Oxygen Therapy

New indications for HBO_2 therapy are considered for acceptance at the meeting of the Hyperbaric Oxygen Therapy Committee during the annual meeting of the Undersea and Hyperbaric Medical Society. This consideration can be initiated from within the Committee itself or may result in response to a written request by a non-Committee member. When a new indication is considered for acceptance, a position paper is written. The information must summarize the in vitro, in vivo, and clinical aspects of the new indication for HBO_2 therapy. Two members of the Hyperbaric Oxygen Committee review the position paper and each writes a critique. The position paper and critiques are presented to the Hyperbaric Oxygen Committee. A consensus of the Hyperbaric Oxygen Committee is required for recommending the indication be moved into the recognized category. If the Committee determines that a new condition merits acceptance, it makes this recommendation to the Executive Committee of the Society, which ultimately votes whether or not to recognize the new indication.

V. List of Abbreviations

ABI	ankle-brachial index
ACGIH	American Conference of Governmental Industrial Hygienists
AGE	arterial gas embolism
AHA	American Heart Association
AKA	above knee amputation
ANAM	automated neuropsychological assessment metric
ARDS	acute respiratory distress syndrome
ATA	atmospheres absolute
ATM	atmosphere
ATP	adenosine triphosphate
AVNFH	avascular necrosis of the femoral head
BCBS	Blue Cross Blue Shield
BCVA	baseline best corrected visual acuity
bFGF	basic fibroblast growth factor
BID	two times a day
BKA	below knee amputation
BMJ	*British Medical Journal*
BP	blood pressure
BRAO	branch retinal artery occlusion
BSA	body surface area
CABG	coronary artery bypass graft
CAGE	cerebral arterial gas embolism
CaO_2	arterial content of oxygen in blood
CAT	catalase
CBC	complete blood count
CDER	Center for Drug Evaluation and Research
CDRH	Center for Devices and Radiological Health
CDSR	Cochrane Database of Systematic Reviews
CEBM	Oxford Centre for Evidence-Based Medicine
CGA	Compressed Gas Association
cGy	centigray
CI	cardiac index
CMS	Centers for Medicare and Medicaid Services
CNS	central nervous system
CO_2	carbon dioxide
COHb	carboxyhemoglobin

CO	carbon monoxide
CONSORT	Consolidated Standards of Reporting Trials
CPA	O_2 stable lecithinase-C alpha toxin
CPB	cardiopulmonary bypass
CPG	clinical practical guidelines
CRA	central retinal artery
CRAO	central retinal artery occlusion
CSF	cerebrospinal fluid
CT	computed tomography
cTnI	troponin I
CV	cardiovascular
CVA	cerebrovascular accident
CvO_2	venous content of oxygen in blood
DAI	diffuse axonal injury
dB	decibel
DCI	decompression illness
DCS	decompression sickness
DFU	diabetic foot ulcer
dL	deciliter
DM	diabetes
DO_2	oxygen delivery
EBI	evidence-based indications
EBM	evidence-based medicine
ECHM	European Committee for Hyperbaric Medicine
EKG	electrocardiogram
EMS	emergency medical services
ENT	ear, nose, and throat
eNOS	endothelial nitric oxide synthase
EPC	endothelial progenitor cells
ESR	erythrocyte sedimentation rate
ESTRO	European Society of Therapeutic Radiology and Oncology
EVA	extravehicular activities
FBF	fibroblast growth factors
FDA	Food and Drug Administration
FiO_2	fraction of inspired oxygen
FMD	flow-mediated dilation

V. List of Abbreviations (continued)

fsw	feet of sea water	IT	intra-tympanic
g	gram	ITT	intention to treat
GAS	group A *streptococcus*	ITS	intratympanic steroid
GCP	good clinical practice	IU	international unit
GCS	Glasgow Coma Scale	IV	intravenous therapy
GI	gastrointestinal	IVFA	intravenous fluorescein angiogram
GMCSF	granulocyte-macrophage colony stimulating factor	IVIG	intravenous immunoglobulin
Gy	gray	IVS	intravenous steroid
H2O$_2$	hydrogen peroxide	KD	ketogenic diet
HBO$_2$	hyperbaric oxygen	kg	kilogram
HCFA	Health Care Financing Administration	kPa	kilopascal
HCIO	hypochlorous acid	LENT-SOMA	late effects in normal tissues subjective, objective, management, and analytic score
HCV	hepatitis C virus	LDL	low density lipoprotein cholesterol
Hgb	hemoglobin	LR	lactated Ringer's solution
HIF	hypoxia-inducible factor	LRINEC	Laboratory Risk Indicator for Necrotizing Fasciitis
HIV	human immunodeficiency virus	MACE	Military Acute Concussion Evaluation
HODFU	hyperbaric oxygen therapy in diabetics with chronic foot ulcers	MBC	minimum bactericidal concentration
HOPPS	Hospital Outpatient Prospective Payment System	MEB	middle ear barotrauma
HTN	hypertension	MESS	mangled extremity severity score
Hz	hertz	mg	milligram
IB	investigator's brochure	MI	myocardial infarction
IBDQ	inflammatory bowel disease questionnaire	MIC	minimum inhibitory concentration
ICA	intracranial abscess	mL	milliliter
ICAM	intracellular adhesion molecule	mmHg	millimeters of mercury
ICG	indocyanine green fluorescence	MMP	matrix metalloproteinase
ICGA	indocyanine green fluorescence angiography	MOF	multiorgan failure
ICU	intensive care unit	MoHC	monoplace hyperbaric chamber
IDE	investigational device exemption	MPa	megapascal
IL	interleukin	MR	magnetic resonance
IM	internal medicine	MRI	magnetic resonance imaging
IMRT	intensity-modulated radiation	mRNA	messenger ribonucleic acid
IND	investigational new drug	MRSA	methicillin-resistant Staphylococcus aureus
INR	in-water recompression	MSAC	Medicare Service Advisory Committee (Australia)
IR	ischemia-reperfusion	msw	meters of sea water
IRB	institutional review board	MT	medical therapy
ISSHL	idiopathic sudden sensorineural hearing loss		

mTBI	mild traumatic brain injury	PCS	post-concussion syndrome
N_2	nitrogen	PDGF	platelet derived growth factor
N_2O	nitrous oxide	PDHA	post-deployment health assessment
NAC	N-acetylcysteine	PDPH	post-dural procedural headache
NAT	nucleic acid testing	PFO	perfringolysin
NATO	North Atlantic Treaty Organization	PET	positron emission tomography
NBA	normobaric air	PG	pyoderma gangrenosum
NBO_2	normobaric oxygen	PM	progressive myopia
NCI-PDQ	National Cancer Institute Patient Data Query	PML	polymorphonuclear leukocytes
NF	nuclear factor	PMN	polymorphonuclear neutrophils
NFPA	National Fire Protection Agency	PMNL	polymorphonuclear leukocytes
NFST	national fire select test	PO_2	partial pressure of oxygen
NIH	National Institute of Health	POS	oral steroid
NIOSH	National Institute for Occupational Safety and Health (U.S.)	ppm	parts per million
NLR	neutrophil-lymphocyte ratio	PTA	pure tone average
NNT	number needed to treat	$PtcO_2$	transcutaneous partial pressure oxygen measurement
NO	nitric oxide	PTCI	percutaneous transluminal coronary intervention
NOS	nitric oxide synthase	PT	prothrombin time
NRC	National Research Council of the National Academies	PTSD	post-traumatic stress disorder
NSAID	nonsteroidal anti-inflammatory drug	PTT	partial prothrombin time
NSF	National Science Foundation	PVR	pulse volume recordings
NSTI	necrotizing soft-tissue infection	QALY	quality adjusted life years
NSE	neuron-specific enolase	QH	every hour
O_2	oxygen	RANKL	receptor activator of nuclear factor-kappa B
ON	osteonecrosis	RBC	red blood cell
OOC	organ of Corti	RCT	randomized controlled trial
OPG	osteoprotegerin	RF	retrolental fibroplasia
ORN	osteoradionecrosis	RNS	reactive nitrogen species
OR	odds ratio	ROS	reactive oxygen species
OSHA	Occupational Safety and Health Administration	SARS	severe acute respiratory syndrome
PAD	Peripheral arterial disease	SCD	sickle cell disease
PAR	percent area reduction	SEK	Swedish kroner currency
paO_2	arterial oxygen tension	SD	standard deviation
PAOD	peripheral arterial occlusive disease	SGB	stellate ganglion block
PBMC	peripheral blood monocytes	SMCS	skeletal muscle compartment syndrome
PCL-M	PTSD checklist – military version	SPC	stem progenitor cell
		SpCO	carboxyhemoglobin saturation

V. List of Abbreviations (continued)

SPECT	single-photon emission computed tomography
SPP	skin perfusion pressure
SSc	systemic scleroderma
SSHL	sudden sensorineural hearing loss
ST	standard therapy
TACO	transfusion associated circulatory overload
TAD	transfusion associated dyspnea
TBSA	total body surface area
TBI	traumatic brain injury
TCOM	transcutaneous oxygen measurement
$TcPO_2$	transcutaneous oxygen partial pressure
TEN	toxic epidermal necrolysis
TGF	transforming growth factor
TIMP	tissue inhibitor of metalloproteinase
TNF	tumor necrosis factor
TRALI	transfusion related acute lung injury
TRAM	transverse rectus abdominis myocutaneous
TRPV	transient receptor potential vanilloid
TTI	transfusion-transmitted infection
TWA	time weighted average
Tx	treatment
UHMS	Undersea and Hyperbaric Medical Society
UMS	Undersea Medical Society
USAF	United States Air Force
USN	United States Navy
USP	United States Pharmacopoeia
VD	vasodilator
VEGF	vascular endothelial growth factor
VGE	venous gas embolism
VLU	venous leg ulcer
VO_2	oxygen consumption
WHO	World Health Organization
WRS	word recognition score
XD	xanthine dehydrogenase
XO	xanthine oxidase

VI. Author Biographies

Caesar A. Anderson MD, MPH, CWS

Dr. Anderson specializes in hyperbaric medicine and limb salvaging with board certification in internal medicine, undersea and hyperbaric medicine and the practice of advanced wound care. He has surgical expertise in the use of bioengineered skin substitutes and advance wound management and serves as medical director of UC San Diego Health's hyperbaric and wound care program in Encinitas. He completed a fellowship in diving and hyperbaric medicine at the University of Pennsylvania Hospital in Philadelphia and a combined residency training program in internal and preventive medicine at Yale-New Haven Hospital and Griffin Hospital in Connecticut. Dr. Anderson did his general surgery residency at the University of Connecticut and earned his medical degree from Howard University College of Medicine in Washington DC, and his master's degree in public health from Yale University School of Medicine.

Dirk J. Bakker MD, PhD, FUHM

Dr. Bakker was a general and transplant surgeon and has been involved in hyperbaric and diving medicine since 1969. Until 1995, he was a professor of surgery at the University of Amsterdam; until 2004, he was medical director of the Academic Medical Center of the University of Amsterdam. His PhD thesis was, "The Influence of Hyperbaric Oxygen Treatment on Aerobic and Anaerobic Soft Tissue Infections." Dr. Bakker is a member of the UHMS, the EUBS, the ICHM, and was a founding member of the European Committee on Hyperbaric Medicine. His awards include the Boerema Award (1987) and the Charles W. Shilling Award of the UHMS (1992). He is a Fellow of the UHMS and an officer in the Order of Orange Nassau in the Netherlands.

Richard C. Baynosa MD, FACS

Associate Professor and Chair, Department of Plastic Surgery, University of Nevada Las Vegas School of Medicine
Program Director, Plastic Surgery Residency Training Program, University of Nevada Las Vegas School of Medicine
Section Head of Breast Surgery, Department of Plastic Surgery, University of Nevada Las Vegas School of Medicine
Vice-Chair, Department of Surgery, University Medical Center of Southern Nevada
Chief, Division of Plastic Surgery, University Medical Center of Southern Nevada

Michael H. Bennett MD, FANZCA, MM(Clin Epi), Dip Advanced DHM (ANZCA)

Professor Bennett is the academic head of the department of anesthesia, a senior staff specialist in diving and hyperbaric medicine at Prince of Wales Hospital, and conjoint professor in the faculty of medicine, University of New South Wales in Sydney, Australia. He graduated from the University of New South Wales in 1979 and spent his early post-graduate training at the Prince Henry/Prince of Wales Hospitals before undertaking training in anesthesia in the UK. He was medical director of the Department of Diving and Hyperbaric Medicine at POWH from 1993 to 2007.

In 2002 he was the recipient of the Behnke Award for outstanding scientific achievement from the Undersea and Hyperbaric Medical Society. He is the author of over 140 peer-reviewed publications including 15 Cochrane reviews of the evidence in diving and hyperbaric medicine. He is an executive member of the Australia and New Zealand College of Anesthetists (ANZCA) special interest group in diving and hyperbaric medicine and chair of the ANZCA DHM subcommittee responsible for the ANZCA Diploma of Advanced DHM. He is a past vice-president of the UHMS and currently the past president of SPUMS. Conjoint Professor, UNSW Medicine, University of NSW. He is also Academic Director, Wales Anesthesia, Prince of Wales Hospital, Randwick, NSW Australia.

VI. Author Biographies (continued)

Gerardo Bosco MD, PhD
Associate Professor, Department of Biomedical Sciences, University of Padova, Italy
Director: Master II level in Diving and Hyperbaric Medicine Course in Technical and Health Management in the Hyperbaric Chamber Department of Biomedical Sciences, University of Padova, Italy

Frank Butler Jr. MD, Capt, MC, USN (Ret)
Dr. Butler is a former U.S. Navy SEAL platoon commander and a pioneer in the field of ophthalmology and diving. He has been a diving medical research officer at the U.S. Navy Experimental Diving Unit where he helped to develop many of the diving techniques and procedures used by Navy SEALs today. His landmark paper, "Diving and Hyperbaric Ophthalmology," was the first comprehensive review of ocular disorders in diving and is now the standard on this topic. His 2008 paper in *Undersea and Hyperbaric Medicine* provided the first comprehensive overview of the use of HBO_2 in ocular disorders. Dr. Butler has volunteered his time as an ophthalmology consultant to UHMS and the Divers' Alert Network since 1995, providing expert advice to divers around the world. He served for three years as a member of the Board of Directors for the Undersea and Hyperbaric Medical Society. He is the Co-Chair of the UHMS Decompression Sickness and Arterial Gas Embolism Committee and is currently spearheading the Society's effort to develop evidence-based best practice guidelines to improve the treatment of these disorders. Dr. Butler has been awarded the U.S. Special Operations Command Medal by Admiral Bill McRaven and the Academy of Underwater Arts and Sciences NOGI Award for Distinguished Service to the diving community. He currently chairs the Department of Defense's Committee on Tactical Combat Casualty Care.

Enrico M. Camporesi MD, FUHM, AB
Enrico M. Camporesi MD (Milan, 1970), FUHM (2000), AB Anesthesiology (1978)
AB Undersea Medicine (2000 and 2009)
HBO Committee (1988, Chair, 1996)
Past President, UHMS (2000-2002)
Treasurer (2012-2014)
Editor in Chief, UHM (2016-present)
Emeritus Professor of Surgery, Department of Surgery, University of South Florida, Tampa, Florida
Attending Anesthesiologist, TeamHealth, Tampa General Hospital, Tampa, Florida
Director of Research, TeamHealth Research Institute
Hyperbaric Medicine Director, Memorial Hospital of Tampa
Research interest in anesthesia, respiration and exercise in extreme environments, diving medicine and hyperbaric oxygen biology

Benjamin Cherng, MBBS, MBBS (National University of Singapore), MRCP (UK)
Consultant, Department of Infectious Diseases, Singapore General Hospital
Program Director, Singhealth Infectious Diseases Residency, Singapore

Paul Cianci MD, FACS, FUHM, FACP
Director, Hyperbaric Medicine Department, Doctors Medical Center, San Pablo, CA
Director Emeritus, Department of Hyperbaric Medicine, John Muir Medical Center, Walnut Creek, CA
Director Emeritus, Department of Hyperbaric Medicine, Saint Francis Memorial Hospital, San Francisco, CA
Diplomate, American Board of Internal Medicine
Fellow, American College of Physicians

Certified by the American Board of Preventative Medicine in the subspecialty of subsea and hyperbaric medicine
Fellow, Undersea and Hyperbaric Medicine
Professor Emeritus of Internal Medicine, University of California, Davis
Past President, Undersea and Hyperbaric Medical Society
Current member of the UHMS Hyperbaric Oxygen Committee
Consultant to the DOD, NOAA, and State of California
Visiting distinguished professor, University of Texas, Houston
Director, Department of Hyperbaric Medicine, Health Science Center, University of Texas, Houston (1998–1990)

Julia Faulkner

Julia Faulkner has been the executive assistant in the Department of Hyperbaric Medicine at Doctors Medical Center, San Pablo, CA, for over 30 years. During that time, she has been an integral part of the preparation and the publishing aspects of many of the peer review papers from this group of doctors.

Laurie Beth Gesell MD, FACEP, FUHM

System Director, Hyperbaric Medicine and Wound Care, Aurora Health Care Medical Group
Section Chair, Undersea and Hyperbaric Medicine, Aurora St. Luke's Medical Center, Milwaukee, Wisconsin

Dr. Gesell is the system director for hyperbaric medicine and wound care with Aurora Health Care Medical Group and section chair for undersea and hyperbaric medicine. She is board certified in emergency medicine and undersea and hyperbaric medicine. Dr. Gesell is a Fellow of the American College of Emergency Physicians, as well as the Undersea and Hyperbaric Medical Society. Dr. Gesell is a past president of the Undersea and Hyperbaric Medical Society, past chair of the UHMS Board of Directors, and former chair of the UHMS Hyperbaric Oxygen Therapy Committee. She currently serves as the UHMS Treasurer. Dr. Gesell also represents the medical specialty as the UHMS Delegate in the AMA House of Delegates.

John J. Feldmeier DO, FACRO, FUHM

Professor Emeritus and Past Chairman, Radiation Oncology, University of Toledo Medical Center

Dr. Feldmeier is Professor Emeritus of Radiation Oncology at the University of Toledo from which he has just retired as the long-term chairman. He has been recognized as a "Best Doctor" since 2007. He is a past president of the Undersea and Hyperbaric Medical Society and recognized as an expert in applying hyperbaric oxygen to the management of radiation injuries. He is board certified in both radiation oncology and hyperbaric medicine.

Catherine E. Hagan MD, MS, CDR MC (UMO) USN

Chief Medical Officer, Staff Ophthalmologist, Anterior Segment & Corneal Refractive Surgeon, Naval Hospital Jacksonville, Florida

Dr. Hagan obtained her undergraduate degree in zoology from the University of Florida and attended medical school at the University of Louisville, KY. In 2007, she became the 11th woman in U.S. history to earn the Submarine Medical Officer Qualification. Upon completion of ophthalmology residency in 2008 at the Naval Medical Center San Diego, CA, she was awarded the departments only Excellence in Research award for her support with the publication, proposal and ultimate approval of Central Retinal Artery Occlusion (CRAO) as an accepted indication for HBO_2 Therapy by the UHMS. Since residency, she has been stationed at Naval Hospital Camp LeJeune, NC, from 2008-2011 and Naval Hospital Jacksonville since 2011, where she has held multiple leadership roles such

VI. Author Biographies (continued)

as Department Head of Ophthalmology and Refractive Surgery, Chair of Credentials Committee, Surgical Physician Advisor of Process Improvement, and Chair of the Medical Executive Committee. She is currently serving as the Chief Medical Officer of Naval Hospital Jacksonville and its five branch health clinics spanning from Key West, FL to Albany, GA. CDR Hagan continues to serve as a consultant on ocular disorders for the U.S. Navy Dive School and is an invited guest lecturer twice a year on the topic of treating CRAO with HBO_2.

Brett B. Hart MD, FUHM

Dr. Hart earned his MD from the Uniformed Services University of the Health Sciences. He completed hyperbaric medicine fellowship training at Duke University and is dual board certified in anesthesiology and undersea and hyperbaric medicine. A former U.S. Navy Undersea Medical Officer, Dr. Hart now serves as a Pharmacovigilance Medical Monitor at Emmes in Rockville, Maryland.

Marvin Heyboer III MD, FACEP, FUHM, FACCWS

Associate Professor, Emergency Medicine
Division Chief, Hyperbaric Medicine & Wound Care
Medical Director, Hyperbaric Medicine & Wound Care Center
Program Director, Fellowship in Undersea & Hyperbaric Medicine
State University of New York, Upstate Medical University, Syracuse, NY
Specialty/Interest: Undersea & Hyperbaric Medicine, Emergency Medicine, Wound Medicine

Marvin Heyboer III is an associate professor at SUNY Upstate Medical University in Syracuse, NY. He is medical director of the Hyperbaric Medicine and Wound Care Center. In addition, he is the program director of the Fellowship in Undersea and Hyperbaric Medicine. He graduated from Case Western Reserve University School of Medicine and completed residency in emergency medicine with Michigan State University at Spectrum Health in Grand Rapids, Michigan. Dr. Heyboer is board certified in emergency medicine and undersea and hyperbaric medicine by the American Board of Emergency Medicine. He is also certified in wound medicine by the American Board of Wound Medicine and Surgery and the American Board of Wound Management. He has presented research in hyperbaric medicine and wound care at multiple national conferences. He is published in national journals including *Undersea and Hyperbaric Medicine, Wound Repair and Regeneration,* and *Journal of the American College of Clinical Wound Specialists.*

Enoch T. Huang MD, MPH&TM, FUHM, FACEP, FACCWS

Dr. Huang is the program medical director for hyperbaric medicine and chronic wound care at Legacy Emanuel Medical Center in Portland, OR. He graduated from Princeton University with a degree in chemistry. He attended medical school at Tulane University School of Medicine where he also obtained a master's degree in public health and tropical medicine. He completed a residency in emergency medicine at the University of California, Irvine and went on to complete a fellowship in undersea and hyperbaric medicine at the University of Pennsylvania. He is board-certified in emergency medicine as well as undersea and hyperbaric medicine. He is the founder and past-president of the Columbia Wound Care Community—a multidisciplinary, multihospital group of wound care providers in the greater Portland metropolitan area. He is the past-president of the Undersea and Hyperbaric Medical Society.

Irving "Jake" Jacoby MD, FACP, FACEP, FAAEM, FUHM

Emeritus Clinical Professor of Medicine and Surgery, Department of Emergency Medicine,
 University of California, San Diego, School of Medicine, La Jolla, California

Attending Physician, Department of Emergency Medicine and Division of Wound Care and Hyperbaric Medicine, University of California, San Diego, Medical Center, San Diego, California

Education: BS (Chemistry), University of Miami, FL; MD, the Johns Hopkins University School of Medicine; IM residency at Boston City Hospital and the Peter Bent Brigham Hospital; Infectious Disease Fellowship, Peter Bent Brigham Hospital in Boston.

He is board certified in internal medicine, infectious diseases, emergency medicine, and undersea and hyperbaric medicine.

Shawna Kleban MD

Chief Resident, Department of Plastic Surgery, University of Nevada Las Vegas School of Medicine

Tracy Leigh LeGros MD, PhD, FAAEM, FACEP, FUHM

Clinical Professor of Emergency Medicine, Program Director, LSU Undersea and Hyperbaric Medicine Fellowship, University Medical Center, New Orleans, Louisiana

Dr. LeGros obtained her Doctorate in Physiology from LSU School of Graduate Studies and her medical doctorate from LSU School of Medicine. She matched to her first choice in residency—the Charity Hospital Emergency Medicine Residency. Tracy graduated as a chief resident and the Lauro Award winner at graduation. Dr. LeGros then completed a fellowship in Undersea and Hyperbaric Medicine with Dr. Keith Van Meter. She has been a clinical and academic attending in both emergency medicine and undersea and hyperbaric medicine for the last 18 years.

Simon J. Mitchell MB ChB, PhD, DipAdvDHM (ANZCA), DipOccMed, FUHM, FANZCA

Professor of Anesthesiology, School of Medicine, University of Auckland

Dr. Mitchell is a physician and scientist with specialist training in diving medicine and anesthesiology. His diving career has included more than 6,000 dives spanning sport, scientific, commercial, and military diving. He was elected to Fellowship of the Explorers' Club of New York in 2006 and was the DAN Rolex Diver of the Year in 2015.

He is widely published with over 150 papers or book chapters. He has twice been vice president of the Undersea and Hyperbaric Medicine Society (USA) and in 2010 received the society's Behnke Award for contributions to the science of diving and hyperbaric medicine. In the past, Simon was a naval diving medical officer and medical director of the Wesley Centre for Hyperbaric Medicine in Brisbane. He now works as a consultant anesthetist at Auckland City Hospital and Professor of Anesthesiology at the University of Auckland.

Richard E. Moon MD, FRCPC, FACP, FCCP, FUHM

Professor of Anesthesiology and Medicine, Medical Director, Center for Hyperbaric Medicine and Environmental Physiology, Duke University Medical Center, Durham, NC

Dr. Moon has served as president of the UHMS. His publications include diving physiology and medicine, hyperbaric oxygen, and monitoring of patients under anesthesia. His research efforts include the study of cardiorespiratory function in humans exposed to environmental conditions ranging from 200 feet of seawater depth to high altitude, gas exchange during diving, the pathophysiology of high-altitude pulmonary edema and the effect of anesthesia and postoperative analgesia on pulmonary function. Ongoing human studies include altitude diving decompression procedures, safety monitoring of rebreather divers, prevention of immersion pulmonary edema, mechanisms of opioid-induced respiratory depression, prevention of complications after leg amputation using HBO$_2$ and optical monitoring of cytochrome redox during ischemia.

Heather Murphy-Lavoie MD, UHM, FACEP, FAAEM

Clinical Professor of Emergency Medicine, LSU Health Sciences Center
University Medical Center, Emergency Department
Emergency Medicine Residency
Undersea and Hyperbaric Medicine Fellowship, New Orleans, Louisiana

Heather Murphy-Lavoie MD, UHM, FACEP, FAAEM is a clinical professor of medicine at the Louisiana State University School of Medicine. She received her undergraduate degree, with honors, in biomedical engineering from Tulane University. She matriculated in the top third of her class from Tulane School of Medicine. She graduated as a chief resident from Charity Hospital's Emergency Medicine residency and completed her Undersea and Hyperbaric Medicine Fellowship under Dr. Keith Van Meter. She is board certified in emergency medicine and in the subspecialty of Undersea and Hyperbaric Medicine. She is a Fellow in the American College of Emergency Physicians (FACEP) and a Fellow in American Academy of Emergency Medicine (FAAEM). She serves on the Education Committee of the American Academy of Emergency Medicine. She has been on the UHMS Education Committee for 13 years, serving as chair for the last six years, and has been on the HBO$_2$ Therapy Committee since 2009. In 2006, she brought forth Central Retinal Artery Occlusion (CRAO) as a proposed new indication before the HBO$_2$ Therapy Committee. It is because of her efforts that CRAO is now an accepted indication. In 2011, she again proposed two new indications before this same august body and coordinated her fellowship team to successfully advocate for the addition of acute idiopathic sensorineural hearing loss as the latest accepted indication. She a nationally recognized lecturer and advocate for the UHM specialty.

Her awards include the following: FUHM status (2014); Paul James Sheffield Education Award for Lifetime Achievement (2012); Caroline Sue Ray Lifetime Achievement Award (2012); Outstanding Lecturer Award for Excellence in Graduate Medical Education; and Hyperbaric Medicine Fellowship (2007 and 2010). She has been instrumental in training 41 UHM fellows to date.

Dr. Murphy-Lavoie has authored numerous scientific publications in emergency medicine and hyperbaric medicine, including over 20 book chapters. She has published extensively on the use of hyperbaric oxygen therapy for ophthalmologic diseases.

Matteo Paganini MD

Emergency Medicine Chief Resident, University of Padova, Italy
Research interests on undersea and hyperbaric medicine, wilderness, prehospital and disaster medicine
Former Italian Navy Cadet, Navy Military School in Venice

Alex Rizzato PhD, MSc

Research fellow, Department of Biomedical Sciences, University of Padova, Italy

Ronald Sato MD

Dr. Sato, a native of Hawaii, received his medical degree from Yale University Medical School and trained as a resident at Stanford University. He has participated as a burn fellow at the University of Texas Health Science Center and has taught at Stanford University. In addition to his work on numerous publications related to burn care and plastic reconstructive surgery, he has served on the advisory board of the American Burn Association and as a member of the editorial staff for the *Journal of Burn Care and Rehabilitation*. Dr. Sato has been the director of the Burn Center at Doctors Medical Center for over 19 years, where he has dedicated a large part of his medical career to the treatment of severely burned patients and those with severely infected and chronic wounds.

Davut J. Savaser MD, MPH, FAAEM, FACEP

Hyperbaric Medicine and Chronic Wound Clinic, Legacy Emanuel Medical Center, Portland, Oregon

Chai Rick Soh MD

Head, Department of Anaesthesiology, Singapore General Hospital (SGH)
Senior Consultant, Hyperbaric and Diving Medicine Centre, SGH
Senior Consultant, Department of Surgical Intensive Care, SGH
Associate Professor, Duke-NUS Medical School.
Deputy Vice Chair, Education, Anaesthesiology Academic Clinical Program
Co-director, Human Structure and Function Course, Duke-NUS Medical School, Singapore

Michael B. Strauss MD

Dr. Strauss has over a 40-year association with hyperbaric medicine focusing on orthopedic, wound care and diving applications of this discipline. He is a board-certified orthopedic surgeon with over 20 years' service as the orthopedic surgeon coordinator for his medical center's Class 2 (no 24/7 onsite neurosurgeon) trauma center. During this time he served as the medical director for his medical center's nationally recognized hyperbaric medicine program. He has over 200 citations in the medical literature on subjects related to his hyperbaric medicine experiences including those on crush injuries and compartment syndromes. Dr. Strauss generated the crush injury section for the first *Hyperbaric Oxygen Therapy Committee Report* and has updated the information with each succeeding report up to and including the present edition.

Edward O. Tomoye DO, MA

Director, North Central Texas Infectious Disease Group, Richland Hills, Texas
Adjunct Associate Professor of Medicine, University of North Texas, Fort worth, Texas
Fellowship in Infectious disease & Immunology, University of Massachusetts
Fellowship in Undersea & Hyperbaric Medicine, Duke University

Research interests: Effects of hyperbaric oxygen in adults with sickle cell crisis
Efficacy of antimicrobial products in chronic wounds
Carbon monoxide levels in mouth smoke: comparing tobacco brands
Analysis of blood pressure elevation during hyperbaric oxygen treatments

Robert A. van Hulst MD, PhD, FUHM, Capt Navy (ret)

Professor of Hyperbaric and Diving Medicine
Captain Royal Dutch Navy (retired)
Director of Diving and Submarine Medicine, Royal Netherlands Navy

Robert van Hulst is a former navy senior undersea medical officer, with his last position as Director Diving and Submarine Medical Center until 2014. Since 2014 he is a full professor in hyperbaric and diving medicine in the Amsterdam University Medical Center, The Netherlands, and head of the hyperbaric department (Boerema chamber). He is a consultant for the Navy for occupational medicine in submarines and escape and rescue. His PhD thesis (2003) is, "Cerebral air embolism and brain metabolism: effects of ventilation and hyperbaric oxygen in healthy and brain traumatized animals." His research interests include cerebral air embolism, pulmonary oxygen toxicity, preconditioning, ventilation/gas exchange during diving and HBO_2 treatment for wound healing and Crohn's disease.

Keith W. Van Meter MD

Louisiana State University-Health Sciences Center, Department of Medicine, Section of Emergency Medicine, New Orleans, Louisiana
Clinical Professor of medicine, LSU School of Medicine
Clinical Professor of Medicine, Tulane University School of Medicine
Chief, Section of Emergency Medicine, LSU School of Medicine
MD at George Washington University School of Medicine
Residency Training Charity Hospital/Tulane School of Medicine
Section Head of Emergency Medicine at LSU HSC/New Orleans
Board certified in emergency medicine, pediatric emergency medicine, hyperbaric medicine, and clinical toxicology

Lindell K. Weaver MD, FACP, FCCP, FCCM, FUHM

Hyperbaric Medicine Division, Intermountain LDS Hospital, Salt Lake City, Utah Hyperbaric Medicine, Intermountain Medical Center, Murray, Utah
University of Utah School of Medicine, Salt Lake City, Utah
Medical Director and Division Chief, Hyperbaric Medicine, LDS Hospital, Salt Lake City, UT and Intermountain Medical Center, Murray, UT
Professor of Medicine, University of Utah School of Medicine.
Training: BS in engineering science, Arizona State University; internship, Naval Hospital San Diego; military, undersea and diving medical officer training followed by undersea medical officer, U.S. Navy; residency in internal medicine, LDS Hospital, Salt Lake City, UT; fellowship in pulmonary/critical care, University of Utah
Undersea and Hyperbaric Medical Society past president
Chair, UHMS Hyperbaric Oxygen Therapy Committee

Head-down position was formerly recommended for the initial treatment of patients with AGE, in order to minimize the risk of additional cerebral embolization because of buoyancy, and shrinkage of bubbles due to increased hydrostatic pressure, and some anecdotal cases support its use.[45] Lateral decubitus position has been recommended in the past for first aid treatment of VGE; however, buoyancy has little if any effect upon arterial[46] or venous[47] distribution of intravascular air. Furthermore, head-down position can worsen cerebral edema.[48] Head-down position is no longer recommended.[49-50] Recommended first aid for AGE includes placing the patient in the supine position. Unconscious patients should ideally be positioned to maximize airway protection and management: the recovery (lateral decubitus) position.[49-50]

Hyperbaric Oxygen. HBO$_2$ to treat gas embolism remains the definitive treatment for arterial gas embolism[51-52] due to the effect of higher ambient pressure to reduce bubble volume, an increase in tissue oxygenation induced by HBO$_2$ and pharmacological effects of hyperbaric hyperoxia that include inhibition of leucocyte adhesion to damaged endothelium.[53-54] Reviews of published cases of arterial gas embolism reveals superior outcomes with the use of HBO$_2$ compared to non-recompression treatment.[32,36,55-65] A short interval between embolism and recompression treatment is associated with a higher probability of good outcome. However, a response to treatment has been observed after 24 or more hours.[66] HBO$_2$ treatment is not required for asymptomatic VGE, however it has produced clinical improvement in patients with the sole manifestation of secondary pulmonary edema.[67]

Because of the tendency for patients with AGE to deteriorate after apparent recovery,[31] early HBO$_2$ is recommended even for patients who appear to have spontaneously recovered. One author has suggested that the presence or absence of air detectable by brain computed tomography should be used as a criterion for HBO$_2$ therapy.[68] However, timely administration of HBO$_2$ usually causes clinical improvement even in the absence of demonstrable air, possibly due to the effect of HBO$_2$ to attenuate leucocyte adherence to damaged endothelium[54] and secondary inflammation, and thus facilitate return of blood flow.

In patients with AGE caused by pulmonary barotrauma there may be a coexisting pneumothorax, which could develop into tension pneumothorax during chamber decompression. Therefore, placement of a chest tube in patients with pneumothorax prior to HBO$_2$ should be considered and is recommended for patients treated in a monoplace chamber. For multiplace chamber treatment, careful monitoring is a feasible option. Coexisting pneumomediastinum does not generally require any specific therapy and will usually resolve during HBO$_2$.

Immediate recompression to 6 atmospheres absolute (ATA) was recommended in the past. However, there is no conclusive evidence that pressures higher than 2.82 ATA (18 msw, 60 fsw) offer any advantage. If possible, an initial compression to 2.82 ATA (60 fsw or 18 msw equivalent depth) breathing 100% oxygen is recommended, using USN Treatment Table 6 or equivalent. The standards against which other treatment schedules ("tables") should be compared are those of the U.S. Navy (*USN Diving Manual*,[69] available at http://www.supsalv.org/) and similar procedures used by other navies and commercial diving operations.[70-71] Shorter tables designed for use in monoplace chambers have been used with success.[72] Significant modification of established HBO$_2$ treatment regimens have been used in facilities and personnel with the necessary expertise and hardware,[70] such that if the clinical response to treatment is judged to be suboptimal, options including deeper recompression or extension of the treatment table can be instituted according to the expertise and resources available.

Administration of repetitive treatments is recommended until there is no further stepwise improvement, typically after no more than one to two hyperbaric treatments, but occasionally up to five to 10.[70-71,73]

More detailed reviews of adjunctive therapies are available in other publications[71,74-76] and a summary can be obtained on the Undersea and Hyperbaric Society website (www.uhms.org/images/Publications/ADJUNCTIVE_THERAPY_FOR_DCI.pdf). Specific adjunctive therapies and their recommendations are listed below.

Adjunctive Therapy

Adjunctive therapies for isolated AGE include the following:

- oxygen administered as a first aid measure (class I, level C)

- lidocaine (class IIa, level B)

- aspirin, NSAIDs (class IIb, level C)

- anticoagulants (class IIb, level C)

- corticosteroids (class III, level C)

- intravenous fluids (D5W class III, level C; isotonic crystalloid, colloid class IIb, level C)

Hyperglycemia should be treated, as it worsens acute CNS injury. Although isolated AGE does not require specific fluid therapy, patients with accompanying decompression sickness may have significant hemoconcentration, and require aggressive fluid resuscitation (see Chapter 7: Decompression Sickness). For patients who are immobilized for 24 hours or greater due to neurological injury, low molecular weight heparin is recommended for prophylaxis against venous thromboembolism (class I, level A). In addition, since hyperthermia can adversely affect neurological outcome, aggressive treatment of fever is recommended. There is a plausible rationale for induced hypothermia, which is not yet standard of care but has been reported for AGE due to lung biopsy[77] and in conjunction with HBO$_2$ for AGE after scuba diving.[78]

For critically ill patients with AGE, no systematic human studies are available. In combination with HBO$_2$, large animal studies support the use of normotension and isocapnia.[44,79-80]

Outcome

While there are no published controlled studies of HBO$_2$ for AGE, in a retrospective review of 656 published AGE cases, Dutka reported full recovery in 78% of 515 individuals who received HBO$_2$ vs. 56% of 141 who did not.[64] In the same series the mortality rates were, respectively, 5% and 42%. Of 19 patients reported by Benson with iatrogenic AGE referred for hyperbaric therapy, after the first treatment five patients (26%) resolved all signs and symptoms, 11 (58%) exhibited improvement, one (5%) had no change and two (11%) were not assessable secondary to medically-induced paralysis.[43] Within two months post-HBO$_2$, three additional patients had resolved completely and six showed further improvement. Eight patients (42%) had complete recovery, six (32%) had partial recovery, and five patients (26%) died of complications of AGE.

In a series of 45 patients treated with HBO$_2$ for AGE within a single institution reported by Beevor, good neurological outcome (extended Glasgow outcome scale 7 or 8) was achieved in 27 (60%).[81] The only statistically significant factor predictive of good outcome was time to HBO$_2$ treatment (good outcome mean 8.8 hours vs. 16.5 hours). However, gas bubbles have been known to persist for several days and there are many reports noting success when HBO$_2$ treatments were begun after delays of hours to days.[61,65,82-83] In the series reported by Benson, one patient had eventual complete recovery despite a 28-hour time from incident to HBO$_2$.[43] In a case report of a 51-year-old diver who lost consciousness within minutes of a 30-meter dive, he remained deeply comatose, intubated and with cardiovascular instability for six days before HBO_2 could be administered. One year after treatment he was leading a functional life.[84]

Evidence-Based Review

The use of HBO_2 for arterial gas embolism and symptomatic venous gas embolism is an AHA class I recommendation (level of evidence C).

Utilization Review

Utilization review is recommended after 10 treatments.

Cost Impact

The primary treatment of choice for air embolism from any cause is HBO_2 therapy. Decreased high mortality rates and prevention or moderation of permanent neurological damage make this modality cost effective.

Table 1. Causes of Arterial Gas Embolism

Direct Arterial Air Entry

Pulmonary barotrauma during ascent from a dive[85]
Mechanical ventilation[86]
Penetrating chest trauma[87]
Chest tube placement[88,89]
Needle biopsy of the lung[90,91]
Bronchoscopy[92]
Cardiopulmonary bypass accident[93-95]
Pulmonary bulla rupture during altitude exposure[96-98]
Accidental air injection into a radial artery catheter[99-102]
Vascular air entry due to necrotizing pneumonia[103]
Pulmonary barotrauma from blast injury[157]
Pulmonary overinflation from inhalation of gas under high pressure[158]

Venous Gas Embolism with Secondary Arterial Entry Via Pulmonary Circulation or Intracardiac Right-to-Left Shunt

Compressed gas diving[7-10,15-16]
Rapid exposure to altitude[17]
Accidental intravenous air injection[104,-105]
Hemodialysis catheter accident[106]
Central venous catheter placement or disconnection[107-108]
Gastrointestinal endoscopy[109-110]
Esophageal ballooning and endoscopic retrograde cholangiopancreatography[111]
Hydrogen peroxide irrigation[89,112-118]
Arthroscopy[119-120]
Cardiopulmonary resuscitation[121]
Percutaneous hepatic puncture[122]
Blowing air into the vagina during orogenital sex[61,123-124]
Sexual intercourse after childbirth[125-126]
Gastric barotrauma following hyperbaric oxygen therapy[127]
Treatment of esophageal cancer[128-129]
Atrial-esophageal fistula following ablation for atrial fibrillation[130-133]

Procedures in which the surgical site is under pressure

Laparoscopy[134-138]
Transurethral surgery[139-140]
Vitrectomy[141]
Endoscopic vein harvesting[142]
Hysteroscopy[143-144]

Passive entry of air into surgical wounds situated above the level of the heart such that venous pressure is subatmospheric[18]

Sitting craniotomy[145]
Cesarean section[146]
Radical perineal prostatectomy[147]
Retropubic prostatectomy[148-149]
Spine surgery[150-151]
Hip replacement[152]
Liver resection[153]
Liver transplantation[154]
Insertion of dental implants[155-156]

Figure 1. Flowchart for Management of Arterial Gas Embolism
Details of management are described in the text.

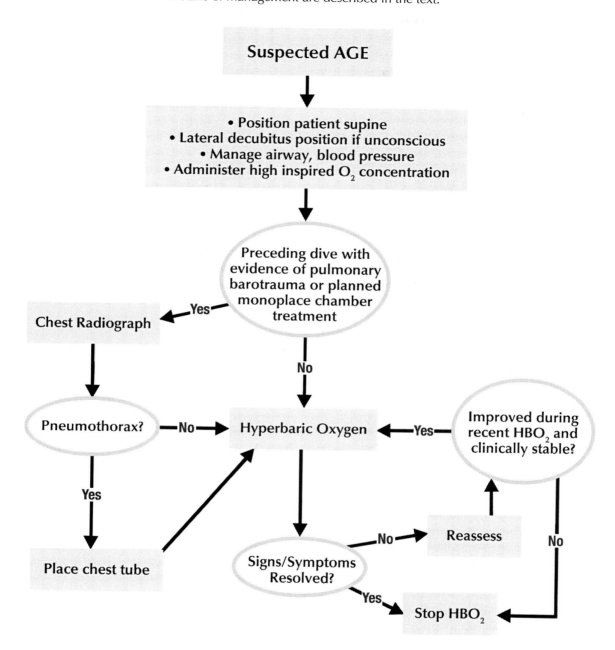

References

1. Benton PJ, Woodfine JD, Westwook PR. Arterial gas embolism following a 1-meter ascent during helicopter escape training: a case report. Aviat Space Environ Med. 1996;67:63-4.
2. Mellem H, Emhjellen S, Horgen O. Pulmonary barotrauma and arterial gas embolism caused by an emphysematous bulla in a SCUBA diver. Aviat Space Environ Med. 1990;61:559-62.
3. Weiss LD, Van Meter KW. Cerebral air embolism in asthmatic scuba divers in a swimming pool. Chest. 1995;107:1653-4.
4. Mason WH, Damon TG, Dickinson AR, Nevison TO, Jr. Arterial gas emboli after blast injury. Proc Soc Exp Biol Med. 1971;136(4):1253-5.
5. Freund U, Kopolovic J, Durst AL. Compressed air emboli of the aorta and renal artery in blast injury. Injury. 1980;12(1):37-8.
6. Guy RJ, Glover MA, Cripps NP. Primary blast injury: pathophysiology and implications for treatment. Part III: Injury to the central nervous system and the limbs. J R Nav Med Serv. 2000;86(1):27-31.
7. Ence TJ, Gong H, Jr. Adult respiratory distress syndrome after venous air embolism. Am Rev Respir Dis. 1979;119:1033-7.
8. Frim DM, Wollman L, Evans AB, Ojemann RG. Acute pulmonary edema after low-level air embolism during craniotomy. Case report. J Neurosurg. 1996;85(5):937-40.
9. Butler BD, Hills BA. Transpulmonary passage of venous air emboli. J Appl Physiol (1985). 1985;59:543-7.
10. Vik A, Brubakk AO, Hennessy TR, Jenssen BM, Ekker M, Slordahl SA. Venous air embolism in swine: transport of gas bubbles through the pulmonary circulation. J Appl Physiol (1985). 1990;69(1):237-44.
11. Messina AG, Leslie J, Gold J, Topkins MJ, Devereux RB. Passage of microbubbles associated with intravenous infusion into the systemic circulation in cyanotic congenital heart disease: documentation by transesophageal echocardiography. Am J Cardiol. 1987;59(9):1013-4.
12. Vik A, Jenssen BM, Brubakk AO. Paradoxical air embolism in pigs with a patent foramen ovale. Undersea Biomed Res. 1992;19(5):361-74.
13. Vik A, Jenssen BM, Brubakk AO. Arterial gas bubbles after decompression in pigs with patent foramen ovale. Undersea Hyperb Med. 1993;20(2):121-31.
14. Ries S, Knauth M, Kern R, Klingmann C, Daffertshofer M, Sartor K, Hennerici M. Arterial gas embolism after decompression: correlation with right-to-left shunting. Neurology. 1999;52(2):401-4.
15. Spencer MP. Decompression limits for compressed air determined by ultrasonically detected bubbles. J Appl Physiol (1985). 1976;40:229-35.
16. Gardette B. Correlation between decompression sickness and circulating bubbles in 232 divers. Undersea Biomed Res. 1979;6(1):99-107.
17. Balldin UI, Pilmanis AA, Webb JT. Central nervous system decompression sickness and venous gas emboli in hypobaric conditions. Aviat Space Environ Med. 2004;75(11):969-72.
18. Majendie F. Sur l'entree accidentelle de l'air dans les veins. J Physiol Exp (Paris). 1821;1:190.
19. Moore RM, Braselton CW. Injections of air and carbon dioxide into a pulmonary vein. Ann Surg. 1940;112:212-8.
20. Tunnicliffe FW, Stebbing GF. Intravenous injection of oxygen gas as therapeutic measure. Lancet. 1916;2:321-3.
21. Yeakel A. Lethal air embolism from plastic blood storage container. JAMA. 1968;204:267-8.
22. Helps SC, Parsons DW, Reilly PL, Gorman DF. The effect of gas emboli on rabbit cerebral blood flow. Stroke. 1990;21:94-9.
23. Helps SC, Meyer-Witting M, Rilley PL, Gorman DF. Increasing doses of intracarotid air and cerebral blood flow in rabbits. Stroke. 1990;21:1340-5.
24. Helps SC, Gorman DF. Air embolism of the brain in rabbits pre-treated with mechlorethamine. Stroke. 1991;22:351-4.
25. Levin LL, Stewart GJ, Lynch PR, Bove AA. Blood and blood vessel wall changes induced by decompression sickness in dogs. J Appl Physiol (1985). 1981;50:944-9.
26. Nossum V, Koteng S, Brubakk AO. Endothelial damage by bubbles in the pulmonary artery of the pig. Undersea Hyperb Med. 1999;26(1):1-8.
27. Nossum V, Hjelde A, Brubakk AO. Small amounts of venous gas embolism cause delayed impairment of endothelial function and increase polymorphonuclear neutrophil infiltration. Eur J Appl Physiol. 2002;86:209-14.
28. Klinger AL, Pichette B, Sobolewski P, Eckmann DM. Mechanotransductional basis of endothelial cell response to intravascular bubbles. Integrative biology : quantitative biosciences from nano to macro. 2011;3(10):1033-42.
29. Sobolewski P, Kandel J, Klinger AL, Eckmann DM. Air bubble contact with endothelial cells in vitro induces calcium influx and IP3-dependent release of calcium stores. Am J Physiol Cell Physiol. 2011;301(3):C679-86.

30. Sobolewski P, Kandel J, Eckmann DM. Air bubble contact with endothelial cells causes a calcium-independent loss in mitochondrial membrane potential. PLoS ONE. 2012;7(10):e47254.

31. Pearson RR, Goad RF. Delayed cerebral edema complicating cerebral arterial gas embolism: Case histories. Undersea Biomed Res. 1982;9:283-96.

32. Elliott DH, Harrison JAB, Barnard EEP. Clinical and radiological features of 88 cases of decompression barotrauma. In: Shilling CW, Beckett MW, editors. Underwater Physiology VI Proceedings of the Sixth Symposium on Underwater Physiology. Bethesda, MD: FASEB; 1978. p. 527-35.

33. Elliott DH, Moon RE. Manifestations of the decompression disorders. In: Bennett PB, Elliott DH, editors. The Physiology and Medicine of Diving. Philadelphia, PA: WB Saunders; 1993. p. 481-505.

34. Lam KK, Hutchinson RC, Gin T. Severe pulmonary oedema after venous air embolism. Can J Anaesth. 1993;40(10):964-7.

35. Fitchet A, Fitzpatrick AP. Central venous air embolism causing pulmonary oedema mimicking left ventricular failure. BMJ. 1998;316(7131):604-6.

36. Blanc P, Boussuges A, Henriette K, Sainty JM, Deleflie M. Iatrogenic cerebral air embolism: importance of an early hyperbaric oxygenation. Intensive Care Med. 2002;28(5):559-63.

37. Francis TJR, Mitchell SJ. Manifestations of decompression disorders. In: Brubakk AO, Neuman TS, editors. Bennett & Elliott's Physiology and Medicine of Diving. New York, NY: Elsevier Science; 2003. p. 578-99.

38. Neuman TS, Bove AA. Combined arterial gas embolism and decompression sickness following no-stop dives. Undersea Biomed Res. 1990;17:429-36.

39. Warren LP, Djang WT, Moon RE, Camporesi EM, Sallee DS, Anthony DC. Neuroimaging of scuba diving injuries to the CNS. AJNR Am J Neuroradiol. 1988;9:933-8.

40. Catron PW, Dutka AJ, Biondi DM, Flynn ET, Hallenbeck JM. Cerebral air embolism treated by pressure and hyperbaric oxygen. Neurology. 1991;41(2 (Pt 1)):314-5.

41. Reuter M, Tetzlaff K, Hutzelmann A, Fritsch G, Steffens JC, Bettinghausen E, Heller M. MR imaging of the central nervous system in diving-related decompression illness. Acta Radiol. 1997;38(6):940-4.

42. Sayama T, Mitani M, Inamura T, Yagi H, Fukui M. Normal diffusion-weighted imaging in cerebral air embolism complicating angiography. Neuroradiology. 2000;42(3):192-4.

43. Benson J, Adkinson C, Collier R. Hyperbaric oxygen therapy of iatrogenic cerebral arterial gas embolism. Undersea Hyperb Med. 2003;30(2):117-26.

44. van Hulst RA, Klein J, Lachmann B. Gas embolism: pathophysiology and treatment. Clin Physiol Funct Imaging. 2003;23(5):237-46.

45. Krivonyak GS, Warren SG. Cerebral arterial air embolism treated by a vertical head-down maneuver. Catheter Cardiovasc Interv. 2000;49(2):185-7.

46. Butler BD, Laine GA, Leiman BC, Warters D, Kurusz M, Sutton T, Katz J. Effects of Trendelenburg position on the distribution of arterial air emboli in dogs. Ann Thorac Surg. 1988;45:198-202.

47. Mehlhorn U, Burke EJ, Butler BD, Davis KL, Katz J, Melamed E, Morris WP, Allen SJ. Body position does not affect the hemodynamic response to venous air embolism in dogs. Anesth Analg. 1994;79:734-9.

48. Dutka AJ. Therapy for dysbaric central nervous system ischemia: adjuncts to recompression. In: Bennett PB, Moon RE, editors. Diving Accident Management. Bethesda, MD: Undersea and Hyperbaric Medical Society; 1990. p. 222-34.

49. Mitchell SJ, Bennett MH, Bryson P, Butler FK, Doolette DJ, Holm JR, Kot J, Lafere P. Pre-hospital management of decompression illness: expert review of key principles and controversies. Diving Hyperb Med. 2018;48(1):45-55.

50. Mitchell SJ, Bennett MH, Bryson P, Butler FK, Doolette DJ, Holm JR, Kot J, Lafere P. Consensus guideline: Pre-hospital management of decompression illness: expert review of key principles and controversies. Undersea Hyperb Med. 2018;45(3):273-86.

51. Navy Department. US Navy Diving Manual. Revision 6. Vol 5 : Diving Medicine and Recompression Chamber Operations. NAVSEA 0910-LP-106-0957. Washington, DC: Naval Sea Systems Command; 2008.

52. Clarke D, Gerard W, Norris T. Pulmonary barotrauma-induced cerebral arterial gas embolism with spontaneous recovery: commentary on the rationale for therapeutic compression. Aviat Space Environ Med. 2002;73(2):139-46.

53. Zamboni WA, Roth AC, Russell RC, Graham B, Suchy H, Kucan JO. Morphological analysis of the microcirculation during reperfusion of ischemic skeletal muscle and the effect of hyperbaric oxygen. Plast Reconstr Surg. 1993;91:1110-23.

54. Martin JD, Thom SR. Vascular leukocyte sequestration in decompression sickness and prophylactic hyperbaric oxygen therapy in rats. Aviat Space Environ Med. 2002;73(6):565-9.

55. Ericsson JA, Gottlieb JD, Sweet RB. Closed-chest cardiac massage in the treatment of venous air embolism. N Engl J Med. 1964;270:1353-4.

56. Moses HL. Casualties in Individual Submarine Escape 1928-1957. Groton, CT: US Naval Submarine Medical Center; 1964. Report No.: Report No. 438.
57. Van Genderen L. Study of Air Embolism and Extra-aveolar Accidents Associated with Submarine Escape Training. Groton, CT: US Naval Submarine Medical Center; 1967. Report No.: 500.
58. Ingvar DH, Adolfson J, Lindemark C. Cerebral air embolism during training of submarine personnel in free escape: an electroencephalographic study. Aerosp Med. 1973;44(6):628-35.
59. Hart GB. Treatment of decompression illness and air embolism with hyperbaric oxygen. Aerosp Med. 1974;45:1190-3.
60. Ah-See AK. Review of arterial air embolism in submarine escape. In: Smith G, editor. Proceedings of the Sixth International Congress on Hyperbaric Medicine. Aberdeen, Scotland: Aberdeen University Press; 1977. p. 349-51.
61. Bray P, Myers RA, Cowley RA. Orogenital sex as a cause of nonfatal air embolism in pregnancy. Obstet Gynecol. 1983;61(5):653-7.
62. Murphy BP, Harford FJ, Cramer FS. Cerebral air embolism resulting from invasive medical procedures. Treatment with hyperbaric oxygen. Ann Surg. 1985;201(2):242-5.
63. Leitch DR, Green RD. Pulmonary barotrauma in divers and the treatment of cerebral arterial gas embolism. Aviat Space Environ Med. 1986;57:931-8.
64. Dutka AJ. Air or gas embolism. In: Camporesi EM, Barker AC, editors. Hyperbaric Oxygen Therapy: A Critical Review. Bethesda, MD: Undersea and Hyperbaric Medical Society; 1991. p. 1-10.
65. Ziser A, Adir Y, Lavon H, Shupak A. Hyperbaric oxygen therapy for massive arterial air embolism during cardiac operations. J Thorac Cardiovasc Surg. 1999;117(4):818-21.
66. Massey EW, Moon RE, Shelton D, Camporesi EM. Hyperbaric oxygen therapy of iatrogenic air embolism. J Hyperb Med. 1990;5:15-21.
67. Zwirewich CV, Müller NL, Abboud RT, Lepawsky M. Noncardiogenic pulmonary edema caused by decompression sickness: rapid resolution following hyperbaric therapy. Radiology. 1987;163:81-2.
68. Dexter F, Hindman BJ. Recommendations for hyperbaric oxygen therapy of cerebral air embolism based on a mathematical model of bubble absorption. Anesth Analg. 1997;84:1203-7.
69. Navy Department. US Navy Diving Manual. Revision 7. Vol 5: Diving Medicine and Recompression Chamber Operations. NAVSEA 0910-LP-115-1921. Washington, DC: Naval Sea Systems Command; 2016.
70. Moon RE, Sheffield PJ. Guidelines for treatment of decompression illness. Aviat Space Environ Med. 1997;68:234-43.
71. Vann RD, Butler FK, Mitchell SJ, Moon RE. Decompression illness. Lancet. 2011;377(9760):153-64.
72. Cianci P, Slade JB, Jr. Delayed treatment of decompression sickness with short, no-air-break tables: review of 140 cases. Aviat Space Environ Med. 2006;77(10):1003-8.
73. Undersea & Hyperbaric Medical Society. UHMS Best Practice Guidelines: Prevention and Treatment of Decompression Sickness and Arterial Gas Embolism. Durham, NC2011.
74. Mitchell SJ. Lidocaine in the treatment of decompression illness: a review of the literature. Undersea Hyperb Med. 2001;28(3):165-74.
75. Bennett M, Mitchell S, Dominguez A. Adjunctive treatment of decompression illness with a non-steroidal anti-inflammatory drug (tenoxicam) reduces compression requirement. Undersea Hyperb Med. 2003;30(3):195-205.
76. Moon RE, editor. Adjunctive Therapy for Decompression Illness. Kensington, MD: Undersea and Hyperbaric Medical Society; 2003.
77. Chang M, Marshall J. Therapeutic hypothermia for acute air embolic stroke. West J Emerg Med. 2012;13(1):111-3.
78. Oh SH, Kang HD, Jung SK, Choi S. Implementation of targeted temperature management in a patient with cerebral arterial gas embolism. Ther Hypothermia Temp Manag. 2018.
79. Dutka AJ, Hallenbeck JM, Kochanek P. A brief episode of severe arterial hypertension induces delayed deterioration of brain function and worsens blood flow after transient multifocal cerebral ischemia. Stroke. 1987;18(2):386-95.
80. van Hulst RA, Haitsma JJ, Lameris TW, Klein J, Lachmann B. Hyperventilation impairs brain function in acute cerebral air embolism in pigs. Intensive Care Med. 2004;30(5):944-50.
81. Beevor H, Frawley G. Iatrogenic cerebral gas embolism: analysis of the presentation, management and outcomes of patients referred to The Alfred Hospital Hyperbaric Unit. Diving Hyperb Med. 2016;46(1):15-21.
82. Takita H, Olszewski W, Schimert G, Lanphier EH. Hyperbaric treatment of cerebral air embolism as a result of open-heart surgery. Report of a case. J Thorac Cardiovasc Surg. 1968;55(5):682-5.
83. Mader JT, Hulet WH. Delayed hyperbaric treatment of cerebral air embolism: report of a case. Arch Neurol. 1979;36(8):504-5.
84. Perez MF, Ongkeko Perez JV, Serrano AR, Andal MP, Aldover MC. Delayed hyperbaric intervention in life-threatening decompression illness. Diving Hyperb Med. 2017;47(4):257-9.

85. Trytko BE, Bennett MH. Arterial gas embolism: a review of cases at Prince of Wales Hospital, Sydney, 1996 to 2006. Anaesth Intensive Care. 2008;36(1):60-4.

86. Morris WP, Butler BD, Tonnesen AS, Allen SJ. Continuous venous air embolism in patients receiving positive end-expiratory pressure. Am Rev Respir Dis. 1993;147:1034-7.

87. Halpern P, Greenstein A, Melamed Y, Taitelman U, Sznajder I, Zveibil F. Arterial air embolism after penetrating lung injury. Crit Care Med. 1983;11(5):392-3.

88. Brownlow HA, Edibam C. Systemic air embolism after intercostal chest drain insertion and positive pressure ventilation in chest trauma. Anaesth Intensive Care. 2002;30(5):660-4.

89. Berlot G, Rinaldi A, Moscheni M, Ferluga M, Rossini P. Uncommon occurrences of air embolism: description of cases and review of the literature. Case Rep Crit Care. 2018;2018:5808390.

90. Lattin G, Jr., O'Brien W, Sr., McCrary B, Kearney P, Gover D. Massive systemic air embolism treated with hyperbaric oxygen therapy following CT-guided transthoracic needle biopsy of a pulmonary nodule. J Vasc Interv Radiol. 2006;17(8):1355-8.

91. Rehwald R, Loizides A, Wiedermann FJ, Grams AE, Djurdjevic T, Glodny B. Systemic air embolism causing acute stroke and myocardial infarction after percutaneous transthoracic lung biopsy - a case report. J Cardiothorac Surg. 2016;11(1):80.

92. Wherrett CG, Mehran RJ, Beaulieu MA. Cerebral arterial gas embolism following diagnostic bronchoscopy: delayed treatment with hyperbaric oxygen. Can J Anaesth. 2002;49(1):96-9.

93. Peirce EC, 2d. Specific therapy for arterial air embolism. Ann Thorac Surg. 1980;29(4):300-3.

94. Niyibizi E, Kembi GE, Lae C, Pignel R, Sologashvili T. Delayed hyperbaric oxygen therapy for air emboli after open heart surgery: case report and review of a success story. J Cardiothorac Surg. 2016;11(1):167.

95. Malik N, Claus PL, Illman JE, Kligerman SJ, Moynagh MR, Levin DL, Woodrum DA, Arani A, Arunachalam SP, Araoz PA. Air embolism: diagnosis and management. Future Cardiol. 2017;13(4):365-78.

96. Closon M, Vivier E, Breynaert C, Duperret S, Branche P, Coulon A, De La Roche E, Delafosse B. Air embolism during an aircraft flight in a passenger with a pulmonary cyst: a favorable outcome with hyperbaric therapy. Anesthesiology. 2004;101(2):539-42.

97. Jung AS, Harrison R, Lee KH, Genut J, Nyhan D, Brooks-Asplund EM, Shoukas AA, Hare JM, Berkowitz DE. Simulated microgravity produces attenuated baroreflex-mediated pressor, chronotropic, and inotropic responses in mice. Am J Physiol Heart Circ Physiol. 2005;289(2):H600-7.

98. Farshchi Zarabi S, Parotto M, Katznelson R, Downar J. Massive ischemic stroke due to pulmonary barotrauma and cerebral artery air embolism during commercial air travel. Am J Case Rep. 2017;18:660-4.

99. Chang C, Dughi J, Shitabata P, Johnson G, Coel M, McNamara JJ. Air embolism and the radial arterial line. Crit Care Med. 1988;16(2):141-3.

100. Dube L, Soltner C, Daenen S, Lemariee J, Asfar P, Alquier P. Gas embolism: an exceptional complication of radial arterial catheterization. Acta Anaesthesiol Scand. 2004;48(9):1208-10.

101. Yang CW, Yang BP. Massive cerebral arterial air embolism following arterial catheterization. Neuroradiology. 2005;47(12):892-4.

102. Murphy GS, Szokol JW, Marymont JH, Avram MJ, Vender JS, Kubasiak J. Retrograde blood flow in the brachial and axillary arteries during routine radial arterial catheter flushing. Anesthesiology. 2006;105(3):492-7.

103. Ceponis PJ, Fox W, Tailor TD, Hurwitz LM, Amrhein TJ, Moon RJ. Non-dysbaric arterial gas embolism associated with chronic necrotizing pneumonia, bullae and coughing: a case report. Undersea Hyperb Med. 2017;44(1):73-7.

104. Abernathy CM, Dickinson TC. Massive air emboli from intravenous infusion pump: etiology and prevention. Am J Surg. 1979;137(2):274-5.

105. Khan M, Schmidt DH, Bajwa T, Shalev Y. Coronary air embolism: incidence, severity, and suggested approaches to treatment. Catheterization & Cardiovascular Diagnosis. 1995;36(4):313-8.

106. Baskin SE, Wozniak RF. Hyperbaric oxygenation in the treatment of hemodialysis-associated air embolism. N Engl J Med. 1975;293(4):184-5.

107. Ordway CB. Air embolus via CVP catheter without positive pressure: presentation of case and review. Ann Surg. 1974;179(4):479-81.

108. Vesely TM. Air embolism during insertion of central venous catheters. J Vasc Interv Radiol. 2001;12(11):1291-5.

109. Raju GS, Bendixen BH, Khan J, Summers RW. Cerebrovascular accident during endoscopy - consider cerebral air embolism, a rapidly reversible event with hyperbaric oxygen therapy. Gastrointest Endosc. 1998;47(1):70-3.

110. Eoh EJ, Derrick B, Moon R. Cerebral arterial gas embolism during upper endoscopy. A A Case Rep. 2015;5(6):93-4.

111. Park S, Ahn JY, Ahn YE, Jeon SB, Lee SS, Jung HY, Kim JH. Two cases of cerebral air embolism that occurred during esophageal ballooning and endoscopic retrograde cholangiopancreatography. Clin Endosc. 2016;49(2):191-6.

112. Bassan MM, Dudai M, Shalev O. Near-fatal systemic oxygen embolism due to wound irrigation with hydrogen peroxide. Postgrad Med J. 1982;58(681):448-50.

113. Tsai SK, Lee TY, Mok MS. Gas embolism produced by hydrogen peroxide irrigation of an anal fistula during anesthesia. Anesthesiology. 1985;63(3):316-7.

114. Rackoff WR, Merton DF. Gas embolism after ingestion of hydrogen peroxide. Pediatrics. 1990;85(4):593-4.

115. Christensen DW, Faught WE, Black RE, Woodward GA, Timmons OD. Fatal oxygen embolization after hydrogen peroxide ingestion. Crit Care Med. 1992;20(4):543-4.

116. Mullins ME, Beltran JT. Acute cerebral gas embolism from hydrogen peroxide ingestion successfully treated with hyperbaric oxygen. J Toxicol Clin Toxicol. 1998;36(3):253-6.

117. Jones PM, Segal SH, Gelb AW. Venous oxygen embolism produced by injection of hydrogen peroxide into an enterocutaneous fistula. Anesth Analg. 2004;99(6):1861-3.

118. Smedley BL, Gault A, Gawthrope IC. Cerebral arterial gas embolism after pre-flight ingestion of hydrogen peroxide. Diving Hyperb Med. 2016;46(2):117-9.

119. Habegger R, Siebenmann R, Kieser C. Lethal air embolism during arthroscopy. A case report. J Bone Joint Surg Br. 1989;71(2):314-6.

120. Faure EAM, Cook RI, Miles D. Air embolism during anesthesia for shoulder arthroscopy. Anesthesiology. 1998;89(3):805-6.

121. Hwang SL, Lieu AS, Lin CL, Liu GC, Howng SL, Kuo TH. Massive cerebral air embolism after cardiopulmonary resuscitation. J Clin Neurosci. 2005;12(4):468-9.

122. Helmberger TK, Roth U, Empen K. Massive air embolism during interventional laser therapy of the liver: successful resuscitation without chest compression. Cardiovasc Intervent Radiol. 2002;25(4):335-6.

123. Kaufman BS, Kaminsky SJ, Rackow EC, Weil MH. Adult respiratory distress syndrome following orogenital sex during pregnancy. Crit Care Med. 1987;15:703-4.

124. Bernhardt TL, Goldmann RW, Thombs PA, Kindwall EP. Hyperbaric oxygen treatment of cerebral air embolism from orogenital sex during pregnancy. Crit Care Med. 1988;16(7):729-30.

125. Batman PA, Thomlinson J, Moore VC, Sykes R. Death due to air embolism during sexual intercourse in the puerperium. Postgrad Med J. 1998;74:612-3.

126. Sadler DW, Pounder DJ. Fatal air embolism occurring during consensual intercourse in a non-pregnant female. J Clin Forensic Med. 1998;5(2):77-9.

127. Gariel C, Delwarde B, Beroud S, Soldner R, Floccard B, Rimmele T. Is decompression illness possible during hyperbaric therapy? a case report. Undersea Hyperb Med. 2017;44(3):283-5.

128. Raja S, Rice TW, Mason DP, Rodriguez C, Tan C, Rodriguez ER, Manno E, Videtic GM, Murthy SC. Fatal cerebral air embolus complicating multimodality treatment of esophageal cancer. Ann Thorac Surg. 2011;92(5):1901-3.

129. Miyamoto S, Mashimo Y, Horimatsu T, Ezoe Y, Morita S, Muto M, Chiba T. Cerebral air embolism caused by chemoradiotherapy for esophageal cancer. J Clin Oncol. 2012;30(25):e237-8.

130. Shim CY, Lee SY, Pak HN. Coronary air embolism associated with atrioesophageal fistula after ablation of atrial fibrillation. Can J Cardiol. 2013;29(10):Pages 1329 e17- e19.

131. Kapur S, Barbhaiya C, Deneke T, Michaud GF. Esophageal injury and atrioesophageal fistula caused by ablation for atrial fibrillation. Circulation. 2017;136(13):1247-55.

132. Thomson M, El Sakr F. Gas in the left atrium and ventricle. N Engl J Med. 2017;376(7):683.

133. Peterson C, Elswick C, Diaz V, Tubbs RS, Moisi M. Delayed presentation of cerebral air embolism from a left atrial-esophageal fistula: a case report and review of the literature. Cureus. 2017;9(11):e1850.

134. Clark CC, Weeks DB, Gusdon JP. Venous carbon dioxide embolism during laparoscopy. Anesth Analg. 1977;56:650-2.

135. Lantz PE, Smith JD. Fatal carbon dioxide embolism complicating attempted laparoscopic cholecystectomy--case report and literature review. J Forensic Sci. 1994;39(6):1468-80.

136. Moskop RJ, Jr, Lubarsky DA. Carbon dioxide embolism during laparoscopic cholecystectomy. South Med J. 1994;87:414-5.

137. Gillart T, Bazin JE, Bonnard M, Schoeffler P. Pulmonary interstitial edema after probable carbon dioxide embolism during laparoscopy. Surg Laparosc Endosc. 1995;5(4):327-9.

138. Cottin V, Delafosse B, Viale JP. Gas embolism during laparoscopy: a report of seven cases in patients with previous abdominal surgical history. Surg Endosc. 1996;10(2):166-9.

139. Vacanti CA, Lodhia KL. Fatal massive air embolism during transurethral resection of the prostate. Anesthesiology. 1991;74(1):186-7.

140. Tsou MY, Teng YH, Chow LH, Ho CM, Tsai SK. Fatal gas embolism during transurethral incision of the bladder neck under spinal anesthesia. Anesth Analg. 2003;97(6):1833-4.

141. Ledowski T, Kiese F, Jeglin S, Scholz J. Possible air embolism during eye surgery. Anesth Analg. 2005;100(6):1651-2.

142. Lin SM, Chang WK, Tsao CM, Ou CH, Chan KH, Tsai SK. Carbon dioxide embolism diagnosed by transesophageal echocardiography during endoscopic vein harvesting for coronary artery bypass grafting. Anesth Analg. 2003;96(3):683-5, table of contents.

143. Sherlock S, Shearer WA, Buist M, Rasiah R, Edwards A. Carbon dioxide embolism following diagnostic hysteroscopy. Anaesth Intensive Care. 1998;26(6):674-6.

144. Imasogie N, Crago R, Leyland NA, Chung F. Probable gas embolism during operative hysteroscopy caused by products of combustion. Can J Anaesth. 2002;49(10):1044-7.

145. Michenfelder JD, Martin JT, Altenburg BM, Rehder K. Air embolism during neurosurgery. An evaluation of right-atrial catheters for diagnosis and treatment. JAMA. 1969;208:1353-8.

146. Fong J, Gadalla F, Gimbel AA. Precordial Doppler diagnosis of haemodynamically compromising air embolism during caesarean section. Can J Anaesth. 1990;37(2):262-4.

147. Jolliffe MP, Lyew MA, Berger IH, Grimaldi T. Venous air embolism during radical perineal prostatectomy. J Clin Anesth. 1996;8(8):659-61.

148. Albin MS, Ritter RR, Reinhart R, Erickson D, Rockwood A. Venous air embolism during radical retropubic prostatectomy. Anesth Analg. 1992;74(1):151-3.

149. Razvi HA, Chin JL, Bhandari R. Fatal air embolism during radical retropubic prostatectomy. J Urol. 1994;151(2):433-4.

150. Lang SA, Duncan PG, Dupuis PR. Fatal air embolism in an adolescent with Duchenne muscular dystrophy during Harrington instrumentation. Anesth Analg. 1989;69(1):132-4.

151. Wills J, Schwend RM, Paterson A, Albin MS. Intraoperative visible bubbling of air may be the first sign of venous air embolism during posterior surgery for scoliosis. Spine. 2005;30(20):E629-35.

152. Andersen KH. Air aspirated from the venous system during total hip replacement. Anaesthesia. 1983;38(12):1175-8.

153. Lee SY, Choi BI, Kim JS, Park KS. Paradoxical air embolism during hepatic resection. Br J Anaesth. 2002;88(1):136-8.

154. Olmedilla L, Garutti I, Perez-Pena J, Sanz J, Teigell E, Avellanal M. Fatal paradoxical air embolism during liver transplantation. Br J Anaesth. 2000;84(1):112-4.

155. Davies JM, Campbell LA. Fatal air embolism during dental implant surgery: a report of three cases. Can J Anaesth. 1990;37(1):112-21.

156. Burrowes P, Wallace C, Davies JM, Campbell L. Pulmonary edema as a radiologic manifestation of venous air embolism secondary to dental implant surgery. Chest. 1992;101(2):561-2.

157. Phillips YY. Primary blast injuries. Ann Emerg Med. 1986;15(12):1446-50.

158. Pao BS, Hayden SR. Cerebral gas embolism resulting from inhalation of pressurized helium [published erratum appears in Ann Emerg Med 1996 Nov;28(5):588]. Ann Emerg Med. 1996;28(3):363-6.

CHAPTER 2A

Arterial Insufficiencies
Central Retinal Artery Occlusion

Heather Murphy-Lavoie MD, Frank Butler MD, Catherine Hagan MD

Background

Central retinal artery occlusion (CRAO) is a relatively rare emergent condition of the eye resulting in sudden painless vision loss. This vision loss is usually dramatic and permanent, and the prognosis for visual recovery is poor. Patients particularly at risk include those with giant cell arteritis, atherosclerosis, and thromboembolic disease. A wide variety of treatment modalities have been tried over the last one hundred years with little to no success, with the exception of hyperbaric oxygen therapy.

Rationale

The arterial blood supply to the eye is provided by the ophthalmic artery, one of the branches of the cavernous portion of the internal carotid artery (Figure 1). Some of the branches of the ophthalmic artery (lacrimal, supraorbital, ethmoidals, medial palpebral, frontal, dorsal nasal) supply orbital structures, while others (central artery of the retina, short and long posterior ciliaries, anterior ciliaries) supply the tissues of the globe.[1] The central retinal artery enters the globe within the substance of the optic nerve and serves the inner layers of the retina through its many branches. The long posterior ciliary arteries provide blood to the choroid and the outer layers of the retina. There are approximately 20 short posterior ciliary arteries and usually two long posterior ciliary arteries. The posterior ciliary vessels originate from the ophthalmic artery and supply the entire uveal tract, cilioretinal arteries, the sclera, the margin of the cornea, and the adjacent conjunctiva. The anterior ciliary arteries also arise from the ophthalmic artery, supply the extraocular muscles, and anastamose with the posterior ciliary vessels to form the major arterial circle of the iris, which supplies the iris and ciliary body.

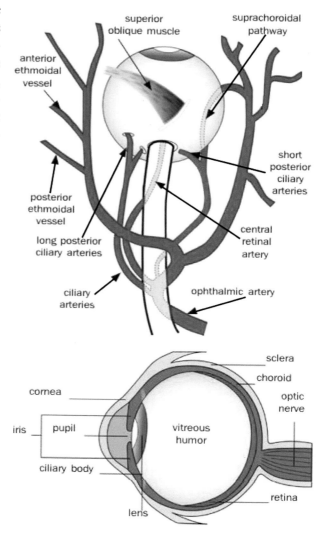

Figure 1. Structural Anatomy of the Eye
Copyright © Best Publishing Company

15

The visual signs and symptoms of vascular occlusive diseases of the retina are dependent on the particular vessel occluded, the degree of occlusion, the location of the occlusion, and the presence or absence of a cilio-retinal artery. In approximately 15-30% of individuals, a cilioretinal artery is present. This artery is part of the ciliary (not retinal) arterial supply but supplies the area of the retina around the macula (central vision area). If a cilio-retinal artery is present, central vision may be preserved in central retinal artery occlusion.

In CRAO, the inner retinal layers (ganglion cell layer and inner nuclear layer) normally served by the retinal circulation will typically lose viability, and this is responsible for the vision loss. These layers may, however, obtain enough oxygen via diffusion from the choroidal circulation to maintain viability if the individual is exposed to elevated partial pressures of oxygen. Animal models have shown that the choroidal vessels may supply sufficient oxygen to the inner layers of the retina to maintain ganglion cell viability even when the retinal vessels have been completely obliterated.[2] Normally, the choroidal circulation supplies the majority of the oxygen to the retina. Under normoxic conditions, approximately 60% of the retina's oxygen comes from the choroidal circulation. Under hyperoxic conditions the choroid is capable of supplying 100% of the oxygen needed by the retina.[3]

In considering the effect of treating CRAO with supplemental oxygen, there are four key factors. First, therapy must be initiated before the retinal tissue is irreparably damaged. For the second factor, the degree of occlusion of the blocked vessel may vary, which may account for why some patients respond to oxygen at lower partial pressures than others. Third, some patients may not respond to HBO$_2$, even if initiated promptly, if the level of occlusion is at the ophthalmic artery. In this event, the blood supply to the posterior ciliary vessels is blocked as well, and there is no collateral circulation to provide oxygenation of the inner layers of the retina. The fourth factor requires an adequate partial pressure of oxygen be maintained to keep the retina viable until circulation is restored via natural recanalization, which usually occurs within 72 hours.

The etiology of the arterial occlusion (thrombosis, embolus, arteritis, vasospasm, foreign material such as filler) has also been described as affecting outcome.[4-5,70] Careful classification of the factors involved in an individual case of CRAO is crucial to understanding the natural outcome and results of therapy. In the largest published series of CRAO patients, Hayreh describes the natural progression of this condition without hyperbaric oxygen therapy. He found that patients with transient CRAO (resolution of symptoms in minutes to hours) and those with cilioretinal arteries had much better outcomes than those who did not. In those patients without cilioretinal arteries or transient presentations, 80% had a final visual outcome of count fingers or less, and only 1.5% of them obtained a final vision of 20/40 or better.[5]

Recanalization occurs in retinal vessels after CRAO.[6-7] In relatively few cases, however, does this angiographic reperfusion lead to an improvement of vision.[7] The retina has the highest rate of oxygen consumption of any organ in the body at 13 mL/100 g/minute.[8-9, 78] Therefore, it is very sensitive to ischemia. In order to be effective, the administration of supplemental oxygen must be continued until such time as flow through the retinal artery has resumed to a level sufficient to maintain inner retinal viability under normoxic conditions.

Patient Selection Criteria

The classic presentation of CRAO is sudden painless loss of vision in the range of light perception to counting fingers. In the case of vision loss to the level of no light perception, the patient may have an ophthalmic artery occlusion and therefore no blood flowing to the choroidal vessels either. If central visual acuity is relatively spared in the presence of a fundus exam consistent with CRAO, the presence of a cilioretinal artery is likely.

On dilated fundoscopic exam, patients with CRAO will classically have a pale yellow/white-appearing retina due to ischemia or necrosis. A cherry-red spot may develop in the macula but this finding may not always be present. The presence of a cherry-red spot is a poor prognostic indicator.[74] Other physical exam findings may include an afferent pupillary defect and boxcarring of arterioles.

Patients presenting within 24 hours of symptom onset should be considered for hyperbaric oxygen therapy. While there are a few case reports of patients presenting after this time interval having positive results when treated with hyperbaric oxygen therapy, the majority of cases do not respond when treated beyond this point.[8,10-14]

While consideration of the pertinent physiology suggests that patients with branch retinal artery occlusions (BRAO) and central retinal vein occlusions may also benefit from hyperbaric oxygen therapy, there is insufficient data in the literature to support this as a routine recommendation.[10,15-16]

Clinical Management

Patients who present with sudden painless loss of vision due to CRAO should be triaged as "emergent" because of the need for immediate oxygen therapy. Visual acuity should be documented as soon as possible. If decreased vision (less than 20/200) is confirmed without improvement with pinhole, the emergency physician should immediately perform a fundoscopic exam using dilation if feasible and not contraindicated. The presence of flashes or floaters preceding the vision loss, pain, history of recent trauma, or age younger than 40 suggests an alternate diagnosis (e.g. retinal detachment/vitreous hemorrhage). An ophthalmologist should be consulted emergently but treatment with supplemental oxygen should not be delayed awaiting his or her arrival. In centers where CRAO is treated by the stroke service, neurology should also be consulted. **Ideally, patients should be admitted to the hospital under the stroke protocol with combined management from ophthalmology and neurology.**[81] Intra-ocular pressure should be measured and treated if elevated. Ocular massage has been anecdotally reported to dislodge clots on occasion.[17]

Diagnostic workup to screen for conditions that may predispose to CRAO should include: Complete blood count (CBC, to screen for platelet disorders or infectious causes); erythrocyte sedimentation rate (ESR) and C-reactive protein (to screen for giant cell arteritis); coagulation panel (fibrinogen, prothrombin time/partial thromboplastin time (PT/PTT); antiphospholipid antibody); lipid panel; EKG; carotid ultrasound; MRI, and echocardiography. Previously undiagnosed vascular risk factors are found in 78% of CRAO patients.[80] MRI of CRAO patients found 32% had an acute or subacute incidental brain infarcts demonstrating the high risk nature of these patients and need for admission from the emergency department.[81] HBO_2 should not be delayed to accomplish any of these diagnostic measures. In cases of suspected arteritic CRAO, treatment with intravenous corticosteroids should be initiated emergently and HBO_2 therapy should still be undertaken.

Fundoscopic findings of CRAO should trigger management as below if symptom onset is within 24 hours or less. Oxygen delivery should be titrated to patient response as follows (also see Figure 2):

1. Deliver oxygen immediately at 1 atmosphere absolute (ATA) (101.325 kPa) at the highest possible fraction of inspired oxygen (FiO_2).

2. If vision improves significantly with normobaric oxygen within 15 minutes, the patient should be admitted to the hospital and given intermittent normobaric oxygen for 15 minutes every hour, alternating with 45 minutes of breathing room air. Visual acuity should be checked at the end of each air-breathing period. This regimen should be continued until a fluorescein angiogram shows patency, the patient's vision remains stable on room air for two hours or a maximum time of 96 hours on intermittent supplemental oxygen therapy has been reached.

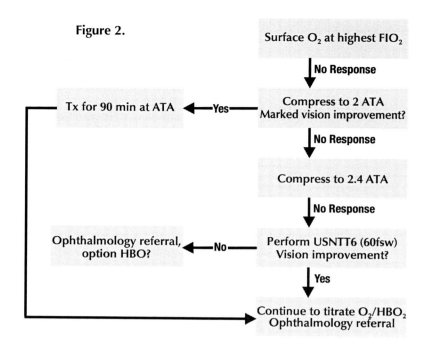

Figure 2.

3. Refer for emergent hyperbaric oxygen therapy if no response within the first 15 minutes. **Hyperbaric oxygen can be delivered for 90 minutes at the depth of return of vision, with a maximum of a USNTT6 for the first treatment.**

4. Compress to 2 ATA (202.65 kPa) on 100% oxygen.

5. Other adjunctive therapies to lower intraocular pressure and/or cause retinal vasodilatation may be performed as well, but should not delay compression. If vision improves significantly at 2 ATA (202.65 kPa), remain at this depth for 90 minutes (air-breathing periods at this depth may not be necessary since the incidence of oxygen toxicity seizures is four times lower at 2 ATA/202.65 kPa than at 2.4 ATA/243.18 kPa),[18] then proceed as outlined in #8 below.

6. If vision fails to improve significantly at 2 ATA (202.65 kPa) by the first air-breathing period (or 30 minutes), compress to 2.4 ATA (243.18 kPa). If vision improves significantly at this depth, conduct a U.S. Navy Treatment Table 9 and then proceed as outlined in #8 below.

7. If vision does not improve significantly at 2.4 ATA (243.18 kPa), compress to 2.8 ATA (283.71 kPa). If no improvement occurs after the first 20-minute breathing period, consider conducting a U.S. Navy Treatment Table 6 (USNTT6). If vision improves significantly, proceed as outlined in Section 8 below. If there is no response to the initial Table 6 treatment, options are to discontinue treatment, continue with normobaric oxygen as in #2, or give two additional treatments for 90 minutes at 2.8 ATA (283.71 kPa) with air-breathing periods on a twice-daily schedule.

8. If the patient has return of vision during hyperbaric treatment, inpatient monitoring and intermittent supplemental oxygen should be considered. Monitoring by a retina specialist should continue. Recovery of vision during the initial treatment of CRAO with HBO$_2$ indicates retinal viability and the potential for return of vision despite the ischemic period suffered prior to treatment. Patients with such a recovery should have their visual status monitored frequently after completion of HBO$_2$.

Patients should be monitored at the chamber for two hours post-treatment. If vision remains normal and hospital admission is not feasible, they can be discharged with instruction to monitor vision every hour. Should vision loss recur, aggressive use of intermittent normobaric oxygen as described in #2 or customized hyperbaric oxygen is indicated to preserve retinal function until CRA recanalization occurs. Hyperbaric treatments twice or three times daily may be necessary until the angiogram normalizes or the patient has no further improvement for three treatments.

Notes

The retina may not tolerate periods of ischemia that persist longer than 90 minutes. Cases of relapse of loss of vision and resultant blindness after discharge have been reported[4,7,12,19,75] and patients should be instructed to return immediately for supplemental oxygen therapy if vision loss recurs after discharge.

One exception to the above regimen is CRAO that results from AGE. In this event, the recommended treatment regimen for AGE should be followed with a minimum of USNTT6. Patients with history of DCI, recent hemodialysis, or general anesthesia should always be treated with HBO_2.

All patients who have lost vision in one eye should be directed to present immediately to a hospital or to their ophthalmologist if vision loss occurs in the fellow eye.

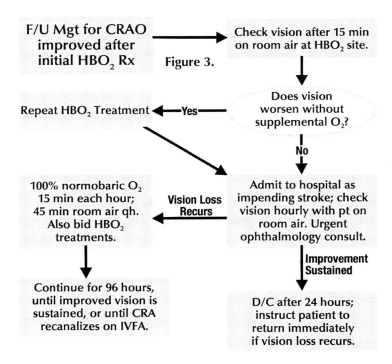

Recommended follow-up management of CRAO patients after initial HBO_2 treatment. Butler 2018.[75]

Key: BID - twice a day CRA- central retinal artery D/C - discharge F/U - follow-up
min - minutes Pt - patient QH - every hour Rx - treatment
IVFA - intravenous fluorescein angiogram

Evidence-Based Review

Possible causes of retinal arterial occlusive disease include atherosclerosis-related thrombus, embolism, vasospasm, and giant cell arteritis. A CRAO with significant visual loss is an ophthalmic emergency. Treatment should be aimed at promptly supplying oxygen to the ischemic retina at a partial pressure sufficient to maintain viability while medically assisted or spontaneous restoration of central retinal artery blood flow occurs. Animal models of retinal injury have shown a reduction in apoptosis from 58% cell loss to 30% and a maintenance of retinal thickness in animals treated with HBO_2 after experimental CRAO.[20, 77]

Traditional therapeutic regimens for CRAO have been aimed at promoting a downstream movement of the embolus by lowering intraocular pressure and producing vasodilatation. These measures include ocular massage, anterior chamber paracentesis, intraocular pressure-lowering medications, vasodilators, and oral diuretics.[4,7-8] These treatment modalities have been generally unsuccessful.[4,7,21] Acute obstruction of the central retinal artery, even when treated promptly, typically results in severe, permanent visual loss.[5,7] Hayreh stated that no currently used therapy is efficacious for CRAO[5,22] but he did not consider the use of HBO_2.

More recent treatment modalities include thrombolytic agents[23-25] and surgical removal of the embolus or thrombus.[26-27] One study reporting the limited success with thrombolytics used in conjunction with intraocular pressure-lowering medications, anterior chamber paracentesis, and methylprednisolone included only patients seen within 48 hours of onset of symptoms and noted that all eight patients in whom visual acuity improved had symptoms for less than 12 hours.[24]

Supplemental oxygen therapy has been used in conjunction with the above regimens. When retinal arterial flow is interrupted, the retinal tissue undergoes a period of ischemia. Blood flow is usually re-established via recanalization, but if ischemia and hypoxia have resulted in cell death and necrosis in the inner layers of the retina, which are areas supplied by the retinal artery, vision may not return when blood flow is re-established.[28] The tissue that is ischemic yet capable of recovery within a certain time frame is called the ischemic penumbra.[28]

Supplemental oxygen need not always be provided at hyperbaric pressures to successfully reverse retinal ischemia in CRAO. One patient suffered a CRAO in his only seeing eye and presented within approximately one hour of vision loss to the emergency department, where he was found to have vision of 20/400 and fundus findings typical of a CRAO. He was treated with oxygen supplied by a non-rebreathing mask at 1 ATM in the ED, and his vision quickly improved to the 20/25 level. After a period of approximately five minutes, the supplemental oxygen was removed, whereupon vision equally quickly returned to 20/400. This process was repeated several times to confirm the efficacy of the supplemental oxygen with the same results. The patient was then hospitalized, anticoagulated, and maintained on supplemental oxygen for approximately 18 hours, after which his central retinal artery presumably recanalized since removal of the supplemental oxygen at that point no longer caused a drop in vision. He was discharged with a visual acuity of 20/25 in his only seeing eye.[29]

Patz reported improvement in two CRAO patients given oxygen at 1 ATA (101.325 kPa). One patient received oxygen after a four-hour delay to therapy, and improvement was maintained after oxygen was discontinued four hours later. The second patient improved significantly after a delay to treatment of 90 minutes and maintained this improvement when oxygen was discontinued three hours later. In both patients, early discontinuation of oxygen was followed by deterioration of vision within minutes and visual recovery when oxygen breathing was resumed shortly thereafter. This phenomenon was observed several times in both patients.[2]

Stone et al. reported two patients with CRAO of greater than six hours duration treated with intermittent carbogen (95% oxygen and 5% carbon dioxide), retrobulbar anesthesia, and anterior chamber paracentesis. The first patient had vision loss of 6 hours duration. His vision improved from hand motion to 20/20 on the above therapy, with carbogen being administered for 10 minutes every hour. The second patient presented eight hours after onset of visual loss and had improvement from finger counting to 20/25. Carbogen was administered 10 minutes every hour for 48 hours.[4]

Of note is that carbon dioxide was added to the oxygen to help prevent retinal vasoconstriction in the cases above. Elevated partial pressures of oxygen cause retinal artery vasoconstriction.[30-32] CO_2 is added to the gas mix in carbogen to counter this effect through its vasodilatation of retinal vessels. If the mechanism of improved oxygenation to the retina is diffusion from the choroidal circulation, however, then the addition of carbon dioxide should be of little benefit since, unlike retinal blood flow, choroidal blood flow is not significantly affected by changes in oxygen tension.[3,32] The hyperoxygenation of the choriocapillaris was noted to more than offset the reduced retinal blood flow as observed by the appearance of arterialized bright-red blood in the retinal veins during HBO_2.[30] Note that carbogen should never be used during HBO because elevated partial pressures of CO_2 potentiate the development of central nervous system oxygen toxicity.

The study published by Augsberger and Magargal in 1980 was notable in that it demonstrated the criticality of the time to oxygen treatment in successful outcome. They used paracentesis, ocular massage, carbogen, acetazolamide, and aspirin to treat 34 consecutive cases of CRAO. Twelve of the 34 patients were successfully treated, with 7 of the 12 having been treated within 24 hours of onset of symptoms. The longest delay to treatment in which treatment was considered successful was 72 hours. The average delay to therapy in the patients with successful outcomes was 21.1 hours, compared to 58.6 hours in those who did not improve. Carbogen inhalation was conducted for 10 minutes every hour during waking hours and 10 minutes every 4 hours at night and continued for 48 to 72 hours in these patients.[12]

One remarkable case report described a patient with angiographically documented obstruction of both the central retinal artery and his temporal posterior ciliary artery.[7] He presented after five hours of visual loss with minimal light perception vision. In addition to ocular massage, anterior chamber paracentesis, timolol, and acetazolamide, he was given carbogen for 10 minutes every hour around the clock. His vision did not improve significantly during his three days of hospitalization, but improved spontaneously approximately 96 hours after onset of vision loss. His vision in the affected eye was documented to be 20/30 one week after discharge. Although the authors of this case report do not necessarily ascribe his recovery to any one of the treatments used,[7] the role of supplemental oxygen in maintaining retinal viability must be considered. Patients with CRAO rarely improve spontaneously.[7]

If hyperoxia at 1 ATM is not effective in reversing vision loss in CRAO, emergent compression and 100% oxygen breathing should be undertaken. Phillips et al. reported a 71-year-old white female patient with CRAO in whom surface oxygen was ineffective in restoring "total" vision loss of approximately two hours duration.[33] Initial treatment with supplemental oxygen at one atmosphere did not reverse this vision loss. Light perception returned as she was compressed on 100% oxygen to 1.45 ATA (146.92 kPa). At the end of the first air-breathing period at 2.8 ATA (283.71 kPa) she had return of vision to her subjective baseline. She was discharged with a visual acuity of 20/30 in her only seeing eye and the 2+ afferent papillary defect noted prior to treatment had resolved after treatment.[33]

The timing of HBO_2 therapy is critical in CRAO. There is a threshold of time beyond which ischemic tissue can no longer recover from a hypoxic event even if reperfusion occurs.[3] Hayreh et al. reported a study in which the ophthalmic artery of rhesus monkeys was completely occluded for varying periods of time. Retinas exposed to periods of greater than 105 minutes without blood flow showed permanent damage. If the duration of occlusion was kept to less than 97 minutes, the retinas returned to normal as evaluated by multiple types of diagnostic testing.[34]

In the clinical setting of CRAO, however, some residual retinal blood flow has been detected by fluorescein angiogram.[6,12] This may help explain the great variability in visual outcome with different time delays to treatment. Ideally, the shorter the time delay until treatment, including HBO_2, the better the likelihood of recovering the ischemic retina that is threatened but viable (penumbra).[3,12,35] Ophthalmology literature includes cases in which humans with a CRAO have regained significant vision even when treatment was delayed for periods of up to two weeks,[36] with the strongest evidence for symptomatic improvement in cases with less than 12 hours delay.[3,8,14,37] See Table 1 for a summary of the cases treated with HBO_2. It is difficult for the clinician to predict which patients will respond to HBO_2 beyond the recognition that minimizing the retinal ischemic time maximizes the potential for visual recovery.[38]

Table 1. Treatment of Retinal Artery Occlusions: Literature Summary

Report	CRAO/ BRAO	Therapy	Delay to Tx	Initial VA	Final VA	Total Patients (n)	Cases Improved (n)
Gool & Jong 1965[40]	BRAO CRAO CRAO BRAO	HBO_2: 3 ATA (303.98 kPa), anticoagulants, Complamin	5 days 2 days Unkn (<24 hr) 10 days	1.5% NLP 125% 1.6%	100% NLP 125% imp VF 1.6%	4	2
Haddad & Leopold 1965[31]	CRAO	HBO_2	Unknown	NLP CF	NLP CF	2	0
Anderson et al. 1965[11]	BRAO CRAO BRAO	HBO_2, retrobulbar lidocaine, ocular massage, nicotinic acid	"several hours" 40+ hrs 6+ days	CF 2-3 ft 20/25 20/200	20/20 20/25 imp VF Unknown	3	2
Takahashi et al. 1977[41]		HBO_2: 2.5 ATA (253.32 kPa), ocular massage, paracentesis, vasodilator	1-6 days	Graph	Graph	9	9
Pallota et al. 1978[42]	CRAO	HBO_2: 2.8 ATA (283.71 kPa)		NLP	10/10	1	1
Sasaki et al. 1978[43]	CRAO	HBO_2, stellate ganglion block				10	7
Szuki et al. 1980[44]	CRAO	HBO_2				6	6
Krasnov et al. 1981[45]	CRAO	HBO_2				39	22
Zhang & Cao 1986[35]	CRAO	HBO_2				80	49
Desola 1987[46]	CRAO	HBO_2				20	11
Miyake et al. 1987[13]	CRAO (53) BRAO (19)	HBO_2 at 2 ATA (202.65 kPa) or 3 ATA (303.98 kPa), varied vasodilators, stellate ganglion block, 2% carbocaine	18 hours to 15 days, all but 3 within 12 days	Graph	Graph	72	32

Report	CRAO/ BRAO	Therapy	Delay to Tx	Initial VA	Final VA	Total Patients (n)	Cases Improved (n)
Kindwall & Goldmann 1988 [47]	CRAO	HBO$_2$				14	7
Hirayama et al. 1990 [48]	CRAO	HBO$_2$; mixtures of urokinase, steroid, bifemelane HCL	<1 month	Graph	Graph	17	12
Hertzog et al. 1992 [8]	CRAO	HBO$_2$: 1.5-2.0 ATA; (151.99-202.65 kPa); mixtures of timolol maleate 0.5%, acetazol-amide, paracentesis, carbogen, vasodilator, steroids, ocular massage, retrobulbar anesthesia	<8 hrs >8, >/=24hrs >24hrs All patients	Graph	Graph	19	14
Beiran et al. 1993 [37]	CRAO	HBO$_2$: 2.5 ATA, (253.32 kPa), ocular massage, SL nifedipine, oral glycerol	2: <100min 1: occluding 1: 6 hrs	LP HM CF 2m HM	6/20 6/6 6/9 CF 60cm	4	4
Yotsukura et al. 1993 [14]	CRAO	HBO$_2$, ocular massage, IV urokinase, and 2/15 with IV prostaglandin	3 hrs to 6 days	Graph	Graph	15	8
Li et al. 1996 [3]	BRAO OS BRAO OD (15mo later)	HBO$_2$: 2.32 ATA (235.07 kPa) HBO$_2$: 2.82 ATA (285.74 kPa)	<24 hours <24 hours	20/200 CF 2ft	20/25 20/25	2	2
Phillips et al. 1999 [33]	CRAO	100% surface O$_2$, HBO$_2$: 2.4 ATA (243.18 kPa)	<2 hrs	NLP	20/30	1	1
Aisenbrey et al. 2000 [49]	CRAO (8) BRAO (10)	HBO$_2$: 240 kPa, ocular massage, paracentesis, IV acetazolamide		Graph	Graph	18	12
Matsuo 2001 [36]	BRAO (OU)	HBO$_2$, IV prostaglandin, urokinase	4 days	20/30 20/600	20/15 20/400	2	2
Beiran et al. 2001 [39]	CRAO (29) BRAO (6)	HBO$_2$: 2.8 ATA (283.71 kPa); mixtures of ocular massage, retrobulbar block, timolol, acetazol-amide, paracentesis	<8 hrs	Graph	Graph	35	29
Weinberger et al. 2002 [50]	CRAO	HBO$_2$, ocular massage, antiglaucoma eyedrops	4-12 hrs	Graph	Graph	21	13
Murphy-Lavoie et al. 2004 [10]	CRAO BRAO	HBO$_2$, 2 ATA (202.65 kPa)	6 hrs - 4 days	Graph	Graph	16	12
Imai et al. 2004 [51]	BRAO	HBO$_2$, stellate ganglion block	2 days	CF	0.08	1	1
Swaby 2005 [52]	CRAO	HBO$_2$: 2.0 ATA, optic nerve sheath fenestration	3 weeks	20/400	Improved	1	1

Table 1. Treatment of Retinal Artery Occlusions: Literature Summary (continued)

Report	CRAO/ BRAO	Therapy	Delay to Tx	Initial VA	Final VA	Total Patients (n)	Cases Improved (n)
Weiss 2009 [53]	CRAO (4) BRAO (1)	HBO$_2$: 1.5 ATA (151.99 kPa), prednisone for the one patient with biopsy proven arteritis	1-21 days	CF 5ft HM LP LP/CF	20/200 20/30 LP LP/CF	4	2
Inoue 2009[54]	CRAO BRAO	HBO$_2$: 1.8 ATA	Hours to 3 days	Graph	Graph	63	30
Weiss 2010 [55]	BRAO	HBO$_2$: 1.5 ATA (151.99 kPa)	1-12 days	CF CF 6ft visual field def	20/70 20/50	5	5
Aten 2011[56]	CRAO	HBO$_2$: 2.4 ATA	7 hours	NR	20/80	1	1
Cope et al. 2011 [57]	CRAO	HBO$_2$: 2.4 ATA (243.18 kPa)	5-144 hours	Graph	Graph	11	8
Telander 2011[19]	CRAO	HBO$_2$ Ocular message Pressure lowering drops	11 hours	CF	20/160	1	1
Menzel et al. 2012 [58]	CRAO	HBO$_2$: 2.4 ATA (243.18 kPa), hemodilution	<12 hours	Graph	Graph	51	30
Canan 2014[64]	CRAO	HBO$_2$: 2.5 ATA, exchange transfusion	<24 hours	CF	20/30	1	1
Hsiao 2014[65]	CRAO	HBO$_2$: 2.5 ATA x 6 Carbogen, pressure lowering eyedrops, hemodilution, corticosteroids	4 hours	CF	20/200	1	1
Masters 2015[66]	CRAO	HBO$_2$: 2.8 ATA	<24 hours	Graph	Graph	29	20
Desola 2015[67]	CRAO	HBO$_2$: 2.3 ATA x 15	<2 months	NR	NR	182	138
Lu 2015[68]	CRAO CRVO	HBO$_2$, ocular massage, anterior paracentesis, aspirin	100min	LP	HM	1	1
Lemos 2015[69]	CRAO	HBO$_2$: 2.4 ATA, aspirin	8 hours	20/400	20/40	1	1
Hwang 2016[70]	CRAO	HBO$_2$	NR	NR	NR	2	0
Olson 2016[71]	CRAO	HBO$_2$: 2.4 ATA - 2.5 ATA x 6 Tx	< 12 hours	CF	20/40	1	1
Tang 2016[72]	CRAO	HBO$_2$ BID x 5 days	>24 hours	20/200	20/200	1	1
Elder 2017[73]	CRAO	HBO$_2$ 2.0-2.8 ATA for 90-120min x 1-7Tx	NR	Graph	Graph	31	23

Table 1. Treatment of Retinal Artery Occlusions: Literature Summary (continued)

Report	CRAO/ BRAO	Therapy	Delay to Tx	Initial VA	Final VA	Total Patients (n)	Cases Improved (n)
Hadanny 2017[74]	CRAO	HBO$_2$: 2-2.4 ATA, ocular massage, anterior chamber paracentesis, ASA, acetazolamide, topical beta-blocker	<20 hours	Graph	Graph	128	86
Butler 2018[75]	CRAO	HBO$_2$: 2.4 ATA for 115min	9.5 hours	HM	CF	1	1
Gunay 2018[76]	CRAO	HBO$_2$: 2.5 ATA for 90min x 10 Tx, ocular message, paracentesis	4 hours	20/400	20/200	1	1

Note: See full graphs of patient results in original papers.

		TOTAL 927 611

OS - left eye
OD - right eye
VA - visual acuity
LP - light perception

VF - visual fields
ED - emergency department
NR - not recorded
NLP - no light perception

CF - counting fingers
HM - hand motion

% IMPROVED   66%

Hertzog et al. reported a series of 17 patients with CRAO treated with HBO$_2$. They retrospectively divided patients into four treatment groups based on the time to onset of treatment and noted that HBO$_2$ seemed useful in preserving visual function when applied within the first eight hours from the onset of visual impairment. The patients in this study were treated for 105 minutes of oxygen at 2 ATA (202.65 kPa) three times a day until they ceased to show improvement in visual acuity or for three to four days if no improvement occurred. They received a mean of 29.3 hours of HBO$_2$ over five to six days early in the data collection period and 34.6 hours over five to six days later in the data collection period. The authors modified their treatment protocol to a 1.5 ATA (151.99 kPa) prolonged exposure midway through the data collection period, accounting for the differences in treatment times. The authors point out that the colloquialism "time is muscle," used in management of myocardial infarctions, can be changed to "time is vision" in CRAO.[8]

Another paper demonstrated success in treating three cases of CRAO in which the patients presented shortly after the onset of symptoms. One patient treated 90 minutes after onset of visual loss had vision improve from light perception to counting fingers after the first 10 minutes of HBO$_2$, with subsequent improvement to 20/70 following five days of two 90-minute HBO$_2$ treatments at 2.5 ATA (253.32 kPa) daily for five days. Another patient presented 40 minutes after visual loss and improved from hand motion to 20/20 after 12 treatments at 2.5 ATA (253.32 kPa) in nine days. A third patient presented four hours after the onset of symptoms with finger-counting vision. He received 10 HBO$_2$ treatments at 2.5 ATA (253.32 kPa) for 90 minutes each, with gradual improvement of visual acuity to the 20/30 level. A last patient who was treated with HBO$_2$ six hours after symptom onset showed no significant improvement in vision.[37]

In 2001, Beiran published a retrospective controlled trial of 35 retinal artery occlusion patients treated with hyper-baric oxygen therapy compared to 37 matched controls from another facility where hyperbaric oxygen was not available.[39] All patients were treated within eight hours of symptom onset, and none of the patients included in the study had a cilioretinal artery. The patients in the hyperbaric group received 2.8 ATA (283.71 kPa) for 90 minutes BID for the first three days and then once daily until no further improvement for three consecutive days.

In the hyperbaric group, 82% of the patients improved compared to only 29.7% of patients in the control group. Improvement was defined as reading at least three lines better on the Snellen chart compared to ability at admission. The mean visual acuity for the hyperbaric group at discharge was 6/20 in meters or about 20/70 in feet.

As with oxygen administration at 1 ATA (101.325 kPa), hyperbaric oxygen must be started within the time interval that retinal tissue can still recover.[7] Reports that describe failure of HBO$_2$ sometimes fail to provide any information concerning the delay to therapy,[31] and HBO therapy in these cases may have been started after the time window for successful treatment had passed. Miyake reported on 53 patients with CRAO and 19 with branch retinal artery occlusions treated with HBO$_2$ over a 13-year period. He found no significant difference between time to treatment and response to HBO$_2$; however, only three of these patients received HBO$_2$ within 24 hours of symptom onset, so most of these individuals were outside the window where HBO$_2$ would have had the best chance of success. A total of 44% of the patients in this study showed improvement of at least two levels on the visual acuity scale after treatment with HBO$_2$ despite this delay to treatment. Unfortunately, no distinction was made between patients with cilioretinal arteries and transient occlusions and those without.[13]

Overall, 66% of cases have shown improvement when treated with HBO$_2$ (see Table 1). These cases of CRAO make it apparent that some patients with CRAO can be treated successfully with hyperoxia, either at 1 ATA (101.325 kPa) or with HBO$_2$. **The sooner the patient is treated, the higher the likelihood of significant improvement in vision** (0.03 logMAR worse for each hour of delay).[74] Patients with a cherry red spot on funduscopic exam have a lower likelihood of significant improvement in vision when treated with HBO$_2$ than those without (49% vs 86%).[74]

Based on the American Heart Association classification of evidence, treatment of CRAO with hyperbaric oxygen therapy is level IIb.[59] There is fair to good evidence to support its use with retrospective controlled case series but no prospective randomized controlled trials. It is acceptable, safe, considered efficacious, but lacks confirmation of efficacy by level I studies. There is no evidence of harm and consistently positive results when HBO$_2$ is begun shortly after onset on vision loss. In addition, there are no alternative therapies with similar outcomes,[21-22] thus presenting ethical considerations for a proposed randomized trial. The relatively rare incidence of this condition does not lend itself to randomized controlled trials as evidenced by the paucity of trials for other therapies in treating this condition. The hopeless and recalcitrant nature of this condition when left untreated mandates we utilize all potentially helpful treatments, including hyperbaric oxygen therapy. Despite this, a recent survey of U.S. centers that have both vascular neurology and retina or neuro-ophthalmology fellowship programs found that only 7% of centers sometimes offer hyperbaric oxygen therapy.[79]

Utilization Review

The optimum number of treatments will vary depending on the severity and duration of the patient's symptoms and the degree of response to treatment. The majority of patients will stabilize within a few days after symptom onset. Utilization review is recommended for patients treated for more than three days after clinical plateau and no further improvement. Stabilization of vision on normoxic breathing and central retinal artery patency on fluorescein angiogram may both be useful in determining when supplemental and/or hyperbaric oxygen may be safely discontinued.[58,60]

Cost Impact

There are no formal cost analyses for this condition in the literature; however, the treatment cost for HBO$_2$ therapy is between $200 and $500 per 90-minute treatment in the clinic/outpatient setting. If each CRAO patient receiving 10 treatments, the cost would be between $2,000 and $5,000 per patient. This is a reasonable price to pay to restore a patient's vision. The cost of long-term care for an individual who has lost useful vision must be weighed in economic impact considerations.

Disclaimer

The opinions expressed in this paper are those of the authors and do not necessarily reflect those of the Department of Defense or the Department of the Navy.

References

1. Cibis GW, Beaver HA, Johns K, et al. Fundamentals and principles of ophthalmology (basic and clinical science course). San Francisco, CA: American Academy of Ophthalmology; 2006. Pp. 38-40.
2. Patz A. Oxygen inhalation in retinal arterial occlusion. Am J Ophthalmol. 1955;40:789-795.
3. Li HK, Dejean BJ, Tang RA. Reversal of visual loss with hyperbaric oxygen treatment in a patient with Susac Syndrome. Ophthalmology. 1996;103(12):2091-2098.
4. Stone R, Zink H, Klingele T, Burde R. Visual recovery after central retinal artery occlusion: two cases. Ann Ophthalmol. 1977;9:445-450.
5. Hayreh SS, Zimmerman MB. Central retinal artery occlusion: visual outcome. Am J Ophthalmol. 2005;140:376-391.
6. David NJ, Norton EWD, Gass JD, Beauchamp J. Fluorescein angiography in central retinal artery occlusion. Arch Ophthal. 1967;77:619-629.
7. Duker JS, Brown GC. Recovery following acute obstruction of the retinal and choroidal circulations. Retina. 1988;8(4):257-260.
8. Hertzog LM, Meyer GW, Carson S, Strauss MB, Hart GB. Central retinal artery occlusion treated with hyperbaric oxygen. J Hyperbaric Medicine. 1992;7:33-42.
9. Jain KK, editor. Textbook of hyperbaric medicine. 4th ed. Cambridge, MA: Hogrefe & Huber Publishers; 2004. Pp. 383- 392.
10. Murphy-Lavoie H, Harch P, VanMeter K. Effect of hyperbaric oxygen on central retinal artery occlusion (abstract). UHMS Scientific Assembly, Australia; 2004.
11. Anderson B, Saltzman H, Heyman A. The effects of hyperbaric oxygenation on retinal arterial occlusion. Arch Ophthal. 1965;73:315-319.
12. Augsburger JJ, Magargal LE. Visual prognosis following treatment of acute central retinal artery obstruction. Br J Ophthalmol. 1980;64:913-917.
13. Miyake Y, Horiguchi M, Matsuura M, et al. Hyperbaric oxygen therapy in 72 eyes with retinal arterial occlusion. In: The 9th international symposium on underwater and hyperbaric physiology. Bethesda, MD: Undersea and Hyperbaric Medical Society; 1987. Pp. 949-953.
14. Yotsukura J, Adachi-Usami E. Correlation of electro-retinographic changes with visual prognosis in central retinal artery occlusion. Ophthalmologica. 1993;207:13-18.
15. Roy M, Bartow W, Ambrus J, Fauci A, Collier B, Titus J. Retinal leakage in retinal vein occlusion: reduction after hyperbaric oxygen. Ophthalmologica. 1989;198:78-83.
16. Miyake Y, Awaya S, Takahashi H, et al. Hyperbaric oxygen and acetazolamide improve visual acuity in patients with cystoid macular edema by different mechanisms. Arch Ophthalmol. 1993;111:1605-1606.
17. Schmidt D. Ocular massage in a case of central retinal artery occlusion the successful treatment of a hitherto undescribed type of embolism. Eur J Med Res. 2000 Apr 19;5(4):157-164.
18. Beard T, Warriner RA, Pascer P, et al. Adverse events during hyperbaric oxygen therapy (HBOT), a retrospective analysis from 25 centers (abstract). Undersea Hyperbaric Medical Society Annual Scientific Meeting, Las Vegas, NV; 2005.
19. Telander G, Hielweil G Schwartz S, Butler F. Diagnostic and therapeutic challenges. Retina. 2011;31(8):1726-1731.
20. Gaydar V, Ezraichi D, Dratviman-Storobinsky O, et al. Invest Ophthalmol Vis Sci. 2011;52:7514-7522.
21. Neubauer AS, Mueller AJ, Schriever S, Gruterich M, Ulbig M, Kampik A. Minimally invasive therapy for clini- cally complete central retinal artery occlusion-results and meta-analysis of literature. Klin Monatsbl Augenheilkd. 2000 Jul;217(1):30-36.
22. Hayreh SS, Podhajsky P. Ocular neovascularization with retinal vascular occlusion: II. Occurrence in central retinal and branch retinal artery occlusion. Arch Ophthalmol. 1982;100:1581-1596.
23. Weber J, Remonda L, Mattle HP, et al. Selective intra-arterial fibrinolysis of acute central retinal artery occlusion. Stroke. 1998;29:2076-2079.
24. Rumelt S, Dorenboim Y, Rehany U. Aggressive systematic treatment for central retinal artery occlusion. Am J Ophthalmol. 1999;128:733-738.
25. Petterson JA, Hill MD, Demchuk AM, et al. Intra-arterial thrombolysis for retinal artery occlusion: The Calgary experience. Can J Neurol Sci. 2005;32:507-511.
26. Garcia-Arumi J, Martinez-Castillo V, Boixadera A, Fonollosa A, Corcostgui B. Surgical embolus removal in retinal artery occlusion. Br J Ophthalmol. 2006;90:1252-1255.
27. Tang WM, Han DP. A study of surgical approaches to retinal vascular occlusions. Arch Ophthalmol. 2000;118:138-143.
28. Mangat HS. Retinal artery occlusion. Surv Ophthalmol. 1995;40:145-156.
29. Butler FK. The eye in the wilderness. In: Auerbach PS, editor. Wilderness medicine. 5th ed. St Louis:MO, Mosby; 2007.

30. Saltzman HA, Hart L, Sieker HO, Duffy EJ. Retinal vascular response to hyperbaric oxygenation. JAMA. 1965;191(4):114-116.
31. Haddad HM, Leopold IH. Effect of hyperbaric oxygenation on microcirculation: Use in therapy of retinal vascular disorders. Invest Ophthalmol. 1965;4:1141-1151.
32. Yu DY, Cringle SJ. Retinal degeneration and local oxygen metabolism. Exp Eye Res. 2005;80:745-751.
33. Phillips D, Diaz C, Atwell G, Chimiak J, Ullman S, et al. Care of sudden blindness: a case report of acute central retinal artery occlusion reversed with hyperbaric oxygen therapy (abstract). Undersea Hyperb Med. 1999;26(suppl):23-24.
34. Hayreh SS, Kolder HE, Weingeist TA. Central retinal artery occlusion and retinal tolerance time. Ophthalmology. 1980;87(1):75-78.
35. Zhang XZ, Cao JQ. Observations on therapeutic results in 80 cases of central serous retinopathy treated with hyperbaric oxygenation. Presented at the 5th Chinese conference on hyperbaric medicine, Fuzhow, China; 1986 Sept 26-29.
36. Matsuo T. Multiple occlusive retinal arteritis in both eyes of a patient with rheumatoid arthritis. Jpn J Ophthalmol. 2001;45:662-664.
37. Beiran I, Reissman P, Scharf J, Nahum Z, Miller B. Hyperbaric oxygenation combined with nifedipine treatment for recent-onset retinal artery occlusion. Eur J Ophthalmol. 1993;3(2):89-94.
38. Perkins SA, Magargal LE, Augsburger JJ, Sanborn GE. The idling retina: reversible visual loss in central retinal artery obstruction. Ann Ophthalmol. 1987;19:3-6.
39. Beiran I, Goldenberg I, Adir Y, Tamir A, Shupak A, Miller B. Early hyperbaric oxygen therapy for retinal artery occlusion. Eur J Ophthalmol. 2001 Oct-Dec;11(4):345-350.
40. Gool VJ, De Jong H. Hyperbaric oxygen treatment in vascular insufficiency of the retina and optic nerve. In: Leding- ham IM, editor. Proceedings of the second international congress on clinical and applied hyperbaric medicine. Edin- burgh: Churchill Livingstone; 1964. Pp. 447-460.
41. Takahashi K, Shima T, Yamamuro M. Hyperbaric oxygenation following stellate ganglion block in patients with retinal artery occlusion. In: Smith G, editor. Proceedings of the sixth international congress on hyperbaric medicine. Aberdeen: University of Aberdeen Press; 1977. Pp. 211-215.
42. Pallotta R, Anceschi S, Costagliola N, et al. Recovery from blindness through hyperbaric oxygen in a case of thrombo- sis on the central retinal artery. Ann Med Nav. 1978;83:591-592.
43. Sasaki K, Fukuda M, Otani S, et al. High pressure oxygen therapy in ocular diseases: With special reference to the effect of concomitantly used stellate ganglion block. Jpn J Anesth. 1978;27:170-176.
44. Suzuki H, Irie J, Horiuchi T, Fukada J, Matsuzaki H. Hyperbaric oxygenation therapy in ophthalmology. Part 1: Incipient insufficiency of the retinal circulation. Jpn Clin Ophthalmol. 1980;34:335-343.
45. Krasnov MM, Kharlap SI, Pereverzina OK, et al. Hyperbaric oxygen in the treatment of vascular disease of the retina. In: Yefunny SN, editor. Abstracts of the seventh international congress on hyperbaric medicine. Moscow: USSR Academy of Sciences; 1981. Pp. 301-302.
46. Desola J. Hyperbaric oxygen therapy in acute occlusive retinopathies. In: Schmutz J, editor. Proceedings of the first Swiss symposium on hyperbaric medicine. Foundation for Hyperbaric Medicine. Basel; 1987. P. 333.
47. Kindwall EP, Goldmann RW. Hyperbaric medicine procedures. Milwaukee, WI: St. Luke's Medical Center; 1988.
48. Hirayama Y, Matsunaga N, Tashiro J, et al. Bifemelane in the treatment of central retinal artery or vein obstruction. Clin Ther. 1990;12:230-235.
49. Aisenbrey S, Krott R, Heller R, et al. Hyperbaric oxygen therapy in retinal artery occlusion. Ophthalmologe. 2000;97:461-467.
50. Weinberger AWA, Siekmann UPF, Wolf S, et al. Treatment of acute central retinal artery occlusion (CRAO) by hyperbaric oxygenation therapy (HBO) - a pilot study with 21 patients. Klin Monatsbl Augenheilkd. 2002;219:728-734.
51. Imai E, Kunikata H, Udono T, et al. Branch artery occlusion: A complication of iron-deficiency anemia in a young adult with a rectal carcinoid. Tohoku J Exp Med. 2004; 203:141-144.
52. Swaby K, Valderrama O, Schiffman J (2005) Treatment of Disc Edema and Retinal Artery Occlusion With Hbo During the Third Trimester of Pregnancy. UHMS Annual Scientific Assembly, Las Vegas, 2005. (Abstract)
53. Weiss JN. Hyperbaric oxygen treatment of nonacute central retinal artery occlusion. Undersea Hyperb Med. 2009;36(6):401-405.
54. Inoue, O; Kajiya, S; Yachimori, (2009) Treatment Of Central Retinal Artery Occlusion(Crao) And Branch Retinal Artery Occlusion (Brao) By Hyperbaric Oxygen Therapy(Hbo) - 107 Eyes Over 20 Years. UHMS Annual Scientific Assembly, Las Vegas, 2009. (Abstract)
55. Weiss JN. Hyperbaric oxygen treatment of retinal artery occlusion. Undersea Hyperb Med. 2010;37(3):167-172.

56. Aten, LA; Stone, JA; Poli, (2011) T. Treatment of a patient with acute central retinal artery occlusion with hyperbaric oxygen therapy. UHMS Annual Scientific Assembly, Ft Worth, 2011. (Abstract)

57. Cope A, Eggert J, O'Brien E. Retinal artery occlusion: visual outcome after treatment with hyperbaric oxygen. Diving Hyperb Med. 2011;40(3)135-138.

58. Menzel-Severing J, Siekmann U, Weinberger A, et al. Early hyperbaric oxygen treatment for nonarteritic central retinal artery obstruction. Am J Ophthalmol. 2012;153:454-459.

59. Oguz H, Sobaci G. The use of hyperbaric oxygen in ophthalmology. Surv Ophthalmol. 2008;53:112-120.

60. Weiss JN. Treatment of central retinal artery occlusions. Undersea Hyperb Med. 2010;37(1):51-53; author reply 54-55.

61. Murphy-Lavoie H, Butler FK. Response to: treatment of central retinal artery occlusions. Undersea Hyperb Med. 2010;37(1):54-55.

62. Gibbons RJ, Smith S, Antman E. American College of Cardiology; American Heart Association: American College of Cardiology/American Heart Association clinical practice guidelines: Part I. Where do they come from? Circulation. 2003;107:2979-2986.

63. Butler FK, Hagan C, Murphy-Lavoie H. Hyperbaric oxygen therapy and the eye. Undersea Hyperb Med. 2008;35:333-387 .

64. Canan H, Ulas B, Altan-Yaycioglu R.(2014) Hyperbaric oxygen therapy in combination with systemic treatment of sickle cell disease presenting as central retinal artery occlusion: a case report. Journal of Medical Case Reports 2014;8:370.

65. Hsaio S, Huang Y. (2014) Partial vision recovery after iatrogenic retinal artery occlusion. Ophthalmology 2014;14:120.

66. Masters T, Westgard B, Hendrikson S (2015) Central Retinal Artery Occulsion Treated with Hyperbaric Oxygen: A Retrospective Review. UHMS Annual Scientific Assembly, perMontreal, 2015. (Abstract)

67. Desola J, Papoutsidakis E, Martos P (2015) Hyperbaric oxygenation in the treatment of Central Retinal Artery Occlusions: An analysis of 214 cases following a prospective protocol. UHMS Annual Scientific Assembly, Montreal, 2015. (Abstract)

68. Lu C, Wang J, Zhou D (2015) Central retinal artery occlusion associated with persistent truncus arteriosus and single atrium: a case report. BMC Ophthalmology 2015; 15:137.

69. Lemos JA, Teixeira C, Carvalho R, et al. (2015) Combined Central Retinal Artery and Vein Occlusion Associated with Factor V Leiden Mutation and Treated with Hyperbaric Oxygen. Case Rep Ophthalmol. 2015 Dec 19;6(3):462-8.

70. Hwang K. (2016) Hyperbaric Oxygen Therapy to Avoid Blindness From Filler Injection. J Craniofac Surg. 2016 Nov; 27(8):2154-2155.

71. Olson EA, Lentz K. (2016) Central Retinal Artery Occlusion: A Literature Review and the Rationale for Hyperbaric Oxygen Therapy. Mo Med. 2016 Jan-Feb;113(1):53-7.

72. Tang P, Engel K, and Parke D (2016) Early Onset of Ocular Neovascularization After Hyperbaric Oxygen Therapy in a Patient with Central Retinal Artery Occlusion. Ophthalmol Ther. 2016; 5:263-269.

73. Elder M, Rawstron J, Davis M. Hyperbaric oxygen in the treatment of acute retinal artery occlusion. Diving Hyperb Med. 2017; 47:4, 233-238.

74. Hadanny A, Maliar A, Fishlev G, et al. (2017) Reversibility of retinal ischemia due to central retinal artery occlusion by hyperbaric oxygen. Clin Ophthalmol. 2017; 11: 115-125.

75. Butler F, Hagan C, Van Hoesen K, et al. Management of Central Retinal Artery Occlusion following successful Hyperbaric Oxygen Therapy: A Case Report. Undersea Hyperb Med. 2018; 45:1. 101-107.

76. Gunay C, Altin G, Kersin B, et al. A Rare Complication after Septoplasty: Visual Loss due to Right Retinal Artery Spasm. J Craniofac Surg 2018; 29: 466-468.

77. Karaman S, Ozkan B, Yazir Y. Comparison of Hyperbaric Oxygen versus Iloprost Treatment in an Experimental Rat Central Retinal Artery Occlusion Model. Graefes Arch Clin Exp Ophthalmol. 2016. 254: 2209-2215.

78. Murphy-Lavoie H, LeGros T, Butler FK, and Jain K. "Hyperbaric Oxygen Therapy and Ophthalmology." In Jain (Ed.), K.K. Jain Textbook of Hyperbaric Medicine, 6th Ed; Springer Publishing. 2016.

79. Youn T, Lavin P, Patrylo M, et al. Current treatment of central retinal artery occlusion: a national survey. J Neuro. 2018; 265: 330-335.

80. Callizo J, Feltgen N, Pantenburg S. Cardiovascular Risk Factors in Central Retinal Artery Occlusion: Results of a Prospective Standardized Medical Exam. Ophthalmology 2015; 122:1881-1888.

81. Wagner B, Lindenbaum E, Logue C. Rethinking the Standard of Care for Patients with Central Retinal Artery Occlusion. Ann Emer Med. 2017; 70:4, Suppl. Pp.S105.

CHAPTER 2B

Arterial Insufficiencies

Hyperbaric Oxygen Therapy for Selected Problem Wounds

Enoch T. Huang MD, MPH&TM, FUHM, FACEP, FACCWS,
Marvin Heyboer III MD, FUHM, FACEP, FACCWS,
Davut J. Savaser MD, MPH, FAAEM, FACEP

Introduction

The field of Undersea and Hyperbaric Medicine has been segregated into those indications related to undersea medicine and those related to wound healing. Historically, though, hyperbaric medicine's role in wound healing owes a debt to Jacques Cousteau's divers working 35 feet under the surface of the Red Sea, who claimed that their wounds healed significantly better when living in an underwater habitat than when they lived on dry land. In 1964, Dr. TK Hunt was asked by the National Science Foundation (NSF) to investigate these divers' claims. Dr. Hunt's work, along with that of his peers and colleagues, provide the scientific evidence and rationale that wound healing is dependent on tissue oxygenation.[1]

The use of hyperbaric oxygen (HBO$_2$) for the treatment of selected problem wounds has focused almost entirely on the diabetic foot ulcer (DFU) in recent years. The prevalence of DFUs in today's patient population and the reimbursement available for the treatment of DFUs have given it priority status in discussions about problem wounds, but there are sound fundamental reasons why additional oxygen may have benefits in the treatment of non-DFU wounds.[2] It is easy to extrapolate that where there is a minimum level of tissue oxygenation required for wound healing, more oxygen in the form of HBO$_2$ would improve healing even further. The challenge is determining whether there is evidence to support this extrapolation. Every wound that takes longer than expected to heal is a problem wound for that patient, so what makes HBO$_2$ acceptable for the treatment of some wounds and not for others?

We provide a systematic approach to guide the wound care practitioner in the selection of HBO$_2$ for the treatment of a problem wound. We begin with a review of the physiology of wound healing and the role of oxygen in wound healing, then discuss means of measuring tissue oxygenation and the mechanisms by which HBO$_2$ has been shown to affect wound healing, and conclude with a breakdown of multiple problem wound types using a standard format including:

- Pathophysiology of disease
- Rationale for HBO$_2$
- Literature Review

- Patient Selection/Treatment Protocol
- Cost Benefit
- Utilization Review

Physiology of Wound Healing

Role of Oxygen in Wound Healing

Oxygen metabolism is a critical co-factor in many cellular processes from collagen deposition to anti-microbial activity.[3-4] Fibroblast replication, collagen deposition,[5] angiogenesis,[6-9] resistance to infection,[10-12] and intracellular leukocyte bacterial killing[10] are all oxygen-sensitive processes that are essential to wound healing. Tissue hypoxia, on the other hand, is a fundamental driver of wound healing inducing several biological processes to adapt and survive in a low-oxygen state. Hypoxia-inducible factors (HIFs) are an integral part of the wound healing cascade and play a central role in hypoxic adaptation, including angiogenesis, anaerobic glycolysis, growth factor signaling, cellular mobility, and erythropoiesis.[13]

Oxygen delivery is a product of cardiac output, peripheral vascular resistance, and oxygen saturation of whole blood. Under normal atmospheric conditions, the amount of O_2 dissolved in plasma is inconsequential, and oxygen delivery is governed by the hemoglobin dissociation curve. Intact skin is generally considered a barrier to oxygen delivery, and the cardiopulmonary system, therefore, is considered the definitive route of oxygenating dermis and subcutaneous tissues.[14] While oxygen carrying capacity is related to hemoglobin, anemia by itself does not inherently inhibit wound healing.[15] Arterial pO_2 is the key factor as to wound healing potential, and this can be modulated through vasodilation, improved cardiac output, and capillary permeability.[2]

The first phase of wound healing is hemostasis, where blood loss is curtailed through a combination of vasoconstriction, platelet aggregation, and the formation of a fibrin clot. Platelets release growth factors that attract various cell types that are critical to the remaining phases of wound healing.[2] In the setting of a chronic wound, blood loss is less of an issue than controlling drainage of serous fluid caused by edema or an ongoing inflammatory process.

The inflammatory phase begins with the migration of polymorphonuclear leukocytes to the wound within the first few days after injury. Neutrophils, monocytes, fibroblasts, and endothelial cells are attracted to the wound and begin the process of breaking down and clearing cellular debris that may prolong inflammation.[2] Monocytes are activated into macrophages, which become the predominant cell type in the inflammatory phase of wound healing. Their role includes tissue debridement, bacterial killing, and secretion of additional cytokines and growth factors that transition the wound into the proliferative phase.[2,16] The killing of bacteria within leukocytes is usually divided into oxidative and non-oxidative pathways. Oxidative killing through production of reactive oxygen species (ROS) is responsible for eliminating bacterial species that commonly infest wounds, while non-oxidative mechanisms are responsible for less virulent bacteria that infest wounds only in the immune-suppressed patient.[17] Killing of certain bacteria by neutrophils is an energy- and oxygen-dependent process that requires glucose for energy production and atmospheric oxygen for production of bactericidal oxygen free radical intermediates and hydrogen peroxide.[18] Neutrophil bacterial killing activity occurs through an oxygen-dependent respiratory burst, where neutrophils convert oxygen to superoxide.[19] Neutrophil phagocytosis of bacteria triggers a series of metabolic changes that can result in a 20-100 fold increase in oxygen consumption.[20-21] A measurable decrease in tissue pO_2 from the normal 60 mmHg to 0-10 mmHg corresponds with the influx of neutrophils.[22] This effect is depressed in patients with local wound ischemia.

Superoxide production showed a half-maximal rate of production with pO_2 between 80-150 mmHg and a maximal rate over 300 mmHg.[4] One of the main mechanisms of efficient phagocyte bacteria killing requires a local pO_2 of 30 mmHg or greater.[11] Neutrophils cultured in zero O_2 killed 37% of organisms in one hour. Raising pO_2 to 5 mmHg resulted in 58% killing rate. Tissue pO_2 of 30 mmHg had a 70% killing rate, and further increases to 150 mmHg had minor increases in killing efficiency.[23] Combining early antibiotic administration and hyperoxia results in more efficient bacterial clearance than delayed antibiotics or oxygen.[12] Increased inspired oxygen decreases the spread of infectious necrosis and increases bacterial clearance.[10]

Collagen deposition, angiogenesis, granulation tissue formation, and epithelialization characterize the proliferative phase of wound healing,[2] and all of these functions are directly related to wound pO_2.[5,24-26] Wound pO_2 initially approaches arterial pO_2 but decreases as vessels thrombose and the number of leukocytes and fibroblasts, which consume oxygen, increase.[27] A healing wound has a higher metabolic demand as evidenced by depression of wound-tissue pO_2 in the first few days after a major surgery.[27] Fibroblast activity is a key component in wound healing, specifically collagen synthesis. Mitosis rate of squamous cells has been shown to be oxygen dependent.[28] Decreased fibroblast activity translates to decreased collagen deposition and slower wound healing. Collagen synthesis requires post-translational hydroxylation with the insertion of an oxygen atom derived from dissolved oxygen via the oxygenase prolyl hydroxylase, and collagen cannot be synthesized without oxygen.[29] The Michaelis constant (K_m) of oxygen for this step was confirmed to be 25 mmHg, so tissue oxygenation below that point would result in decreased collagen deposition.[1] Similarly, the quality of collagen deposition is also O_2 dependent as tensile strength increases with high pO_2 and decreases with high pCO_2.[5] Oxygen in high concentrations has been shown to stimulate angiogenesis.[6,9] Neovascularization occurs through angiogenesis and vasculogenesis, two processes that are increased through hyperoxia.[30-31] A number of studies suggest that HIF-1 plays an important role in homing of circulating SPCs to ischemic tissue, promoting vasculogenesis.[13] Epithelialization has been shown to increase with hyperoxia and decrease with hypoxia.[25,32-33]

Remodeling occurs weeks to months after a wound is epithelialized and describes the process by which newly deposited collagen is reorganized into a more structurally sound lattice. The initial collagen deposited in a wound is thinner than mature collagen and lies parallel to the skin.[34] Wound strength increases over the next four to five weeks with the production of additional collagen and crosslinking of collagen fibers.[2] A newly healed wound is still quite fragile, with a tensile strength of about 3% at one week, 20% after three weeks, and only 80% after three months. The newly healed skin never reaches 100% of uninjured tissue,[2,35] and the ultimate strength of the wound is dependent on the quantity and quality of collagen.[2]

To summarize, hypoxia initiates the wound healing cascade through the stabilization of HIF, which then stimulates multiple gene transcription sequences involved in wound healing. The result of HIF stimulation is the migration of multiple cell types to the wound bed, all of which consume oxygen and lower the already depleted wound of oxygen. The wound oxygen extraction fraction is about 0.7 to 1.0 vol% (1 mL of O_2 is extracted per 100 mL of O_2 delivered to a wound), and the amount extracted rises with increased oxygen breathing. Oxygen extraction fraction increases with oxygen delivery, which is evidence that oxygenases involved in wound healing are upregulating their activity with the amount of available O_2.[1] Intermittent hypoxia may stimulate a latent capability for increased collagen synthesis, which is then fulfilled by increasing available energy during normoxia.[36]

Defining a Problem Wound

The crux of this diagnosis is what exactly qualifies a wound as a "problem" wound. Tissue hypoxia is a final common pathway to poor wound healing, so any nonhealing wound may potentially be considered a problem wound that would benefit from hyperoxic exposure if it were hypoxic. One would hope that objective demonstration of hypoxia would be sufficient to qualify a wound for hyperbaric oxygen therapy, but this has not always been borne out in clinical practice.

There are several tests available to identify the presence of local tissue hypoxia. Local tissue hypoxia may be the result of macrovascular arterial insufficiency and/or microvascular arterial insufficiency. Evaluation of macrovascular status may be performed using ankle-brachial index (ABI), pulse volume recordings (PVR), arterial Doppler, CT/MR angiogram, and angiography. Microvascular disease may be evaluated using skin perfusion pressure (SPP), transcutaneous oxygen measurement (TCOM), or indocyanine green fluorescence angiography (ICGA).

TCOM measures the transcutaneous oxygen pressure ($TcPO_2$) through intact skin. $TcPO_2$ values are an estimation of the partial pressure of oxygen in the local tissues being measured using noninvasive heated electrodes.[37] This provides an objective means of evaluating local tissue hypoxia and identifying wounds at risk of nonhealing and amputation. Typically, electrodes are placed adjacent to the ulcer in the periwound skin, and one is placed as a control (e.g., chest wall). The $TcPO_2$ values can be used to both predict wound healing and response to HBO_2 therapy.

First, the $TcPO_2$ measured while breathing normobaric room air can be used to predict healing and response to HBO_2.[37-40] Measurements less than 40 mmHg are defined as hypoxic and are associated with a reduced likelihood of healing. Second, $TcPO_2$ values that are less than 35 mmHg while breathing 100% normobaric oxygen are associated with a 41% failure rate with HBO_2.[39] Third, wounds that are hypoxic on room air ($TcPO_2$ <40 mmHg) and have a $TcPO_2$ increase while breathing 100% normobaric oxygen that is both above 35 mmHg and >50% above the normobaric air value are likely to benefit from HBO_2 (associated with a 69% chance of beneficial response).[39] Finally, the most valuable predictor of response to HBO_2 is an in-chamber $TcPO_2$.[38] In-chamber $TcPO_2$ values of 200-299 mmHg and higher had significantly reduced failure rates.[38] In-chamber values > 200 mmHg had an 84% likelihood of benefit from HBO_2.[39] In-chamber values < 100 mmHg had only a 14% likelihood of benefit from HBO_2.[37]

Appropriate patient selection is important in assuring efficacious use of HBO_2. While clinical evidence supports the use of HBO_2 in the treatment of advanced nonhealing diabetic foot ulcers to increase healing rates and decrease major amputation rates,[41-42] there have been studies that have questioned the efficacy of HBO_2 in clinical practice.[43] Patient selection becomes even more important when considering HBO_2 for less established problem wound types. As such, evidence of tissue hypoxia or hypoperfusion should be used in the patient selection process of problem wounds that are to receive HBO_2.[44] This should include both normobaric and hyperbaric measurements. Nonetheless, local tissue oxygen measurements should not be the sole determinate in deciding to use HBO_2 for a problem wound. One must be aware of both the local effects and the systemic effects from HBO_2 that result in neovasculogenesis and wound healing.[31,45] While these modalities measure the local tissue changes, it does not account for the systemic effects as a result of endothelial progenitor stem cell mobilization.[45-46]

In-chamber $TcPO_2$ may be used to determine optimal treatment pressure. A study by Heyboer et al. indicated that the in-chamber $TcPO_2$ can be used to determine whether 2 atmospheres absolute (ATA) or 2.4 ATA is the best treatment pressure for a patient undergoing HBO_2 for a lower extremity wound.[47] The study used $TcPO_2$ levels previously mentioned that indicate a likely response to HBO_2. Based off that information, the study used an in-chamber $TcPO_2$ cut-off of 250 mmHg. They demonstrated that nearly 80% of patients reached a $TcPO_2$ >250 mmHg at 2 ATA. Meanwhile, among those with a $TcPO_2$ <250 mmHg at 2 ATA, nearly half (41%) reached levels >250 mmHg when chamber pressure was increased to 2.4 ATA. This allows for objective choice of treatment pressure that can maximize benefit while minimizing risk.[47]

There has been much interest in utilizing other means of assessing tissue perfusion. Indocyanine green fluorescence angiography (ICGA) is able to detect and monitor microvascular skin perfusion using an intravenous injection of ICG followed by imaging with a near-infrared laser camera. It has been used extensively by surgeons in the operating room.[48-52] Recent publications have reported its use for HBO$_2$ patients with soft tissue radionecrosis,[53-54] and for assessing perfusion in chronic wounds being treated with HBO$_2$.[55] While this is a very promising tool, Huang and Nichols presented their experience that shows there is more work that needs to be done to determine clinical decision-making parameters surrounding ICGA.[56]

The Role of Hyperbaric Oxygen in Wound Healing

Physiology of HBO$_2$

The most obvious role of HBO$_2$ in wound healing is its ability to provide oxygen to ischemic wounds. Henry's Law states that the amount of gas dissolved in a liquid is directly proportional to the partial pressure of the gas above the liquid. When breathing 100% O$_2$ at 3 ATA, enough oxygen is dissolved in plasma to support the body's metabolic demands without requiring dissociation of O$_2$ that is bound to hemoglobin.[57] Practically speaking, this increases O$_2$ diffusion distance from capillary beds tenfold and loads skin and subcutaneous tissue with supranormal levels of oxygen. Arterial PO$_2$ elevations to 1500 mmHg or greater are achieved at 2-2.5 ATA. Soft tissue and muscle PO$_2$ levels are correspondingly elevated. Oxygen diffusion at the tissue level varies in a direct linear relationship to the increased partial pressure of oxygen present in the circulating plasma.[58] Previously ischemic tissue beds may now be oxygenated—at least temporarily—giving the tissue the much-needed substrate to fuel some of the processes of wound healing.

While reversing tissue hypoxia ameliorates many of the ill effects of tissue ischemia, the role of HBO$_2$ is more than just providing the oxygen required to support wound healing. Otherwise, patients breathing 100% O$_2$ should see increased healing of their wounds. Rather, HBO$_2$ affords several advantages when compared to breathing normobaric oxygen such as amelioration of ischemia-reperfusion injury, stimulation of circulating stem progenitor cells (SPCs), augmentation of neutrophil bacterial killing activity, and production of reactive oxygen and nitrogen species.[59]

Reactive oxygen species (ROS) and reactive nitrogen species (RNS) are important signaling molecules in the production of various growth factors, cytokines, and hormones.[60] ROS are the natural byproducts of metabolism and may include superoxide (O$_2^{\bullet-}$), hydrogen peroxide (H$_2$O$_2$), hypochlorous acid (HClO), and hydroxyl (HO$^{\bullet}$). RNS include nitric oxide (NO) and peroxynitrite (ONOO$^{\bullet}$), the product of NO and O$_2^{\bullet-}$. There are three NO synthase enzymes responsible for synthesizing NO: NOS-1 (neuronal NO synthase, nNOS), NOS-2 (inducible/inflammatory NO synthase, iNOS), and NOS-3 (endothelial NO synthase, eNOS). Reactive species may have either positive or negative effects, depending on their concentration and intracellular localization.[60] ROS are generated as a part of normal metabolism and are opposed by antioxidant defenses. There is a balance that must be achieved between too little and too much ROS in the wound. For instance, chronic wounds have been shown to have an overproduction of ROS, resulting in oxidative stress within the tissues.[61] Oxidative stress is not synonymous with oxygen toxicity,[59] however, and the body's antioxidant defenses are capable of handling the oxidative stress from the use of intermittent HBO$_2$.[62-68]

HBO$_2$ has been shown to ameliorate the effects of ischemia-reperfusion (IR) injury caused by adherence of circulating neutrophils to the vascular endothelium. HBO$_2$ has been shown in both animals and humans to inhibit the ability of circulating neutrophils to bind to vascular endothelium via the ß$_2$ integrin adhesion molecule, reducing

IR-related inflammation and edema. It is important to note that HBO_2 does not inhibit the antimicrobial functions of neutrophils, such as degranulation, phagocytosis, or the respiratory burst.[69-71]

While hyperbaric oxygen's role in stimulating angiogenesis has been demonstrated most convincingly for irradiated tissue,[72-74] it has been demonstrated to be involved in vasculogenesis through the recruitment and differentiation of circulating SPCs to form vessels de novo.[30,59] Thom demonstrated that a single exposure to HBO_2 doubles the concentration of SPCs, and a course of 20 HBO_2 sessions resulted in an eightfold increase in SPCs.[45] Knowing that HIF-1 helps circulating SPCs to home into ischemic tissue,[13] Thom's finding that HBO_2 increased stem cell HIF content in diabetic patients suggests that this may be the basis for improved healing.[75] Conversely, previous researchers showed that HIF-1 is rapidly broken down in nonhypoxic environments.[76] In addition, Zhang et al. have demonstrated that hyperbaric oxygen improves wound healing by down-regulating HIF-1α, attenuating cell apoptosis and reducing inflammation.[77] These conflicting findings illustrate that our understanding of the interactions between HIF and HBO_2 are incomplete.

HBO_2 has been shown to increase synthesis of a long list of growth factors and receptors such as vascular endothelial growth factor (VEGF),[78] basic fibroblast growth factor (bFGF),[79] transforming growth factor-ß$_1$ (TGF-ß$_1$),[79] angiopoietin-2,[80] matrix metalloproteinase-2 (MMP-2), matrix metalloproteinase-9 (MMP-9), tissue inhibitor of metalloproteinase-1 (TIMP-1),[81] and platelet-derived growth factor (PDGF) receptors.[82] Extracellular matrix production and collagen synthesis are also linked with HBO_2.[6] HBO_2 is reported to accelerate epithelialization by about 30%,[32] while wound contraction appears to be independent of ambient oxygen tensions.[25] Boykin et al. demonstrated increases in NO levels in wound fluid taken from diabetic ulcers that showed increased granulation tissue formation and healing of wounds after a course of 20 HBO_2 treatments at 2.0 ATA for 90 minutes.[83] Over 8,000 genes and molecular chaperones have been shown at the molecular and cellular level to be up- and down-regulation in microvascular cell cultures.[84] In all of the genes tested, the cell cultures showed large responses when exposed to HBO_2 but not when they were exposed to 100% oxygen at 1 ATA.[84]

Diabetic Foot Ulcers

Pathophysiology of Disease

The diabetic foot ulcer is the result of multi-organ system dysfunction linked to hyperglycemia and its myriad downstream effects. On a cellular level, diabetes mellitus affects certain cell subtypes that are unable to down-regulate glucose transport into the cell in the face of hyperglycemia.[85] Hyperglycemia causes a chronic increase in superoxide, which suppresses eNOS, a potent vasodilator, and results in vasoconstriction and peripheral hypoxia.[85] Hyperglycemia also leads to thickening of capillary basement membranes, reducing oxygen diffusion from capillary beds to surrounding tissues,[86] decreased bone marrow eNOS activity required for SPC mobilization,[60] and repression of HIF-1 production.[87-88] Autonomic neuropathy reduces the diabetic patient's ability to mount a hyperemic response to injury, leading to a functional ischemia on top of anatomical ischemia.[86] Neuropathy in all of its forms (i.e., sensory, motor, and autonomic) is responsible for the majority of the pathology of the diabetic foot. Clawfoot deformity, hammertoes, and Charcot arthropathy predispose the diabetic patient to initial ulceration. Dermatologic changes from autonomic neuropathy leads to dry, cracking, callused skin that is a gateway for bacterial invasion. Increased pressure from the callus, paired with sensory neuropathy, is a deadly combination of symptoms initiating the diabetic foot ulcer.[89]

Rationale for HBO$_2$

Diabetic foot ulcers (DFUs) are prone to hypoxia and infection. HBO$_2$ delivers oxygen at higher than atmospheric pressure, resulting in increased arterial oxygen tensions in the plasma and drives the oxygen into hypoxic injured tissue.[38,90-91] HBO$_2$ has both local and systemic effects.[59] The result is neovascularization and collagen deposition at the site of hypoxic tissue such as those in DFUs.[30,92] Local tissue microangiopathy and host SPC mobilization dysfunction are present in diabetics with nonhealing DFUs.[93] HBO$_2$ directly addresses these deficiencies by reversing the hypoxia caused by diabetes mellitus and stimulating growth factors including vascular endothelial growth factor (VEGF), basic fibroblast growth factor (FGF), transforming growth factor beta-1 (TGF-β), nitric oxide (NO), and platelet derived growth factor (PDGF).[78-79,82-83] HBO$_2$ systemically stimulates mobilization of endothelial stem progenitor cells (SPC) through endothelial nitric oxide synthase (eNOS), increasing NO$^-$ without the need for the cytokine + receptor complex. Along with the effects of HIF-1a, this bypasses the missing step in diabetics, resulting in elevated levels of serum SPCs (CD 34+ and CD45-dim) and improved homing to the site of injury. The recruitment of SPCs results in *de novo* neovasculogenesis, increased collagen formation at the site of the DFU, improved granulation tissue formation, and better healing.[45,59,94-96]

Literature Review

Huang and Heyboer published a detailed analysis of the hyperbaric literature published through 2017 regarding DFUs.[97] Here, we provide a synopsis of the most pertinent studies and refer you to the previous analysis for a more detailed discussion of each study. Table 1 includes a list of all currently published trials investigating HBO$_2$ for the treatment of DFU.

The first report of the effectiveness of HBO$_2$ for the treatment of DFUs was published in 1979.[98] Since then, there have been nine randomized controlled trials, over 20 observational studies, and over a dozen systematic reviews on the subject. This body of work has established the DFU as the prototypical "problem wound" that has a positive outcome when treated with HBO$_2$. Despite a plethora of research, HBO$_2$ is still not widely accepted for the treatment of DFU and has been the target of health systems and agencies around the world seeking to restrict reimbursement for HBO$_2$ therapy. In the US, this added scrutiny is the result of an exponential rise in the number of hyperbaric facilities with a dramatic rise in the number of patients being treated with HBO$_2$.[99]

When looking at study design, the body of literature can be broken down into three blocks:

- Nonrandomized, observational studies (prospective and retrospective)
- Randomized controlled trials (RCTs)
- Systematic reviews and meta-analyses

Some studies had comparison groups that either did not receive a hyperbaric exposure at all (referred to as a control group) or received a combination of increased pressure and lower fraction of inspired oxygen (FiO$_2$ ≤ 0.21) to simulate HBO$_2$ and preserve blinding of the study group (referred to as a sham group).

We assume a simple set of best practice management principles of DFUs *prior* to utilization of HBO$_2$ termed VOIDS (vascular optimization, offloading of the neuropathic ulcer, infection control, diabetes control, and surgical debridement) in order to extract the most relevant takeaway messages from each study. A chronological breakdown of the literature allows us to put each of the lessons learned into historical perspective and to appreciate how each piece of the puzzle fits into the big picture. Because the inclusion/exclusion criteria of the published trials differ, it is important to understand which population of DFU was studied and what question each study was designed to answer. Although there are many grading systems in use, all of the studies that categorized the severity of the ulcer used the Wagner grading system for patient selection, requiring us to utilize this classification system above others when considering patient risk stratification.

- **Early Studies on DFU**

  The first published study of treating diabetic ulcers with HBO_2 was in 1979. Hart and Strauss published a retrospective report of 35 patients with "previously refractive skin ulcerations" that were treated with HBO_2. Ten out of 11 DFUs improved (73%) or healed (18%), but they did mention the severity of the ulcers or the hyperbaric protocol employed.[100] Davis et al. published the next case series that focused on response of DFUs to HBO_2 in 1987.[101] They reported a 70% healing rate among 168 patients who underwent HBO_2 for a nonhealing DFU and a major amputation rate (above the ankle) of 30% (and a corresponding limb salvage rate of 70%), but there was no control group or information about the severity of ulcers. They recognized that revascularization should be prioritized, and they recommended HBO_2 post-revascularization in order to support wound healing. Most of their treatment failures were in older diabetic patients without palpable pedal pulses who also had angiographic demonstration of large vessel occlusion at or above the ankle. This study found that HBO_2 was usually futile in elderly diabetics with large-vessel occlusion.[101]

- **HBO_2 and Limb Salvage**

  A series of prospective and retrospective studies out of Italy provided the first insights into the role of HBO_2 in limb salvage, a term that had not yet been popularized. This group also provided a seminal RCT looking at the effects of HBO_2 on the healing of DFUs. A prospective study published by Baroni et al. in 1987[102] admitted 28 patients with DFUs to the hospital. Twenty-three patients had gangrene (most closely corresponding to a Wagner Grade 4 DFU) while five had a perforating ulcer (most closely corresponding to a Wagner Grade 2 or 3 DFU). Eighteen patients received HBO_2. Ten patients declined to have HBO_2 because of "psychological reasons," such as confinement anxiety and "fear of earache" and were assigned to the control group, which received the same wound care treatment. HBO_2 was delivered at 2.5-2.8 ATA for 90 minutes. Baroni et al. used 2.8 ATA initially for an "antibacterial effect" before switching to 2.5 ATA for a "reparative effect." The HBO_2 group received a mean of 34 ± 21 treatments and had a healing rate of 89% (16/18) compared to 10% (1/10) in the control group (p=0.001). In addition, the amputation rate in the HBO_2 group was 11% (2/18) compared to 40% (4/10) in the control group (p=0.001). The study noted that the HBO_2 group had faster healing and a decreased hospital length of stay (62 days versus 82 days, p=NS). Baroni et al. theorized that there was alteration of the microcirculation (i.e., arteriovenous shunts, obstruction of small vessels by platelet plugs, red blood cell thrombi or albumin deposits in basement membranes) even with normal macrovascular function.[102] Their historical above-knee amputation (AKA) rate from 1979-1981 (before utilization of HBO_2) was 40%, while their AKA rate from 1982-1984 was 8.4% for patients receiving HBO_2 and 40% for the control group.[102]

  Oriani et al. continued the work above and published a retrospective review in 1982 that included 80 patients (62 HBO_2, 18 controls) that were admitted to the hospital with advanced ulcers and gangrene.[103] They maintained the same protocol of lengthy hospital admissions, strict glycemic control, aggressive daily surgical debridement, and culture-driven antibiotics. The HBO_2 group received 72 ± 29 treatments at 2.5-2.8 ATA x 90 minutes and had a healing rate of 95% (59/62) compared to 67% (12/18) healing in the control group (p<0.001). The major amputation rate was only 5% (3/62) in the HBO_2 group compared to 33% (6/18) in the control group (p<0.001). Their updated limb salvage statistics boasted a 4.8% (3/62) AKA rate in the HBO_2 group compared to a 33% (6/18) AKA rate in the non-HBO_2 group between 1983-1987.[103]

A third report from this group summarized their 10-year experience between 1982-1992, now numbering 172 patients with DFU that were treated with HBO_2.[104] Patients were being treating earlier, for longer periods of time, and were given HBO_2 as part of a systematic effort to assist demarcation, improve debridement, and repair damaged tissue rather than a last-ditch effort to halt wet gangrene. Limb salvage success included a transmetatarsal amputation that allowed weight bearing, as amputation of the leg or the thigh was not required. They reported an 86% success rate out of 151 patients that completed at least 12 HBO_2 sessions. They also promoted the following tenets of therapy that are valid today: HBO_2 should be used as early as possible; a multidisciplinary team needs to be involved in the care of the patient; and there should be periodic re-evaluation of the response to therapy. They were also the first to recommend that HBO_2 be stopped if there were no signs of improvement on the basis of clinical or oximetric testing.[104]

- **The First Randomized Control Trials**

  In 1992, Doctor et al. published the first randomized trial on the use of HBO_2 for DFU, but the study protocol did not bear many similarities to protocols in use at the time or now. They studied 30 hospitalized patients with chronic DFU, but they did not report on the severity of the DFUs other than that some had gangrene requiring immediate amputation above the ankle. The manuscript did not specify the patient enrollment process, but one assumes there was an even distribution of 15 patients who received HBO_2 and 15 who served as controls. Their only documentation of vascular status was the presence or absence of distal pulses. Using a nonstandard HBO_2 protocol—3 ATA of 100% oxygen x 45 minutes for a total of four treatments over a two-week period—their reported major amputation rate was only 13% in the HBO_2 group compared to 47% in the control group ($p<0.05$). They also documented a decrease in positive wound cultures (19 pre-HBO_2 vs. two post-HBO_2, $p<0.05$) for patients receiving HBO_2 compared to the control group (16 vs. 12, $p=NS$).[105] Despite the atypical HBO_2 protocol, this study demonstrated efficacy for HBO_2 and raised the question whether a prolonged course of HBO_2 for DFU was mandatory or whether a shortened course of HBO_2 immediately after surgery might be sufficient.

  Faglia et al. published a nonblinded randomized control trial of 68 hospitalized patients with DFUs in 1996.[106] They admitted all patients that presented to their center with Grade 3 or 4 DFU, as were those with Wagner Grade 2 ulcers that were large and infected and showed a defective healing in 30 days of outpatient therapy. The HBO_2 group received treatment at 2.2-2.5 ATA x 90 minutes (reduced from the 2.5-2.8 ATA used in previous publications by the Italian researchers above) for 38 ± 8 treatments. Their protocol included an aggressive pre-HBO_2 revascularization protocol, and both groups had patients that required angioplasty (25.7% of HBO_2 group vs. 24.2% of controls) and bypass grafts (11.4% of HBO_2 group vs. 15.1% of controls). Despite intervention, post-revascularization ABI and $TcPO_2$ measurements showed that both groups still exhibited peripheral arterial disease (PAD) and wound hypoxia (ABI of 0.65 ± 0.28 and 23.25 ± 10.6 mmHg in the HBO_2 group vs. 0.64 ± 0.25 and 21.29 ± 10.7 mmHg in controls). One of the key highlights of this study was the role of aggressive revascularization and glycemic control. It included vasculopaths that other studies regularly exclude, essentially showing that HBO_2 was effective for the diabetic *and* ischemic/hypoxic foot. Faglia et al. found that HBO_2 reduced major amputations (9% in HBO_2 group vs. 33% in controls, $p=0.002$) and increased tissue oxygenation as measured by $TcPO_2$ (increase of 14 mmHg in the HBO_2 group vs. 5 mmHg in the controls, $p=0.002$). The major amputation rate for those with a Wagner 4 diabetic foot ulcer in the HBO_2 group was 9.1% compared to 55% in the control group ($p=0.002$), but there was no statistically significant difference between the 2 groups when comparing Wagner 2 or Wagner 3 ulcers.[106] This marks the first time that a study explicitly reported wound demographics using the Wagner classification system, and the Centers for Medicare and Medicaid Services (CMS) considered this the pivotal study to approve the use of HBO_2 for DFU in the United States.[107] It is important to note that the CMS criteria does not mirror the Faglia inclusion criteria, as the current (as of 2018) coverage determination restricts HBO_2 to patients with a Wagner 3 of higher DFU that has failed to respond to 30 days of standard wound care.[108] A critical reading of the protocol shows that Faglia used HBO_2 on all Wagner 3 or 4 DFUs immediately after hospital admission and only included Wagner 2 DFUs if there was no response to therapy for 30 days (showing least benefit with HBO_2).[106] There are many criticisms of the use of the Wagner scale, and other classifications may be superior in predicting wound healing potential,[109] but the CMS criteria for HBO_2 reimbursement are tied to the use of the Wagner classification because of this paper.

- **Determining Criteria for Patient Selection**

  In 1991, Wattel et al. published a case series of 59 patients with DFUs who underwent HBO_2 in hopes of identifying factors that would predict which patients would heal and which would not.[110] They reported a healing rate of 81.4% and an amputation rate of 18.6% (11/59). The only factor that was associated with a healed DFU was the wound $TcPO_2$ while breathing oxygen under pressure. Patients who healed had an in-chamber $TcPO_2$ of 786 ± 258 mmHg compared with 323 ± 214 mmHg in those who did not heal (p<0.005).[110]

  Faglia et al. published a retrospective cohort in 1998 that reported a major amputation rate of 14% in the HBO_2 group and 31% in the control group (p=0.012). They determined that independent variables associated with major amputation were prior major amputation, higher Wagner Grade, prior stroke, ABI, and $TcPO_2$ level. They found that HBO_2 had an independent protective role. When comparing the three time periods, the major amputation rate decreased from 40.5% (1979-1981) to 33.3% (1986-1987) to 23.5% (1990-1993) in spite of a population with statistically significant greater PAD, Wagner Grade, and infection. They concluded the decreasing amputation rate was due to evaluation by a "foot team" and a new dedicated "foot clinic," and treating complicated DFUs with a multidisciplinary foot team cannot be overlooked.[111]

  Two case series reported by Fife et al. in 2002 and 2007 helped to clarify the question of patient selection in terms of tissue oxygen measurements.[37-38] The 2002 study focused on the use of $TcPO_2$ to predict healing response with HBO_2 and included 774 patients, of which 629 had adjunctive HBO_2. They reported that 65% healed or improved but did not report an actual healing rate. Patients with an in-chamber $TcPO_2$ of <100 mmHg had a low likelihood of healing, while a $TcPO_2$ > 200 mmHg provided the best single discriminator (reliability of 74% and positive predictive value [PPV] of 58%) for healing.[38] On the other hand, combining 1 ATA air $TcPO_2$ < 15 mmHg and in-chamber $TcPO_2$ < 400 mmHg predicts wound healing failure with a reliability of 75.8% and PPV of 73.3%.[38] The 2007 study analyzed 971 patients who had adjunctive HBO_2 for a DFU. The endpoint of this study was "improvement" rather than an actual healing rate and again found that an in-chamber $TcPO_2$ < 100 mmHg had a response rate of only 14% while an in-chamber $TcPO_2$ > 200 mmHg had a response rate of 84%. Factors that significantly impacted outcome included renal failure with dialysis, pack-year smoking history, number of HBO_2 treatments, and interruption of the treatment regimen. It was necessary to separate renal failure patients from statistical analysis because there was such a large difference between the outcomes of renal failure (n=136) and nonrenal failure patients (n=835).[37]

  Strauss also published work in 2002 on the use of $TcPO_2$ to predict response to HBO_2.[112] His findings mirrored those of Fife and showed that $TcPO_2$ measurements > 200 mmHg under hyperbaric conditions defined a responder group (healing of wound) with 80% sensitivity and 88% specificity regardless of room air $TcPO_2$.[112] An analysis of the combined Fife and Strauss data confirmed that nearly 90% of DFUs with a $TcPO_2$ > 200 mmHg under hyperbaric conditions progressed to healing.[113] The UHMS published a clinical practice guideline on the use of $TcPO_2$ for wound healing in 2009.[39]

In 2001, Kalani et al. published a prospective cohort trial on 38 patients with chronic diabetic foot ulcers that could be inferred to be only Wagner Grade 1 or 2 ulcers as none of the patients had a deep infection or full thickness gangrene.[114] Unlike the Italian studies that admitted and treated patients immediately, this was the first prospective study of HBO_2 for a chronic ulcer that had been present for more than two months. Only the first 14 subjects were randomized before the hyperbaric facility became unavailable for a two-year period. The final 14 patients only received HBO_2 when the hyperbaric facility was available. By the conclusion of the study, 17 patients were enrolled in the HBO_2 group and 21 patients in the control group. The HBO_2 group received a typical treatment at 2.5 ATA x 90 minutes for 40-60 treatments. At the three-year follow-up period, the HBO_2 group had a 76% healing rate and 12% major amputation rate compared to a 48% healing rate and 33% amputation rate in controls, but this was not statistically significant. The only difference between groups was the $TcPO_2$ while breathing oxygen at 2.5 ATA, which was nearly 60% higher in the group that healed (234 ± 110 mmHg in the healed group vs. 142 ± 65 mmHg in the major amputation group, p = 0.3),[114] which was consistent with the Fife and Strauss studies. Despite a lack of statistical significance and incomplete randomization, this study showed that HBO_2 was helpful for hypoxic Wagner Grade 1 and 2 DFUs even after three years.

- **Recent Randomized Controlled Trials**

Recent researchers began to apply more rigorous study design methodology in answering questions about adjunctive HBO_2 for DFU; however, there was a distinct change in the type of patient that was being investigated. All of the recent studies required ulcer age of at least four weeks before entering the patient into the study. As a result, this excluded the more acute DFUs that had been included by the Italian researchers a decade prior and focused on the more clinically stable outpatient population.

The first randomized double-blinded placebo-controlled study on 18 patients with DFU and concomitant PAD was published by Abidia et al. in 2003.[115] Like Kalani et al., they only included Wagner Grade 1 or 2 patients with DFUs that had not healed for at least six weeks. Nine patients in the HBO_2 group received 100% oxygen at 2.4 ATA x 90 minutes for 30 treatments while the control group received 21% oxygen (air) at 2.4 ATA x 90 minutes for 30 treatments. All patients were screened for PAD. Occlusive arterial disease was confirmed if their ABI was < 0.8 or great toe TBI was < 0.7. As opposed to the Faglia study, anyone for whom vascular intervention was planned was excluded from the study. The primary endpoint of the study was whether there was a significant reduction in ulcer size six weeks after completion of HBO_2, at six months, and at one year after healing. There was no difference in healing rate at six weeks, but the healing rate at one-year follow-up was 63% in the HBO_2 group compared to 0% in the control group (p=0.027). There was no statistically significant difference in minor or major amputation rates between groups. There was evidence of continued healing following completion of HBO_2 that suggested a persistent benefit following completion of treatment.[115] This supports the theory that HBO_2 initiates the process of healing, which can then continue even under normoxic conditions.

Kessler et al. published an unblinded randomized controlled trial on 27 patients with Wagner Grade 1-3 DFUs in 2003.[116] These ulcers were chronic and had to have been present for at least three months despite stabilization of blood sugars, offloading of the ulcers, and control of infection. This group excluded patients with significant PAD by screening out 22 patients with a dorsal foot $TcPO_2$ < 30 mmHg. After these patients were screened out, 14 patients were randomized to the HBO_2 group and 13 patients to the control group. Both groups were hospitalized for the first two weeks before being discharged. While hospitalized, the HBO_2 group received treatment at 2.5 ATA x 90 minutes twice daily for 20 treatments, and the control group received no additional therapy. During the two-week period after discharge, all patients were given an offloading shoe to wear, culture-directed antibiotics, and glycemic control using insulin. Measurements were taken at three time points: the time of enrollment, immediately after the hospitalization period (two weeks) and two weeks after discharge (four weeks). The HBO$_2$ group had a significantly larger reduction in wound size than the control group (41.8% vs. 21.7%, p = 0.037) at the time of discharge, but there was no significant difference (61.9% vs. 55.1%) by the four-week follow-up.[116] There was no statistically significant difference in healing rate or amputation rate two weeks after completion of HBO$_2$, but one criticism of this study was that this is a very short time frame based on the nature of the disease, and most other studies were considering healing durability at the one-year mark. The design of the study also allowed both groups to be discharged home after two weeks, where they would have to comply with use of an offloading shoe. It is possible that the early gains in the HBO$_2$ group may have been voided if the deleterious effects of inadequate offloading outweighed the benefits of HBO$_2$.

In the first large scale study of HBO$_2$ for DFU, Duzgun et al. published an unblinded randomized controlled trial on 100 patients with Wagner Grade 2-4 DFUs that had not healed with at least four weeks of appropriate care.[117] A subtlety of their inclusion criteria was that they used a modified Wagner Grading scale, where a Wagner Grade 2 DFU reached the level of tendon or joint and a Wagner Grade 3 DFU reached bone but did not have a requirement for infection. Patients were randomized evenly with 50 patients in the HBO$_2$ group and control group respectively. The HBO$_2$ group had a higher percentage of males, obesity, and tobacco use—all high-risk factors for poor wound healing. The HBO$_2$ protocol was 100% oxygen at 2-3 ATA x 90 minutes either once or twice daily for 20-30 treatments. The HBO$_2$ group had a higher rate of healing without surgery (66% vs. 0%, p < 0.05), fewer major amputations (0% vs. 34%, p < 0.05), and fewer minor amputations (8% vs. 48%, p < 0.05) when compared to control patients. The decision to perform an amputation was made by an unblinded surgeon, leaving room for selection bias.[117] The definition of healing in this study—spontaneous healing without surgical intervention in the operating room—is different than what most clinicians would consider a relevant statistic, which may explain why the healing rate of the control group was zero. If we look at the actual reported figures, it is possible to extrapolate that there were nine patients in the control group that healed with surgery but without amputation, while four patients in the HBO$_2$ group healed with surgery but without amputation, giving a more realistic "healing rate" of 74% in the HBO$_2$ group vs. 18% in the control group.

Löndahl et al.[118] published a rigorous randomized double-blinded sham-controlled trial on 75 patients with chronic Wagner Grade 2-4 DFUs in 2010. All patients had a chronic DFU > three months duration and had been treated at a diabetic foot clinic for > two months. There were 38 patients in the HBO$_2$ group and 37 patients in the control group. The HBO$_2$ protocol was 100% oxygen at 2.5 ATA x 90 minutes for up to 40 treatments while the control group received treatment on air at 2.5 ATA x 90 minutes for up to 40 treatments. While this protocol excluded anyone who had been re-vascularized < two months before study, it did not prevent patients from being re-vascularized after inclusion (no patient received open bypass after inclusion, but percutaneous angioplasty was performed in six HBO$_2$ patients and four control patients). Patient randomization was stratified on a toe blood pressure cutoff of 35 mmHg (33 in HBO$_2$ group had pressure ≤ 35 mmHg vs. 29 in control group). Offloading, infection control, metabolic control, and wound debridement were performed according to a standard protocol for both groups. The one-year healing rate based on intention-to-treat analysis was significantly higher in the HBO$_2$ group than in the control group (52% vs. 29%, p=0.03, NNT 4.2) and was even higher using per-protocol analysis for patients who received > 35 treatments (61% vs. 27, p=0.009, NNT 3.1). Of note, the HBO$_2$ group had a nonsignificant increase in major amputation rate (5% vs. 2%).[118] Subgroup analysis of TcPO$_2$ showed that baseline TcPO$_2$ correlated with healing rates following HBO$_2$.[40]

- $TcPO_2$ < 25 mmHg - 0% healed
- $TcPO_2$ 26 - 50 mmHg - 50% healed
- $TcPO_2$ 51-75 mmHg - 73% healed
- $TcPO_2$ > 75 mmHg - 100% healed

A follow-up paper from Löndahl et al. reported long-term health related quality of life using a short form (SF)-36 assessment 12 months after treatment was improved for patients who received HBO_2 in the categories of role limitation due to physical health, role limitation due to emotional health, and social function.[119]

Ma et al. published a prospective, nonblinded, randomized controlled trial of 36 hospitalized patients with Wagner 1-3 diabetic foot ulcers in 2013.[120] Patients were evenly randomized between the HBO_2 and control groups. Patients were included if they had a chronic DFU for >3 months duration and had received standard care for >2 months. Patients were excluded if they had a dorsal foot $TcPO_2$ <30 mmHg. The HBO_2 protocol was 100% oxygen at 2.5 ATA x 90 minutes twice daily for only 20 treatments (two weeks), and both groups had strict offloading with custom molded footwear and strict nonweight-bearing instructions, treatment of infection with culture-directed antibiotics, and tight glycemic control (< 8 mmol/L or 144 mg/dL) using subcutaneous insulin. They reported greater reduction in ulcer size at day 14 (42% in the HBO group vs. 18% in the control group, p<0.05) but did not have any long-term reporting past day 14.[120]

- **Evidence Against HBO_2**

  In 2013, Margolis et al. published a large longitudinal observational cohort study of 6,259 patients with a plantar DFU that called into question the effectiveness of adjunctive HBO_2 in the treatment of DFUs.[43] The data came from a clinical database that included roughly 11,000 subjects with a DFU of all Wagner Grades. Eighty-three percent of patients were removed from analysis because they had healed or had an amputation within 28 days. Of the remaining patients, 6,259 had <40% healing at four weeks and were included in the study (793 patients received HBO_2 and 5,466 did not receive HBO_2). The HBO_2 group received 100% oxygen at 2-2.4 ATA for 90 minutes, but the average number of treatments was not reported. Margolis used a statistical technique called propensity scoring to compensate for the lack of randomization.[43] All analysis was dependent upon the assumption that providers had strictly adhered to clinical practice guidelines in these areas, but this turned out to be erroneous in several instances.[121] The database only reported whether patients had "adequate lower extremity perfusion" and "standard care," but neither of these were defined. The clinical practice of the participating facilities in the database purportedly followed CMS guidelines for use – restricting HBO_2 for Wagner Grade 3 or higher DFUs – but 54.3% of patient who received HBO_2 were classified as Wagner Grade 2 DFUs and should not have been eligible for HBO_2.[43] There were only two outcomes that were considered: a fully epithelialized (healed) wound and any level of lower extremity amputation (LEA). The results at 16 weeks showed that the patients who received HBO_2 had a lower healing rate (42.3% vs. 49.6%), higher overall amputation rate (6.7% vs. 2.1%), and higher major amputation rate (3.3% vs. 1.3%) than those who did not receive HBO_2. The hazard ratio for patients receiving HBO_2 was actually higher for amputation (2.37) and lower for healing (0.68) when compared to patients who did not receive HBO_2. Even when looking at patients with Wagner Grade 3 or higher DFUs, the hazard ratio for amputation was still higher (1.41) for the HBO_2 patients.

The HBO_2 group had a much higher percentage of Wagner 3-5 DFUs compared with the non-HBO_2 group (45.7% vs. 18.4%) as a result of the non-randomized nature of the database. The authors describe propensity scoring in their statistical analysis to adjust for these factors, but if performed inappropriately, may lead to increased rather than decreased bias.[121] In response to criticism of the paper, Margolis clarified that this paper was a study of the *effectiveness* of HBO_2 in clinical practice opposed to the *efficacy* studies that had previously been performed.[41,105-106,115,117,120] When contacted directly, Margolis stated that a confounder in patient selection of sufficient magnitude could invalidate propensity scoring if it was not taken into account,[122] but secondary analyses that were performed showed that the likelihood of an unaccounted confounder was unlikely.[123] We have already described multiple studies that demonstrate the efficacy of HBO_2 in the treatment of a DFU under standardized conditions, yet the results of this study call into question whether this can be translated into clinical practice. The lesson from this study emphasizes the importance of proper patient selection and avoiding HBO_2 overuse in cases that are futile, cases where the DFU will heal without HBO_2, or cases with inadequate wound care prior to initiation of HBO_2.

Fedorko et al. published the results of a double-blinded placebo-controlled randomized controlled trial analyzing 107 patients with Wagner 2–4 DFUs in 2016.[124] There were 51 patients in the HBO_2 group and 56 patients in the sham group. All ulcers were present for at least four weeks. Patients were excluded if they were candidates for revascularization or had undergone revascularization within the prior three months. The HBO_2 group received 100% oxygen at 2.4 ATA x 90 minutes while the sham group received air at 1.2 ATA x 90 minutes. Both groups received a total of 30 treatments, although only 61% of the HBO_2 group completed all 30 treatments (20% had < 11 treatments). Patient outcome was assessed at completion of HBO_2 and at six-week follow-up after completion of treatment.[124] Unfortunately, this study deviates from previous studies in its defined outcomes, making it problematic to make direct comparisons. They did not report actual amputation rates as endpoints; instead, their primary endpoint was the efficacy of HBO_2 in reducing predefined *indications* for amputation, which included a lack of significant progress in wound healing, persistent deep infection in bone and tendon, inability to bear weight on the affected limb, or pain causing significant disability. Furthermore, while it was the adjudicating surgeon's prerogative to examine the patient, none of the subjects underwent physical examination to make the determination of whether a patient actually required amputation. All decisions were made using chart review and a photograph of the index ulcer. They reported no difference in the number of patients that met criteria for amputation (22.4% [11/49] of the HBO_2 group vs. 24% [13/54] in the control group). Just under half of patients were Wagner 2 DFUs (Wagner Grades 2, 3, and 4 ulcers in HBO_2 group: 47%, 45%, 8% vs. control group: 43%, 54% and 4%). After publication, there was much additional criticism of the study[125-127] and even some allegations of irregularities with the research protocol.[128] The fact that this paper did not report actual amputation rates and used a surrogate of meeting indications for amputation (there is evidence that at least one patient in the "amputation group" is walking around on healed feet without amputation[129]) raises the specter that there was an ulterior motive in over-reporting amputations in the HBO_2 group.[127] Despite the controversy around the study, the takeaway lesson is that HBO_2 may potentially be over-used in the treatment of DFUs. Fedorko et al. acknowledged that there may be a subset of DFU patients that would benefit from HBO_2 but did not recommend its use until that subset could be elucidated with further research.[124]

In the most recent publication (2018) on the subject, Santema et al. published a multicenter randomized clinical trial in the Netherlands looking at the use of HBO_2 for ischemic DFUs.[130] They included 60 patients in each group and compared HBO_2 (100% oxygen at 2.4-2.5 ATA for 90 minutes) plus standard care versus standard care alone. Inclusion criteria were Wagner Grade 2-4 DFUs that had been present for at least four weeks, had limb ischemia as evidenced by ankle blood pressure < 70 mmHg, toe blood pressure <40 mmHg, or forefoot $TcPO_2$ <40 mmHg, and had undergone assessment for revascularization prior to randomization. Their primary outcome measure was limb salvage and wound healing at 12 months, as well as the time to achieve wound healing. Their secondary endpoints were amputation free survival (AFS) and mortality. Using intention-to-treat analysis, they reported no difference between groups for wound healing, limb salvage, or amputation free survival. After 12 months, 30 index wounds were healed in the SC+ HBO$_2$ group vs. 28 in the SC group. Limb salvage was achieved in 47 patients in the SC group vs. 53 patients in the SC+HBO$_2$. AFS was achieved in 41 patients in the SC group and 49 patients in the SC+ HBO$_2$ group.[130]

A per-protocol analysis on patients who completed the prescribed course of 30 HBO$_2$ sessions showed significantly fewer major amputations and higher AFS in the HBO$_2$ group. In this per-protocol analysis, 18 patients (22%) in the SC group underwent a major amputation while only two (5%) in the SC+HBO$_2$ group underwent major amputation. Using the per-protocol analysis, the number needed to treat was determined to be six patients (95% CI 3 to 33). They noted that 21 patients (35%) did not complete the HBO$_2$ protocol – 11 in the SC+ HBO$_2$ group did not start HBO$_2$ and 10 did not complete the course of HBO$_2$ as planned. Out of the 11 who did not start HBO$_2$, five patients declined to undergo HBO$_2$, four were excluded by the physician, and two patients healed before starting therapy. Out of the 10 who did not complete HBO$_2$, four were deceased, three were admitted to the hospital or had surgery, and three stopped on their own. Additionally, four patients that were randomized to the SC group insisted on receiving HBO$_2$ on their own.[130] While intention-to-treat provides the most scientifically rigorous analysis of the data, some have criticized the study design for allowing patients who were not willing to undergo HBO$_2$ to be enrolled in the study.[131] An important takeaway from this study is that proper patient selection is a critical part of treating patients with DFU. A full course of HBO$_2$ is not always practical, and patients with advanced morbidity may have increased difficulty completing the prescribed therapy.[132]

- **Systematic Reviews and Meta-Analyses**

There have been almost twice as many systematic reviews[41-42,133-143] than randomized clinical trials[105-106,115-118,120,124] in the area of adjunctive HBO$_2$ for DFUs. Early reviews had fewer studies for consideration than later reviews, the sophistication of the research protocols improved over time as researchers better understood both the questions to ask and the relevance of the answers, and the methodology for systematic review itself has evolved. A common theme among the early reviews was the paucity of quality research in sufficient numbers to convincingly answer whether HBO$_2$ was effective at either healing DFUs or preventing major lower limb amputation, and there were many that recommended further high quality studies of the diabetic foot.[133,144] Later reviews that included randomized clinical trials were more positive, with some showing a reduction in major lower extremity amputations,[140] some showing improved healing of DFUs,[136,141] and some showing both.[134-135,137,143] In contrast, the systematic review generated by the Canadian Programs for Assessment of Technology in Health (PATH) came to a different conclusion when reviewing the same literature, showing that there is still bias in how the data can be interpreted. Despite finding that "pooled analysis of the RCT and observational data showed that treatment with HBO$_2$ reduced the risk of major amputation by 60 percent (p = .29) and 61 percent (p = .003) compared with standard wound care, respectively, they concluded that due to the limited RCT evidence, it is not possible to conclusively establish the benefits and harms of treating diabetic lower limb ulcers with HBO$_2$. No significant effects on amputation rates were found in the RCT evidence and in the high quality studies, no difference was found.[139]

The biggest variable in the HBO$_2$/DFU literature is the heterogeneity of the patient population with DFUs. When looking at the types of patients included, some studies included vasculopaths while others excluded them; some included patients who were revascularized, while others did not; some had acute surgical wounds and others had ulcers that had been present for months. Since the Wagner Grading system was first mentioned by Faglia et al.,[106] it has been applied inconsistently throughout the literature. It is clear that all DFUs are not equal, and the approach to analyze this data becomes difficult.

- **Clinical Practice Guidelines**

   Clinical practice guidelines (CPGs) have appeared with greater frequency in the literature since being promoted by the Institute of Medicine.[145] While there are many guidelines on the management of the diabetic foot ulcer, only a few briefly mention hyperbaric oxygen therapy. The 2012 Infectious Disease Society of America (IDSA) concluded that studies have not adequately defined the role of most adjunctive therapies for diabetic foot infections, but systematic reviews suggest that granulocyte colony-stimulating factors and systemic HBO_2 may help prevent amputations.[146] The National Institute for Health and Care Excellence (NICE) in 2015 updated their singular recommendation *against* hyperbaric oxygen therapy unless as part of a clinical trial.[147] The International Working Group on the Diabetic Foot (IWGDF) published their 2016 recommendation to consider the use of systemic hyperbaric oxygen therapy and recommended further blinded and randomized trials to confirm cost effectiveness, as well as to identify the population most likely to benefit from its use.[148]

   In 2016, The Society of Vascular Surgery CPG recommended HBO_2 for DFUs that fail to demonstrate improvement (>50% wound area reduction) after a minimum of four weeks of standard wound therapy.[149]

   For all of the CPGs above, DFUs were homogenized into a single entity. Given that not all DFUs are of the same severity, these recommendations were inadequate for clinicians to make nuanced clinical decisions. The Undersea and Hyperbaric Medical Society (UHMS) completed a hyperbaric-centric systematic review and generated its own set of CPGs regarding the use of HBO_2 for DFU. The UHMS used the Grading of Recommendations Assessment, Development and Evaluation (GRADE) methodology[150] – adopted by over 70 organizations including the Cochrane Collaboration, the World Health Organization (WHO), the Centers for Disease Control (CDC), and the Agency for Healthcare Research and Quality (AHRQ) – and attempted to homogenize the literature based on severity of the DFUs.

   While we attempted to include classification systems other than the Wagner Grade, none of the analyzed studies used an alternative system. Similarly, we were unable to group studies that stratified patients into treatment and control groups based on $TcPO_2$, vascular status, or severity of infection. We were ultimately able to define patients using three criteria:

   - Wagner Grade ≤ 2 DFU with wounds older than 30 days
   - Wagner Grade ≥ 3 DFU with wounds older than 30 days
   - Wagner Grade ≥ 3 DFU with acute wounds that required urgent surgery.

   Based on these patient populations, we were able to generate three recommendations.

   Recommendation 1: In patients with Wagner Grade 2 or lower DFUs, we suggest against using HBO_2 (very low-level evidence in support of HBO_2, conditional recommendation).[42]

   We did not find enough evidence to support the use of HBO_2 in patients with mild DFUs. This is in keeping with many of the other systematic reviews and challenges the liberal use of HBO_2 for Wagner Grade 2 DFUs.

Recommendation 2: In patients with Wagner Grade 3 or higher DFUs that have not shown significant improvement after 30 days of treatment, we suggest adding HBO$_2$ to the standard of care to reduce the risks of major amputation and incomplete healing (moderate-level evidence, conditional recommendation).[42]

When looking at the population of patient most often treated with HBO$_2$—chronic Wagner Grade 3 or higher DFU—we found more evidence in support of adjunctive HBO$_2$ and were able to make a recommendation for its use.

Recommendation 3: In patients with Wagner Grade 3 or higher DFUs who have just had a surgical debridement of an infected foot (e.g., partial toe or ray amputation; debridement of ulcer with underlying bursa, cicatrix or bone; foot amputation; incision and drainage [I&D] of deep space abscess; or necrotizing soft tissue infection), we suggest adding acute postoperative HBO$_2$ to standard wound care in order to reduce the risk of major amputation (moderate level evidence, conditional recommendation).[42]

When looking at the acute DFUs requiring emergent surgery—a population that is not explicitly covered by CMS guidelines—we found that there was a benefit in starting HBO$_2$ immediately rather than waiting the CMS-mandated 30 days of care. Whether this is a cost-effective therapy is not known because the majority of the patients in this analysis remained inpatients for 60-90 days.[106] A shorter, concentrated course of HBO$_2$ may be beneficial,[105,116] but this would have to be proven in a future randomized controlled trial.

Patient Selection/Treatment Protocol

Patient selection is the most critical factor with regard to effective and efficient use of HBO$_2$. There are patients with DFUs that will heal without HBO$_2$, there are patients who are not going to heal even with the addition of HBO$_2$, and then there are patients who may heal if HBO$_2$ is added to their comprehensive treatment plan. A fundamental tenet of this treatment plan is that HBO$_2$ is an adjunct to best practices that include vascular assessment and intervention, offloading of neuropathic ulcers, infection control, diabetes control, and surgical debridement of devitalized tissue. Without these, HBO$_2$ cannot be expected to be successful; yet, HBO$_2$ should not be delayed if there is rapid, ongoing tissue loss. The timing of HBO$_2$ is also critical in its ability to affect a change. Tissue that has already succumbed to ischemia is unable to be saved, so HBO$_2$ must be utilized when there is still a chance to ameliorate the effects of hypoxia in the ischemic penumbra.

For patients with DFU, the UHMS Clinical Practice Guideline suggests against using HBO$_2$ for the treatment of Wagner Grade 2 DFUs. It suggests using HBO$_2$ for Wagner Grade 3 DFUs that have not healed for 30 days or more, and it suggests using HBO$_2$ for Wagner Grade 3 DFUs that have just had surgical intervention. Clinical judgment is required to determine whether exceptions to the recommendations should be made.[42]

For diabetic patients who have an acutely infected Wagner Grade 3 DFU that have required surgical intervention, HBO$_2$ should be initiated urgently if there is a concern of tissue malperfusion and hypoxia (Figure 1). This should occur even if the offending infected tissue (e.g., infected bone, necrotic tissue) has been excised. Unfortunately, amputation of a toe (and subsequent "unchecking" of the qualifying box of having infected bone) is a common argument for why HBO$_2$ is no longer indicated, but this simplistic argument misses the crucial role of oxygen in wound healing. From our discussion of wound healing physiology, we know that tissue hypoxia *increases* in the first 3-4 days following surgery, placing greater metabolic demand on tissue that is already compromised. It is the ability of HBO$_2$ to hyperoxygenate this compromised tissue in the postoperative phase that warrants its use even after the toe has been amputated. With that understanding, a postoperative course of HBO$_2$ may not require as many sessions if the tissue's metabolic demand has normalized.

Proper patient selection for DFUs that do not require acute surgical intervention depends on whether or not the fundamental tenets of wound healing have been addressed. Providers should document their attempts to optimized vascular status, offloading of weight-bearing ulcers, control infection, improve nutrition, correct hyperglycemia, and debride devitalized tissue, understanding that HBO_2 alone will not heal DFUs. It should also be understood that inability to normalize all of these parameters is not a reason to exclude HBO_2 from the treatment plan. There have been attempts by insurance providers to deny coverage of HBO_2 for patients with poorly controlled diabetes mellitus (i.e., Hba1c >7.0%). However, Moffat et al. reviewed 25 studies looking at Hba1c and healing and found no direct correlation between the two. There was no RCT that demonstrated Hba1c <7.0% improved DFU healing, and they found that every study included patients with Hba1c >7.0% that have successfully healed their wounds.[151] The decision to initiate HBO_2 as an adjunctive therapy should always be based on the best clinical judgement of the provider, not whether all variables have been normalized.

Because $TcPO_2$ at pressure (2.0-2.5 ATA) may be most predictive of response to HBO_2,[38-39,44,112] it is reasonable to make a $TcPO_2$ measurement under hyperbaric conditions, especially if there are no other alternatives to amputation. If the values obtained suggest a lack of efficacy, but no alternative to amputation exists, it is appropriate to treat a patient 10-15 times in order to determine whether they will respond. By two to three weeks into treatment, one should begin to see the effects of neovascularization. Lack of response corroborates the $TcPO_2$ findings and should discourage further HBO_2.[104]

Treatment protocols range from pressures of 2.0 to 2.5 ATA depending on facility practice. Treatment lengths are for 90-120 minutes with or without air breaks. Acute surgical wounds may require fewer than 30 sessions of HBO_2 if there are clinical indications that tissue hypoxia is no longer a significant factor and the wound is healing. A course of outpatient therapy is usually 30 sessions, although many patients will require up to 40 sessions.[118] One has to realize that it is often very difficult for patients to commit to the demands of coming for daily HBO_2 therapy. Several studies have demonstrated an association between completion of the prescribed HBO_2 sessions with improved healing.[118,130,152] Löndahl et al. and Santema et al. reported that 20% and 35% of their patients, respectively, were unable to complete at least 35 treatments, but the ones that did had significantly better outcomes.[118,130] Few patients will require more than 40 sessions, but it is still within acceptable practice parameters provided there is objective utilization review. This should include periodic re-evaluation and documentation of the continued adherence to the fundamental tenets described above, as well as documentation of signs of clinical progress.

A frequent criticism of all of the studies mentioned above is the small sample size of each study and the large percentage of patients with Wagner Grade 2 DFUs. In an effort to report data at a population level, Ennis et al. published an observational study reviewing over two million Wagner Grade 3 or 4 DFUs that showed an overall healing rate of 56.04%. The use of any amount of HBO_2 improved the healing rate to 60.01%, while those patients who completed a full course of HBO_2 had a healing rate of 75.24%.[152] It is not clear whether this is because completing the course of HBO_2 increased healing rates or whether it is a reflection that healthier patients, who would likely go on to heal, are able to complete a course of therapy while sicker patients, who are less likely to heal, cannot make the daily trips to the hyperbaric department.

Cost Benefit

HBO_2 as an adjunct to treatment of selected problem wounds has been shown to be cost-effective when compared to major lower extremity amputation[1,53-155] Preventing a below the knee amputation by salvaging a ray resection or transmetatarsal amputation of the foot, or preventing an above the knee amputation by preserving a below the knee amputation, represents a satisfactory outcome in these high-risk patients. Guo et al. used economic modeling of previously published outcomes to determine that HBO_2 produced long-term cost benefits of treatment in diabetic limb salvage.[156] In a 1,000 wound cohort model, 155 cases of major lower extremity amputation would be averted with approximately 50.2, 265.3, and 608.7 Quality-adjusted-life-years (QALY) are gained in years 1, 5, and 12 respectively due to use of HBO_2. In this 2003 publication, the incremental cost per additional QALY gained $27,310, $5,166, and $2,255 (US) at the 1, 5, and 12 year periods making HBO_2 more cost-effective based on a long-term perspective.[156] Relatively broad variations in cost-effectiveness ratios across different scenarios of application of HBO_2 point out the need for proper clinical practice guidelines.

The Canadian Agency for Drugs and Technologies in Health reviewed HBO_2 in DFU care and concluded that HBO_2 was more effective than standard care alone, reduced major lower extremity amputations from 32% to 11% in those receiving HBO_2, and decreased the proportion of unhealed wounds with an acceptable 12-year cost-to-outcome compared to standard care.[157] Recent cost estimates for a course of HBO_2 to treat a DFU in the United States approaches $50,000.[158] Chuck et al. performed an extensive economic analysis comparing HBO_2 against standard treatment for DFU. They adjusted the model to include data significant to Canada and typical outcomes from a known data source. The model was adjusted for initial cost per patient as well as for downstream costs. This study shows that initial costs are similar, but HBO_2 provides a higher potential for healed foot ulcers and significantly increases QALY.[159]

Santema et al. published an economic analysis of HBO_2 for a variety of indications but could only identify one RCT (Abidia) that reported both economic and clinical outcome data on the use of HBO_2 for the treatment of DFUs.[160] Abidia reported a 37% reduction in cost in the HBO_2 cohort when compared to the sham group. Patients who received a course of 30 HBO_2 treatments incurred a cost of £3,000, which was offset by fewer post-treatment office visits per year (33.75±62 in HBO_2 group vs. 136.5±126 in control group) and associated charges (£1,972 in HBO_2 group vs. £7,946 in control group), leaving a balance in favor of HBO_2 by £2,960 for each patient treated.[115] Santema collected economic data with their $DAMO_2CLES$ study, but the results were not published with the clinical outcomes and will be included in a future publication.[130]

Eggert et al. reported cost and mortality data on 106 patients between 2005-2013 who were treated on a comprehensive limb salvage protocol (LSP) including HBO_2 versus 53 historical controls who were not enrolled in the LSP and had either an below-knee amputation (BKA) or above-knee amputation (AKA).[155] Ninety-six of the 106 patients completed the LSP with an average cost of $33,100. The costs of lower extremity amputation for the historical controls ranged from $66,300 (BKA) to $73,000 (AKA). Out of those 96 patients who completed the protocol, 88 (91.7%) had an intact lower extremity at the one-year mark with 35.4% mortality during the follow-up period compared to a 47.2% mortality rate for the historical control group.[155]

Utilization Review

Utilization review should be performed after the initial 30 days of treatment and at least that frequently thereafter. The key elements of review should include documentation of wound dimensions, presence or absence of improvement in wound healing, confounding factors to explain absence of improvement (e.g., surgical debridement of wound causing enlargement), status of VOIDS efforts (e.g., glycemic control, offloading efforts, antibiotic therapy), and a rationale and plan for further HBO_2 if needed. For patients who have had tissue hypoxia documented by $TcPO_2$, one should begin to see the effects of neovascularization by two to three weeks. A lack of improvement in $TcPO_2$ measurements should discourage further HBO_2.[104]

Arterial Insufficiency Ulcers

Pathophysiology of Disease

Peripheral arterial disease (PAD) affects 8-12 million people over the age of 40 years in the United States.[161] PAD results in tissue ischemia due to atherosclerosis of the aorta, iliac, and lower extremity arteries.[162] The 10-year mortality rate nears 60% and is dependent on age and arterial insufficiency (AI) severity.[163] Many patients who have AI develop arterial insufficiency ulcers (AIU). AIUs often fail to heal despite standard management that includes revascularization, addressing systemic factors (e.g., tobacco use, diabetes, hypertension, hyperlipidemia, obesity), offloading, treatment of infection, appropriate local wound care, and appropriate debridement in the setting of adequate tissue oxygen perfusion.[162-166]

Many of these patients are not candidates for revascularization. The result of nonhealing in many cases is above-ankle amputation, which increases patient morbidity and mortality risks. The overall prognosis is dependent on the location and degree of arterial stenosis and ability to revascularize. With revascularization, the healing rates have been reported at 50-90% and amputation rates of <20%.[164-165] Without revascularization, the results change dramatically with healing rates of only 40-50% and amputation rates increasing to 25-40%.[164-165]

Rationale for HBO$_2$

HBO$_2$ is one adjunctive therapy to consider in patients with a nonhealing AIU despite standard care. The delivery of oxygen at higher than atmospheric pressure results in increased arterial oxygen tensions and increased concentrations of oxygen in the plasma, thus driving oxygen into otherwise hypoxic injured tissue.[38,90-91] HBO$_2$ has both local and systemic effects. Locally, HBO$_2$ increases multiple growth factors including local nitric oxide (NO).[78-79,82-83,92] Systemically, HBO$_2$ induces bone marrow NO production and results in progenitor stem cell release from bone marrow.[31,45,83,94,167] As a result, there is neovascularization at the site of hypoxic tissue such as nonhealing ischemic lower extremity ulcers.[30-31,168] Notably, there is evidence patients with advanced PAD have a decrease in NO bioactivity and nitrate metabolism which is likely the result of inhibition of nitric oxide synthase (NOS). HBO$_2$ has been found to increase NO levels through direct activation of NOS.[169]

Literature Review

Previous studies addressing the benefit of HBO$_2$ for nonhealing lower extremity ulcers have focused on advanced DFUs. Determining clinical outcomes for true AIUs is made more difficult due to the fact that most published studies assessing AIUs also have concomitant diabetes. This may call into question mixed etiology wounds (arterial insufficiency ulcer and diabetic foot ulcer).[106,163-165] The Wound Healing Society's Clinical Practice Guideline recommends consideration of HBO$_2$ in patients with an AIU who fail to heal despite revascularization or are not a candidate for revascularization.[163]

Heyboer et al. evaluated the use of adjunctive HBO$_2$ for recalcitrant AIU in the absence of diabetes.[170] The study evaluated 82 patients with a primary diagnosis of AIU who underwent HBO$_2$. Patients evaluated had failed to heal despite revascularization or were not candidates for revascularization. These were patients who had exhausted all means for healing and were anticipating nonhealing and above-ankle amputation. Addition of HBO$_2$ resulted in healing rates nearing 50%, 0% major amputation rate, and an overall above-ankle amputation rate of only 17.1%. The healing rate reached 56% in patients who were not candidates for revascularization, which was higher than traditionally reported with standard therapy alone.[164-166] In addition, the major amputation rate in this group was 21%, which is below rates previously reported with standard therapy alone.[119,126,164] In patients who failed to heal despite revascularization, HBO$_2$ resulted in healing rates near 50%.[170]

Patient Selection/Treatment Protocol

Patients with an AIU may be considered for HBO_2 if their wound has failed to heal despite standard wound care that includes either revascularization or who have been evaluated by vascular surgery and are not a candidate for revascularization. HBO_2 treatments are delivered at 2–2.5 ATA for 90 to 120 minutes once or twice daily for five to seven days a week. It is recommended that a room air normobaric $TcPO_2$ measurement be completed to determine baseline level of ongoing ischemia. If using a monoplace chamber, an in-chamber $TcPO_2$ may be used to guide treatment pressure with a goal to reach a therapeutic $TcPO_2$, and an in-chamber $TcPO_2$ may be used to identify those who are unable to reach adequate $TcPO_2$ levels predictive of healing despite maximum treatment pressures.

Utilization Review

Utilization review should be undertaken after the initial 30 treatments have been completed and at least that frequently thereafter. If the initial in-chamber $TcPO_2$ levels suggest a lack of efficacy but there is no alternative other than amputation, it is reasonable to complete a trial of 10-15 HBO_2 treatments to determine whether there is a response. If there is a lack of clinical response by this time, further HBO_2 should be discouraged.

Calciphylaxis

Pathophysiology of Disease

Calciphylaxis (or calcific uremic arteriolopathy) is a rare and potentially life-threatening syndrome. It causes small vessel calcification of unknown etiology, subsequent painful skin lesions, and finally chronic, nonhealing ulcers and gangrene. It is associated with end-stage renal disease (ESRD) patients on dialysis with a prevalence of 1-4%.[171-172] The incidence has been reported as increasing.[173] It has a high mortality of 60-80% with most patient deaths as a result of complications of infection of the calciphylaxis wounds and sepsis.[174] While the exact pathogenesis is unclear, it involves vascular calcification from calcium deposition in the media of the dermal and subcutaneous arterioles resulting in hypovascularity, fibrosis, and dermal necrosis. The lower extremities are the most commonly involved although various sites have been reported.[175]

Rationale for HBO_2

HBO_2 delivers oxygen at higher than atmospheric pressure resulting in increased arterial oxygen tensions in the plasma and drives the oxygen into hypoxic injured tissue.[38,90-91] HBO_2 has both local and systemic effects.[59] The result is neovascularization and collagen deposition at the site of hypoxic tissue such as those in calciphylaxis.[30,92]

Literature Review

Treatments available include discontinuation of oral calcium supplementation, lower serum phosphorous with a noncalcium-based oral binder, decreased dialysate calcium concentrations, parathyroidectomy, sodium thiosulfate provided at time of dialysis treatment, and HBO_2 therapy. Despite the supplementation and dialysate changes, mortality rates remain high. There have been promising results reported with addition of sodium thiosulfate and/or HBO_2 therapy.

The benefits of HBO_2 in the treatment of calciphylaxis have been reported in many case reports and a few retrospective case series.[172,176-183] An et al. reported on 34 patients with calciphylaxis who underwent an average of 44 HBO_2 treatments. There were 11 patients with complete healing, 9 with improvement in their wound/ wound score, 2 with no change, and 12 with deterioration.[176] In Podymow et al., two out of five patients showed complete resolution of extensive necrotic ulcers and improvement in wound area transcutaneous oxygen pressure.[172] Basile et al. reported on 11 patients with calciphylaxis who underwent HBO$_2$. Eight patients had healing of their ulcers.[177] Arenas et al. reported on two patients treated successfully with HBO$_2$.[178] Don et al. reported on the successful treatment of two patients with HBO$_2$.[179] Dean and Werman reported a case of a female patient with end-stage renal disease and diabetes mellitus who presented with lower extremity calciphylaxis who responded to seven weeks of HBO$_2$ treatments after failing to respond to standard care including parathyroidectomy and wound debridement.[180] Vassa et al. reported on a case of a woman on continuous ambulatory peritoneal dialysis who presented with lower extremity calciphylaxis who also failed standard care but showed resolution of her skin lesions after 38 HBO$_2$ therapy sessions.[181]

There have been promising results when both sodium thiosulfate and HBO$_2$ are used together. McCulloch et al. reported on five patients with calciphylaxis who underwent HBO$_2$. There were two patients with >20 HBO$_2$ treatments who had resolution of their ulcers while the other three had <15 HBO$_2$ treatments with one stopped early by primary service, one withdrawn to palliative care, and one who died of sepsis. The patients with resolution received both HBO$_2$ and thiosulfate.[182] Baldwin et al. reported on seven patients treated with a multi-interventional approach that included both thiosulfate and HBO$_2$. Six of the patients had complete recovery.[183]

Patient Selection/Treatment Protocol

Patients with calciphylaxis may be considered for HBO$_2$. Biopsy confirmed diagnosis is recommended, but multidisciplinary consensus of clinical diagnosis is acceptable. HBO$_2$ treatments are delivered at 2–2.5 ATA for 90 to 120 minutes once or twice daily for five to seven days a week for a minimum of 20 treatments. It is recommended that patients also receive thiosulfate while undergoing HBO$_2$ to maximize benefit and chances for a successful outcome.

Utilization Review

Utilization review should be undertaken after the initial 30 treatments have been completed and at least that frequently thereafter. It is important to recognize that patients who receive a subtherapeutic number of HBO$_2$ treatments (<20) are unlikely to benefit from HBO$_2$.

Graft Versus Host Disease

Pathophysiology of Disease

Allogeneic stem cell transplantation in the treatment of hematopoietic and lymphatic malignancies may result in the known complication of graft-versus-host disease (GvHD). The most common findings of GvHD are cutaneous manifestations. They can range from pruritus, to rash, to chronic wound development.[184] The process of GvHD is mediated by the donor T cells. In addition, chronic GvHD appears pathologically related to autoimmune disorders, often accompanied by nonspecific autoantibodies.[184] Locally the process leads to dermal/subcutaneous endothelial damage and micro-angiopathy in the course GvHD which results in local tissue ischemia and fibrosis.[185-186]

Rationale for HBO$_2$

HBO$_2$ delivers oxygen at higher than atmospheric pressure resulting in increased arterial oxygen tensions in the plasma and drives the oxygen into hypoxic injured tissue.[38,90-91] HBO$_2$ has both local and systemic effects.[59] The result is neovascularization and collagen deposition at the site of hypoxic tissue such as those in GvHD,[30,59] It is

In the same year of 2013, Fakhar et al. describe a case of a 41-year old female with Beckwith-Wiedemann who suffered third-degree burns to her left breast from spilling coffee at the age of 22. After multiple episodes of recurrent graft dehiscence and infections, she ultimately underwent elective bilateral reduction mammoplasty at the age of 37. She subsequently developed recurrent ulcerations at the suture margins which were determined to be postsurgical pyoderma gangrenosum. She was treated over the course of a year with hydroxychloroquine, minocycline, dapsone, and chronic steroids without significant improvement. She ultimately required bilateral mastectomy at the age of 39 because of the recalcitrant wounds. She developed ulcers over her left chest wall two months after surgery that extended to her deep muscles and vasculature and was associated with intermittent profuse bleeding. She required multiple blood transfusions and IV iron for anemia that ensued. She failed treatment with cyclosporine, colchicine, IVIG, and MMF and required prednisone dosed up to 120 mg/day with occasional IV steroid pulses. Surgical closure and negative pressure device implementation were unsuccessful. Local steroid injections led to pathergy as well. She remained on high-dose steroids for two years and developed a Cushingoid habitus with obstructive sleep apnea (OSA) and steroid-induced dysglycemia. The patient was ultimately started on an anti-TNF-alpha inhibitor of adalimumab, MMF, and prednisone which helped to decrease the size of the ulcer. HBO_2 was also implemented with 60 treatments of 100% oxygen at 2.0 ATA that led to further clinical improvement, per the authors. This was the first case of PG described with Beckwith-Wiedemann syndrome successfully treated with HBO_2.[198]

In a case report from Korea in 2014, Seo et al. describe a 65-year-old male with a 17-year history of ulcerative colitis (UC) with bilateral and painful pretibial ulcerations who was placed on mesalazine alone for treatment of UC. She underwent debridement of the lesions along with 29 sessions of HBO_2 for 120 minutes at 2.4 ATA over three months with 100% resolution of lesions.[213]

In 2016, Chiang et al. reported on a 54-year-old woman with type 2 diabetes mellitus, peptic ulcer disease, and hypertension who presented with a two-week history of multiple painful ulcers on her buttocks, hands, and lower extremities. The patient had an extensive work-up and was ultimately determined to have PG. The patient was treated with HBO_2 at 2.5 ATA for 90 minutes total daily for a total of 12 sessions. Pain decreased, and the wounds were healed with some scarring within the span of two weeks. This also allowed a decrease in her steroid regimen as well.[214]

In 2016, Feitosa et al. examined the adjunctive effect of HBO_2 in patients with pharmaco-refractory perineal Crohn's disease, enterocutaneous fistulas and pyoderma gangrenosum. It was a prospective IRB-approved study from 2008-2015 with patients treated with HBO_2 consisting of breathing 100% oxygen at 2.4 ATA for two hours. Number of treatments varied from individual to individual with a median of 20 treatments (range 10-86). Standard wound care was performed with cleaning, topical dressings, antibiotics, and surgical debridement when needed. No complications related to HBO_2 were reported. Only 10.3% (n=3) of the total 29 patients enrolled in this study were patients with a sole diagnosis of pyoderma gangrenosum. One patient had concomitant PG with enterocutaneous fistula and another had PG, ECF and perineal Crohn's disease (PCD). Patients with a diagnosis of PG (n=5) had a 100% healing rate following HBO_2.[215]

Patient Selection/Treatment Protocol

As pyoderma gangrenosum can cause select problem wounds that are often refractory to conventional therapy with oral, intramuscular or parenteral steroids, immune-modulating therapies, various topical dressings and applications, negative pressure wound therapy, and other systemic and topical drug therapies or regimens, it is recommended that hyperbaric oxygen therapy be used as a helpful adjunct, given the current literature review above. If therapy is refractory to the above trialed conventional remedies, HBO_2 is a viable option and may assist with healing of these problematic wounds.

Most data and/or protocols have consisted of hyperbaric oxygen therapy being administered in the 2.0-2.5 ATA range for anywhere from 30-120 minutes while breathing 100% oxygen. A reasonable protocol would be to treat these patients at 2.4 ATA for 90 minutes with 100% oxygen for a total of 30 treatments.

Utilization Review

Utilization review should be performed after an initial 30 treatments are utilized or after complete healing of the wound is achieved, whichever comes first. Continuation of HBO_2 should be carefully weighed with conventional drug regimens provided to the patient. Ideally, every effort should be made to wean the patient off conventional therapy while receiving HBO_2 in order to mitigate the side effects of dysglycemia and immune suppression that are associated with many of the steroids, monoclonal antibody or immune-modulating therapies. One should also consider possible concomitant surgical interventions during HBO_2. A multidisciplinary approach should be sought when determining the goals and milestones of therapy.

Scleroderma, Systemic Sclerosis and Raynaud's Phenomenon

Pathophysiology of Disease

Systemic Scleroderma (SSc), also referred to as systemic sclerosis or diffuse scleroderma, is an autoimmune disease of the connective tissue of the human body that involves the hands and face with late involvement of the internal organs. It is a direct result of an abnormal thickening of skin that is caused by the accumulation of collagen and subsequent damage to smaller arteries. It can be divided into two categories: localized and systemic. Localized SSc affects the skin of the face, hands and feet. Diffuse or systemic scleroderma affects the face, hands, and feet, as well as visceral organs, specifically the heart, lungs, kidneys and GI tract.[216]

The pathophysiology of scleroderma is an underlying overproduction of collagen due to autoimmune dysfunction. This subsequent deposition in subcutaneous tissues and various other parts of the body creates a physiologically hypoxic environment by restricting blood flow to the skin. This impairs wound healing and causes wounds that eventually become infected, which further reduces oxygen delivery to the periphery of tissues.

Rationale for HBO_2

HBO_2 delivers oxygen at higher than atmospheric pressure resulting in increased arterial oxygen tensions in the plasma and drives the oxygen into hypoxic injured tissue.[38,90-91] HBO_2 has both local and systemic effects.[59] The result is neovascularization and collagen deposition at the site of hypoxic tissue such as those in SSc.[30,59] Systemic scleroderma is an autoimmune disease, and HBO_2 may play a role in immune modulation. Studies have demonstrated the beneficial effects of HBO_2 in minimizing the proliferation of damaging lymphocytes and modulating the biology of cytokines and inflammatory mediators.[187-188]

Literature Review

The literature is comprised mainly of case reports. In 1967, there was a case series of six women between the ages of 46 and 71 that were treated with 2 ATA of HBO_2 twice daily for 10-14 days with subsequent improvement in symptoms.[217] The improvements in symptoms were reported to have lasted for longer than one month with skin mobility being commented on as being more mobile. They followed the occurrence and symptoms associated with body ulcers, classified as both ischemic and infected in these patients, and noted that subjects had subjective pain relief within 48 hours of initiation of hyperbaric oxygen therapy. They observed that the ulcers healed in one to three weeks, which was faster than what was to be expected for the natural course of the disease.[217] The mechanism theorized behind this improved outcome in these patients was thought to be secondary to increased oxygen supply to the arterial wall resulting in less spasm and increased peripheral tissue oxygenation. The authors do mention the occurrence of the side effect of a transient myopia in one of the patients, lasting three weeks. In response to this particular case series, some have stipulated that improvement in this condition may even be achieved with a raising of temperature in the hyperbaric environment, for which a rise in ambient temperature has been anecdotally reported to be as effective in lasting mitigation of symptoms. Therefore, it was speculated that this "warming" could be a confounder in the improvement of pain in these patients.

In another case from Korea in 1976, a patient with SSc underwent HBO_2 therapy at 2.5 ATA over 16 weeks of therapy for a skin contraction with ultimate regression of the skin contraction after completion of therapy. However, there was no report of skin ulceration or wound.[218]

In an abstract publication in 1991 by Slade, patients with CVD (collagen vascular disease) ranging from rheumatoid arthritis to scleroderma to Sjogren's and Raynaud's and others, were treated with HBO_2 therapy with improvement in outcomes observed, suggesting benefit in patients with wounds secondary to collagen disorders. However, no specific data is offered on number of patients treated or number of treatments received.[219]

In 1995, there was report of improvement in cognitive function in a lupus/scleroderma crossover patient with hyperbaric oxygen therapy. This case did not exhibit any wounds.[220]

In 1997, there is publication of a negative case report from Zurich, Switzerland, revealing a large recalcitrant leg ulcer, failing hyperbaric oxygen therapy, and ultimately responding after undergoing femoropopliteal bypass surgery and radical debridement with skin grafting, in order to avoid amputation. The article reports the patient undergoing prior hyperbaric oxygen therapy for one hour daily but does not report the duration or the treatment pressure at which the patient was treated.[221]

A 2006 article by Markus et al. includes two cases of scleroderma treated with HBO_2 at 2.4 ATA that resulted in complete wound healing for both cases as the primary outcome. In the first case of a 37-year-old male, local ischemia was established via transcutaneous oximetry for the wounds of his bilateral medial malleoli. The patient underwent 30 treatments of HBO_2 in a monoplace chamber at 2.4 ATA with resultant complete wound healing. Follow-up $TcPO_2$ measurements at four months showed increased perfusion to the distal extremities with no ulcer recurrence at six months postconsultation. The second case reported was a 41-year-old female with digital ulcerations to the tips of the second and third digits of her right hand and the tip of the third digit of her left hand. $TcPO_2$ measurements were recorded and the patient underwent an identical HBO_2 regimen, as noted above, with complete healing of her right third digit ulceration and left second digit ulceration. The left third digit ulceration improved but did not completely heal after HBO_2. Follow-up $TcPO_2$ levels at six months showed increased perfusion as well.[222]

There is a case report in 2013, in Greece, of a patient with both systemic sclerosis and Raynaud's phenomenon who was successfully treated for intractable ulcers from systemic sclerosis. The case report describes a 75-year-old female with right great toe and left medial ankle ulcers who had $TcPO_2$ measurements obtained and subsequently treated with 34 treatments of HBO_2 at 2.4 ATA for 90 minutes of oxygen with each treatment. She underwent daily ulcer debridement and achieved complete healing of both ulcers. The treatment was reported to prevent the consulting vascular surgeon from amputating the right great toe.[223]

Moran et al. in 2014 searched English language studies from 2000-2013 examining nonpharmacologic interventions for the treatment of SSc and found only two cases treated with HBO_2. He concluded that the use of HBO_2 demonstrated some effectiveness in the treatment of scleroderma patients,[216] but these were the same two cases reported in the Markus et al. study above.[222] Although there were very few cases of SSc treated with HBO_2 reported in the English language literature, the Chinese literature does have a retrospective study of 90 SSc patients that were treated with HBO_2 between September 2008 and March 2011. After undergoing HBO_2 at 2.0 ATA for an unclear number of sessions, the patient population exhibited a 91.1% significantly improved rate, 6.7% improved rate, and only 2.2% not-cured rate.[224]

A 2017 case report by Poirier et al. describes a patient with refractory ulcers of the toes that developed as a consequence of systemic sclerosis. After refusing treatment with iloprost, a prostacyclin analog, the patient underwent 30 treatments with HBO_2 at 2.5 ATA over a 10-week period and achieved complete healing after eight months. The authors suggest HBO_2 as an alternative to failed or contraindicated conventional medical therapies for systemic sclerosis.[225]

A retrospective analysis out of Turkey in 2017 reported on six patients with SSc that underwent HBO_2 for their ulcers, with three patients exhibiting digital ulcers of the hands and the other three with leg ulcers. Three of the six patients had bilateral lesions as well (two leg ulcers and one digital ulcer patient). Once HBO_2 was applied, four patients healed completely while two patients were nearly healed with none requiring amputation. The mean number of HBO_2 treatments was 41 overall with 53 for digital ulcer patients and 28 for leg ulcer patients. There were no adverse events reported.[226]

In a case report from 2018 in Japan, Sato et al. describe an 84-year-old woman who had painful digital ulcers with Raynaud's disease who was hospitalized and underwent HBO_2 at 2.0 ATA for 60 minutes of oxygen for a total of 10 treatments. Complete healing of her digital ulcers was achieved after six weeks, four weeks after reception of 10 treatments of HBO_2.

Patient Selection/Treatment Protocol

There are multiple case reports that suggest potential benefit of use of HBO_2 in the treatment of SSc. There are no randomized, controlled studies that demonstrate HBO_2 to be a validated treatment for SSc or Raynaud's disease. Any potential research and/or use should be weighed with the relative risks/benefits of therapy. Approval for HBO_2 should be obtained prior to initiating treatment. Typical treatment pressures range from 2.0-2.5 ATA for up to 30 sessions.

Utilization Review

Utilization review should be undertaken after the initial 30 treatments have been completed and at least that frequently thereafter.

Sickle Cell Ulcers

Pathophysiology of Disease

Sickle cell disease (SCD) is a genetic disorder characterized by the inheritance of sickle-cell hemoglobin (HbS), which causes red blood cells (erythrocytes) to deform and take a sickled shape. This sickled shape impairs binding of oxygen to the heme group, which compromises circulation, produces ischemia, and may cause permanent damage or hemolysis of the red blood cells causing a resultant anemia, or sickle cell anemia.[227] In a large study of 2,075 patients with SCD, it was shown that patients will have an approximate prevalence of 2.5% for lower extremity ulcers in patients with SCD.[228] However there is a paucity of literature examining the treatment of wounds or skin ulcers caused by sickle cell disease. In addition to skin ulcers, sickle cell disease causes other manifestations of ischemic disease (e.g., pain crisis) that have been treated using HBO_2.

Rationale for HBO_2

There has been evidence attributed to the treatment of patients with HBO_2 in order to raise pO_2 in SCD patients and reducing the potential for sickling of red blood cells.[229] In 1969, Laszlo et al. first showed in five patients that exposure of sickle cell disease patients to HBO_2 at 2 ATA lowered the percentage of circulating sickle cells and maintained this effect for a period thereafter, as well.[230]

Wallyn et al., in 1985, studied the effect of HBO_2 on sickle cell hyphema and showed that when the eyes of adult albino rabbits were injected with anticoagulated sickle cell blood, the pO_2 of the aqueous humor of the eyes increased significantly under HBO_2 conditions (p<0.0001). They also showed that the percentage of sickled cells in the anterior chamber decreased from an average of 35.7% to 4.1% in rabbits who were exposed to HBO_2 at 2.0 ATA for 2 hours. It was hypothesized, based on these results from this animal study, that HBO_2 may be of use in treating patients who suffer from hyphema as a complication from SCD.[231]

Contrary to the above, Mychaskiw et al., in 2001, via a rather simple in vitro study, showed that HBO_2 did not have an effect on sickled cells in vitro and that there may be another process involved, in vivo, that would account for observed clinical effects from other studies.[232]

Literature Review

Rudge reported the only two cases of cutaneous ulcers secondary to SCD in 1991 with a 50% response rate. The first case was an 18-year-old male with a left malleolar ulcer that had originally healed 2 weeks after an insect bite. The ulcer recurred a month later and was refractive to antibiotics and local wound care. Osteomyelitis was ruled out, and the patient was given 100% oxygen at 2.4 ATA for 90 minutes, 6 days a week. The ulcer began to heal two weeks after starting HBO_2 and had healed in four weeks. There was no ulcer recurrence at the two 2-year follow-up. The second case was a 36-year-old female with a left medial malleolus ulcer of eight-month duration. The patient failed local wound therapy and a trial of pentoxyfilline. After macrovascular disease was ruled out, the patient was given 100% oxygen at 2.4 ATA for 90 minutes, five days a week. The patient had no evidence of healing after 32 treatments and HBO_2 was discontinued.[233]

Desforges and Wang reported a negative case series in 1966, noting a lack of improvement in a series of six patients with painful sickle cell crises. None showed improvement after one hour of treatment, but they did exhibit a decrease in the number of circulating sickled cells.[234]

The first reported case of sickle cell crisis successfully treated with HBO_2 was published in 1971 by Reynolds, who was able to showcase improvement in a 25-year-old female patient with acute abdominal crisis symptoms (reticulocyte count 10.3%) while undergoing HBO_2 at 2 ATA for 90 minutes with each treatment. The patient's abdominal pain resolved within the first 30 minutes at 2.0 ATA, and she remained asymptomatic for about three hours. After recurrence of symptoms, she was treated a second time within that same 24-hour period and remained symptom-free for eight hours subsequently. She received a total of four treatments during her hospital stay and remained free of pain for the remainder of her hospitalization.[235]

In 1973, Freilich et al. published three case reports of scleral buckling procedures performed under HBO_2 conditions for retinal detachment without the development of anterior segment ischemia, a frequent complication of this procedure without HBO_2.[229]

Stirnemann et al. showed that nine patients treated for vaso-occlusive crises from 2006-2007 had a reduction of their visual analog scale (VAS) pain scores from 3.3 to 1.9 out of 10 after the first day of HBO_2. They treated patients at a treatment pressure of 2.5 ATA for total of 90 minutes and 60 minutes on HBO_2. There was also a downward trend in pain-controlling dose of analgesic (morphine), albeit not statistically significant (P=0.08), for one day after HBO_2; however, the analgesic dose required two days after HBO_2 was noted to be zero, which was statistically significant (P=0.004). Two patients did suffer otalgia during the treatment sessions; however, none suffered permanent sequelae.[236]

Azik et al. in 2012 describe a case of successful treatment of a priapism in an 11-year-old male with SCD that was treated with both automated red cell exchange and HBO_2, as the patient had a priapism for 72 hours. Conventional treatment with IV fluid hydration, sedation, oxygenation and transfusion of packed red blood cells (PRBCs), along with a surgical intervention of a corpora cavernosa-glans penis shunt. Despite this, detumescence did not occur. The patient was then treated with HBO_2 for a total of 90 minutes at 2.5 ATA with 5 sessions weekly for a total of 11 sessions. This successfully treated the priapism.[237]

Canan et al. in 2014 describe successful treatment of a 25-year-old male with central retinal artery occlusion of the left eye (OS) secondary to SCD with 120 minutes of HBO_2 at 2.5 ATA twice daily for the first seven days and then once daily for the following six days for a total of 20 sessions. Baseline best corrected visual acuity (BCVA) in OS was being able to count fingers. BCVA after two treatments was 20/200 OS, and 20/60 at the end of 20 sessions. On his three-month follow-up visit, he was noted to have 20/30 BCVA OS.[238]

Patient Selection/Treatment Protocol

There are many case reports of various presentations of SCD, with the same underlying mechanism of vaso-occlusion, that would suggest the potential benefit of use of HBO_2 in treatment of these ailments, especially when conventional therapies are of no benefit. There are no randomized, controlled studies that demonstrate HBO_2 to be a validated treatment for SCD or crises or wounds related to SCD. There is insufficient evidence to support the routine use of HBO_2 to treat cutaneous manifestations of SCD. Approval for HBO_2 should be obtained prior to initiating treatment. Typical treatment pressures range from 2.0-2.5 ATA for up to 30 sessions.

Utilization Review

There are a variety of reasons for using HBO_2 in the treatment of complications of SCD, and each has its own rationale for why HBO_2 is being used. From a wound care perspective, utilization review should generally be undertaken after the initial 30 treatments have been completed and at least that frequently thereafter. For other manifestations of SCD, the length of treatment should correlate with the severity of symptoms.

Venous Stasis Ulcers

Pathophysiology of Disease

Venous ulcer disease or venostasis ulcers dominate the differential diagnosis for lower extremity ulcers, accounting for up to 90% of all chronic wounds of the lower extremity. They are chronic nonhealing ulcers that occur in

60. Thom SR. Oxidative stress is fundamental to hyperbaric oxygen therapy. J Appl Physiol (1985). 2009;106(3):988-995.
61. Schafer M, Werner S. Oxidative stress in normal and impaired wound repair. Pharmacol Res. 2008;58(2):165-171.
62. Dennog C, Gedik C, Wood S, Speit G. Analysis of oxidative DNA damage and HPRT mutations in humans after hyperbaric oxygen treatment. Mutat Res. 1999;431(2):351-359.
63. Dennog C, Hartmann A, Frey G, Speit G. Detection of DNA damage after hyperbaric oxygen (HBO) therapy. Mutagenesis. 1996;11(6):605-609.
64. Dennog C, Radermacher P, Barnett YA, Speit G. Antioxidant status in humans after exposure to hyperbaric oxygen. Mutat Res. 1999;428(1-2):83-89.
65. Rothfuss A, Dennog C, Speit G. Adaptive protection against the induction of oxidative DNA damage after hyperbaric oxygen treatment. Carcinogenesis. 1998;19(11):1913-1917.
66. Speit G, Dennog C, Eichhorn U, Rothfuss A, Kaina B. Induction of heme oxygenase-1 and adaptive protection against the induction of DNA damage after hyperbaric oxygen treatment. Carcinogenesis. 2000;21(10):1795-1799.
67. Speit G, Dennog C, Lampl L. Biological significance of DNA damage induced by hyperbaric oxygen. Mutagenesis. 1998;13(1):85-87.
68. Speit G, Dennog C, Radermacher P, Rothfuss A. Genotoxicity of hyperbaric oxygen. Mutat Res. 2002;512(2-3):111-119.
69. Juttner B, Scheinichen D, Bartsch S, et al. Lack of toxic side effects in neutrophils following hyperbaric oxygen. Undersea Hyperb Med. 2003;30(4):305-311.
70. Thom SR, Mendiguren I, Hardy K, et al. Inhibition of human neutrophil beta2-integrin-dependent adherence by hyperbaric O2. Am J Physiol. 1997;272(3 Pt 1):C770-777.
71. Thom SR. Functional inhibition of leukocyte B2 integrins by hyperbaric oxygen in carbon monoxide-mediated brain injury in rats. Toxicol Appl Pharmacol. 1993;123(2):248-256.
72. Marx RE, Ehler WJ, Tayapongsak P, Pierce LW. Relationship of oxygen dose to angiogenesis induction in irradiated tissue. Am J Surg. 1990;160(5):519-524.
73. Svalestad J, Hellem S, Thorsen E, Johannessen AC. Effect of hyperbaric oxygen treatment on irradiated oral mucosa: microvessel density. Int J Oral Maxillofac Surg. 2015;44(3):301-307.
74. Svalestad J, Thorsen E, Vaagbo G, Hellem S. Effect of hyperbaric oxygen treatment on oxygen tension and vascular capacity in irradiated skin and mucosa. Int J Oral Maxillofac Surg. 2014;43(1):107-112.
75. Thom SR, Milavonova T. Hyperbaric oxygen therapy increases stem cell number and HIF-1 content in diabetics (Abstract). Undersea Hyperb Med. 2008;35(4):1.
76. Berra E, Roux D, Richard DE, Pouyssegur J. Hypoxia-inducible factor-1 alpha (HIF-1 alpha) escapes O(2)-driven proteasomal degradation irrespective of its subcellular localization: nucleus or cytoplasm. EMBO Rep. 2001;2(7):615-620.
77. Zhang Q, Chang Q, Cox RA, Gong X, Gould LJ. Hyperbaric oxygen attenuates apoptosis and decreases inflammation in an ischemic wound model. J Invest Dermatol. 2008;128(8):2102-2112.
78. Sheikh AY, Gibson JJ, Rollins MD, Hopf HW, Hussain Z, Hunt TK. Effect of hyperoxia on vascular endothelial growth factor levels in a wound model. Arch Surg. 2000;135(11):1293-1297.
79. Kang TS, Gorti GK, Quan SY, Ho M, Koch RJ. Effect of hyperbaric oxygen on the growth factor profile of fibroblasts. Arch Facial Plast Surg. 2004;6(1):31-35.
80. Lin S, Shyu KG, Lee CC, et al. Hyperbaric oxygen selectively induces angiopoietin-2 in human umbilical vein endothelial cells. Biochem Biophys Res Commun. 2002;296(3):710-715.
81. Sander AL, Henrich D, Muth CM, Marzi I, Barker JH, Frank JM. In vivo effect of hyperbaric oxygen on wound angiogenesis and epithelialization. Wound Repair Regen. 2009;17(2):179-184.
82. Bonomo SR, Davidson JD, Yu Y, Xia Y, Lin X, Mustoe TA. Hyperbaric oxygen as a signal transducer: upregulation of platelet derived growth factor-beta receptor in the presence of HBO2 and PDGF. Undersea Hyperb Med. 1998;25(4):211-216.
83. Boykin JV, Jr., Baylis C. Hyperbaric oxygen therapy mediates increased nitric oxide production associated with wound healing: a preliminary study. Adv Skin Wound Care. 2007;20(7):382-388.
84. Godman CA, Chheda KP, Hightower LE, Perdrizet G, Shin DG, Giardina C. Hyperbaric oxygen induces a cytoprotective and angiogenic response in human microvascular endothelial cells. Cell Stress Chaperones. 2010;15(4):431-442.
85. Brownlee M. The pathobiology of diabetic complications: a unifying mechanism. Diabetes. 2005;54(6):1615-1625.
86. Dinh TL, Veves A. A review of the mechanisms implicated in the pathogenesis of the diabetic foot. Int J Low Extrem Wounds. 2005;4(3):154-159.
87. Catrina SB, Okamoto K, Pereira T, Brismar K, Poellinger L. Hyperglycemia regulates hypoxia-inducible factor-1alpha protein stability and function. Diabetes. 2004;53(12):3226-3232.

88. Gao W, Ferguson G, Connell P, et al. High glucose concentrations alter hypoxia-induced control of vascular smooth muscle cell growth via a HIF-1alpha-dependent pathway. J Mol Cell Cardiol. 2007;42(3):609-619.

89. Vinik AI, Maser RE, Mitchell BD, Freeman R. Diabetic autonomic neuropathy. Diabetes Care. 2003;26(5):1553-1579.

90. Rollins MD, Gibson JJ, Hunt TK, Hopf HW. Wound oxygen levels during hyperbaric oxygen treatment in healing wounds. Undersea Hyperb Med. 2006;33(1):17-25.

91. Tibbles PM, Edelsberg JS. Hyperbaric-oxygen therapy. N Engl J Med. 1996;334(25):1642-1648.

92. Asano T, Kaneko E, Shinozaki S, et al. Hyperbaric oxygen induces basic fibroblast growth factor and hepatocyte growth factor expression, and enhances blood perfusion and muscle regeneration in mouse ischemic hind limbs. Circ J. 2007;71(3):405-411.

93. Gallagher KA, Liu ZJ, Xiao M, et al. Diabetic impairments in NO-mediated endothelial progenitor cell mobilization and homing are reversed by hyperoxia and SDF-1 alpha. J Clin Invest. 2007;117(5):1249-1259.

94. Goldstein LJ, Gallagher KA, Bauer SM, et al. Endothelial progenitor cell release into circulation is triggered by hyperoxia-induced increases in bone marrow nitric oxide. Stem Cells. 2006;24(10):2309-2318.

95. Liu ZJ, Velazquez OC. Hyperoxia, endothelial progenitor cell mobilization, and diabetic wound healing. Antioxid Redox Signal. 2008;10(11):1869-1882.

96. Camporesi, EM, Bosco,G. Mechanisms of action. In: Weaver, LK, ed. Hyperbaric Oxygen Therapy Committee Indications. 13th ed. North Palm Beach, Florida: Best Publishing Company. 2014;241-246.

97. Huang E, Heyboer M. Adjunctive hyperbaric oxygen therapy for diabetic foot ulcers. In: Whelan H, Kindwall E, eds. Hyperbaric Medicine Practice. 4th ed. North Palm Beach, Florida: Best Publishing Company; 2018.

98. Hart G, Strauss MB. Responses of ischaemic ulcerative conditions to OHP. Paper presented at: Sixth International Congress on Hyperbaric Medicine 1979; Aberdeen, Scotland.

99. Huang ET. Hyperbaric medicine today: an historically noble discipline challenged by loss of critical access and overutilization—an introduction to invited commentary. Undersea Hyperb Med. 2017;44(1):1-3.

100. Hart G, Strauss M. Responses of ischaemic ulcerative conditions to OHP. Proceedings of the Sixth International Congress on Hyperbaric Medicine. 1979:312-314.

101. Davis JC. The use of adjuvant hyperbaric oxygen in treatment of the diabetic foot. Clin Podiatr Med Surg. 1987;4(2):429-437.

102. Baroni G, Porro T, Faglia E, et al. Hyperbaric oxygen in diabetic gangrene treatment. Diabetes Care. 1987;10(1):81-86.

103. Oriani G, Meazza D, Favales F, Pizzi G, Aldeghi A, Faglia E. Hyperbaric Oxygen Therapy in Diabetic Gangrene. Journal of Hyperbaric Medicine. 1990;5(3):171-175.

104. Oriani G, Michael M, Meazza D, et al. Diabetic Foot and Hyperbaric Oxygen Therapy: A Ten-Year Experience. Journal of Hyperbaric Medicine. 1992;7(4):213-221.

105. Doctor N, Pandya S, Supe A. Hyperbaric oxygen therapy in diabetic foot. Journal of postgraduate medicine. 1992;38(3):112-114, 111.

106. Faglia E, Favales F, Aldeghi A, et al. Adjunctive systemic hyperbaric oxygen therapy in treatment of severe prevalently ischemic diabetic foot ulcer. A randomized study. Diabetes Care. 1996;19(12):1338-1343.

107. Fife C. Personal Communication about CMS approval of hyperbaric oxygen therapy for diabetic foot ulcers. 2014.

108. National Coverage Determination (NCD) for Hyperbaric Oxygen Therapy (20.29). In. Version 3 ed: Centers for Medicare and Medicaid Services; 1996.

109. Game F. Classification of diabetic foot ulcers. Diabetes Metab Res Rev. 2016;32 Suppl 1:186-194.

110. Wattel F, Mathieu D, Fossati P, Neviere R, Coget JM. Hyperbaric Oxygen in the Treatment of Diabetic Foot Lesions: Search for Predictive Healing Factors. Journal of Hyperbaric Medicine. 1991;6(4):263-268.

111. Faglia E, Favales F, Aldeghi A, et al. Change in major amputation rate in a center dedicated to diabetic foot care during the 1980s: prognostic determinants for major amputation. Journal of diabetes and its complications. 1998;12(2):96-102.

112. Strauss MB, Bryant BJ, Hart GB. Transcutaneous oxygen measurements under hyperbaric oxygen conditions as a predictor for healing of problem wounds. Foot Ankle Int. 2002;23(10):933-937.

113. Moon H, Strauss M, La S, Miller S. The validity of transcutaneous oxygen measurements in predicting healing of diabetic foot ulcers. Undersea Hyperb Med. 2016;43(6).

114. Kalani M, Jorneskog G, Naderi N, Lind F, Brismar K. Hyperbaric oxygen (HBO) therapy in treatment of diabetic foot ulcers. Long-term follow-up. Journal of diabetes and its complications. 2002;16(2):153-158.

115. Abidia A, Laden G, Kuhan G, et al. The role of hyperbaric oxygen therapy in ischaemic diabetic lower extremity ulcers: a double-blind randomised-controlled trial. Eur J Vasc Endovasc Surg. 2003;25(6):513-518.

116. Kessler L, Bilbault P, Ortega F, et al. Hyperbaric oxygenation accelerates the healing rate of nonischemic chronic diabetic foot ulcers: a prospective randomized study. Diabetes Care. 2003;26(8):2378-2382.

117. Duzgun AP, Satir HZ, Ozozan O, Saylam B, Kulah B, Coskun F. Effect of hyperbaric oxygen therapy on healing of diabetic foot ulcers. J Foot Ankle Surg. 2008;47(6):515-519.

118. Londahl M, Katzman P, Nilsson A, Hammarlund C. Hyperbaric oxygen therapy facilitates healing of chronic foot ulcers in patients with diabetes. Diabetes Care. 2010;33(5):998-1003.

119. Londahl M, Landin-Olsson M, Katzman P. Hyperbaric oxygen therapy improves health-related quality of life in patients with diabetes and chronic foot ulcer. Diabet Med. 2011;28(2):186-190.

120. Ma L, Li P, Shi Z, Hou T, Chen X, Du J. A prospective, randomized, controlled study of hyperbaric oxygen therapy: effects on healing and oxidative stress of ulcer tissue in patients with a diabetic foot ulcer. Ostomy Wound Manage. 2013;59(3):18-24.

121. Carter MJ, Fife CE, Bennett M. Comment on: Margolis et al. lack of effectiveness of hyperbaric oxygen therapy for the treatment of diabetic foot ulcer and the prevention of amputation: a cohort study. Diabetes Care. 2013;36:1961-1966. Diabetes Care. 2013;36(8):e131.

122. Margolis D. Personal communication about propensity scoring. 2013.

123. Margolis DJ, Gupta J, Hoffstad O, Papdopoulos M, Thom SR, Mitra N. Response to comments on: Margolis et al. Lack of effectiveness of hyperbaric oxygen therapy for the treatment of diabetic foot ulcer and the prevention of amputation: a cohort study. Diabetes Care. 2013;36:1961-1966. Diabetes Care. 2013;36(8):e132-133.

124. Fedorko L, Bowen JM, Jones W, et al. Hyperbaric oxygen therapy does not reduce indications for amputation in patients with diabetes with nonhealing ulcers of the lower limb: a prospective, double-blind, randomized controlled clinical trial. Diabetes Care. 2016.

125. Londahl M, Fagher K, Katzman P. Comment on Fedorko et al. Hyperbaric oxygen therapy does not reduce indications for amputation in patients with diabetes with nonhealing ulcers of the lower limb: a prospective, double-blind, randomized controlled clinical trial. Diabetes Care. 2016;39:392-399. Diabetes Care. 2016;39(8):e131-132.

126. Murad MH. Comment on Fedorko et al. Hyperbaric oxygen therapy does not reduce indications for amputation in patients with diabetes with nonhealing ulcers of the lower limb: a prospective, double-blind, randomized controlled clinical trial. Diabetes Care. 2016;39:392-399. Diabetes Care. 2016;39(8):e135.

127. Huang ET. Comment on Fedorko et al. Hyperbaric oxygen therapy does not reduce indications for amputation in patients with diabetes with nonhealing ulcers of the lower limb: a prospective, double-blind, randomized controlled clinical trial. Diabetes Care. 2016;39:392-399. Diabetes Care. 2016;39(8):e133-134.

128. LeDez K. Serious concerns about the Toronto hyperbaric oxygen for diabetic foot ulcer study. Undersea Hyperb Med. 2016;43(6):737-741.

129. Fedorko Study Subject #1121 Testimonial. https://www.youtube.com/watch?v=1TPNBRHZe1Q2016.

130. Santema KTB, Stoekenbroek RM, Koelemay MJW, et al. Hyperbaric oxygen therapy in the treatment of ischemic lower- extremity ulcers in patients with diabetes: Results of the DAMO2CLES multicenter randomized clinical trial. Diabetes Care. 2018;41(1):112-119.

131. Huang E. Comment on Santema et al. Hyperbaric oxygen therapy in the treatment of ischemic lower-extremity ulcers in patients with diabetes: results of the DAMO2CLES multicenter randomized clinical trial. Diabetes Care. 2018;41:112-119. Diabetes Care. 2018;41(4):e61.

132. Santema KTB, Stoekenbroek RM, Koelemay MJW, Ubbink DT, Group DCS. Response to comments on Santema et al. Hyperbaric oxygen therapy in the treatment of ischemic lower-extremity ulcers in patients with diabetes: results of the DAMO2CLES multicenter randomized clinical trial. Diabetes Care. 2018;41:112-119. Diabetes Care. 2018;41(4):e62-e63.

133. Wunderlich RP, Peters EJ, Lavery LA. Systemic hyperbaric oxygen therapy: lower-extremity wound healing and the diabetic foot. Diabetes Care. 2000;23(10):1551-1555.

134. Bishop AJ, Mudge E. Diabetic foot ulcers treated with hyperbaric oxygen therapy: a review of the literature. Int Wound J. 2014;11(1):28-34.

135. Goldman RJ. Hyperbaric oxygen therapy for wound healing and limb salvage: a systematic review. PM & R : the journal of injury, function, and rehabilitation. 2009;1(5):471-489.

136. Kranke P, Bennett MH, Martyn-St James M, Schnabel A, Debus SE. Hyperbaric oxygen therapy for chronic wounds. Cochrane Database Syst Rev. 2012;4:CD004123.

137. Liu R, Li L, Yang M, Boden G, Yang G. Systematic review of the effectiveness of hyperbaric oxygenation therapy in the management of chronic diabetic foot ulcers. Mayo Clinic Proceedings. 2013;88(2):166-175.

138. Murad MH, Altayar O, Bennett M, et al. Using GRADE for evaluating the quality of evidence in hyperbaric oxygen therapy clarifies evidence limitations. J Clin Epidemiol. 2014;67(1):65-72.

139. O'Reilly D, Pasricha A, Campbell K, et al. Hyperbaric Oxygen Therapy for Diabetic Ulcers: Systematic Review and Meta-Analysis. International Journal of Technology Assessment in Health Care. 2013;29(3):269-281.

140. Roeckl-Wiedmann I, Bennett M, Kranke P. Systematic review of hyperbaric oxygen in the management of chronic wounds. The British Journal of Surgery. 2005;92(1):24-32.
141. Stoekenbroek RM, Santema TB, Legemate DA, Ubbink DT, van den Brink A, Koelemay MJ. Hyperbaric oxygen for the treatment of diabetic foot ulcers: a systematic review. Eur J Vasc Endovasc Surg. 2014;47(6):647-655.
142. Wang Z, Hasan R, Firwana B, et al. A systematic review and meta-analysis of tests to predict wound healing in diabetic foot. J Vasc Surg. 2016;63(2 Suppl):29S-36S e21-22.
143. Game FL, Hinchliffe RJ, Apelqvist J, et al. A systematic review of interventions to enhance the healing of chronic ulcers of the foot in diabetes. Diabetes Metab Res Rev. 2012;28 Suppl 1:119-141.
144. Wang C, Schwaitzberg S, Berliner E, Zarin DA, Lau J. Hyperbaric oxygen for treating wounds: a systematic review of the literature. Arch Surg. 2003;138(3):272-279; discussion 280.
145. Clinical Practice Guidelines We Can Trust. In: Institute of Medicine of the National Academies; 2011.
146. Lipsky BA, Berendt AR, Cornia PB, et al. 2012 Infectious Diseases Society of America clinical practice guideline for the diagnosis and treatment of diabetic foot infections. Clin Infect Dis. 2012;54(12):e132-173.
147. Diabetic foot problems: prevention and management. In. London: National Institute for Health and Care Excellence; 2015.
148. Game FL, Attinger C, Hartemann A, et al. IWGDF guidance on use of interventions to enhance the healing of chronic ulcers of the foot in diabetes. Diabetes Metab Res Rev. 2016;32 Suppl 1:75-83.
149. Hingorani A, LaMuraglia GM, Henke P, et al. The management of diabetic foot: a clinical practice guideline by the Society for Vascular Surgery in collaboration with the American Podiatric Medical Association and the Society for Vascular Medicine. J Vasc Surg. 2016;63(2 Suppl):3S-21S.
150. Guyatt GH, Oxman AD, Vist GE, et al. GRADE: an emerging consensus on rating quality of evidence and strength of recommendations. BMJ. 2008;336(7650):924-926.
151. Moffat AD, Worth ER, Weaver LK. Glycosylated hemoglobin and hyperbaric oxygen coverage denials. Undersea Hyperb Med. 2015;42(3):197-204.
152. Ennis W, Huang E, Gordon H. Impact of hyperbaric oxygen on more advanced Wagner Grades 3 and 4 diabetic foot ulcers: matching therapy to specific wound conditions. Advances in Wound Care. 2018;7(12):11.
153. Cianci P, Petrone G, Drager S, Lueders H, Lee H, Shapiro R. Salvage of the problem wound and potential amputation with wound care and adjunctive hyperbaric oxygen therapy: An economic analysis. Journal of Hyperbaric Medicine. 1988;3(3):127-141.
154. Cianci P, Petrone G, Green B. Adjunctive hyperbaric oxygen in the salvage of the diabetic foot. Undersea Biomed Res. 1991;18(Suppl):109.
155. Eggert JV, Worth ER, Van Gils CC. Cost and mortality data of a regional limb salvage and hyperbaric medicine program for Wagner Grade 3 or 4 diabetic foot ulcers. Undersea Hyperb Med. 2016;43(1):1-8.
156. Guo S, Counte MA, Gillespie KN, Schmitz H. Cost-effectiveness of adjunctive hyperbaric oxygen in the treatment of diabetic ulcers. Int J Technol Assess Health Care. 2003;19(4):731-737.
157. Hailey D, Jacobs P, Perry D, Chuck A, Morrison A, Boudreau R. Adjunctive hyperbaric oxygen therapy for diabetic foot ulcer: an economic analysis. Canadian Agency for Drugs and Technologies in Health; March 2007.
158. Lipsky BA, Berendt AR. Hyperbaric oxygen therapy for diabetic foot wounds: has hope hurdled hype? Diabetes Care. 2010;33(5):1143-1145.
159. Chuck AW, Hailey D, Jacobs P, Perry DC. Cost-effectiveness and budget impact of adjunctive hyperbaric oxygen therapy for diabetic foot ulcers. Int J Technol Assess Health Care. 2008;24(2):178-183.
160. Santema TB, Stoekenbroek RM, van Steekelenburg KC, van Hulst RA, Koelemay MJ, Ubbink DT. Economic outcomes in clinical studies assessing hyperbaric oxygen in the treatment of acute and chronic wounds. Diving Hyperb Med. 2015;45(4):228-234.
161. Rosamond W, Flegal K, Furie K, et al. Heart disease and stroke statistics—2008 update: a report from the American Heart Association Statistics Committee and Stroke Statistics Subcommittee. Circulation. 2008;117(4):e25-146.
162. Thomas DR. Managing peripheral arterial disease and vascular ulcers. Clin Geriatr Med. 2013;29(2):425-431.
163. Hopf HW, Ueno C, Aslam R, et al. Guidelines for the treatment of arterial insufficiency ulcers. Wound Repair Regen. 2006;14(6):693-710.
164. Tautenhahn J, Lobmann R, Koenig B, Halloul Z, Lippert H, Buerger T. The influence of polymorbidity, revascularization, and wound therapy on the healing of arterial ulceration. Vasc Health Risk Manag. 2008;4(3):683-689.
165. Marston WA, Davies SW, Armstrong B, et al. Natural history of limbs with arterial insufficiency and chronic ulceration treated without revascularization. J Vasc Surg. 2006;44(1):108-114.
166. Mlekusch W, Schillinger M, Sabeti S, Maca T, Ahmadi R, Minar E. Clinical outcome and prognostic factors for ischaemic ulcers treated with PTA in lower limbs. Eur J Vasc Endovasc Surg. 2002;24(2):176-181.

167. Milovanova TN, Bhopale VM, Sorokina EM, et al. Hyperbaric oxygen stimulates vasculogenic stem cell growth and differentiation in vivo. J Appl Physiol (1985). 2009;106(2):711-728.

168. Capla JM, Ceradini DJ, Tepper OM, et al. Skin graft vascularization involves precisely regulated regression and replacement of endothelial cells through both angiogenesis and vasculogenesis. Plast Reconstr Surg. 2006;117(3):836-844.

169. Boger RH, Bode-Boger SM, Thiele W, Junker W, Alexander K, Frolich JC. Biochemical evidence for impaired nitric oxide synthesis in patients with peripheral arterial occlusive disease. Circulation. 1997;95(8):2068-2074.

170. Heyboer M, 3rd, Grant WD, Byrne J, et al. Hyperbaric oxygen for the treatment of nonhealing arterial insufficiency ulcers. Wound Repair Regen. 2014;22(3):351-355.

171. Angelis M, Wong LL, Myers SA, Wong LM. Calciphylaxis in patients on hemodialysis: a prevalence study. Surgery. 1997;122(6):1083-1089; discussion 1089-1090.

172. Podymow T, Wherrett C, Burns KD. Hyperbaric oxygen in the treatment of calciphylaxis: a case series. Nephrol Dial Transplant. 2001;16(11):2176-2180.

173. Coates T, Kirkland GS, Dymock RB, et al. Cutaneous necrosis from calcific uremic arteriolopathy. Am J Kidney Dis. 1998;32(3):384-391.

174. Budisavljevic MN, Cheek D, Ploth DW. Calciphylaxis in chronic renal failure. J Am Soc Nephrol. 1996;7(7):978-982.

175. Bhambri A, Del Rosso JQ. Calciphylaxis: a review. J Clin Aesthet Dermatol. 2008;1(2):38-41.

176. An J, Devaney B, Ooi KY, Ford S, Frawley G, Menahem S. Hyperbaric oxygen in the treatment of calciphylaxis: A case series and literature review. Nephrology (Carlton). 2015;20(7):444-450.

177. Basile C, Montanaro A, Masi M, Pati G, De Maio P, Gismondi A. Hyperbaric oxygen therapy for calcific uremic arteriolopathy: a case series. J Nephrol. 2002;15(6):676-680.

178. Arenas MD, Gil MT, Gutierrez MD, et al. Management of calcific uremic arteriolopathy (calciphylaxis) with a combination of treatments, including hyperbaric oxygen therapy. Clin Nephrol. 2008;70(3):261-264.

179. Don BR, Chin AI. A strategy for the treatment of calcific uremic arteriolopathy (calciphylaxis) employing a combination of therapies. Clin Nephrol. 2003;59(6):463-470.

180. Dean SM, Werman H. Calciphylaxis: a favorable outcome with hyperbaric oxygen. Vasc Med. 1998;3(2):115-120.

181. Vassa N, Twardowski ZJ, Campbell J. Hyperbaric oxygen therapy in calciphylaxis-induced skin necrosis in a peritoneal dialysis patient. Am J Kidney Dis. 1994;23(6):878-881.

182. McCulloch N, Wojcik SM, Heyboer M, 3rd. Patient outcomes and factors associated with healing in calciphylaxis patients undergoing adjunctive hyperbaric oxygen therapy. J Am Coll Clin Wound Spec. 2015;7(1-3):8-12.

183. Baldwin C, Farah M, Leung M, et al. Multi-intervention management of calciphylaxis: a report of 7 cases. Am J Kidney Dis. 2011;58(6):988-991.

184. Hymes SR, Alousi AM, Cowen EW. Graft-versus-host disease: part I. Pathogenesis and clinical manifestations of graft-versus-host disease. J Am Acad Dermatol. 2012;66(4):515 e511-518; quiz 533-514.

185. Stussi G, Tsakiris DA. Late effects on haemostasis after haematopoietic stem cell transplantation. Hamostaseologie. 2012;32(1):63-66.

186. Biedermann BC, Sahner S, Gregor M, et al. Endothelial injury mediated by cytotoxic T lymphocytes and loss of microvessels in chronic graft versus host disease. Lancet. 2002;359(9323):2078-2083.

187. Gassas A, Wayne Evans A, Armstrong C, Doyle JJ. Open wound chronic skin graft-vs-host disease. Are these wounds ischemic? Pediatr Transplant. 2007;11(1):101-104.

188. Al-Waili NS, Butler GJ. Effects of hyperbaric oxygen on inflammatory response to wound and trauma: possible mechanism of action. ScientificWorldJournal. 2006;6:425-441.

189. Song XY, Sun LN, Zheng NN, Zhang HP. Effect of hyperbaric oxygen on acute graft-versus-host disease after allogeneic bone marrow transplantation. Zhongguo Shi Yan Xue Ye Xue Za Zhi. 2008;16(3):623-626.

190. Heyboer M, 3rd, Taylor J, Morgan M, Mariani P, Jennings S. The use of hyperbaric oxygen therapy in the treatment of non-healing ulcers secondary to graft-versus-host disease. J Am Coll Clin Wound Spec. 2013;5(1):14-18.

191. Tutrone WD, Green K, Weinberg JM, Caglar S, Clarke D. Pyoderma gangrenosum: dermatologic application of hyperbaric oxygen therapy. J Drugs Dermatol. 2007;6(12):1214-1219.

192. Hickman JG, Lazarus GS. Pyoderma gangrenosum: a reappraisal of associated systemic diseases. Br J Dermatol. 1980;102(2):235-237.

193. Powell FC, Su WP, Perry HO. Pyoderma gangrenosum: classification and management. J Am Acad Dermatol. 1996;34(3):395-409; quiz 410-392.

194. Brooklyn T, Dunnill G, Probert C. Diagnosis and treatment of pyoderma gangrenosum. BMJ. 2006;333(7560):181-184.

195. Prystowsky JH, Kahn SN, Lazarus GS. Present status of pyoderma gangrenosum. Review of 21 cases. Arch Dermatol. 1989;125(1):57-64.

196. Wolff K, Stingl G. Pyoderma gangrenosum. In: Freedberg E, ed. Fitzpatrick's dermatology in general medicine. New York, NY: McGraw-Hill, Health Professions Division; 2003:969-975.
197. Hurwitz RM, Haseman JH. The evolution of pyoderma gangrenosum. A clinicopathologic correlation. Am J Dermatopathol. 1993;15(1):28-33.
198. Fakhar F, Memon S, Deitz D, Abramowitz R, Alpert DR. Refractory postsurgical pyoderma gangrenosum in a patient with Beckwith Wiedemann syndrome: response to multimodal therapy. BMJ Case Rep. 2013;2013.
199. Niezgoda JA, Cabigas EB, Allen HK, Simanonok JP, Kindwall EP, Krumenauer J. Managing pyoderma gangrenosum: a synergistic approach combining surgical debridement, vacuum-assisted closure, and hyperbaric oxygen therapy. Plast Reconstr Surg. 2006;117(2):24e-28e.
200. Thomas CY, Jr., Crouch JA, Guastello J. Hyperbaric oxygen therapy for pyoderma gangrenosum. Arch Dermatol. 1974;110(3):445-446.
201. Fuhrman DL. Letter: Hyperbaric oxygen therapy. Arch Dermatol. 1975;111(5):657.
202. Wyrick WJ, Mader JT, Butler ME, Hulet WH. Hyperbaric oxygen treatment of pyoderma gangrenosum. Arch Dermatol. 1978;114(8):1232-1233.
203. Davis JC, Landeen JM, Levine RA. Pyoderma gangrenosum: skin grafting after preparation with hyperbaric oxygen. Plast Reconstr Surg. 1987;79(2):200-207.
204. Wasserteil V, Bruce S, Sessoms SL, Guntupalli KK. Pyoderma gangrenosum treated with hyperbaric oxygen therapy. Int J Dermatol. 1992;31(8):594-596.
205. Fitzpatrick D. Primary treatment of pyoderma gangrenosum with hyperbaric oxygen therapy: a case report. Wounds. 1997;9:4.
206. Jacobs P, Wood L, Van Niekerk GD. Therapy: hyperbaric oxygen as the only effective treatment in mutilating and resistant systemic vasculitis. Hematology. 2000;5(2):167-172.
207. Vieira WA, Barbosa LR, Martin LM. Hyperbaric oxygen therapy as an adjuvant treatment for pyoderma gangrenosum. An Bras Dermatol. 2011;86(6):1193-1196.
208. Hill DS, O'Neill JK, Toms A, Watts AM. Pyoderma gangrenosum: a report of a rare complication after knee arthroplasty requiring muscle flap cover supplemented by negative pressure therapy and hyperbaric oxygen. J Plast Reconstr Aesthet Surg. 2011;64(11):1528-1532.
209. Mazokopakis EE, Kofteridis DP, Pateromihelaki AT, Vytiniotis SD, Karastergiou PG. Improvement of ulcerative pyoderma gangrenosum with hyperbaric oxygen therapy. Dermatol Ther. 2011;24(1):134-136.
210. Altunay I, Kucukunal A, Sarikaya S, Tukenmez Demirci G. A favourable response to surgical intervention and hyperbaric oxygen therapy in pyoderma gangrenosum. Int Wound J. 2014;11(4):350-353.
211. Araujo FM, Kondo RN, Minelli L. Pyoderma gangrenosum: skin grafting and hyperbaric oxygen as adjuvants in the treatment of a deep and extensive ulcer. An Bras Dermatol. 2013;88(6 Suppl 1):176-178.
212. Ratnagobal S, Sinha S. Pyoderma gangrenosum: guideline for wound practitioners. J Wound Care. 2013;22(2):68-73.
213. Seo HI, Lee HJ, Han KH. Hyperbaric oxygen therapy for pyoderma gangrenosum associated with ulcerative colitis. Intest Res. 2018;16(1):155-157.
214. Chiang IH, Liao YS, Dai NT, et al. Hyperbaric oxygen therapy for the adjunctive treatment of pyoderma gangrenosum: a case report. Ostomy Wound Manage. 2016;62(5):32-36.
215. Feitosa MR, Feres Filho O, Tamaki CM, et al. Adjunctive hyperbaric oxygen therapy promotes successful healing in patients with refractory Crohn's disease. Acta Cir Bras. 2016;31 Suppl 1:19-23.
216. Moran ME. Scleroderma and evidence based non-pharmaceutical treatment modalities for digital ulcers: a systematic review. J Wound Care. 2014;23(10):510-516.
217. Dowling GB, Copeman PW, Ashfield R. Raynaud's phenomenon in scleroderma treated with hyperbaric oxygen. Proc R Soc Med. 1967;60(12):1268-1269.
218. Chun W, Kim S, Seong H, Chong T. Hyperbaric oxygen therapy in systemic scleroderma. Korean J Dermatol. 1974;12(1):4.
219. Slade B. The Effect of hyperbaric oxygen therapy (HBO) on wound healing in patients with collagen-vascular disease: a retrospective analysis. Undersea Biomed Res. 1991;18(Suppl):1.
220. Wallace DJ, Silverman S, Goldstein J, Hughes D. Use of hyperbaric oxygen in rheumatic diseases: case report and critical analysis. Lupus. 1995;4(3):172-175.
221. Hafner J, Kohler A, Enzler M, Brunner U. Successful treatment of an extended leg ulcer in systemic sclerosis. Vasa. 1997;26(4):302-304.
222. Markus YM, Bell MJ, Evans AW. Ischemic scleroderma wounds successfully treated with hyperbaric oxygen therapy. J Rheumatol. 2006;33(8):1694-1696.
223. Gerodimos C, Stefanidou S, Kotsiou M, Melekos T, Mesimeris T. Hyperbaric oxygen treatment of intractable ulcers in a systemic sclerosis patient. Aristotle University Medical Journal. 2013;40(3):4.

Table 2. Response Time Requirements for CO Alarms [26]

CO Concentration (ppm)	Response Time
30±3	Not sooner than 30 days
70±5	60–240 minutes
150±5	10–50 minutes
400±10	4–15 minutes

Exposures to high levels of CO (e.g. greater than 10,000 to 20,000 ppm) may rapidly result in death, possibly without symptoms as loss of consciousness can occur before symptom onset.[27] Carbon monoxide exposure for several hours to concentrations of 500 to 1000 ppm can be lethal to humans. At lower ambient levels of CO exposure (less than 500 ppm), common symptoms are headaches, nausea and vomiting, dizziness, general malaise, and altered mental status.[9,11-12] Some patients may have chest pain, shortness of breath, and myocardial ischemia, and may require mechanical ventilation and treatment of shock.[9]

Poisoning can occur from brief exposures to high levels of CO or from longer exposures to lower levels. Some patients with occult CO poisoning have manifested symptoms for weeks, months, or even years of time.[28] Symptoms are similar to those with acute poisoning, although those with chronic CO poisoning often have more fatigue, affective problems, and neurological abnormalities.[29-30] Often the poisoning etiology is discovered when a heating appliance or water heater is identified as faulty. Some patients have an acute episode of poisoning that draws attention to prior unrecognized CO exposure.[11] Any patient with CO poisoning can develop permanent sequelae regardless of the exposure duration.[14,29,31]

Carbon monoxide poisoning is a clinical diagnosis based upon the presence of symptoms and the CO exposure conditions (i.e., history of inhalation of CO or elevated ambient CO levels). Exposure can be confirmed by an elevated COHb, however, the half-life of COHb is relatively short, particularly when breathing supplemental oxygen, and some CO-poisoned patients will have normal COHb levels at the time of evaluation.[32-34] A COHb level of at least 3-4% in non-smokers or 10% in smokers indicates likely exogenous CO exposure.[35]

Carboxyhemoglobin can be measured by blood gas oximeter (spectrophotometer) from arterial or venous blood.[36] Traditional non-invasive pulse oximeters cannot discriminate COHb from HbO_2,[37] but a newer multi wavelength pulse oximeter can do so.[38-39] In a prospective study conducted in the emergency department setting, the false positive rate for SpCO by this monitor was 9% and the false negative rate was 18%.[40] Those authors recommend the results from this monitor could broaden the differential diagnosis to consider CO exposure, but the monitor should not be used to rule out CO poisoning.[40] In the correct clinical setting, SpCO results can confirm the diagnosis of CO poisoning.

CO Pathophysiology and HBO_2

The injuries caused by CO traditionally have been viewed as due to a hypoxic stress brought on by an elevated COHb level and leftward shift of the oxyhemoglobin curve.[41] Carbon monoxide preferentially binds to hemoglobin in place of oxygen and CO in the blood distributes via diffusion through the extravascular tissues. There, CO binds to heme proteins responsible for the production of adenosine triphosphate and interrupts cellular metabolism. However, perivascular and neuronal injuries arise by mechanisms other than hypoxia.[42-43] Neuropathology is due to a complex cascade of biochemical events involving several immunological and inflammatory pathophysiologic processes,[11,44-50] many independent of pure hypoxic stress,[51-53] that can evolve over weeks of time.[54] Endothelial-derived microparticles may be the initial stimulus for a subsequent cascade of immunological effects.[55] Some biochemical changes are independent of poisoning severity.[56]

The two organ systems most susceptible to injury from CO are the cardiovascular and central nervous systems. The COHb level is not predictive as a risk factor for CO mediated morbidity or mortality.[57-65] In some animal models CO-mediated hypoxia plus a decrease in perfusion due to an associated cardiovascular insult are required to precipitate CNS pathology,[43-44,66-68] yet loss of consciousness is not required for cognitive sequelae.[64,69,70] Exposure to relatively low levels of CO (50–90 ppm for 60 minutes) causes vascular oxidative stress in animal studies.[42,71-72]

Human and animal data indicate that major cardiac injury at the time of poisoning is due primarily to CO-induced hypoxic stress.[66,73,74] Carbon monoxide may increase the risk for cardiovascular-related death in patients with initial CO-induced cardiac injury over the 10 years following injury,[75] although another study suggests that increased mortality due to psychosocial factors and accidents is more likely.[76] As with brain injury from other causes, many neurological problems can follow CO poisoning including cognitive sequelae, anxiety and depression, persistent headaches, dizziness, sleep problems, motor weakness, vestibular and balance problems, gaze abnormalities, peripheral neuropathies, hearing loss, tinnitus, somatic complaints, and Parkinsonian-like syndrome. Neuropsychological sequelae following CO poisoning are common.[10,31,77-79] The incidence of anxiety and depression is high following acute CO poisoning and may not be favorably influenced by HBO_2.[80]

Breathing oxygen hastens the removal of COHb. The half-life of COHb in adults breathing air at sea level is approximately five to six hours[32] but reduced alveolar ventilation would lengthen the half-life. With administration of normobaric oxygen, the COHb half-life in adults is 74 ±25 minutes (mean ±1 SD).[33] Hyperbaric oxygen accelerates COHb dissociation compared to breathing pure oxygen at sea-level pressure.[32,34,81-83] Additionally, HBO_2, but not ambient pressure oxygen, has several actions that are beneficial in ameliorating CNS injuries. These include an improvement in mitochondrial function,[67,84] inhibition of lipid peroxidation,[85] impairment of leukocyte adhesion to injured microvasculature,[86] and reduction in brain inflammation caused by the CO-induced adduct formation of myelin basic protein.[87] Animals poisoned with CO and treated with HBO_2 have a more rapid improvement in cardiovascular status,[81] lower mortality,[88] and lower incidence of neurological sequelae.[87-89] Table 3 describes the pathophysiology of CO poisoning and the mechanisms of action by which HBO_2 can favorably influence this pathophysiology.

Table 3. CO Pathophysiology and Effects of HBO$_2$

CO Pathophysiology	Effect of HBO$_2$
Formation of COHb[90-91]	Rapid clearance of CO from blood and tissues[34]
Increased Hb affinity for oxygen and leftward shift of oxyhemoglobin dissociation curve[41,91]	Sufficient dissolved oxygen in blood that O$_2$Hb is unnecessary[92-96]
Tissue hypoxia[97-100]	Normalization of tissue oxygenation[101]
Binding to cellular proteins (i.e., cytochromes, myoglobin) and increased steady-state concentration of nitric oxide[102-113]	Reversal of cytochrome binding[67,114]
Inhibition of cellular metabolism[104,115-117]	Preservation of adenosine triphosphate production[84,118-120]
Oxidative stress (i.e., due to mitochondrial production of reactive oxygen species and free radical production from heme degradation)[43-44,46,105,110,113,121-122]	Adaptive/protective oxidative stress response through increased heme oxygenase-1[123-124] Upregulation and modulation of various antioxidant enzymes[125-131] Induction of heat shock protein, which protects against oxidative stress[132-133]
Dopamine/catecholamine hyperexciteability via gene upregulation,[134] hypothesized to damage the globus pallidus/deep white matter[135]	Favorable modulation of gene expression to regulate dopamine[134]
Impaired astrocyte neurotrophic function[136-137]	Preservation of astrocyte ability to synthesize and secrete neurotrophins[136-137]
Elevation of microparticles[55]	
Activation of platelet adhesion molecules and platelet-neutrophil aggregation, resulting in neutrophil degranulation, release of myeloperoxidase, and endothelial cell oxidative stress[42,48,51,71,112-113]	Reduced myeloperoxidase activity[127,138-139]
Neutrophil adherence to vasculature, leukocyte immune response, and conversion of xanthine dehydrogenase (XD) to xanthine oxidase (XO)[47,51,86,111,140-141]	Reduced leukocyte adhesion[142-143] Inhibition of immune response[86,144] Blocking XD conversion to XO[86]
Lipid peroxidation[46,141]	Prevention of brain lipid peroxidation[85]
Alteration in the structure of myelin basic protein and subsequent lymphocyte proliferation[52]	Muted adduct formation and blocked inflammatory response to altered myelin basic protein[51,87]
Excitatory neurotransmitter toxicity[45,68,145-148]	
Activation of hypoxia-inducible factor-1alpha[149,150]	Decrease in hypoxia-inducible factor-1 expression[151-153]
Neuronal necrosis and apoptosis[49,154]	Reduction of necrosis and protection against accelerated apoptosis[119,153,155-157]

Patient Selection Criteria

Patients manifesting signs of serious poisoning (e.g. transient or prolonged unconsciousness, neurologic signs, cardiovascular dysfunction, or severe acidosis) should be referred for HBO_2 regardless of the COHb level. Epidemiologic studies suggest that prognosis is poorer for patients who have underlying cardiovascular disease, are older than 60 years of age, have suffered any interval of unconsciousness due to the CO poisoning, or demonstrate severe acidosis.[58-59]

Despite many texts and articles claiming the contrary, the COHb level does not correlate with signs and symptoms,[9] nor with the development of neurological or cognitive sequelae after poisoning.[31,57-59,64,158] Nevertheless, referral of patients with COHb ≥25% for HBO_2 is reasonable.[159] A majority of hyperbaric physicians use HBO_2 for patients with less severe symptoms when COHb levels are elevated to the range of 25–30% or when neuropsychological testing is abnormal,[160] even though the role of neuropsychological tests in patient selection for HBO_2 therapy is not clear.[10,79,161-165]

One study's univariate analysis of patients not treated with HBO_2 which inspected potential risk factors for six-week cognitive sequelae revealed that age ≥36 years, loss of consciousness, COHb levels ≥25%, or with CO exposure intervals ≥24 hours were at increased risk for cognitive sequelae without HBO_2. However, the multivariable logistic regression, which included patients receiving HBO_2, revealed that patients ≥36 years old treated with HBO_2 had reduced six-week cognitive sequelae rates. Although the multivariable logistic regression showed that longer CO exposure duration was associated with increased cognitive sequelae rates, the sample size was underpowered regarding an HBO_2 effect.[31] However, of 5 patients with CO exposure duration > 24 hours, none treated with HBO_2 had cognitive sequelae. Cerebellar dysfunction (e.g. abnormal finger-to-nose, rapid alternating movements, or heel-shin testing) at the time of evaluation may also indicate increased risk for cognitive sequelae.[10] In this regard, it is important to recognize that HBO_2 can reduce 6-week cognitive sequelae in patients without initial cerebellar dysfunction (p=0.05).[10,166] When other risk factors are present, the absence of cerebellar abnormalities should not dissuade a physician from using HBO_2.

No risk factor is fully predictive of long-term outcome. In another study, individuals with no loss of consciousness and COHb ≤15% shared the same risk for cognitive sequelae as those with more severe poisoning.[64] Even mildly poisoned patients demonstrate many biochemical changes in blood.[56] Research suggest that patients who do not carry the apolipoprotein E4 allele, a genetic marker associated with worse outcome after brain injury,[167-168] may respond much more favorably to HBO_2 following CO poisoning than E4 carriers.[169] However, only 14–25% of humans carry the E4 allele[170] and genetic information is not available at the time of acute evaluation. Based on all the above factors, it is recommended that HBO_2 be considered for all cases of acute symptomatic CO poisoning.[10,12,31]

Clinical Management

Administration of supplemental oxygen is recommended to treat CO poisoning although there are no clinical trials demonstrating improved outcomes using oxygen therapy administered at atmospheric pressure. Nevertheless, supplemental oxygen inhalation will hasten dissociation of CO from hemoglobin and provide enhanced tissue oxygenation.[33]

The optimal HBO_2 dosing (pressure, duration, and frequency) is not known, but the optimal benefit from HBO_2 occurs in those treated with the least delay after exposure.[61] The majority of HBO_2 facilities offer a single HBO_2 session to CO-poisoned patients.[171] However, in selected patients repeated treatments may yield a better outcome than a single treatment.[77] Randomized trials demonstrating improved outcomes have offered two protocols:

1. Initial compression to 3 atmospheres absolute (ATA) (303.98 kPa), then 2 ATA (202.65 kPa) for 140 minutes, followed by two HBO$_2$ sessions at 2 ATA (202.65 kPa) for 90 minutes (five-minute air-breathing periods were used periodically to reduce oxygen toxicity) in 6 to 12 hour intervals.[10]

2. Initial compression to 2.8 ATA (283.71 kPa), then 2 ATA (202.65 kPa) for 120 minutes, without further HBO$_2$.[79]

A blinded randomized trial testing the first protocol compared neuropsychological outcomes in patients who received only the first HBO$_2$ session to outcomes in patients who received all three sessions in 24 hours. This trial found no difference between groups in cognitive sequelae rates at six weeks and six months (available in abstract form).[172]

Two review papers have offered guidance for medical management beyond HBO$_2$.[11-12] Of note, poisoned patients should have an electrocardiogram and serial measurement of cardiac enzymes such as the creatinine kinase MB fraction and troponin I. If there is evidence of cardiac injury, further cardiac evaluation and follow-up is advisable.[75,173]

Although the frequency is reduced by HBO$_2$,[10-11,31,79] some patients will develop cognitive or other adverse sequelae. As clinical investigations involving neuro-imaging and neuropsychiatric assessment become more sophisticated, they seem to demonstrate that some cognitive and cerebral vascular abnormalities from CO persist despite aggressive therapy,[10,80,160,174-176] although the incidence is lower with HBO$_2$ treatment.[10,31,79,177] Follow-up of poisoned patients and referral of those with sequelae to the appropriate resource is important.

Children with CO poisoning may be safely treated with HBO$_2$.[178] Children can have an uneventful recovery following poisoning or can have long-term problems.[179-180] A recent small prospective study found that all enrolled children had neuropsychological test results in the average range at six weeks and six months after poisoning, although many had symptoms suggesting CO-related problems. Additionally, most had vestibular and balance abnormalities consistent with brain injury.[181-182]

In contrast, CO can be teratogenic and toxic to the developing fetus, particularly in cases of serious poisoning.[183-185] Based upon mathematical modeling derived from animal experiments, the half-life of fetal COHb is 1.5 times the half-life of adult COHb.[186] One prospective study concluded that mild exposures are likely to result in normal fetal outcome but severe CO poisoning carries serious risk to the fetus in terms of viability and development and that HBO$_2$ may decrease fetal hypoxia and improve outcome.[183] Pregnant women can be safely treated with HBO$_2$ for acute CO poisoning without fetal harm.[187-188] If there is evidence of fetal distress, HBO$_2$ may be considered even if the mother is asymptomatic.

Although not approved for human use, a novel human engineered human neuroglobin that displaces CO from COHb, then is excreted by the kidneys, may hold promise as an antidote for acute CO poisoning.[189] In vitro, this agent reduced COHb half-life from >500 minutes to 25 seconds, while in mice, COHb elimination was 35% faster than breathing 100% oxygen. It has not been tested in humans and may not reduce the immune-mediated aspects of CO poisoning. Clinical trials are necessary to determine whether this potential antidote is safe and effective in humans.[190]

Patients with CO poisoning should be followed after discharge. Even with hyperbaric oxygen, they may have persistent problems after CO poisoning[10] or even develop new problems weeks to months later.[191-192] Common complaints in patients with these problems are headaches, dizziness, imbalance, fatigue, sleep disturbance, and neuropsychological and affective symptoms,[193] similar to those reported in post-concussive syndrome.[194] Treatment is supportive. Some patients have cardiac problems after CO poisoning that require intervention.[195]

Studies that have followed CO-poisoned patients to a year and beyond have documented long-term adverse effects on cognitive function, quality of life, and general health.[10,31,80,196-199] From three-year follow-up of 84 accidental and intentional CO-poisoned patients, Smith and Brandon[196] reported that 11% had "gross neuropsychiatric sequelae" directly attributable to the poisoning, while 30-40% had memory, personality, or affective changes. In long-term follow-up of 52 CO-poisoned patients (mean six years from poisoning, range 3.4-10.8 years), 13-19% had cognitive impairments in memory, attention, and executive function and 38% had neurological deficits.[197-198] In another study that followed poisoned patients for 30 years after a mass casualty mining accident, investigators found cognitive dysfunction in 69% of survivors. In the subgroup of 129 who had brain MRI, 83% had structural neuroimaging abnormalities.[199] From the Taiwan National Insurance database, patients with CO poisoning appear to have a higher risk for developing dementia, Parkinson's disease, diabetes mellitus, and cardiovascular disease.[200-203] Those treated with HBO_2 had reduced short-term and long-term mortality.[204] From the University of Pittsburg, a retrospective analysis of 1099 CO-poisoned patients showed a reduction of inpatient and one-year mortality with HBO_2.[65]

Some case reports and series report benefit with HBO_2 administration weeks, months, or even years after poisoning,[205-212] but this has not been studied in randomized, controlled trials. In this circumstance, HBO_2 is used to treat brain injury from CO poisoning, which is likely analogous to other types of brain injury.[213-214]

Evidence-Based Review

More than 16,000 CO-poisoned patients were treated in North American hyperbaric chambers from 1992–2002.[171] However, researchers estimate more than 50,000 CO-poisoned patients are evaluated in emergency departments annually in the United States.[215] Among patients treated with HBO_2, both mortality and neurocognitive morbidity are improved beyond that expected with ambient pressure supplemental oxygen therapy.[10-12,31,60-62,77,79,216-218]

There are six published randomized clinical trials in acute CO poisoning with conflicting results[10,79,161-162,219,220] In the study by Raphael et al., no statistically significant benefit was observed when HBO_2 was compared with normobaric oxygen therapy.[161] However, the lack of benefit with HBO_2 may be attributed to nearly half of the study group being treated more than six hours after exposure and use of HBO_2 at only 2 ATA (202.65 kPa).[221] Conclusions from this study are further compromised by the lack of neuropsychological outcome measures and because only mildly poisoned patients were used in the comparative trial (no patients had loss of consciousness).

In follow-up to this clinical trial, the study group conducted a similar study that enrolled 385 CO-poisoned patients over 11 years.[220] Patients without loss of consciousness were randomized to six hours of normobaric oxygen or four hours of normobaric oxygen plus one HBO_2 session (Trial A). Patients with loss of consciousness were randomized to four hours of normobaric oxygen plus one HBO_2 session versus four hours normobaric oxygen plus two HBO_2 sessions (Trial B). Patients receiving HBO_2 were compressed to 2 ATA (202.65 kPa) at 100% oxygen over 30 minutes, remained at 2 ATA (202.65 kPa) for 60 minutes, then decompressed over 30 minutes to atmospheric pressure. All HBO_2 patients received 10 mg intramuscular diazepam prior to compression. In patients without loss of consciousness, recovery rates were similar between groups (58% vs. 61%). In patients with loss of consciousness, recovery was lower in those receiving two HBO_2 sessions compared to one HBO_2 session (47% vs. 68%).

These trials have been criticized for under-dosing HBO_2.[221-222] In mechanistic terms, the lower 2 ATA (202.65 kPa) treatment pressure may not have promoted recovery of mitochondrial metabolism.[84] A partial pressure of oxygen greater than 2 ATA (202.65 kPa) is necessary to achieve maximum inhibition of adhesion molecules in human polymorphonuclear leukocytes.[223] The latter mechanism is an important HBO_2 related beneficial property modulating CO-mediated oxidative injury (Table 3).[86]

The studies by Ducasse et al. and Thom et al. were both prospective, randomized clinical trials involving treatment at 2.5–2.8 ATA (253.32–283.71 kPa) within six hours of poisoning, and both studies found significantly better outcomes with HBO_2 vs. normobaric pressure oxygen treatment.[79,162] The lack of blinding potentially limits the strength of inferences one can draw from these two studies.

A blinded, randomized clinical trial from Australia demonstrated that HBO_2 therapy did not improve outcome at hospital discharge (approximately three days after poisoning) as compared to three to six days of O_2 via high-flow mask (or endotracheal tube).[219] This trial has several important methodological issues that limit confidence in the conclusions including:

1. One-month cognitive outcomes were not reported. Rather, only cognitive outcomes after a few days after poisoning were reported.

2. Poor one-month follow-up. Only 46% of enrolled patient returned for one-month evaluation.

3. Patients in the control group were treated unconventionally (all were admitted to the hospital and received three to six days of high concentrations of supplemental normobaric O_2).

4. Cluster randomization was employed which might have biased the results.

5. No intention-to-treat analysis was performed, although with a low follow-up rate the results probably would be similar.

6. The neuropsychological testing instrument could not discern depression from cognitive dysfunction.[163] Over half the patients had attempted suicide, raising a major question about the true incidence of neurological sequelae in this trial.

A double-blind randomized clinical trial[10] meeting all elements of the CONSORT statement for reporting clinical trials[166,224] demonstrated a significant reduction in six-week neuropsychological sequelae rates in patients treated with HBO_2 (25% vs. 46%; $p=0.007$). In this study, patients randomized to HBO_2 received three sessions—an initial session of 150 minutes, with 60 minutes at 3 ATA (303.98 kPa), followed by two sessions of 120 minutes at 2 ATA (202.65 kPa) in a 24-hour period. Pre-chamber cerebellar dysfunction was strongly associated with cognitive sequelae, but even after correction for pre-chamber cerebellar dysfunction and stratification variables (age, loss of consciousness, time to chamber) HBO_2 remained the more effective therapy. The favorable influence of HBO_2 was maintained through 12-month follow-up.

Based on the American Heart Association (AHA) recommendation classification system,[225] HBO_2 is recommended for patients with acute CO poisoning (Class I – Strong). This recommendation is made based upon Level B-R evidence, supported by one high-quality randomized trial, two moderate quality randomized trials, a supportive meta-analysis,[226] and significant animal research.

Some advocate treating CO-poisoned patients who have continued symptoms with HBO_2 daily, until a clinical plateau is achieved (personal communication), analogous to HBO_2 recommendations in patients with decompression illness.[227] Case series may support this recommendation.[205-212]

Utilization Review

Determination of the optimal pressure and number of hyperbaric oxygen treatments will require additional study, as will the time following poisoning after which therapy is no longer effective. Based on favorable evidence from randomized trials, dosing between 2.5 and 3 ATA (253.32–303.98 kPa) is recommended.[10,79,162,221] While the majority of hyperbaric centers treat with a single HBO_2 session, the best evidence for reduced cognitive sequelae after CO poisoning is for three HBO_2 treatments within 24 hours,[10] and some practitioners follow this recommendation.[171] Preliminary results from a blinded, randomized trial of one vs. three HBO_2 sessions revealed that three sessions did not confer advantage over one session in preventing neuropsychological sequelae. Enrollment in this study was limited to non-intubated, English-speaking patients with accidental CO poisoning at a single institution.

Currently, there is no clear consensus among hyperbaric practitioners as to the length of delay from poisoning beyond which there is little chance for benefit from HBO_2.[171,228] One animal study found the optimal time to HBO_2 treatment was five hours from CO exposure.[155] In the randomized trial by Weaver et al., more than 60% of enrolled patients were treated with HBO_2 in less than six hours following poisoning, the remainder within six to 24 hours. Therefore, this trial was not powered to determine the role of HBO_2 after six hours.[10] Whether HBO_2 confers clinical improvement or a reduced rate of neurocognitive sequelae if administered beyond six hours from poisoning is unknown; however, because brain injury can follow CO poisoning, it is reasonable to treat CO-poisoned patients as soon as possible, up to 24 hours after poisoning. Most hyperbaric oxygen practitioners do not offer HBO_2 when the interval from CO poisoning to HBO_2 is more than 24 hours,[171] though some have reported successful outcomes with this practice.[205,207,209,212,229] A CO treatment strategy is offered in Figure 1.

The Divers Alert Network can provide a referral to a hyperbaric chamber capable of caring for CO-poisoned patients (1-919-684-9111). A list of accredited hyperbaric facilities can be found on the UHMS website (www.uhms.org).

Cost Impact

The cost of HBO_2 as a primary therapy in CO poisoning is modest; however, prevention of morbidity from neurologic and cognitive sequelae represents a substantial cost savings to the health care system and society.

CO Poisoning Complicated by Cyanide Poisoning

Rationale

Individuals with CO poisoning from fires may also have been exposed to cyanide,[230] from the burning of synthetic hydrocarbon products. In combination these two agents may exhibit synergistic toxicity.[231-233] Severe cyanide poisoning is rapidly fatal; symptoms of mild or moderate cyanide exposure can be similar to that of CO poisoning and include headache, nausea, confusion, altered mental status, and cardiac problems.[230,234] While CO poisoning can be rapidly diagnosed by COHb via co-oximetry, currently laboratory testing for cyanide cannot be performed quickly enough to confirm diagnosis before initiating treatment.[230] Carbon monoxide poisoning complicated by cyanide should be considered in patients presenting from fires who manifest altered mental status and those patients with soot in the mouth or mucous membranes.[235]

Once in the body, cyanide binds to the enzyme cytochrome c oxidase and blocks production of adenosine triphosphate (ATP). The result is cellular hypoxia and metabolic acidosis.[236] Patients with cyanide poisoning often require life support measures such as assisted ventilation, supplemental oxygen, and blood pressure support.[230,235]

After supportive care has been established, a cyanide antidote can be administered. A number of antidotes exist but vary in their regional availability.[237] If available, hydroxocobalamin with or without sodium thiosulfate is considered the antidote of choice[230,237-239] as these agents appear to be effective and have a lower risk of serious side effects than other pharmacotherapies.[240] Amyl nitrite and sodium nitrite induce methemoglobinemia to bind cyanide to methemoglobin, facilitating the binding of cyanide, forming cyanomethemoglobin. However, methemoglobinemia potentially impairs the oxygen-carrying capacity of hemoglobin and those treatments are now considered contraindicated in the setting of concomitant CO poisoning.[235-241] Caregivers should be aware that administration of hydroxocobalamin before COHb measurement may yield unreliable co-oximetry results.[242-244]

Clinical reports involving the use of HBO_2 in pure cyanide poisoning are infrequent; however, some reports suggest a benefit.[245-247] There are no controlled clinical trials examining HBO_2 for pure cyanide poisoning or CO poisoning complicated by cyanide. A clinical trial evaluating hydroxocobalamin also treated patients with HBO_2 and no adverse interactions were reported.[248]

Theoretically, HBO_2 may be of benefit in cyanide poisoning as it is known to preserve ATP production.[67] However, the interplay of CO, cyanide, and nitric oxide regarding cytochrome c oxidase is complicated[249] and the role of HBO_2 is not known. Early animal work examining HBO_2 for pure cyanide poisoning found that animals receiving HBO_2 immediately after potassium cyanide injection had improved survival.[250-251] Hyperbaric oxygen also restored brain electrical activity in mice [250] and protected mitochondrial function in rabbits.[252] However, in another murine experiment, HBO_2 was not better than atmospheric oxygen in enhancing the effect of the cyanide antidotes sodium nitrite and sodium thiosulfate.[253]

More recent animal work has shown that in rats with elevated interstitial brain lactate and glucose concentration after cyanide poisoning, HBO_2 and hydroxocobalamin comparably reduced these markers.[254] In this experiment, HBO_2 conferred the added benefits of increased cerebral tissue oxygen partial pressure and reduced respiratory distress and cyanosis.[254] Hydroxocobalamin is predominantly active in the extracellular space[255] and in a rat model HBO_2 increased the concentration of cyanide in circulating blood when administered both immediately and five hours after cyanide exposure.[256] The mechanism of action for this process is not fully understood[256] and this effect has not been reliably observed in humans with cyanide poisoning,[257] perhaps due to variability in patient management and presentation.

Evidence-Based Review of HBO_2 for Cyanide Poisoning

See the section on carbon monoxide poisoning above. At this time, the evidence does not support HBO_2 for pure cyanide poisoning but HBO_2 is indicated for acute CO poisoning including mixed poisoning. Clinically, HBO_2 has been widely applied for CO poisoning complicated by cyanide.[235,248,258]

Utilization Review of HBO_2 for Cyanide Poisoning

The treatment protocol is the same as for CO poisoning.

Cost Impact of HBO₂ for Cyanide Poisoning

Since most patients with CO poisoning complicated by cyanide poisoning will receive a few treatments, the cost of HBO$_2$ for this condition is justifiable. In this serious condition, a reduction in mortality and possibly morbidity reduces health care cost.

Smoke Inhalation

Based on anecdotal clinical reports and controlled animal trials,[259-262] HBO$_2$ is of possible benefit for the pulmonary injury related to smoke inhalation. However, there is currently insufficient evidence to support HBO$_2$ for smoke inhalation unless the patient has concomitant CO poisoning. Smoke inhalation patients are often critically ill, and only hyperbaric medicine centers with critical care expertise can treat them.[263]

Acknowledgments

I thank Claude Piantadosi MD of Duke University for his review of Table 3, and Kayla Deru of Intermountain Healthcare for writing assistance.

Figure 1. Flowchart for Carbon Monoxide Poisoning Treatment
Details of management are described in the text.

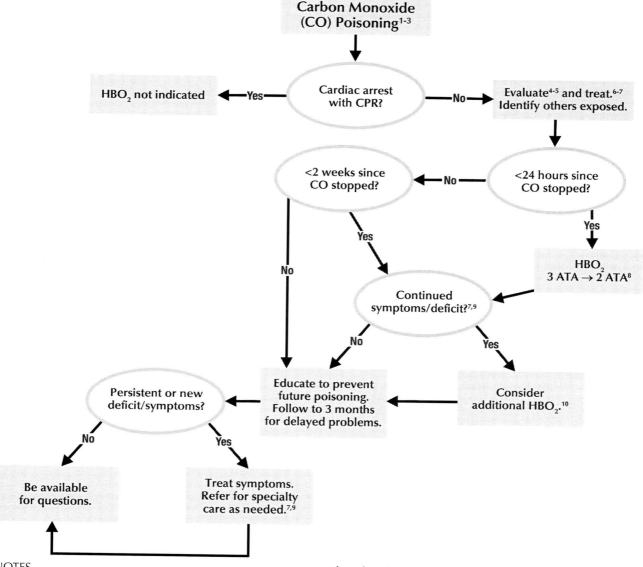

NOTES

[1] CO Poisoning = CO Exposure + Symptoms.

[2] May be acute or chronic (>24 hours exposure, typically intermittent).

[3] COHb and SpCO may be elevated or normal due to time from poisoning and oxygen administration

[4] Neurological evaluation: rapid alternating movements, finger-to-nose, heel/shin; if able to stand, tandem gait, Sharpened Romberg test.

[5] Laboratory evaluation: COHb, pregnancy test, Troponin I, electrocardiogram. As indicated, CBC, lactate, CMP, CK, drug screen, liver function tests, chest radiograph, echocardiogram. Do not delay HBO$_2$.

[6] Non-rebreather facemask oxygen, high flow nasal cannula oxygen (heated, humidified oxygen at up to 60 liters per minute), or 100% oxygen by endotracheal tube if indicated.

If smoke inhalation, consider cyanide antidote, rapid intubation, and treatment of thermal injuries.

[7] For shortness of breath, palpitations, chest pain, or fatigue, refer for cardiac evaluation.

[8] This protocol has been shown to reduce sequelae (Weaver LK, et al. N Engl J Med. 2002;347:1057 -67): 3.0 ATA for 60 minutes with two 5-minute air-breathing periods, then 2.0 ATA for 60 minutes with one 5-minute air-breathing period. Other treatment schedules at 2.5-3.0 ATA may be similarly effective.

[9] For cognitive, affective, somatic, or neurological complaints, refer for neurological, neuropsychological, or psychological evaluation as indicated.

[10] Some advocate daily HBO$_2$ to a clinical plateau.

References

1. Benzon HT, Claybon L, Brunner EA. Elevated carbon monoxide levels from exposure to methylene chloride. JAMA. 1978 Jun 2;239(22):2341.

2. Rioux JP, Myers RA. Hyperbaric oxygen for methylene chloride poisoning: report on two cases. Ann Emerg Med. 1989 Jun;18(6):691-695.

3. Huff JS, Kardon E. Carbon monoxide toxicity in a man working outdoors with a gasoline-powered hydraulic machine. N Engl J Med. 1989 Jun 8;320(23):1564.

4. DiMaio VJ, Dana SE. Deaths caused by carbon monoxide poisoning in an open environment (outdoors). J Forensic Sci. 1987 Nov;32(6):1794-1795.

5. Jumbelic MI. Open air carbon monoxide poisoning. J Forensic Sci. 1998 Jan;43(1):228-230.

6. Easley RB. Open air carbon monoxide poisoning in a child swimming behind a boat. South Med J. 2000 Apr;93(4):430-432.

7. Hampson NB, Holm JR, Courtney TG. Garage carbon monoxide levels from sources commonly used in intentional poisoning. Undersea Hyperb Med. 2017 Jan-Feb;44(1):11-15.

8. Winder C. Carbon monoxide-induced death and toxicity from charcoal briquettes. Med J Aust. 2012 Sep 17;197(6):349-350.

9. Hampson NB, Dunn SL, UHMS CDC CO Poisoning Surveillance Group. Symptoms of carbon monoxide poisoning do not correlate with the initial carboxyhemoglobin level. Undersea Hyperb Med. 2012 Mar-Apr;39(2):657-665.

10. Weaver LK, Hopkins RO, Chan KJ, et al. Hyperbaric oxygen for acute carbon monoxide poisoning. N Engl J Med. 2002 Oct 3;347(14):1057-1067.

11. Weaver LK. Clinical practice. Carbon monoxide poisoning. N Engl J Med. 2009 Mar 19;360(12):1217-1225.

12. Hampson NB, Piantadosi CA, Thom SR, Weaver LK. Practice recommendations in the diagnosis, management, and prevention of carbon monoxide poisoning. Am J Respir Crit Care Med. 2012 Dec 1;186(11):1095-1101.

13. Rose JJ, Wang L, Xu Q, et al. Carbon Monoxide Poisoning: Pathogenesis, Management, and Future Directions of Therapy. Am J Respir Crit Care Med. 2017 Mar 1;195(5):596-606.

14. Penney D, Benignus V, Kephalopoulos S, Kotzias D, Kleinman M, Verrier A. Carbon monoxide. WHO guidelines for indoor air quality: selected pollutants. Bonn, Germany: WHO Regional Office for Europe; 2010. Pp. 55-102.

15. EPA. Air quality criteria for carbon monoxide. Research Triangle Park, NC: U.S. Environmental Protection Agency; 2000.

16. McGrath JJ. The interacting effects of altitude and carbon monoxide. In: Penney DG, editor. Carbon monoxide toxicity. Boca Raton, FL: CRC Press LLC; 2000. Pp. 135-156.

17. Reh CM, Deitchman SD. Health Hazard Evaluation HETA 88-320-2176. U.S. National Institute for Occupational Safety and Health; 1992.

18. NIOSH. Criteria for a recommended standard occupational exposure to carbon monoxide. Cincinnati, OH: National Institute for Occupational Safety and Health; 1972.

19. 29 CFR 1910.1000.

20. NIOSH. 1988 OSHA PEL project documentation. Carbon monoxide. 1988 [updated September 28, 2011]. Available from: http://www.cdc.gov/niosh/pel88/630-08.html.

21. ACGIH. Threshold limit values for chemical substances and physical agents and biological exposure indices. Cincinnati, OH: American Conference of Governmental Industrial Hygienists; 2005.

22. National Research Council. Carbon monoxide. Emergency and continuous exposure guidance levels for selected submarine contaminants. Washington, D.C.: The National Academies Press; 2007. Pp. 67-702.

23. Yoon SS, Macdonald SC, Parrish RG. Deaths from unintentional carbon monoxide poisoning and potential for prevention with carbon monoxide detectors. JAMA. 1998 Mar 4;279(9):685-687.

24. Hampson NB, Courtney TG, Holm JR. Should the placement of carbon monoxide (CO) detectors be influenced by CO's weight relative to air? J Emerg Med. 2012 Apr;42(4):478-482.

25. Hampson NB, Courtney TG, Holm JR. Diffusion of carbon monoxide through gypsum wallboard. JAMA. 2013 Aug 21;310(7):745-746.

26. Underwriters Laboratories. UL 2034. Standard for safety. Single and multiple station carbon monoxide alarms. 4 ed. Northbrook, IL: Underwriters Laboratories, Inc.; 2017 March 31.

27. Penney DG. Essential reference tables, graphs, and other data. In: Penney DG, editor. Carbon Monoxide Poisoning. Boca Raton, FL: CRC Press; 2008. Pp. 753-764.

28. Kirkpatrick JN. Occult carbon monoxide poisoning. West J Med. 1987 Jan;146(1):52-56.

29. Penney DG. Chronic carbon monoxide poisoning: a case series. In: Penney DG, editor. Carbon monoxide poisoning. Boca Raton, FL: CRC Press; 2008. Pp. 551-567.

30. Penney DG. Chronic carbon monoxide poisoning. In: Penney DG, editor. Carbon monoxide toxicity. Boca Raton, FL: CRC Press; 2000. Pp. 393-418.

31. Weaver LK, Valentine KJ, Hopkins RO. Carbon monoxide poisoning: risk factors for cognitive sequelae and the role of hyperbaric oxygen. Am J Respir Crit Care Med. 2007 Sep 1;176(5):491-497.

32. Peterson JE, Stewart RD. Absorption and elimination of carbon monoxide by inactive young men. Arch Environ Health. 1970 Aug;21(2):165-171.

33. Weaver LK, Howe S, Hopkins R, Chan KJ. Carboxyhemoglobin half-life in carbon monoxide-poisoned patients treated with 100% oxygen at atmospheric pressure. Chest. 2000 Mar;117(3):801-808.

34. Pace N, Strajman E, Walker EL. Acceleration of carbon monoxide elimination in man by high pressure oxygen. Science. 1950 Jun 16;111(2894):652-654.

35. Radford EP, Drizd TA. Blood carbon monoxide levels in persons 3-74 years of age: United States, 1976-80. Adv Data. 1982 Mar 17(76):1-24.

36. Touger M, Gallagher EJ, Tyrell J. Relationship between venous and arterial carboxyhemoglobin levels in patients with suspected carbon monoxide poisoning. Ann Emerg Med. 1995 Apr;25(4):481-483.

37. Hampson NB. Pulse oximetry in severe carbon monoxide poisoning. Chest. 1998 Oct;114(4):1036-1041.

38. Suner S, Partridge R, Sucov A, et al. Non-invasive pulse CO-oximetry screening in the emergency department identifies occult carbon monoxide toxicity. J Emerg Med. 2008 May;34(4):441-450.

39. Chee KJ, Nilson D, Partridge R, et al. Finding needles in a haystack: a case series of carbon monoxide poisoning detected using new technology in the emergency department. Clin Toxicol (Phila). 2008 Jun;46(5):461-469.

40. Weaver LK, Churchill SK, Deru K, Cooney D. False positive rate of carbon monoxide saturation by pulse oximetry of emergency department patients. Respir Care. 2013 Feb;58(2):232-240.

41. Roughton F, Darling R. The effect of carbon monoxide on oxyhemoglobin dissociation curve. Am J Physiol. 1944;141:17-31.

42. Thom SR, Ohnishi ST, Fisher D, Xu YA, Ischiropoulos H. Pulmonary vascular stress from carbon monoxide. Toxicol Appl Pharmacol. 1999 Jan 1;154(1):12-19.

43. Piantadosi CA, Zhang J, Demchenko IT. Production of hydroxyl radical in the hippocampus after CO hypoxia or hypoxic hypoxia in the rat. Free Radic Biol Med. 1997;22(4):725-732.

44. Zhang J, Piantadosi CA. Mitochondrial oxidative stress after carbon monoxide hypoxia in the rat brain. J Clin Invest. 1992 Oct;90(4):1193-1199.

45. Ishimaru H, Katoh A, Suzuki H, Fukuta T, Kameyama T, Nabeshima T. Effects of N-methyl-D-aspartate receptor antagonists on carbon monoxide-induced brain damage in mice. J Pharmacol Exp Ther. 1992 Apr;261(1):349-352.

46. Thom SR. Carbon monoxide-mediated brain lipid peroxidation in the rat. J Appl Physiol. 1990 Mar;68(3):997-1003.

47. Thom SR. Leukocytes in carbon monoxide-mediated brain oxidative injury. Toxicol Appl Pharmacol. 1993 Dec;123(2):234-247.

48. Ischiropoulos H, Beers MF, Ohnishi ST, Fisher D, Garner SE, Thom SR. Nitric oxide production and perivascular nitration in brain after carbon monoxide poisoning in the rat. J Clin Invest. 1996 May 15;97(10):2260-2267.

49. Piantadosi CA, Zhang J, Levin ED, Folz RJ, Schmechel DE. Apoptosis and delayed neuronal damage after carbon monoxide poisoning in the rat. Exp Neurol. 1997 Sep;147(1):103-114.

50. Meilin S, Rogatsky GG, Thom SR, Zarchin N, Guggenheimer-Furman E, Mayevsky A. Effects of carbon monoxide on the brain may be mediated by nitric oxide. J Appl Physiol. 1996 Sep;81(3):1078-1083.

51. Thom SR, Bhopale VM, Han ST, Clark JM, Hardy KR. Intravascular neutrophil activation due to carbon monoxide poisoning. Am J Respir Crit Care Med. 2006 Dec 1;174(11):1239-1248.

52. Thom SR, Bhopale VM, Fisher D, Zhang J, Gimotty P. Delayed neuropathology after carbon monoxide poisoning is immune-mediated. Proc Natl Acad Sci USA. 2004 Sep 14;101(37):13660-13665.

53. Gorman DF, Huang YL, Williams C. Prolonged exposure to one percent carbon monoxide causes a leucoencephalopathy in un-anaesthetised sheep. Toxicology. 2001 Aug 28;165(2-3):97-107.

54. Beppu T, Fujiwara S, Nishimoto H, et al. Fractional anisotropy in the centrum semiovale as a quantitative indicator of cerebral white matter damage in the subacute phase in patients with carbon monoxide poisoning: correlation with the concentration of myelin basic protein in cerebrospinal fluid. J Neurol. 2012 Aug;259(8):1698-1705.

55. Xu J, Yang M, Kosterin P, et al. Carbon monoxide inhalation increases microparticles causing vascular and CNS dysfunction. Toxicol Appl Pharmacol. 2013 Dec 1;273(2):410-417.

56. Thom SR, Bhopale VM, Milovanova TM, et al. Plasma biomarkers in carbon monoxide poisoning. Clin Toxicol (Phila). 2010 Jan;48(1):47-56.

57. Winter PM, Miller JN. Carbon monoxide poisoning. JAMA. 1976 Sep 27;236(13):1502.

58. Choi IS. Delayed neurologic sequelae in carbon monoxide intoxication. Arch Neurol. 1983 Jul;40(7):433-435.

59. Min SK. A brain syndrome associated with delayed neuropsychiatric sequelae following acute carbon monoxide intoxication. Acta Psychiatr Scand. 1986 Jan;73(1):80-86.

60. Smith G, Sharp GR. Treatment of carbon-monoxide poisoning with oxygen under pressure. Lancet. 1960;276(7156):905-906.

61. Goulon M, Barios A, Rapin M, Nouailhat F, Grosbuis S, Labrousse J. Carbon monoxide poisoning and acute anoxia due to breathing coal gas and hydrocarbons. J Hyperb Med. 1986;1(1):23-41.

62. Myers RA, Snyder SK, Emhoff TA. Subacute sequelae of carbon monoxide poisoning. Ann Emerg Med. 1985 Dec;14(12):1163-1167.

63. Mathieu D, Wattel F, Mathieu-Nolf M, et al. Randomized prospective study comparing the effect of HBO versus 12 hours NBO in non comatose CO poisoned patients: results of the interim analysis. Undersea Hyperb Med. 1996;23(Suppl):7.

64. Chambers CA, Hopkins RO, Weaver LK, Key C. Cognitive and affective outcomes of more severe compared to less severe carbon monoxide poisoning. Brain Inj. 2008 May;22(5):387-395.

65. Rose JJ, Nouraie M, Gauthier MC, et al. Clinical Outcomes and Mortality Impact of Hyperbaric Oxygen Therapy in Patients With Carbon Monoxide Poisoning. Crit Care Med. 2018 Jul;46(7):e649-e655.

66. Ginsberg MD, Myers RE. Experimental carbon monoxide encephalopathy in the primate I. Physiologic and metabolic aspects. Arch Neurol. 1974 Mar;30(3):202-208.

67. Brown SD, Piantadosi CA. Recovery of energy metabolism in rat brain after carbon monoxide hypoxia. J Clin Invest. 1992 Feb;89(2):666-672.

68. Okeda R, Funata N, Song SJ, Higashino F, Takano T, Yokoyama K. Comparative study on pathogenesis of selective cerebral lesions in carbon monoxide poisoning and nitrogen hypoxia in cats. Acta Neuropathol. 1982;56(4):265-272.

69. Mayevsky A, Meilin S, Rogatsky GG, Zarchin N, Thom SR. Multiparametric monitoring of the awake brain exposed to carbon monoxide. J Appl Physiol. 1995 Mar;78(3):1188-1196.

70. Hopkins RO, Weaver LK, Larson LV, Howe S. Loss of consciousness (LOC) is not required for neurological sequelae due to CO poisoning. Undersea Hyperb Med. 1995;22(Suppl):14.

71. Thom SR, Fisher D, Xu YA, Garner S, Ischiropoulos H. Role of nitric oxide-derived oxidants in vascular injury from carbon monoxide in the rat. Am J Physiol. 1999 Mar;276(3 Pt 2):H984-992.

72. Thom SR, Garner S, Fisher D, Ischiropoulos H. Vascular nitrosative stress from CO exposure. Undersea Hyperb Med. 1998;25(Suppl):47.

73. Cramlet SH, Erickson HH, Gorman HA. Ventricular function following acute carbon monoxide exposure. J Appl Physiol. 1975 Sep;39(3):482-486.

74. Anderson EW, Andelman RJ, Strauch JM, Fortuin NJ, Knelson JH. Effect of low-level carbon monoxide exposure on onset and duration of angina pectoris. A study in ten patients with ischemic heart disease. Ann Intern Med. 1973 Jul;79(1):46-50.

75. Henry CR, Satran D, Lindgren B, Adkinson C, Nicholson CI, Henry TD. Myocardial injury and long-term mortality following moderate to severe carbon monoxide poisoning. JAMA. 2006 Jan 25;295(4):398-402.

76. Hampson NB, Rudd RA, Hauff NM. Increased long-term mortality among survivors of acute carbon monoxide poisoning. Crit Care Med. 2009 Jun;37(6):1941-1947.

77. Gorman DF, Clayton D, Gilligan JE, Webb RK. A longitudinal study of 100 consecutive admissions for carbon monoxide poisoning to the Royal Adelaide Hospital. Anaesth Intensive Care. 1992 Aug;20(3):311-316.

78. Hardy KR, Thom SR. Pathophysiology and treatment of carbon monoxide poisoning. J Toxicol Clin Toxicol. 1994;32(6):613-629.

79. Thom SR, Taber RL, Mendiguren, II, Clark JM, Hardy KR, Fisher AB. Delayed neuropsychologic sequelae after carbon monoxide poisoning: prevention by treatment with hyperbaric oxygen. Ann Emerg Med. 1995 Apr;25(4):474-480.

80. Jasper BW, Hopkins RO, Duker HV, Weaver LK. Affective outcome following carbon monoxide poisoning: a prospective longitudinal study. Cogn Behav Neurol. 2005 Jun;18(2):127-134.

81. End E, Long CW. Oxygen under pressure in carbon monoxide poisoning. J Ind Hyg Toxicol. 1942;20(10):302-306.

82. Britten JS, Myers RA. Effects of hyperbaric treatment on carbon monoxide elimination in humans. Undersea Biomed Res. 1985 Dec;12(4):431-438.

83. Myers RAM, Jones DW, Britten JS. Carbon monoxide half life study. Flagstaff, AZ: Best Publishing Company Co.; 1987. Pp.263-266.

84. Cardellach F, Miro O, Casademont J. Hyperbaric oxygen for acute carbon monoxide poisoning. N Engl J Med. 2003 Feb 6;348(6):557-560; author reply 557-560.

85. Thom SR. Antagonism of carbon monoxide-mediated brain lipid peroxidation by hyperbaric oxygen. Toxicol Appl Pharmacol. 1990 Sep 1;105(2):340-344.

86. Thom SR. Functional inhibition of leukocyte B2 integrins by hyperbaric oxygen in carbon monoxide-mediated brain injury in rats. Toxicol Appl Pharmacol. 1993 Dec;123(2):248-256.

87. Thom SR, Bhopale VM, Fisher D. Hyperbaric oxygen reduces delayed immune-mediated neuropathology in experimental carbon monoxide toxicity. Toxicol Appl Pharmacol. 2006 Jun 1;213(2):152-159.

88. Peirce EC, 2nd, Zacharias A, Alday JM, Jr., Hoffman BA, Jacobson JH, 2nd. Carbon monoxide poisoning: experimental hypothermic and hyperbaric studies. Surgery. 1972 Aug;72(2):229-237.

89. Tomaszewski CA, Rudy J, Wathen J, Brent J, Rosenberg N, Kulig K. Prevention of neurologic sequelae from carbon monoxide by hyperbaric oxygen in rats. Ann Emerg Med. 1992;21(5):631-632.

90. Haldane J. The relation of the action of carbonic oxide to oxygen tension. J Physiol. 1895 Jul 18;18(3):201-217.

91. Douglas CG, Haldane JS, Haldane JB. The laws of combination of haemoglobin with carbon monoxide and oxygen. J Physiol. 1912 Jun 12;44(4):275-304.

92. Haldane JB. Carbon monoxide as a tissue poison. Biochem J. 1927;21(5):1068-1075.

93. Haldane JS. Respiration. New Haven: Yale University Press; 1922.

94. Boerema I, Meyne NG, Brummelkamp WK, et al. Life without blood (a study of the influence of high atmospheric pressure and hypothermia on dilution of the blood). J Cardiovasc Surg. 1960;13:133-146.

95. Weaver LK. Technique of Swan-Ganz catheter monitoring in patients treated in the monoplace hyperbaric chamber. J Hyperb Med. 1992;7(1):1-18.

96. Weaver LK, Howe S, Snow GL, Deru K. Arterial and pulmonary arterial hemodynamics and oxygen delivery/extraction in normal humans exposed to hyperbaric air and oxygen. J Appl Physiol. 2009 Jul;107(1):336-345.

97. Koehler RC, Jones MD, Jr., Traystman RJ. Cerebral circulatory response to carbon monoxide and hypoxic hypoxia in the lamb. Am J Physiol. 1982 Jul;243(1):H27-32.

98. Koehler RC, Traystman RJ, Jones MD, Jr. Regional blood flow and O2 transport during hypoxic and CO hypoxia in neonatal and adult sheep. Am J Physiol. 1985 Jan;248(1 Pt 2):H118-124.

99. Koehler RC, Traystman RJ, Rosenberg AA, Hudak ML, Jones MD, Jr. Role of O2-hemoglobin affinity on cerebrovascular response to carbon monoxide hypoxia. Am J Physiol. 1983 Dec;245(6):H1019-1023.

100. Barker SJ, Tremper KK. The effect of carbon monoxide inhalation on pulse oximetry and transcutaneous PO2. Anesthesiology. 1987 May;66(5):677-679.

101. Fuson RL, Saltzman HA, Boineau JP, Smith WW, Spach MS, Brown IW, Jr. Oxygenation and carbonic acidosis in cyanotic dogs exposed to hyperbaric oxygenation. Surg Gynecol Obstet. 1966 Feb;122(2):340-352.

102. Keilin D, Hartree EF. Cytochrome and cytochrome oxidase. Proc R Soc Lond B. 1939;127(3):167-191.

103. Ball EG, Strittmatter CF, Cooper O. The reaction of cytochrome oxidase with carbon monoxide. J Biol Chem. 1951 Dec;193(2):635-647.

104. Chance B, Erecinska M, Wagner M. Mitochondrial responses to carbon monoxide toxicity. Ann N Y Acad Sci. 1970 Oct 5;174(1):193-204.

105. Caughey WS. Carbon monoxide bonding in hemeproteins. Ann N Y Acad Sci. 1970 Oct 5;174(1):148-153.

106. Wald G, Allen DW. The equilibrium between cytochrome oxidase and carbon monoxide. J Gen Physiol. 1957 Mar 20;40(4):593-608.

107. Penney DG, Zak R, Aschenbrenner V. Carbon monoxide inhalation: effect on heart cytochrome c in the neonatal and adult rat. J Toxicol Environ Health. 1983 Aug-Sep;12(2-3):395-406.

108. Piantadosi CA. Carbon monoxide, oxygen transport, and oxygen metabolism. J Hyperb Med. 1987;2(1):27-44.

109. Coburn RF, Mayers LB. Myoglobin O2 tension determined from measurement of carboxymyoglobin in skeletal muscle. Am J Physiol. 1971 Jan;220(1):66-74.

110. Brown SD, Piantadosi CA. In vivo binding of carbon monoxide to cytochrome c oxidase in rat brain. J Appl Physiol. 1990 Feb;68(2):604-610.

111. Thom SR, Ohnishi ST, Ischiropoulos H. Nitric oxide released by platelets inhibits neutrophil B2 integrin function following acute carbon monoxide poisoning. Toxicol Appl Pharmacol. 1994 Sep;128(1):105-110.

112. Thom SR, Ischiropoulos H. Mechanism of oxidative stress from low levels of carbon monoxide. Res Rep Health Eff Inst. 1997 Dec(80):1-19; discussion 21-17.

113. Thom SR, Xu YA, Ischiropoulos H. Vascular endothelial cells generate peroxynitrite in response to carbon monoxide exposure. Chem Res Toxicol. 1997 Sep;10(9):1023-1031.

114. Brown SD, Piantadosi CA. Reversal of carbon monoxide-cytochrome c oxidase binding by hyperbaric oxygen in vivo. Adv Exp Med Biol. 1989;248:747-754.

115. D'Amico G, Lam F, Hagen T, Moncada S. Inhibition of cellular respiration by endogenously produced carbon monoxide. J Cell Sci. 2006 Jun 1;119(Pt 11):2291-2298.

116. Chance B, Williams GR. The respiratory chain and oxidative phosphorylation. Adv Enzymol Relat Subj Biochem. 1956;17:65-134.
117. Alonso JR, Cardellach F, Lopez S, Casademont J, Miro O. Carbon monoxide specifically inhibits cytochrome c oxidase of human mitochondrial respiratory chain. Pharmacol Toxicol. 2003 Sep;93(3):142-146.
118. Daugherty WP, Levasseur JE, Sun D, Rockswold GL, Bullock MR. Effects of hyperbaric oxygen therapy on cerebral oxygenation and mitochondrial function following moderate lateral fluid-percussion injury in rats. J Neurosurg. 2004 Sep;101(3):499-504.
119. Lou M, Chen Y, Ding M, Eschenfelder CC, Deuschl G. Involvement of the mitochondrial ATP-sensitive potassium channel in the neuroprotective effect of hyperbaric oxygenation after cerebral ischemia. Brain Res Bull. 2006 Mar 31;69(2):109-116.
120. Stewart RJ, Yamaguchi KT, Mason SW, Roshdieh BB, Dabassi NI, Ness NT. Tissue ATP levels in burn injured skin treated with hyperbaric oxygen. Undersea Biomed Res. 1989;16(Suppl):53.
121. Piantadosi CA, Tatro L, Zhang J. Hydroxyl radical production in the brain after CO hypoxia in rats. Free Radic Biol Med. 1995 Mar;18(3):603-609.
122. Cronje FJ, Carraway MS, Freiberger JJ, Suliman HB, Piantadosi CA. Carbon monoxide actuates O(2)-limited heme degradation in the rat brain. Free Radic Biol Med. 2004 Dec 1;37(11):1802-1812.
123. Rothfuss A, Radermacher P, Speit G. Involvement of heme oxygenase-1 (HO-1) in the adaptive protection of human lymphocytes after hyperbaric oxygen (HBO) treatment. Carcinogenesis. 2001 Dec;22(12):1979-1985.
124. Speit G, Dennog C, Eichhorn U, Rothfuss A, Kaina B. Induction of heme oxygenase-1 and adaptive protection against the induction of DNA damage after hyperbaric oxygen treatment. Carcinogenesis. 2000 Oct;21(10):1795-1799.
125. Gregorevic P, Lynch GS, Williams DA. Hyperbaric oxygen modulates antioxidant enzyme activity in rat skeletal muscles. Eur J Appl Physiol. 2001 Nov;86(1):24-27.
126. Kim CH, Choi H, Chun YS, Kim GT, Park JW, Kim MS. Hyperbaric oxygenation pretreatment induces catalase and reduces infarct size in ischemic rat myocardium. Pflugers Arch. 2001 Jul;442(4):519-525.
127. Ayvaz S, Kanter M, Aksu B, et al. The effects of hyperbaric oxygen application against cholestatic oxidative stress and hepatic damage after bile duct ligation in rats. J Surg Res. 2013 Jul;183(1):146-155.
128. Bosco G, Yang ZJ, Nandi J, Wang J, Chen C, Camporesi EM. Effects of hyperbaric oxygen on glucose, lactate, glycerol and anti-oxidant enzymes in the skeletal muscle of rats during ischaemia and reperfusion. Clin Exp Pharmacol Physiol. 2007 Jan-Feb;34(1-2):70-76.
129. Godman CA, Joshi R, Giardina C, Perdrizet G, Hightower LE. Hyperbaric oxygen treatment induces antioxidant gene expression. Ann N Y Acad Sci. 2010 Jun;1197:178-183.
130. Ozden TA, Uzun H, Bohloli M, et al. The effects of hyperbaric oxygen treatment on oxidant and antioxidants levels during liver regeneration in rats. Tohoku J Exp Med. 2004 Aug;203(4):253-265.
131. Yasar M, Yildiz S, Mas R, et al. The effect of hyperbaric oxygen treatment on oxidative stress in experimental acute necrotizing pancreatitis. Physiol Res. 2003;52(1):111-116.
132. Dennog C, Radermacher P, Barnett YA, Speit G. Antioxidant status in humans after exposure to hyperbaric oxygen. Mutat Res. 1999 Jul 16;428(1-2):83-89.
133. Shyu WC, Lin SZ, Saeki K, et al. Hyperbaric oxygen enhances the expression of prion protein and heat shock protein 70 in a mouse neuroblastoma cell line. Cell Mol Neurobiol. 2004 Apr;24(2):257-268.
134. Wang W, Xue L, Li Y, et al. RNA sequencing analysis reveals new findings of hyperbaric oxygen treatment on rats with acute carbon monoxide poisoning. Undersea Hyperb Med. 2016 Nov-Dec;43(7):759-770.
135. Park EJ, Min YG, Kim GW, Cho JP, Maeng WJ, Choi SC. Pathophysiology of brain injuries in acute carbon monoxide poisoning: a novel hypothesis. Med Hypotheses. 2014 Aug;83(2):186-189.
136. Juric DM, Finderle Z, Suput D, Brvar M. The effectiveness of oxygen therapy in carbon monoxide poisoning is pressure- and time-dependent: a study on cultured astrocytes. Toxicol Lett. 2015 Feb 17;233(1):16-23.
137. Juric DM, Suput D, Brvar M. Hyperbaric oxygen preserves neurotrophic activity of carbon monoxide-exposed astrocytes. Toxicol Lett. 2016 Jun 24;253:1-6.
138. Zhang Y, Lv Y, Liu YJ, et al. Hyperbaric oxygen therapy in rats attenuates ischemia-reperfusion testicular injury through blockade of oxidative stress, suppression of inflammation, and reduction of nitric oxide formation. Urology. 2013 Aug;82(2):489 e489-489 e415.
139. Miljkovic-Lolic M, Silbergleit R, Fiskum G, Rosenthal RE. Neuroprotective effects of hyperbaric oxygen treatment in experimental focal cerebral ischemia are associated with reduced brain leukocyte myeloperoxidase activity. Brain Res. 2003 May 2;971(1):90-94.
140. Thom SR, Fisher D, Manevich Y. Roles for platelet-activating factor and *NO-derived oxidants causing neutrophil adherence after CO poisoning. Am J Physiol Heart Circ Physiol. 2001 Aug;281(2):H923-930.

141. Thom SR. Dehydrogenase conversion to oxidase and lipid peroxidation in brain after carbon monoxide poisoning. J Appl Physiol. 1992 Oct;73(4):1584-1589.

142. Thom SR. Effects of hyperoxia on neutrophil adhesion. Undersea Hyperb Med. 2004 Spring;31(1):123-131.

143. Zamboni WA, Roth AC, Russell RC, Graham B, Suchy H, Kucan JO. Morphologic analysis of the microcirculation during reperfusion of ischemic skeletal muscle and the effect of hyperbaric oxygen. Plast Reconstr Surg. 1993 May;91(6):1110-1123.

144. Vlodavsky E, Palzur E, Soustiel JF. Hyperbaric oxygen therapy reduces neuroinflammation and expression of matrix metalloproteinase-9 in the rat model of traumatic brain injury. Neuropathol Appl Neurobiol. 2006 Feb;32(1):40-50.

145. Hara S, Mukai T, Kurosaki K, Kuriiwa F, Endo T. Characterization of hydroxyl radical generation in the striatum of free-moving rats due to carbon monoxide poisoning, as determined by in vivo microdialysis. Brain Res. 2004 Aug 6;1016(2):281-284.

146. Hiramatsu M, Yokoyama S, Nabeshima T, Kameyama T. Changes in concentrations of dopamine, serotonin, and their metabolites induced by carbon monoxide (CO) in the rat striatum as determined by in vivo microdialysis. Pharmacol Biochem Behav. 1994 May;48(1):9-15.

147. Newby MB, Roberts RJ, Bhatnagar RK. Carbon monoxide- and hypoxia-induced effects on catecholamines in the mature and developing rat brain. J Pharmacol Exp Ther. 1978 Jul;206(1):61-68.

148. Thom SR, Fisher D, Zhang J, Bhopale VM, Cameron B, Buerk DG. Neuronal nitric oxide synthase and N-methyl-D-aspartate neurons in experimental carbon monoxide poisoning. Toxicol Appl Pharmacol. 2004 Feb 1;194(3):280-295.

149. Chin BY, Jiang G, Wegiel B, et al. Hypoxia-inducible factor 1alpha stabilization by carbon monoxide results in cytoprotective preconditioning. Proc Natl Acad Sci U S A. 2007 Mar 20;104(12):5109-5114.

150. Choi YK, Kim CK, Lee H, et al. Carbon monoxide promotes VEGF expression by increasing HIF-1alpha protein level via two distinct mechanisms, translational activation and stabilization of HIF-1alpha protein. J Biol Chem. 2010 Oct 15;285(42):32116-32125.

151. Calvert JW, Cahill J, Yamaguchi-Okada M, Zhang JH. Oxygen treatment after experimental hypoxia-ischemia in neonatal rats alters the expression of HIF-1alpha and its downstream target genes. J Appl Physiol. 2006 Sep;101(3):853-865.

152. Li Y, Zhou C, Calvert JW, Colohan AR, Zhang JH. Multiple effects of hyperbaric oxygen on the expression of HIF-1 alpha and apoptotic genes in a global ischemia-hypotension rat model. Exp Neurol. 2005 Jan;191(1):198-210.

153. Ostrowski RP, Colohan AR, Zhang JH. Mechanisms of hyperbaric oxygen-induced neuroprotection in a rat model of subarachnoid hemorrhage. J Cereb Blood Flow Metab. 2005 May;25(5):554-571.

154. Tofighi R, Tillmark N, Dare E, Aberg AM, Larsson JE, Ceccatelli S. Hypoxia-independent apoptosis in neural cells exposed to carbon monoxide in vitro. Brain Res. 2006 Jul 7;1098(1):1-8.

155. Brvar M, Luzar B, Finderle Z, Suput D, Bunc M. The time-dependent protective effect of hyperbaric oxygen on neuronal cell apoptosis in carbon monoxide poisoning. Inhal Toxicol. 2010 Oct;22(12):1026-1031.

156. Calvert JW, Zhou C, Nanda A, Zhang JH. Effect of hyperbaric oxygen on apoptosis in neonatal hypoxia-ischemia rat model. J Appl Physiol. 2003 Nov;95(5):2072-2080.

157. Rosenthal RE, Silbergleit R, Hof PR, Haywood Y, Fiskum G. Hyperbaric oxygen reduces neuronal death and improves neurological outcome after canine cardiac arrest. Stroke. 2003 May;34(5):1311-1316.

158. Garland H, Pearce J. Neurological complications of carbon monoxide poisoning. Q J Med. 1967 Oct;36(144):445-455.

159. Thom SR. Hyperbaric-oxygen therapy for acute carbon monoxide poisoning. N Engl J Med. 2002 Oct 3;347(14):1105-1106.

160. Hampson NB, Dunford RG, Kramer CC, Norkool DM. Selection criteria utilized for hyperbaric oxygen treatment of carbon monoxide poisoning. J Emerg Med. 1995 Mar-Apr;13(2):227-231.

161. Raphael JC, Elkharrat D, Jars-Guincestre MC, et al. Trial of normobaric and hyperbaric oxygen for acute carbon monoxide intoxication. Lancet. 1989 Aug 19;2(8660):414-419.

162. Ducasse JL, Celsis P, Marc-Vergnes JP. Non-comatose patients with acute carbon monoxide poisoning: hyperbaric or normobaric oxygenation? Undersea Hyperb Med. 1995 Mar;22(1):9-15.

163. Schiltz KL. Failure to assess motivation, need to consider psychiatric variables, and absence of comprehensive examination: a skeptical review of neuropsychologic assessment in carbon monoxide research. Undersea Hyperb Med. 2000 Spring;27(1):48-50.

164. Amitai Y, Zlotogorski Z, Golan-Katzav V, Wexler A, Gross D. Neuropsychological impairment from acute low-level exposure to carbon monoxide. Arch Neurol. 1998 Jun;55(6):845-848.

165. Hampson NB, Mathieu D, Piantadosi CA, Thom SR, Weaver LK. Carbon monoxide poisoning: interpretation of randomized clinical trials and unresolved treatment issues. Undersea Hyperb Med. 2001 Fall;28(3):157-164.

166. Weaver LK, Hopkins RO, Chan KJ, et al. Carbon Monoxide Research Group, LDS Hospital, Utah in reply to Scheinkestel et al. and Emerson: the role of hyperbaric oxygen in carbon monoxide poisoning. Emerg Med Australas. 2004 Oct-Dec;16(5-6):394-399; discussion 481-392.

167. Jordan BD, Relkin NR, Ravdin LD, Jacobs AR, Bennett A, Gandy S. Apolipoprotein E epsilon4 associated with chronic traumatic brain injury in boxing. JAMA. 1997 Jul 9;278(2):136-140.

168. Li L, Bao Y, He S, et al. The Association Between Apolipoprotein E and Functional Outcome After Traumatic Brain Injury: A Meta-Analysis. Medicine (Baltimore). 2015 Nov;94(46):e2028.

169. Hopkins RO, Weaver LK, Valentine KJ, Mower C, Churchill S, Carlquist J. Apolipoprotein E genotype and response of carbon monoxide poisoning to hyperbaric oxygen treatment. Am J Respir Crit Care Med. 2007 Nov 15;176(10):1001-1006.

170. Tsuang D, Kukull W, Sheppard L, et al. Impact of sample selection on APOE epsilon 4 allele frequency: a comparison of two Alzheimer's disease samples. J Am Geriatr Soc. 1996 Jun;44(6):704-707.

171. Hampson NB, Little CE. Hyperbaric treatment of patients with carbon monoxide poisoning in the United States. Undersea Hyperb Med. 2005 Jan-Feb;32(1):21-26.

172. Weaver LK, Churchill S, Deru K, Handrahan D. A randomized trial of one v. three hyperbaric oxygen sessions for acute carbon monoxide poisoning. Undersea Hyperb Med. 2018;45(5):579.

173. Satran D, Henry CR, Adkinson C, Nicholson CI, Bracha Y, Henry TD. Cardiovascular manifestations of moderate to severe carbon monoxide poisoning. J Am Coll Cardiol. 2005 May 3;45(9):1513-1516.

174. De Reuck J, Decoo D, Lemahieu I, et al. A positron emission tomography study of patients with acute carbon monoxide poisoning treated by hyperbaric oxygen. J Neurol. 1993 Jul;240(7):430-434.

175. Maeda Y, Kawasaki Y, Jibiki I, Yamaguchi N, Matsuda H, Hisada K. Effect of therapy with oxygen under high pressure on regional cerebral blood flow in the interval form of carbon monoxide poisoning: observation from subtraction of technetium-99m HMPAO SPECT brain imaging. Eur Neurol. 1991;31(6):380-383.

176. Murata T, Koshino Y, Nishio M, et al. Serial proton magnetic resonance spectroscopy in a patient with acute carbon monoxide poisoning. Biol Psychiatry. 1995 Apr 15;37(8):541-545.

177. Haberstock D, Hopkins RO, Weaver LK, Churchill S. Prospective longitudinal assessment of symptoms in acute carbon monoxide (CO) poisoning. Undersea Hyperb Med. 1998;25(Suppl):48.

178. Waisman D, Shupak A, Weisz G, Melamed Y. Hyperbaric oxygen therapy in the pediatric patient: the experience of the Israel Naval Medical Institute. Pediatrics. 1998 Nov;102(5):E53.

179. Kim JK, Coe CJ. Clinical study on carbon monoxide intoxication in children. Yonsei Med J. 1987;28(4):266-273.

180. Klees M, Heremans M, Dougan S. Psychological sequelae to carbon monoxide intoxication in the child. Sci Total Environ. 1985 Aug;44(2):165-176.

181. Cunningham SD, Weaver LK, Deru K, Jensen J, Petty L. Prospective neuropsychological assessment of children with carbon monoxide poisoning. Undersea Hyperb Med. 2012;39(5):981-982.

182. Weaver LK, Cunningham SD, Farnsworth K, Layton B, Deru K, Petty L. Prospective vestibular outcomes of children with carbon monoxide poisoning. Undersea Hyperb Med. 2012;39(5):982.

183. Koren G, Sharav T, Pastuszak A, et al. A multicenter, prospective study of fetal outcome following accidental carbon monoxide poisoning in pregnancy. Reprod Toxicol. 1991;5(5):397-403.

184. Penney DG. Effects of carbon monoxide exposure on developing animals and humans. In: Penney DG, editor. Carbon monoxide. Boca Raton, FL: CRC Press, Inc.; 1996. Pp. 109-144.

185. Norman CA, Halton DM. Is carbon monoxide a workplace teratogen? A review and evaluation of the literature. Ann Occup Hyg. 1990 Aug;34(4):335-347.

186. Longo LD. The biological effects of carbon monoxide on the pregnant woman, fetus, and newborn infant. Am J Obstet Gynecol. 1977 Sep 1;129(1):69-103.

187. Van Hoesen KB, Camporesi EM, Moon RE, Hage ML, Piantadosi CA. Should hyperbaric oxygen be used to treat the pregnant patient for acute carbon monoxide poisoning? A case report and literature review. JAMA. 1989 Feb 17;261(7):1039-1043.

188. Elkharrat D, Raphael JC, Korach JM, et al. Acute carbon monoxide intoxication and hyperbaric oxygen in pregnancy. Intensive Care Med. 1991;17(5):289-292.

189. Azarov I, Wang L, Rose JJ, et al. Five-coordinate H64Q neuroglobin as a ligand-trap antidote for carbon monoxide poisoning. Sci Transl Med. 2016 Dec 7;8(368):368ra173.

190. Weaver LK. Engineered proteins: A carbon monoxide antidote. Nature Biomedical Engineering. 2017 02/10/online;1:0030.

191. Kitamoto T, Tsuda M, Kato M, Saito F, Kamijo Y, Kinoshita T. Risk factors for the delayed onset of neuropsychologic sequelae following carbon monoxide poisoning. Acute Med Surg. 2016 Oct;3(4):315-319.

192. Kuroda H, Fujihara K, Kushimoto S, Aoki M. Novel clinical grading of delayed neurologic sequelae after carbon monoxide poisoning and factors associated with outcome. Neurotoxicology. 2015 May;48:35-43.

193. Pepe G, Castelli M, Nazerian P, et al. Delayed neuropsychological sequelae after carbon monoxide poisoning: predictive risk factors in the Emergency Department. A retrospective study. Scand J Trauma Resusc Emerg Med. 2011 Mar 17;19:16.

194. Ruff RM, Iverson GL, Barth JT, et al. Recommendations for diagnosing a mild traumatic brain injury: a National Academy of Neuropsychology education paper. Arch Clin Neuropsychol. 2009 Feb;24(1):3-10.

195. Alvarez VM, Parikh M, Weaver LK, Deru K. Cardiac MRI findings in patients with CO poisoning. Undersea Hyperb Med. 2015;42(5):468-469.

196. Smith JS, Brandon S. Morbidity from acute carbon monoxide poisoning at three-year follow-up. Br Med J. 1973 Feb 10;1(5849):318-321.

197. Hopkins RO, Weaver LK. Cognitive outcomes 6 years after acute carbon monoxide poisoning. Undersea Hyperb Med. 2008;35(4):258.

198. Weaver LK, Hopkins RO, Churchill S, Deru K. Neurological outcomes 6 years after acute carbon monoxide poisoning. Undersea Hyperb Med. 2008;35(4):258-259.

199. Mimura K, Harada M, Sumiyoshi S, et al. [Long-term follow-up study on sequelae of carbon monoxide poisoning; serial investigation 33 years after poisoning]. Seishin Shinkeigaku Zasshi. 1999;101(7):592-618.

200. Huang CC, Ho CH, Chen YC, et al. Increased risk for diabetes mellitus in patients with carbon monoxide poisoning. Oncotarget. 2017 Sep 8;8(38):63680-63690.

201. Wong CS, Lin YC, Hong LY, et al. Increased Long-Term Risk of Dementia in Patients With Carbon Monoxide Poisoning: A Population-Based Study. Medicine (Baltimore). 2016 Jan;95(3):e2549.

202. Wong CS, Lin YC, Sung LC, et al. Increased long-term risk of major adverse cardiovascular events in patients with carbon monoxide poisoning: A population-based study in Taiwan. PLoS One. 2017;12(4):e0176465.

203. Lai CY, Chou MC, Lin CL, Kao CH. Increased risk of Parkinson disease in patients with carbon monoxide intoxication: a population-based cohort study. Medicine (Baltimore). 2015 May;94(19):e869.

204. Huang CC, Ho CH, Chen YC, et al. Hyperbaric Oxygen Therapy Is Associated With Lower Short- and Long-Term Mortality in Patients With Carbon Monoxide Poisoning. Chest. 2017 Nov;152(5):943-953.

205. Keim L, Koneru S, Ramos VFM, et al. Hyperbaric oxygen for late sequelae of carbon monoxide poisoning enhances neurological recovery: case report. Undersea Hyperb Med. 2018 Jan-Feb;45(1):83-87.

206. Chang DC, Lee JT, Lo CP, et al. Hyperbaric oxygen ameliorates delayed neuropsychiatric syndrome of carbon monoxide poisoning. Undersea Hyperb Med. 2010 Jan-Feb;37(1):23-33.

207. Coric V, Oren DA, Wolkenberg FA, Kravitz RE. Carbon monoxide poisoning and treatment with hyperbaric oxygen in the subacute phase. J Neurol Neurosurg Psychiatry. 1998 Aug;65(2):245-247.

208. Myers RA, DeFazio A, Kelly MP. Chronic carbon monoxide exposure: a clinical syndrome detected by neuropsychological tests. J Clin Psychol. 1998 Aug;54(5):555-567.

209. Spagnolo F, Costa M, Impellizzeri M, et al. Delayed hyperbaric oxygen treatment after acute carbon monoxide poisoning. J Neurol. 2011 Aug;258(8):1553-1554.

210. Vila JF, Meli FJ, Serqueira OE, Pisarello J, Lylyk P. Diffusion tensor magnetic resonance imaging: a promising technique to characterize and track delayed encephalopathy after acute carbon monoxide poisoning. Undersea Hyperb Med. 2005 May-Jun;32(3):151-156.

211. Watanuki T, Matsubara T, Higuchi N, et al. [Clinical examination of 3 patients with delayed neuropsychiatric encephalopathy induced by carbon monoxide poisoning, who recovered from severe neurocognitive impairment by repetitive hyperbaric oxygen therapy]. Seishin Shinkeigaku Zasshi. 2014;116(8):659-669.

212. Koita N, Mitsuhashi M, Maki T, et al. Two case reports : improvement of delayed leukoencephalopathy after carbon monoxide poisoning more than one month after onset with hyperbaric oxygen therapy. J Neurol Sci. 2017;381:499.

213. Weaver LK, Wilson SH, Lindblad AS, et al. Hyperbaric oxygen for post-concussive symptoms in United States military service members: a randomized clinical trial. Undersea Hyperb Med. 2018;45(2):129-156.

214. Boussi-Gross R, Golan H, Fishlev G, et al. Hyperbaric oxygen therapy can improve post concussion syndrome years after mild traumatic brain injury - randomized prospective trial. PLoS One. 2013;8(11):e79995.

215. Hampson NB, Weaver LK. Carbon monoxide poisoning: a new incidence for an old disease. Undersea Hyperb Med. 2007 May-Jun;34(3):163-168.

216. Mathieu D, Nolf M, Durocher A, et al. Acute carbon monoxide poisoning. Risk of late sequelae and treatment by hyperbaric oxygen. J Toxicol Clin Toxicol. 1985;23(4-6):315-324.

217. Norkool DM, Kirkpatrick JN. Treatment of acute carbon monoxide poisoning with hyperbaric oxygen: a review of 115 cases. Ann Emerg Med. 1985 Dec;14(12):1168-1171.

218. Huang ET, Hardy KR, Stubbs JM, Lowe RA, Thom SR. Ventriculo-peritoneal shunt performance under hyperbaric conditions. Undersea Hyperb Med. 2000 Winter;27(4):191-194.

219. Scheinkestel CD, Bailey M, Myles PS, et al. Hyperbaric or normobaric oxygen for acute carbon monoxide poisoning: a randomised controlled clinical trial. Med J Aust. 1999 Mar 1;170(5):203-210.

220. Annane D, Chadda K, Gajdos P, Jars-Guincestre MC, Chevret S, Raphael JC. Hyperbaric oxygen therapy for acute domestic carbon monoxide poisoning: two randomized controlled trials. Intensive Care Med. 2011 Mar;37(3):486-492.

221. Brown SD, Piantadosi CA. Hyperbaric for carbon monoxide poisoning. Lancet. 1989 Oct 28;2(8670):1032-1033.

222. Birmingham CM, Hoffman RS. Hyperbaric oxygen therapy for acute domestic carbon monoxide poisoning: two randomized controlled trials. Intensive Care Med. 2011 Jul;37(7):1218; author reply 1219.

223. Thom SR, Mendiguren I, Hardy K, et al. Inhibition of human neutrophil beta2-integrin-dependent adherence by hyperbaric O2. Am J Physiol. 1997 Mar;272(3 Pt 1):C770-777.

224. Moher D, Schulz KF, Altman D, Group C. The CONSORT statement: revised recommendations for improving the quality of reports of parallel-group randomized trials. JAMA. 2001 Apr 18;285(15):1987-1991.

225. Halperin JL, Levine GN, Al-Khatib SM, et al. Further Evolution of the ACC/AHA Clinical Practice Guideline Recommendation Classification System: A Report of the American College of Cardiology/American Heart Association Task Force on Clinical Practice Guidelines. J Am Coll Cardiol. 2016 Apr 5;67(13):1572-1574.

226. Lin CH, Su WH, Chen YC, et al. Treatment with normobaric or hyperbaric oxygen and its effect on neuropsychometric dysfunction after carbon monoxide poisoning: A systematic review and meta-analysis of randomized controlled trials. Medicine (Baltimore). 2018 Sep;97(39):e12456.

227. Moon RE. Hyperbaric oxygen treatment for decompression sickness. Undersea Hyperb Med. 2014 Mar-Apr;41(2):151-157.

228. Hampson NB, Dunn SL, Yip FY, Clower JH, Weaver LK. The UHMS/CDC carbon monoxide poisoning surveillance program: three-year data. Undersea Hyperb Med. 2012 Mar-Apr;39(2):667-685.

229. Stoller KP. Hyperbaric oxygen and carbon monoxide poisoning: a critical review. Neurol Res. 2007 Mar;29(2):146-155.

230. Anseeuw K, Delvau N, Burillo-Putze G, et al. Cyanide poisoning by fire smoke inhalation: a European expert consensus. Eur J Emerg Med. 2013 Feb;20(1):2-9.

231. Norris JC, Moore SJ, Hume AS. Synergistic lethality induced by the combination of carbon monoxide and cyanide. Toxicology. 1986 Aug;40(2):121-129.

232. Moore SJ, Ho IK, Hume AS. Severe hypoxia produced by concomitant intoxication with sublethal doses of carbon monoxide and cyanide. Toxicol Appl Pharmacol. 1991 Jul;109(3):412-420.

233. Pitt BR, Radford EP, Gurtner GH, Traystman RJ. Interaction of carbon monoxide and cyanide on cerebral circulation and metabolism. Arch Environ Health. 1979 Sep-Oct;34(5):345-349.

234. Baud FJ. Cyanide: critical issues in diagnosis and treatment. Hum Exp Toxicol. 2007 Mar;26(3):191-201.

235. Lawson-Smith P, Jansen EC, Hyldegaard O. Cyanide intoxication as part of smoke inhalation--a review on diagnosis and treatment from the emergency perspective. Scand J Trauma Resusc Emerg Med. 2011;19:14.

236. Beasley DM, Glass WI. Cyanide poisoning: pathophysiology and treatment recommendations. Occup Med (Lond). 1998 Oct;48(7):427-431.

237. Borron SW, Baud FJ. Antidotes for acute cyanide poisoning. Curr Pharm Biotechnol. 2012 Aug;13(10):1940-1948.

238. Toon MH, Maybauer MO, Greenwood JE, Maybauer DM, Fraser JF. Management of acute smoke inhalation injury. Crit Care Resusc. 2010 Mar;12(1):53-61.

239. Reade MC, Davies SR, Morley PT, Dennett J, Jacobs IC, Australian Resuscitation C. Review article: management of cyanide poisoning. Emerg Med Australas. 2012 Jun;24(3):225-238.

240. Thompson JP, Marrs TC. Hydroxocobalamin in cyanide poisoning. Clin Toxicol (Phila). 2012 Dec;50(10):875-885.

241. Desai SS, M. Cyanide poisoning. In: Basow DS, editor. UpToDate. Waltham, MA: UpToDate; 2013.

242. Lee J, Mukai D, Kreuter K, Mahon S, Tromberg B, Brenner M. Potential interference by hydroxocobalamin on cooximetry hemoglobin measurements during cyanide and smoke inhalation treatments. Ann Emerg Med. 2007 Jun;49(6):802-805.

243. Pamidi PV, DeAbreu M, Kim D, Mansouri S. Hydroxocobalamin and cyanocobalamin interference on co-oximetry based hemoglobin measurements. Clin Chim Acta. 2009 Mar;401(1-2):63-67.

244. Livshits Z, Lugassy DM, Shawn LK, Hoffman RS. Falsely low carboxyhemoglobin level after hydroxocobalamin therapy. N Engl J Med. 2012 Sep 27;367(13):1270-1271.

245. Trapp WG. Massive cyanide poisoning with recovery: a boxing-day story. Can Med Assoc J. 1970 Mar 14;102(5):517.

In earlier papers, Stevens et al.[1,25] already described the lethal effects and cardiovascular effects of purified alpha- and theta-toxins from *C. perfringens*.

The other toxins are ancillary to CPA and PFO, which gives rise to hemoglobinuria, hemolysis, jaundice, anemia, tissue necrosis, renal failure, and serious systemic effects such as cardiotoxicity and brain dysfunction. The other exotoxins are synergistic and enhance the rapid spread of infection by destroying, liquefying, and dissecting healthy tissue. The clostridial organisms surround themselves with toxins. Local host defense mechanisms are abolished when the toxin production is sufficiently high. This results in fulminating tissue destruction and further clostridial growth. Alpha-toxin can be fixed to susceptible skin cells in 20–30 minutes, is detoxified within hours after its elaboration, and causes active immunity with production of a specific antitoxin.[19,28] The infection, however, is so progressive with continuous production of alpha-toxin that the patient dies before any immunity can develop.

Toxin gene expression in *C. perfringens* is regulated by the VirR/VirS-VR-RNA cascade together with two cell-to-cell signaling systems, the agr-system and AI-2 signaling.[29]

An extensive and updated review about the role of clostridial toxins in the pathogenesis of gas gangrene was given by Stevens and Bryant.[30]

Bryant and Stevens[31] recently updated this again. They still do not mention hyperbaric oxygen in the treatment and report mortality between 30% and 100%. They hope that novel prevention, diagnostic, and treatment modalities may be on the horizon.

Awad et al.[32] showed genetic evidence for the essential role of alpha-toxin in gas gangrene.

Eaton et al.[33] have further described the crystal structure in combination with the working mechanisms of alpha-toxin. In conjunction with previous findings, almost the whole working mechanism with the structure of their toxin is now known.

Stevens et al.[34] also showed evidence that CPA and PFO differentially modulate the immune response and induce acute tissue necrosis in clostridial gas gangrene.

Much more has become known in recent years about the action and also the interaction between the various clostridial toxins in the onset and progression of gas gangrene. A very informative review on a cellular and molecular model of the pathogenesis of clostridial myonecrosis is given by Stevens[1] and Titball.[35]

In atraumatic clostridial myonecrosis from C. septicum, its virulence is largely mediated by four exotoxins; alpha, beta, gamma and delta toxins. Not to be confused with CPA, the alpha toxin produced by C. septicum is a lethal and necrotizing pore-forming toxin that inserts into cell membranes causing an influx of Ca^{2+} ions into the cell that eventually results in cell death.[6]

The Role of Hyperbaric Oxygen Treatment for Gas Gangrene

The action of HBO_2 on clostridia (and other anaerobes) is based on the formation of O_2 free radicals in the relative absence of free radical degrading enzymes such as superoxide dismutases, catalases, and peroxidases. Van Unnik[36] showed that an O_2 tension of 250 mmHg is necessary to stop alpha-toxin production. Although it does not kill all clostridia, it is bacteriostatic both *in vivo* and *in vitro*.(35-39) Tissue O_2 measurements made by

Schoemaker,[41] Kivisaari and Niinikoski,[42] and Sheffield[43] have shown that treatment with HBO$_2$ at 3 atmospheres absolute (ATA) (303.98 kPa) is required to achieve tissue partial pressures above 300 mmHg. Free-circulating toxins and/or tissue-bound toxins are not affected by high O$_2$ levels but they are rapidly detoxified by normal host factors.[18,37,44-45] If further toxin elaboration is prevented by the addition of hyperbaric oxygen, a very sick patient can rapidly be made nontoxic.

Diagnosis

The diagnosis of clostridial myonecrosis is based primarily on clinical data, supported by the demonstration of Gram-positive rods from the fluids of the involved tissues as well as a virtual absence of leukocytes. A leukocytosis indicates a mixed infection. Roggentin et al.[46] developed an immunoassay for rapid and specific detection of *C. perfringens*, *C. septicum*, and *C. sordelli* by determining their sialidase activity (neuraminidase) in serum and tissue homogenates. Sialidases produced by these three clostridia were bound to polyclonal antibodies raised against the respective enzymes and immobilized onto microtiter plates. Applied to nine samples from patients, there was a high correlation between the results of the immunoassay and the bacteriological analysis of the infection.[46] Scheven[47] described identification of *C. perfringens* in mixed-infected clinical materials by means of a modified reversed CAMP test.

The onset of gas gangrene may occur between one to six hours after injury or an operation and begins with severe and sudden pain in the infected area before the clinical signs appear. In atraumatic clostridial myonecrosis, no trauma is apparent and in its stead are certain predisposing risks such as colonic and gynecologic malignancy, radiation or chemotherapy and neutropenia.

This seemingly disproportionate pain in a clinically still-normal area must make the clinician highly suspicious for a developing gas gangrene, especially after trauma or an operation. The body temperature is initially normal but then rises very quickly. In the early phases the skin overlying the wound appears shiny and tense and then becomes dusky and progresses to a bronze discoloration. The infection can advance at a rate of six inches per hour. Any delay in recognition or treatment may be fatal. Hemorrhagic bullae or vesicles may also be noted. A thin, sero-sanguinolent exudate with a sickly, sweet odor is present. Swelling and edema of the infected area is pronounced. The muscles appear dark red to black or greenish. They are non-contractile and do not bleed when cut. The tissue gas seen on radiographs appears as featherlike figures between muscle fibers and is an early and highly characteristic sign of clostridial myonecrosis. Crepitus is usually present as well.

Therapy

The acute problem in gas gangrene is not normal tissue or already necrotic tissue, but the rapidly advancing phlegmon in between, which is caused by the continuous production of alpha-toxin in infected but still-viable tissue. It is essential to stop alpha-toxin production as soon as possible and to continue therapy until the advance of the disease process has been clearly arrested. Since van Unnik showed that a tissue PO$_2$ of 250 mmHg is necessary to stop toxin production completely, the only way to achieve this is to start hyperbaric oxygen therapy (HBO$_2$) as soon as possible.[36] A minimum of three to four HBO$_2$ treatments is necessary for this response. Treatment starts on the basis of the clinical picture and the positive-Gram stained smear of the wound fluid (without leukocytes). HBO$_2$ treatment stops alpha-toxin production and inhibits bacterial growth, thus enabling the body to utilize its own host defense mechanisms.[36-40]

Although a three-pronged approach consisting of HBO$_2$, surgery, and antibiotics is essential in treating gas gangrene, initial surgery can be restricted to opening of the wound. An initial fasciotomy may be undertaken but lengthy and extensive procedures in these very ill patients can usually be postponed, depending on how rapidly HBO$_2$ therapy can be initiated. Debridement of necrotic tissue can be performed between HBO$_2$ treatments and should be delayed until clear demarcation between dead and viable tissues can be seen.

Treatment Results

The first clinical results in gas gangrene were remarkable but difficult to reproduce in the animal model.[38-39,48] Despite wide variations in O$_2$ tolerance between small and large laboratory animals and human beings, HBO$_2$ therapy has been used to treat experimental clostridial infections in animals. The greatest reduction in mortality in dogs was achieved by a combination of HBO$_2$, surgery, and antibiotics.[40] In general, studies of several investigators[38-39,48-51] have shown that HBO$_2$ substantially reduced mortality and morbidity in animals following clostridial infections when used in combination with surgery and antibiotics.

Major retrospective clinical studies indicate that the lowest morbidity and mortality are achieved with initial conservative surgery and rapid initiation of HBO$_2$ therapy. Results decline progressively when HBO$_2$ therapy is delayed. Early aggressive surgery and delayed HBO$_2$ treatment led to a significantly higher mortality and morbidity than when HBO$_2$ is administered promptly.[52-54]

Ertmann and Havemann indicate, on the basis of their experience in a series of 136 patients treated over a 20-year period, the necessity for a combined treatment approach. However, they place surgery earlier in the protocol, sometimes after the first hyperbaric session. All patients who were treated without hyperbaric oxygen or only once or twice, died.[55]

The work by Brummelkamp et al.[56-57] updated by Bakker[5,58] totaling 409 cases of clostridial gas gangrene showed a mortality directly related to the clostridial infection of 11.7%. All 48 patients who died did so within 26 hours after the start of HBO$_2$ therapy. HBO$_2$ therapy also greatly reduced the amputation rate: Only 18% required amputation post-hyperbaric therapy vs. 50–55% following primary surgery.[5,52-53]

Hart et al.[59] reported a 17% amputation rate with combined therapeutic management. Reduced mortality rates were also demonstrated by Hart et al.,[59] Hitchcock et al.,[19] Holland et al.,[60] Van Zijl,[61] and Heimbach.[62]

Hitchcock[19] showed a 5.1% mortality rate among 58 patients whose HBO$_2$ therapy began within the first 24 hours; these results reinforce results of earlier clinical trials.

Mortality in the series of Hirn[48] was 28%. He concluded that mortality and morbidity could be reduced if the disease is recognized early and appropriate therapy applied promptly. He recommends adequate and operative debridement, antibiotics, HBO$_2$ and surgical intensive care.

In experimental monomicrobial gas gangrene, the combination therapy of surgery and HBO$_2$ started 45 minutes after the inoculation of bacteria reduced mortality to 13% compared with 38% with surgery alone. The combination therapy appeared to be especially effective in wound healing and in prevention of morbidity compared with surgical debridement alone. The effectiveness of the combination therapy was strongly time-dependent.

In the multimicrobial gas gangrene model, the addition of HBO$_2$ to surgery tended to reduce mortality, but the difference between the groups was not statistically significant. However, the combined therapy with surgery and HBO$_2$ was highly effective in reducing morbidity and mortality and improving wound healing compared with surgical debridement alone.[61]

Early HBO₂ treatment in gas gangrene is lifesaving because less heroic surgery needs to be performed in gravely ill patients and the cessation of alpha-toxin production is rapid. It is also limb and tissue saving because no major amputations or excisions are done prematurely (except opening of wounds). It clarifies the demarcation so that within 24–30 hours there is a clear distinction between dead and still-living tissue. In this way, both the number and the extent of amputations are reduced.

In 1984, Peirce already concluded that the modern treatment of gas gangrene involves the simultaneous use of antibiotics, surgical debridement, and hyperbaric oxygen.[63] He also believed that, even at that time, it would be unethical to carry out a randomized clinical study to compare these three modalities. This opinion was based on the results published until 1984.[58,63]

Subsequent experience continues to support the approach he recommended. With the same therapy these results have been consistent over the years, and the outcome has been further improved with advanced intensive care medicine.

Utilization Review

The recommended treatment profile consists of O₂ at 3 ATA (303.98 kPa) pressure for 90 minutes, three times in the first 24 hours and then twice per day for the next two to five days. The actual decision on termination of treatment depends on the patient's response to HBO₂ therapy.

In Bakker's series[5] there was no mortality after the third hyperbaric session. This is confirmed by Ertmann and Havemann.[55] If the patient remains toxic, the treatment profile needs to be extended. Utilization review is indicated after 10 treatments.

Cost Impact

Hyperbaric oxygen reduces morbidity and prevents or lowers the level of amputation necessitated by limb gas gangrene, thereby justifying the costs.[64] HBO₂ is generally not used longer than five to seven days.

Evidence Grading of the Efficacy of Treatment

The first *Report of the Hyperbaric Oxygen Therapy Committee* (1977) put gas gangrene in Category I, where HBO₂ was considered a primary therapeutic intervention to be included with surgery and antibiotics.

The justification for this was the following: "Since 1956 the efficacy of hyperbaric oxygen in the treatment of clostridial gas gangrene has been amply demonstrated by numerous clinical series. Both mortality and morbidity have been greatly reduced. Reduction of morbidity, salvage of additional major joints in limb gangrene, and the saving of life in severe cases justify the costs. Treatment beyond a few days is seldom if ever required."[65]

In 1960, the randomized clinical trial was an oddity.[66] Not much has changed in the pathophysiology or experimental or clinical results of gas gangrene, except in the way we are establishing the evidence of our results.[67] The microbiological background of gas gangrene is continually better understood, but that did not change our therapeutic approach. Also, the results of our therapy remain remarkably constant through the years.[5]

The concept of evidence-based medicine (EBM) is dynamic rather than static. Clinical expertise and patient choices are incorporated more and more in clinical decision making.[67]

We do not know of any RCT in gas gangrene and HBO_2 therapy because this was judged unethical in 1984[63] considering the published results and, more important, the consistency of the results through the years.

Tibbles and Edelsberg[68] classify gas gangrene as a disease for which the weight of scientific evidence supports hyperbaric oxygen as effective adjunctive therapy. The discovery of beneficial cellular and biochemical effects strengthened the rationale for this, although they recognize the paucity of RCTs. However, this is also true for many other therapies in many indications in clinical medicine from those years (e.g. appendectomy for acute appendicitis).

Mitton and Hailey[69] conclude from retrospective reviews and one level IV study that there is a strong rationale for the use of hyperbaric oxygen treatment because of evidence suggesting significant reductions in both mortality and morbidity.

Heimbach[20] found more than 1,200 cases of gas gangrene treated with hyperbaric oxygen in 117 articles in the literature. After adding the 600 cases from Bakker's series (until 2003) we can safely assume that about 2,000 patients have been treated. The results in Bakker's published series[5] indicate a significant reduction in mortality and morbidity by the use of adjunctive hyperbaric oxygen.

A systematic review by the Cochrane group could not show any beneficial effect of HBO_2 on treating gas gangrene.[70] The European Committee for Hyperbaric Medicine (ECHM) has also evaluated the evidence supporting hyperbaric oxygen in the treatment of gas gangrene. The lack of RCTs place the evidence supporting HBO_2 therapy for gas gangrene in level C (Consensus opinion of experts), but for the 2016 European Consensus Conference, the ECHM used the modified GRADE system for evidence analysis, together with the DELPHI system for consensus evaluation and classified HBO_2 for gas gangrene as a Type 1 recommendation (strongly recommended).[71]

Figure 1. Flowchart for Gas Gangrene
Details of management are described in the text.

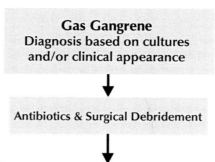

Gas Gangrene
Diagnosis based on cultures and/or clinical appearance

Antibiotics & Surgical Debridement

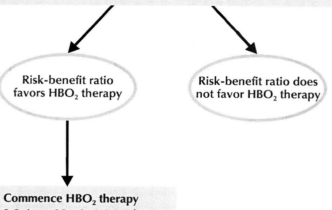

Consider risks versus benefits for HBO_2 therapy

Increased Benefit
- Extensive tissue involvement
- Inadequate response to antibiotics and surgery
- Patient with diminished reserves
- Immune-compromised patients

Increased Risk
- High vasopressor/inotrope/ ventilatory requirement
- Multi-organ failure
- Environment hyperbaric chamber (IC facility prerequisite)

Risk-benefit ratio favors HBO_2 therapy

Risk-benefit ratio does not favor HBO_2 therapy

Commence HBO_2 therapy
Day 1: 2-3 times 90 min 2.8-3.0 bar
Day 2 and 3: 2 times 90 min 2.8-3.0 bar
Day 4-7: 1 session 90 min 2.8-3.0 bar

References

1. Stevens DL. The pathogenesis of clostridial myonecrosis. Int J Med Microbiol. 2000;290(4-5):497-502.
2. Van Hulst RA, Bakker DJ. Selected aerobic and anaerobic soft-tissue infections. In: Whelan HT, Kindwall EP, editors. Hyperbaric Medicine Practice. North Palm Beach, FL: Best Publishing Company; 2017. Pp. 435-63.
3. Lucey BP, Hutchins GM. William H. Welch, MD, and the discovery of Bacillus welchii. Arch Pathol Lab Med. 2004;128(10):1193-5.
4. Weinstein L, Barza MA. Gas gangrene. N Engl J Med. 1973;289(21):1129-31.
5. Bakker D. Clostridial myonecrosis. In: Bakker DJ, Cramer FS, eds. Hyperbaric surgery: perioperative care: Flagstaff, AZ: Best Publishing Co.; 2002:283-316.
6. Srivastava I, Aldape MJ, Bryant AE, Stevens DL. Spontaneous C. septicum gas gangrene: A literature review. Anaerobe. 2017;48:165-71.
7. Abella BS, Kuchinic P, Hiraoka T, Howes DS. Atraumatic Clostridial myonecrosis: case report and literature review. J Emerg Med. 2003;24(4):401-5.
8. Sutton SS, Jumper M, Shah A, Edun B. Clostridium tertium Peritonitis and Concurrent Bacteremia in a Patient With a History of Alcoholic Cirrhosis. J Investig Med High Impact Case Rep. 2017;5(3):2324709617731457.
9. Kelesidis T, Tsiodras S. Clostridium sphenoides bloodstream infection in man. Emerg Infect Dis. 2011;17(1):156-8.
10. Aldape MJ, Bryant AE, Stevens DL. Clostridium sordellii infection: epidemiology, clinical findings, and current perspectives on diagnosis and treatment. Clin Infect Dis. 2006;43(11):1436-46.
11. Williamson ED, Titball RW. A genetically engineered vaccine against the alpha-toxin of Clostridium perfringens protects mice against experimental gas gangrene. Vaccine. 1993;11(12):1253-8.
12. Stevens DL, Titball RW, Jepson M, Bayer CR, Hayes-Schroer SM, Bryant AE. Immunization with the C-Domain of alpha -Toxin prevents lethal infection, localizes tissue injury, and promotes host response to challenge with Clostridium perfringens. J Infect Dis. 2004;190(4):767-73.
13. Shreya D, Uppalapati SR, Kingston JJ, Sripathy MH, Batra HV. Immunization with recombinant bivalent chimera r-Cpae confers protection against alpha toxin and enterotoxin of Clostridium perfringens type A in murine model. Mol Immunol. 2015;65(1):51-7.
14. Titball RW. Clostridium perfringens vaccines. Vaccine. 2009;27 Suppl 4:D44-7.
15. McLeod JW. Variations in the periods of exposure to air and oxygen necessary to kill anaerobic bacteria. Acta Pathol Microbiol Scand. 1930;3(suppl):255.
16. Shimizu T, Ohtani K, Hirakawa H, Ohshima K, Yamashita A, Shiba T, et al. Complete genome sequence of Clostridium perfringens, an anaerobic flesh-eater. Proc Natl Acad Sci U S A. 2002;99(2):996-1001.
17. Benamar S, Cassir N, Caputo A, Cadoret F, La Scola B. Complete Genome Sequence of Clostridium septicum Strain CSUR P1044, Isolated from the Human Gut Microbiota. Genome Announc. 2016;4(5).
18. Maclennan JD. The histotoxic clostridial infections of man. Bacteriol Rev. 1962;26:177-276.
19. Hitchcock CR, Demello FJ, Haglin JJ. Gangrene infection: new approaches to an old disease. The Surgical clinics of North America. 1975;55(6):1403-10.
20. Heimbach RD. Gas gangrene. In: Kindwall EP, ed. Hyperbaric medicine practice: Flagstaff, AZ: Best Publishing Co.; 1994:373-94.
21. Kiu R, Hall LJ. An update on the human and animal enteric pathogen Clostridium perfringens. Emerg Microbes Infect. 2018;7(1):141.
22. Navarro MA, McClane BA, Uzal FA. Mechanisms of Action and Cell Death Associated with Clostridium perfringens Toxins. Toxins (Basel). 2018;10(5).
23. Takehara M, Takagishi T, Seike S, Ohtani K, Kobayashi K, Miyamoto K, et al. Clostridium perfringens alpha-Toxin Impairs Innate Immunity via Inhibition of Neutrophil Differentiation. Sci Rep. 2016;6:28192.
24. Takagishi T, Takehara M, Seike S, Miyamoto K, Kobayashi K, Nagahama M. Clostridium perfringens alpha-toxin impairs erythropoiesis by inhibition of erythroid differentiation. Sci Rep. 2017;7(1):5217.
25. Stevens DL, Troyer BE, Merrick DT, Mitten JE, Olson RD. Lethal effects and cardiovascular effects of purified alpha- and theta-toxins from Clostridium perfringens. J Infect Dis. 1988;157(2):272-9.
26. Stevens DL, Bryant AE, Adams K, Mader JT. Evaluation of therapy with hyperbaric oxygen for experimental infection with Clostridium perfringens. Clin Infect Dis. 1993;17(2):231-7.
27. Verherstraeten S, Goossens E, Valgaeren B, Pardon B, Timbermont L, Haesebrouck F, et al. Perfringolysin O: The Underrated Clostridium perfringens Toxin? Toxins (Basel). 2015;7(5):1702-21.
28. Willis AT. Clostridia of wound infection. London: Butterworth; 1969:490.
29. Ohtani K. Gene regulation by the VirS/VirR system in Clostridium perfringens. Anaerobe. 2016;41:5-9.

30. Stevens DL, Bryant AE. The role of clostridial toxins in the pathogenesis of gas gangrene. Clin Infect Dis. 2002;35(Suppl 1):S93-S100.

31. Bryant AE, Stevens DL. Clostridial myonecrosis: new insights in pathogenesis and management. Curr Infect Dis Rep. 2010;12(5):383-91.

32. Awad MM, Bryant AE, Stevens DL, Rood JI. Virulence studies on chromosomal alpha-toxin and theta-toxin mutants constructed by allelic exchange provide genetic evidence for the essential role of alpha-toxin in Clostridium perfringens-mediated gas gangrene. Mol Microbiol. 1995;15(2):191-202.

33. Eaton JT, Naylor CE, Howells AM, Moss DS, Titball RW, Basak AK. Crystal structure of the C. perfringens alpha-toxin with the active site closed by a flexible loop region. J Mol Biol. 2002;319(2):275-81.

34. Stevens DL, Tweten RK, Awad MM, Rood JI, Bryant AE. Clostridial gas gangrene: evidence that alpha and theta toxins differentially modulate the immune response and induce acute tissue necrosis. J Infect Dis. 1997;176(1):189-95.

35. Titball RW, Naylor CE, Basak AK. The Clostridium perfringens alpha-toxin. Anaerobe. 1999;5(2):51-64.

36. Van U. Inhibition of Toxin Production in Clostridium Perfringens in Vitro by Hyperbaric Oxygen. Antonie Van Leeuwenhoek. 1965;31:181-6.

37. Kaye D. Effect of hyperbaric oxygen on Clostridia in vitro and in vivo. Proc Soc Exp Biol Med. 1967;124(2):360-6.

38. Hill GB, Osterhout S. Experimental effects of hyperbaric oxygen on selected clostridial species. II. In-vitro studies in mice. J Infect Dis. 1972;125(1):26-35.

39. Muhvich KH, Anderson LH, Mehm WJ. Evaluation of antimicrobials combined with hyperbaric oxygen in a mouse model of clostridial myonecrosis. J Trauma. 1994;36(1):7-10.

40. Demello FJ, Hashimoto T, Hitchcock CR, Haglin JJ. The effect of hyperbaric oxygen on the germination and toxin production of Clostridium perfringens spores. In: Wada J, Iwa JT, editors. Proceedings of the fourth international congress on hyperbaric medicine. Baltimore, MD: Williams and Wilkins, 1970. 270.

41. Schoemaker G. Oxygen tension measurements under hyperbaric conditions In: Boerema I, Brummelkamp WH, Meijne NG, eds. Clinical application of hyperbaric oxygen: Amsterdam: Elsevier; 1964:330-5.

42. Kivisaari J, Niinikoski J. Use of silastic tube and capillary sampling technic in the measurement of tissue PO 2 and PCO 2. Am J Surg. 1973;125(5):623-7.

43. Sheffield PJ. Tissue oxygen measurements. In: Davis JC, Hunt TK, eds. Problem wounds: the role of oxygen. New York, NY: Elsevier; 1988:17-51.

44. Nora PF, Mousavipour M, Laufman H. Mechanisms of action of high pressure oxygen in Clostridium perfringens exotoxin toxicity. In: Brown IW, Cox BG, eds. Hyperbaric medicine, publ 1404. Washington, DC: National Academy of Science National Research Council; 1966:544-51.

45. Nora PF, Mousavipour M, Mittelpunkt A, Rosenberg M, Laufman H. Brain as target organ in Clostridium perfringens exotoxin toxicity. Arch Surg. 1966;92(2):243-6.

46. Roggentin T, Kleineidam RG, Majewski DM, Tirpitz D, Roggentin P, Schauer R. An immunoassay for the rapid and specific detection of three sialidase-producing clostridia causing gas gangrene. J Immunol Methods. 1993;157(1-2):125-33.

47. Scheven M. [Detection of Clostridium perfringens in mixed infection patient samples using a modified reverse CAMP test]. Z Gesamte Hyg. 1991;37(2):90-1.

48. Hirn M. Hyperbaric oxygen in the treatment of gas gangrene and perineal necrotizing fasciitis. A clinical and experimental study. Eur J Surg Suppl. 1993(570):1-36.

49. Demello FJ, Haglin JJ, Hitchcock CR. Comparative study of experimental Clostridium perfringens infection in dogs treated with antibiotics, surgery, and hyperbaric oxygen. Surgery. 1973;73(6):936-41.

50. Kelley HG, Jr., Pace WG, 3rd. Treatment of Anaerobic Infections in Mice with Hyperpressure Oxygen. Surg Forum. 1963;14:46-7.

51. Klopper PJ. Hyperbaric oxygen treatment after ligation of the hepatic artery in rabbits. In: Boerema I, Brummelkamp WH, Meijne NG, eds. Clinical application of hyperbaric oxygen. Amsterdam: Elsevier; 1964:31-5.

52. Schott H. [Gas gangrene (principles of treatment, results)]. Hefte Unfallheilkd. 1979;138:179-86.

53. Nier H, Kremer K. [Gas gangrene--still a diagnostic and therapeutic problem]. Zentralbl Chir. 1984;109(6):402-17.

54. Pailler JL, Labeeu F. [Gas gangrene: a military disease?]. Acta Chir Belg. 1986;86(2):63-71.

55. Erttmann M, Havemann D. [Treatment of gas gangrene. Results of a retro- and prospective analysis of a traumatologic patient sample over 20 years]. Unfallchirurg. 1992;95(10):471-6.

56. Brummelkamp WH, Hogendijk J, Boerema I. Treatment of anaerobic infections (clostridial myositis) by drenching the tissues with oxygen under high atmospheric pressure. Surgery. 1961;49:299-302.

57. Brummelkamp WH. Considerations on Hyperbaric Oxygen Therapy at Three Atmospheres Absolute for Clostridial Infections Type Welchii. Ann N Y Acad Sci. 1965;117:688-99.

58. Bakker DJ. The use of hyperbaric oxygen in the treatment of certain infectious diseases, especially gas gangrene and acute dermal gangrene. Wageningen, Holland: Drukkerij Veenman BV; 1984.
59. Hart GB, Lamb RC, Strauss MB. Gas gangrene. J Trauma. 1983;23(11):991-1000.
60. Holland JA, Hill GB, Wolfe WG, Osterhout S, Saltzman HA, Brown IW, Jr. Experimental and clinical experience with hyperbaric oxygen in the treatment of clostridial myonecrosis. Surgery. 1975;77(1):75-85.
61. Van Zijl JJW. Discussion of hyperbaric oxygen. In: Brown IW, Cox BG, eds. Hyperbaric medicine. publ 1404. Washington, DC: National Academy of Science National Research Council; 1966:552-4.
62. Heimbach RD. Gas gangrene. Review and update. HBO Rev. 1980;1:41-6.
63. Peirce EC. Gas gangrene: a critique of therapy. Surg Rounds. 1984;7:17-25.
64. Marroni A, Longobardi P, Cali-Corleo R. Cost-Effectiveness Evaluation of HBO Therapy. In: Mathieu D, ed. Handbook on Hyperbaric Medicine. Dordrecht, The Netherlands: Springer; 2006:674-7.
65. Kindwall EP, chairman. Hyperbaric oxygen therapy committee report. UMS Report Number 5-23-77; 1977:4.
66. Evidence-Based Medicine Working G. Evidence-based medicine. A new approach to teaching the practice of medicine. JAMA. 1992;268(17):2420-5.
67. Haynes RB, Devereaux PJ, Guyatt GH. Clinical expertise in the era of evidence-based medicine and patient choice. Evid Based Med. 2002;7:36-8.
68. Tibbles PM, Edelsberg JS. Hyperbaric-oxygen therapy. N Engl J Med. 1996;334(25):1642-8.
69. Mitton C, Hailey D. Health technology assessment and policy decisions on hyperbaric oxygen treatment. Int J Technol Assess Health Care. 1999;15(4):661-70.
70. Yang Z, Hu J, Qu Y, Sun F, Leng X, Li H, et al. Interventions for treating gas gangrene. Cochrane Database Syst Rev. 2015(12):CD010577.
71. Mathieu D, Marroni A, Kot J. Tenth European Consensus Conference on Hyperbaric Medicine: recommendations for accepted and non-accepted clinical indications and practice of hyperbaric oxygen treatment. Diving Hyperb Med. 2017;47(1):24-32.

CHAPTER 5

The Effect of Hyperbaric Oxygen on Compromised Grafts and Flaps

Shawna Kleban MD, Richard C. Baynosa MD (corresponding author)

Abstract

The use of grafts and flaps serves as an integral tool in the armamentarium of the reconstructive surgeon. Proper planning and surgical judgment are critical in the ultimate success of these procedures.

However, there are situations when grafts and/or flaps can become compromised and require urgent intervention for salvage. These instances can include irradiated or otherwise hypoxic wound beds, excessively large harvested grafts, random flap ischemia, venous or arterial insufficiency, and ischemia-reperfusion injury. Alternatively, compromised grafts and flaps can be inadvertently created secondary to trauma. It is in these types of cases, HBO_2 therapy can serve as a useful adjunct in the salvage of compromised flaps and grafts.

This review outlines the extensive basic science and clinical evidence available in support of the use of HBO_2 therapy for compromised grafts and flaps. The literature demonstrates the benefit of adjunctive HBO_2 therapy for multiple types of grafts and flaps with various etiologies of compromise. HBO_2 therapy can enhance graft and flap survival by several methods including decreasing the hypoxic insult, enhancing fibroblast function and collagen synthesis, stimulating angiogenesis and inhibiting ischemia-reperfusion injury. The expedient initiation of hyperbaric oxygen therapy as soon as flap or graft compromise is identified maximizes tissue viability and ultimately graft/flap salvage.

Rationale

Hyperbaric oxygen therapy is neither necessary nor recommended for the support of normal, uncompromised grafts or flaps. However, in tissue compromised by irradiation or in other cases where there is decreased perfusion or hypoxia, as in traumatic amputations and degloving injuries, HBO_2 therapy has been shown to be extremely useful in flap salvage. Hyperbaric oxygen can help maximize the viability of the compromised tissue, thereby reducing the need for regrafting or repeat flap procedures.

The criteria for selecting the proper patients who are likely to benefit from adjunctive hyperbaric oxygen for graft or flap compromise are crucial for a successful outcome. Identification of the underlying cause for graft or flap compromise can assist in determining the proper clinical management and use of HBO_2 therapy. A number of studies have shown the efficacy of HBO_2 therapy on enhancement of flap and graft survival in a variety of experimental and clinical situations.

Patient Selection Criteria

As hyperbaric oxygen therapy is indicated only in certain pathologic disorders, proper patient selection criteria begins by recognizing the underlying cause of the compromise of the flap or graft. While compromised skin grafts and composite grafts are often classified with compromised flaps, these two entities are distinctly different from a physiologic standpoint. All flaps, by definition, have an inherent blood supply, whereas grafts are avascular tissues that rely on the quality of the recipient bed for survival and revascularization. Because of this dependence, the diagnosis of a compromised graft begins with proper assessment of the recipient wound bed.

The most effective solution for the compromised graft is prevention. By ensuring an appropriate recipient bed for a given graft size, a compromised graft can be avoided altogether. There are instances, however, when a questionable recipient bed goes unrecognized or when the size of the harvested graft exceeds the dimensions that can be sustained by the recipient bed. Traumatic avulsions of the soft tissues of the nose, ear and fingertips or poor surgical planning/judgement can lead to excessively large composite grafts. These compromised grafts become hypoxic and may be salvaged with prompt institution of HBO_2 therapy. Hyperbaric oxygen can help maximize the viability of the compromised graft while revascularization takes place, thereby reducing the need for repeat grafting procedures, which incur further operations and increased donor site morbidity.

There are many etiologies of flap compromise. These can range from random ischemia, to venous congestion/ occlusion, to arterial occlusion, even after meticulous harvest and inset. Similarly, traumatic accidents can result in significant avulsion of soft tissues, extensive degloving injuries, and open fractures with poorly perfused skin flaps.

In addition, free tissue transfers, flaps in which the arterial and venous blood supply is divided and reattached to another location by microsurgical anastomosis, can have their own special problems. Free flaps can be exposed to both ischemia-reperfusion injury and secondary ischemic insults, which can compromise the viability of the flap.

In many cases, surgical re-exploration will identify and treat the etiology of flap compromise. However, in some instances there is no correctable mechanical cause of decreased flap perfusion. Moreover, in skin flaps created by trauma, the compromised perfusion is typically the result of crush injury or the development of exceptionally large random flaps that do not follow the classic 3:1 length-to-width ratio, resulting in poor perfusion to the distal flap. In these cases, HBO_2 therapy can play an important role in flap salvage. The key to successful salvage is the prompt institution of HBO_2 therapy, which can help maximize tissue viability while perfusion is restored. Similar to its use in compromised grafts, HBO_2 therapy can reduce the need for repeat flap procedures, thus decreasing overall patient morbidity.

Evidence-Based Review

An evidence-based review of the benefits of hyperbaric oxygen therapy on compromised grafts and flaps encompasses a variety of experimental trials. These studies can be classified into animal studies and clinical studies. A recent review of these topics was conducted by Francis and Baynosa.[1] Here we provide a more in-depth review of the current literature.

Animal Studies

Although basic science and animal studies are classified by the Oxford Centre for Evidence-Based Medicine (CEBM) as Level 5 evidence and are no longer valued as highly as they once were, they still present one of the best scientific methods to maintain complete control of the experimental study population. The main benefit in examining these studies that evaluate the use of HBO_2 therapy for compromised flaps and grafts is not only the sheer volume of controlled experiments that have been conducted, but also the overwhelmingly positive results of HBO$_2$ therapy in these studies. A recent review of the cellular mechanisms of hyperbaric oxygen pathways and ischemia reperfusion injury provides a summary of the basic science to support the use of HBO$_2$ therapy in compromised flaps and grafts.[2]

The role of HBO$_2$ therapy in compromised wound beds *vs.* non-compromised wound beds has been examined experimentally in animal models. Kivisaari and Niinikoski[3] showed that HBO$_2$ therapy in rats at 2 atmospheres absolute (ATA) had no effect on the healing rate of non-compromised open wounds in which the circulation was left intact. However, when the wound edges were devascularized, HBO$_2$ therapy significantly enhanced wound closure rates over control groups.

Shulman and Krohn,[4] in a study of full-thickness and partial-thickness wounds in rats, found that HBO$_2$ therapy shortened healing time significantly. Further, the combination of repeated skin grafting and HBO$_2$ therapy reduced the healing time of partial-thickness wounds to one-half that of non-treated controls. No attempt at wound sterilization was made in performing these surgeries. Superficial contamination did occur in all animals, but infection was entirely absent in the groups treated with HBO$_2$ therapy.

There are a number of experimental studies describing the effect of HBO$_2$ therapy on compromised skin grafts and composite grafts. Erdmann et al.[5-6] evaluated the effect of HBO$_2$ therapy as treatment for skin allograft rejection. Using a mouse skin allograft rejection model, these authors demonstrated that treatment with HBO$_2$ therapy alone[5] or in combination with cyclosporine[6] lengthened the time to allograft rejection. This effect was more profound in animals receiving more frequent HBO$_2$ therapy compared to animals receiving less frequent HBO$_2$ therapy.

Renner et al.[7] investigated the efficacy of HBO$_2$ therapy in improving survival of reattached auricular composite grafts. A prospective randomized double-blind study used 20 New Zealand albino rabbits randomized to a treatment or control group. Their study was a continuation of a pilot study suggesting some enhancement of composite graft survival with the use of HBO$_2$ therapy in the rabbit ear. Both experiments have demonstrated a slight survival benefit using HBO$_2$ therapy in auricular composite grafts in the rabbit model.

Rubin et al.[8] studied the hyperoxic effects of composite skin grafts in rabbit ears. Experimental animals received 100% oxygen at 2 ATA twice daily for 21 treatments. Grafts in HBO$_2$ therapy-treated animals demonstrated significantly greater survival than grafts in control animals. Similarly, Zhang et al.[9] examined the effects of HBO$_2$ therapy on composite skin grafts in the rabbit ear model. Experimental animals received HBO$_2$ therapy at 2 ATA daily for five days and demonstrated a significantly increased survival area compared to the control group, 82% vs. 26.5%.

Li et al.[10] investigated the efficacy of HBO$_2$ therapy on rabbit auricular composite graft survival of different sizes. Circular chondrocutaneous composite grafts of 0.5, 1.0 or 2.0 cm in diameter were harvested and reattached to the rabbit ears. Experimental animals received HBO$_2$ therapy for 90 minutes at 2.4 ATA for five days. Three weeks post-operatively, the 2.0-cm composite grafts treated with HBO$_2$ therapy had a mean graft survival rate of 85.8% compared to the control group's 51.3% survival rate. There was no benefit seen in the smaller grafts. This suggests a benefit of HBO$_2$ therapy for the larger-size composite grafts, which could be considered compromised and hypoxic.

More recently, Fodor et al.[11] looked at the effect of HBO$_2$ therapy on the survival of relatively large 3.0 x 3.0 cm composite grafts including skin, subcutaneous tissue and fascia harvested from the upper back of rats. The experimental group was treated with HBO$_2$ therapy for 90 minutes at 2.0 ATA daily for two weeks. After this time, they examined both the internal and external surfaces of the grafts comparing the experimental group and controls. After two weeks of HBO$_2$ therapy, the internal surface of the experimental composite grafts had a mean survival rate of 62% comared to 41% survival rate in controls (p=0.001). The external surface of the HBO$_2$ therapy-treated grafts had a 31% survival rate compared to 25% survival in the control group, but this was not statistically significant. Although complete survival was not achieved, this study suggests that composite grafts that are harvested or traumatically created and much larger than the classically recommended size of 1.5cm can benefit from HBO$_2$ therapy, even if only to preserve the deep layer as a suitable bed for subsequent skin grafting.

Several early studies have demonstrated the benefits of HBO$_2$ therapy on experimental skin flaps.[12-14] The effects of HBO$_2$ therapy on compromised and ischemic random flaps have been studied experimentally as well. Niinikoski[15] found a 51% improvement in the length of the viable portion of tubed random skin flaps in rats treated with HBO$_2$ therapy (2.5 ATA for two hours twice daily for two days) compared to air-breathing controls ($p<0.001$). The author suggested that enhanced diffusion of oxygen into the area of disturbed circulation was the mechanism for improvement of tissue viability. Gruber et al.[16] showed that in skin flaps in rats, HBO$_2$ therapy at 3 ATA raised mean tissue oxygen tensions to 600 mmHg, whereas 100% oxygen at sea level did not raise mean flap oxygen tension.

Pellitteri et al.[17] demonstrated the effect of HBO$_2$ therapy in a pig model of random skin flap survival. Random skin flaps in swine were designed to result in a predictable length of necrosis, and the experimental animals were treated with HBO$_2$ therapy for 90 minutes at 2.0 ATA over six days. The compromised flaps in the treatment animals demonstrated a mean survival of 77%, which correlated to 35% less necrosis when compared to the control animals.

Arturson and Khanna,[18] in an experimental study on standard dorsal random skin flaps in rats designed to give a predictable and a constant degree of necrosis, revealed that HBO$_2$ therapy had a significant improvement in flap survival over untreated controls ($p<0.05$). Other flap-enhancing agents were studied, and in some cases these agents enhanced flap survival. However, the best results were found in rats treated with HBO$_2$ therapy.

Similarly, Esclamado et al.[19] studied the effect of HBO$_2$ therapy on survival of dorsal random skin flaps in rats in comparison to another adjunctive therapy – steroids. The random skin flaps were divided into four groups: control, steroids only, HBO$_2$ therapy only, and combined steroids plus HBO$_2$ therapy. HBO$_2$ therapy consisted of 90-minute treatments at 2.4 ATA twice daily for three days. Each of the experimental groups showed a statistically significant ($p<0.01$) improvement in flap survival. However, the best results were seen in the HBO$_2$ therapy-only group, which showed a 36% improvement compared to controls.

Stewart et al.[20] demonstrated the positive effect of HBO$_2$ therapy in combination with free-radical scavengers in increased random skin flap survival. HBO$_2$ therapy for 90 minutes at 2.5 ATA daily was combined with one of several different free-radical scavengers, including superoxide dismutase, catalase and alpha-tocopherol acetate, and each combination demonstrated significantly greater flap survival ($p<0.05$) compared to controls.

Conversely, da Rocha et al.[21-22] suggested that the addition of the antioxidant N-acetylcysteine (NAC), a precursor to the potent free radical scavenger glutathione, to HBO$_2$ therapy does not improve flap survival above HBO$_2$ therapy alone. Dorsal random skin flaps in rats were divided into four groups including sham, NAC,

HBO$_2$ therapy, and HBO$_2$ therapy plus NAC. The group treated with HBO$_2$ therapy demonstrated significantly increased survival and decreased molecular markers for apoptosis in comparison to the NAC group and sham. However, the combination of HBO$_2$ plus NAC did not significantly improve on the results of the NAC group alone and the best results were seen in the HBO$_2$ therapy-only group.

Greenwood and Gilchrist[23] demonstrated the effectiveness of HBO$_2$ therapy in reducing the extent of ischemic necrosis of skin flaps created in previously irradiated rats. Mean flap necrosis was significantly greater ($p<0.05$) in the control (air) group vs. the HBO$_2$ therapy group.

A controlled, randomized study on the effects of HBO$_2$ therapy and irradiation on experimental random skin flaps has been performed by Nemiroff et al.[24-25] One hundred eighty-five rats were randomly assigned to one of 15 conditions, including possible sequencing effects of HBO$_2$ therapy, irradiation and flap creation, as well as controls that included flap creation only, irradiation only and HBO$_2$ therapy groups. Results showed that all groups receiving HBO$_2$ therapy within four hours after flap elevation had significantly greater flap survival time ($p<0.05$), with as much as a 22% increase in flap survival.

Other studies have also looked at the benefit of HBO$_2$ therapy in improving survival of random pattern skin flaps complicated by other factors known to compromise wound healing. Zhang et al.[26] demonstrated the beneficial effects of HBO$_2$ therapy in improving dorsal random skin flap survival in diabetic rats. They demonstrated a significant ($p<0.01$) reduction in necrosis in the diabetic rats treated with HBO$_2$ therapy for 90 minutes at 2.5 ATA daily for seven days compared to the untreated diabetic rats (50.5% vs. 38.5%).

Selcuk et al.[27] revealed a positive effect of HBO$_2$ therapy on random dorsal skin flap survival in nicotine-treated rats. While the HBO$_2$ therapy group demonstrated significantly better survival than the control group (63.80% vs. 56.98%, $p=0.007$) and the control group had significantly better survival than the nicotine group (56.98% vs. 36.15%, $p<0.01$), there was no significant difference between the control group and the nicotine group treated with HBO$_2$ therapy (56.98% vs. 54.08%). Similarly, Demirtas et al.[28] used a degloving injury model in the tails of nicotine-treated rats to demonstrate that HBO$_2$ therapy treatment could not only significantly improve the survival rate compared to controls and nicotine-treated rats, but also mitigate the detrimental effects in the nicotine-treated rats and increase survival rate to the level of controls. These studies suggest that HBO$_2$ therapy may have a role in increasing random flap survival even in cases where there are multiple etiologies of flap compromise.

Further work by Nemiroff and Lungu[29] elucidated some of the mechanisms whereby HBO$_2$ therapy enhanced random flap survival. Skin flaps from animals treated with HBO$_2$ therapy vs. controls were analyzed in a controlled, standardized method. The number and size of blood vessels in the microvasculature was significantly greater for all of the HBO$_2$ therapy groups when compared with that in controls ($p<0.01$). The mean surface area of vessels of the flap-HBO$_2$ therapy groups was also significantly greater than in controls in all but one group ($p<0.01$). The authors concluded that HBO$_2$ therapy significantly enhanced flap survival by increasing and/or maintaining the number and possibly the size of vessels within the microvasculature. The authors stated that, to be most efficacious, HBO$_2$ therapy must be administered as soon as possible after surgery. Other investigators have shown that HBO$_2$ therapy can enhance healing and flap survival by promoting angiogenesis.[30-33]

Manson and associates,[30] in studies using histochemical staining with ATPase to visualize small blood vessels, demonstrated that capillaries grew distally almost three times further in pedicle flaps of pigs that were treated with HBO$_2$ therapy, compared with age-matched controls.

Further studies using pedicle flap models have also demonstrated a beneficial effect of HBO₂ therapy. Champion and colleagues,[34] using a pedicle flap model in rabbits, were able to obtain 100% survival of HBO₂ therapy-treated flaps (2 ATA for two hours twice a day for five days), whereas all control flaps had significant areas of necrosis to greater than 40%. Similarly, work by McFarlane and Wermuth[35] concluded that HBO₂ therapy was of definite value in preventing necrosis in a pedicle flap in the rat and also had limited the extent of necrosis in a free-composite graft. The authors noted that their particular experimental design was a severe test of treatment and attests to the value of HBO₂ therapy in preventing necrosis.[35]

Jurell and Kaijser,[36] using a cranially based pedicle flap in a rat, showed that rats treated with HBO₂ therapy had a significantly greater flap survival compared with controls ($p<0.001$). The surviving area of the HBO₂ therapy group was approximately twice that of the control group. Even when the start of HBO₂ therapy was delayed for 24 hours after surgery, there was still a significantly greater survival area of HBO₂ therapy-treated flaps when compared with controls ($p<0.01$). However, the increase in surviving area was greater if the HBO₂ therapy was begun immediately after surgery. This emphasizes the importance of initiating HBO₂ therapy as soon as a flap problem is suspected.

Tan et al.[37] studied the effect of HBO₂ therapy and air under pressure on skin survival in acute neurovascular island flaps in rats. Skin flaps treated with hyperbaric 8% oxygen (equivalent to room air at standard HBO₂ therapy treatment pressure) exhibited no improvement in skin survival. Skin flaps treated with hyperbaric 100% oxygen exhibited significant increases in survival.

Similarly, Ramon et al.[38] studied the effects of HBO₂ therapy in a rat transverse rectus abdominis myocutaneous (TRAM) pedicle flap skin paddles in comparison to a control group, a normobaric 100% oxygen group and a hyperbaric air-equivalent mixture in prevention of TRAM flap necrosis. The areas of surviving skin paddles in the rat TRAM flaps treated with HBO₂ therapy showed a significant improvement compared to the control group ($p<0.05$).

Prada et al.[39] compared the effect of allopurinol, superoxide-dismutase, and HBO₂ therapy on axial pattern skin flap survival after eight hours of warm ischemia. All treatments demonstrated significantly improved survival compared to controls with mean survival percentages of 63.53%, 83.03%, and 55.98% respectively for allopurinol, superoxide-dismutase and HBO₂ therapy (2.8 ATA for 45 minutes every 12 hours for three days). Unfortunately, this study did not examine the potential benefit of combination therapy using these beneficial interventions.

Nemiroff and colleagues, in controlled animal studies using random and axial flap models, have clearly shown that HBO₂ therapy can significantly enhance flap survival.[24-25,40] Nemiroff's[40] study investigated the effects of pentoxifylline and HBO₂ therapy on skin flaps in rats under four conditions. Pentoxifylline is a rheologic agent, which enhances capillary circulation by increasing the flexibility of red blood cells. Sixty animals were randomly divided into one of four groups:

1. a control group
2. pentoxifylline
3. HBO₂ therapy-treated group
4. a pentoxifylline plus HBO₂ therapy-treated group

Rats that were treated with HBO_2 therapy received a total of 14 two-hour treatments at 2.5 ATA in divided doses. Results indicated that the surviving length of flaps in the pentoxifylline or HBO_2 therapy-treated groups were significantly greater than those in the control group. However, animals treated with both pentoxifylline and HBO_2 therapy had significantly greater flap survival than animals in any of the other three groups ($p<0.001$). This reflected a 30-39% improvement over animals treated with pentoxifylline alone or HBO_2 therapy alone and an 86% improvement over control animals.

Other experiments combining HBO_2 therapy with other therapies in pedicle flap models have had positive results. Collins et al.[41] examined the effects of HBO_2 therapy and nicotinamide on 7 x 7 cm inferior epigastric pedicle skin flaps in rats. The HBO_2 therapy groups had a mean survival of 76.7% in comparison to the control group survival of 45.7%. However, the combination of HBO_2 therapy and nicotinamide demonstrated a mean survival of 90.9% with a statistical significance of $p<0.01$.

Total venous occlusion can occur in axial flaps secondary to mechanical obstruction or in free flaps secondary to venous anastomotic thrombosis. Lozano et al.[42] evaluated the effect of HBO_2 therapy and medicinal leeching on axial skin flaps subjected to total venous occlusion. Hyperbaric oxygen protocol consisted of 90-minute treatments, twice daily, with 100% oxygen at 2.5 ATA for four days. The leeching protocol consisted of placing medicinal leeches on the congested flaps for 15 minutes, once daily, for four days. Laser Doppler measurements of flap perfusion and the percentage of flap necrosis were evaluated. The flaps in the sham group (elevation of the flap only) demonstrated 99% survival, whereas the flaps in the venous occlusion-only group demonstrated 100% necrosis. The flaps in the occlusion with HBO_2 therapy, the occlusion with leeching, and the occlusion with HBO_2 therapy and leeching groups demonstrated 1, 25 and 67% survival, respectively. This study demonstrated that HBO_2 therapy alone was not an effective treatment for skin flaps compromised by total venous occlusion. The combination of leeching and HBO_2 therapy treatment of total venous occlusion resulted in a significant increase in flap survival above that found with leeching alone.

Yucel and Bayramicli[43] investigated the effects of HBO_2 therapy and heparin on the survival of the rat inferior epigastric venous flap. They concluded that the rat inferior epigastric venous flap may be an ischemic flap with capillary circulation through a single venous pedicle, but it needs HBO_2 therapy to survive, especially during the acute period. Heparin treatment, reducing the flap size, and the presence of a vascular wound bed also improve survival rates.

In addition to total venous occlusion, compromised pedicle flaps may suffer from partial venous congestion or arterial insufficiency. Ulkur et al.[44] evaluated the effect of HBO_2 therapy on pedicle flaps with arterial, venous, and combined arteriovenous insufficiency. Their findings indicated that HBO_2 therapy increased the percentage of survival length and mean laser Doppler flows of axial pattern skin flaps with all types of vascular insufficiency. This effect, however, was greatest in the arterial insufficiency flaps.

Ischemia-reperfusion injury can be a significant cause of compromise for free flaps or pedicle flaps subjected to prolonged ischemia either intra-operatively or post-operatively. Several experimental studies have demonstrated the beneficial effects of HBO_2 therapy in ischemia-reperfusion injury of both skin and muscle flaps. Zamboni et al.[45] examined the effect of HBO_2 therapy administered during prolonged total ischemia and immediately following ischemia during reperfusion in axial pattern skin flaps in a rat model. The animals were divided into four experimental groups:

1. Control Group exposed to eight-hour flap ischemia without HBO_2 therapy

2. Group 1 treated with HBO_2 therapy during the ischemia

3. Group 2 treated with HBO_2 therapy following the ischemia

4. Group 3 treated with HBO_2 therapy during ischemia but with the flap contained in a metal-coated Mylar bag to prevent oxygen diffusion

Mean flap necrosis for controls was 28%, while HBO_2 therapy during ischemia or during reperfusion significantly reduced this necrosis to 9 and 12%, respectively ($p<0.01$). The percentage of necrosis for Group 3, with any local effect of HBO_2 therapy on the flap being blocked by the diffusion barrier was 5%. This was also significantly better than the controls ($p<0.0005$) but no different from the other two HBO_2 therapy groups. Thus, HBO_2 therapy significantly increased the percentage of axial pattern skin flap survival when administered during or immediately after total flap ischemia. This beneficial effect was opposite to the author's original hypothesis that HBO_2 therapy would exacerbate reperfusion injury. In a follow-up study, the same skin flap model was used to show that HBO_2 therapy increased microvascular blood flow during reperfusion compared to untreated ischemic controls.[46] Kaelin et al.[47] have shown that HBO_2 therapy during reperfusion significantly improved the survival of free skin flaps following microvascular reattachment and ischemia times of up to 24 hours. The skin flap studies have been corroborated by skeletal muscle experiments, which are more important from a clinical standpoint since muscle is more sensitive to ischemia and reperfusion injury.

An observation of a skeletal muscle microcirculatory flap model of ischemia-reperfusion injury has given some insight into potential mechanisms for this beneficial response.[48] HBO_2 therapy administered during and up to one hour following a four-hour global ischemia significantly reduced neutrophil endothelial adherence in venules and also blocked the progressive arteriolar vasoconstriction associated with reperfusion injury. The fact that neutrophil endothelial adherence is dependent on CD18 function in this model provides indirect evidence that HBO_2 therapy is affecting the neutrophil CD18 adhesion molecule. Subsequent studies by Jones et al.[49] have suggested that effects of HBO_2 therapy on CD18 neutrophil adherence are dependent on nitric oxide via a nitric oxide synthase (NOS) pathway. More recently, Baynosa et al.[50] have used this skeletal muscle model of ischemia-reperfusion injury to demonstrate that the benefits of HBO_2 therapy may result from an early increase in NOS activity followed by a delayed increase in NOS expression. In addition, the effects of HBO_2 therapy on CD18 polarization and neutrophil adhesion were found to be mediated by a vascular endothelial growth factor (VEGF) pathway involving the extracellular matrix plasminogen system.[51]

Hong et al.[52] demonstrated the effects of HBO_2 therapy on ischemia-reperfusion injury of a superior epigastric-based TRAM flap in a rat model. These studies demonstrated a significant increase in survival in the groups treated with HBO_2 therapy ($p<0.05$), which was similar whether the HBO_2 therapy was initiated before or after reperfusion. The results of this study suggest a possible decreased expression of the adhesion molecule ICAM-1 on endothelial cells secondary to HBO_2 therapy.

Focusing on the role of free oxygen radicals on ischemia-reperfusion injury, Tomur et al.[53] studied the effects of HBO_2 therapy and/or an antioxidant vitamin combination (Vitamins E and C) in a rat epigastric island skin-flap model of ischemia-reperfusion injury. These authors demonstrated a significant increase in flap survival in the HBO_2 therapy, the antioxidant, and the combined therapy groups ($p<0.05$) after eight hours of ischemia and subsequent reperfusion.

A beneficial effect of HBO_2 therapy in situations of secondary flap ischemia has been demonstrated in experimental studies. Stevens et al., using a rat axial skin flap model, induced a primary ischemia of six hours followed by two hours of reperfusion and then a secondary ischemia time of 6, 10 and 14 hours.[54] The secondary ischemic time at which 50% of the flaps survived (D50) in both air and 100% oxygen groups was six hours. The secondary ischemic time to D50 in the HBO_2 group was significantly increased to 10 hours.

In a separate experiment, Wong et al. used an axial skeletal muscle flap model in rats. Percent necrosis following a two-hour primary ischemia was significantly reduced from 40% to 24% by HBO_2 therapy.[55] Adding a secondary two-hour ischemia time significantly increased necrosis in controls to 85%, which was significantly reduced in the HBO_2 therapy group to 58%.

These studies have important implications in free tissue transfer complicated by postoperative thrombosis, with the thrombosis effectively acting as a secondary ischemia.

Gampper et al.[56] studied the beneficial effect of HBO_2 therapy on island flaps subjected to secondary venous ischemia in the rat superficial epigastric flap model. They concluded that HBO_2 therapy significantly increased the survival of flaps subjected to a secondary ischemia, even if administered before primary ischemia. The effect of administering HBO_2 therapy prior to secondary venous ischemia was marginal, which may be due to the effect of HBO_2 therapy not lasting longer than five hours.

Figure 1. The Levels of Clinical Evidence Based on Study Design
Adapted from the Oxford Centre for Evidence-Based Medicine (CEBM).

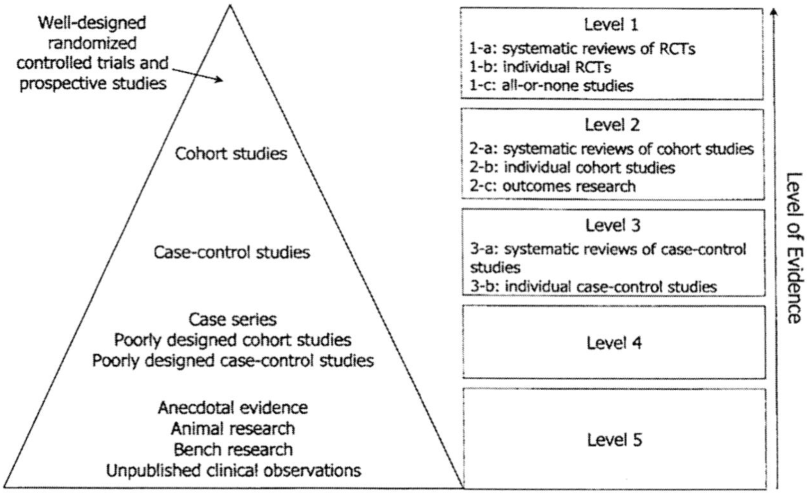

Clinical Studies

With the current emphasis on evidence-based medicine and practice, the clinical data available in the literature plays a tremendous role in the decision to recommend or institute a treatment. The levels of evidence according to the Oxford CEBM are outlined in Figure 1. A review of the literature examining the clinical evidence available for the use of HBO_2 therapy for compromised flaps and/or grafts reveals no less than 23 studies involving over 2,200 different flaps or grafts, with the available clinical evidence ranging from level 1 to level 4 type studies.

Perrins and colleagues were among the first clinicians to examine the benefit of HBO$_2$ therapy in compromised flaps and grafts. Their initial work[57] was first published in 1966 and demonstrated preliminary results of the value of HBO$_2$ therapy in ischemic skin flaps. Later, this group demonstrated the value of adjunctive HBO$_2$ therapy for compromised skin grafts in a controlled clinical study. In this blinded prospective, randomized controlled trial[58] involving 48 patients, half of the patients were treated with HBO$_2$ therapy and half served as controls. Experimental patients received HBO$_2$ therapy at 2.0 ATA for 120 minutes twice a day for three days. Complete graft take was defined as >95% total surface area survival. A significant 29% improvement in graft survival was seen in the HBO$_2$ therapy group compared to controls. Complete survival of grafts occurred in 64% of the treated group as opposed to only 17% of the controls ($p<0.01$). 100% of the HBO$_2$ therapy patients achieved >60% graft survival while only 64% of controls achieved at least 60% graft survival. Although the etiology of graft compromise in this study is not defined, the patients in this study clearly manifest an etiology for graft compromise given the low success rates in the control population. Results of this study suggested that whole-body exposure of HBO$_2$ therapy significantly enhanced compromised graft healing. This remains the single level 1 prospective, randomized controlled trial evaluating the use of HBO$_2$ therapy for compromised grafts to date.

Level 2 evidence is also available in a study published by Roje et al.[59] in 2008. This retrospective, controlled cohort study evaluated the effect of adjunctive HBO$_2$ therapy on short-term complications for war injury reconstructions. They studied a total of 388 patients with 289 patients in the control group and 99 patients in the HBO$_2$ therapy group, which received treatments ranging from 2.2–2.8 ATA with the frequency and number of sessions based on the clinical scenario. Outcome measures for this study included skin graft lyses and flap necrosis as well as soft tissue infection and osteomyelitis. The study revealed a significantly higher incidence of skin graft lyses in the control group (52%) compared to the HBO$_2$ therapy group (23%) ($p<0.001$). Similarly, flap necrosis was also significantly higher in the control group (51%) compared to the HBO$_2$ therapy group (15%) ($p<0.001$).

In order to determine if the beneficial effects seen in this study were related to injury severity, the authors scrutinized their data and further stratified the patients into four subgroups based on severity with group I patients having the most severe and complex injuries and group IV patients having the least severe injuries. Compromising factors for injuries in group IV included ischemia, compartment syndrome, complex soft tissue injury or open fracture while group I injuries were further complicated by blood vessel injury, nerve injury, crush syndrome, and guillotine amputation of an extremity. Group II and III injuries were further characterized by initial soft tissue infection with group II injuries having a neurovascular injury present while group III injuries did not. This further substratification of the patients based on injury severity continued to demonstrate a statistically significant beneficial effect of HBO$_2$ therapy across each of the injury groups, which held true in the preservation and salvage of both compromised grafts and flaps.

Other favorable case series have been reported in the literature involving both compromised flaps and grafts. Gonnering et al.[60] used adjunctive HBO$_2$ therapy (2.0 ATA for 120 minutes twice a day for five days) in six patients undergoing periorbital reconstruction. This study demonstrated complete survival of two ischemic random flaps and four composite grafts ranging in size from 1.7–2.2cm. Similarly, Bowersox et al.[61] demonstrated a benefit to adjunctive HBO$_2$ therapy in their series of 105 patients with compromised grafts or ischemic skin flaps where 90% of patients had risk factors considered to be poor prognostic indicators of flap/graft survival. Adjunctive HBO$_2$ therapy was performed at 2.0 ATA for 90 minutes twice a day for five to seven days followed by 120 minutes daily once sustained clinical improvement was noted. Patients received an average of 16 + 4 treatments overall. Eighty-nine percent of compromised flaps and 91% of threatened skin grafts were salvaged using this protocol. Failed flaps and grafts were associated with two or more risk factors for poor wound healing. In addition, compromised flap failure was associated with a delay in the initiation of HBO$_2$ therapy of over 2 weeks (19.8 days post-op for failed flaps vs. 4.6 days post-op for salvaged flaps, $p<0.01$).

Several other case series [62-65] have suggested a benefit of HBO$_2$ therapy for compromised grafts. These studies involved both skin grafts as well as composite grafts used in a wide variety of reconstructive scenarios including nasal reconstructions, chronic non-healing leg ulcers and periorbital reconstruction. Likewise, there have been several case series[66-68] that have demonstrated the benefit of HBO$_2$ therapy in the treatment and salvage of compromised flaps. Ueda et al.[66] studied 26 compromised flaps (23 axial and three random flaps) treated with HBO$_2$ therapy and noted an average improvement of 92.1%. Mathieu et al.[67] examined the use of HBO$_2$ therapy in 15 pedicle flaps where seven flaps survived while eight flaps failed. They noted a positive correlation between transcutaneous PO$_2$ (TCOM) readings and defined a value of 50 mmHg at pressure as the critical cutoff for success when deciding whether to treat with HBO$_2$ therapy for compromised flaps. Waterhouse et al.[68] studied the value of HBO$_2$ therapy in 14 free flaps and two replantations compromised by prolonged ischemia, a secondary ischemia, or radiation history. This study demonstrated that the benefit of HBO$_2$ therapy was related to the time to initiation of treatment with 89% of patients (eight of nine) treated within 24 hours having complete salvage, with partial necrosis (< 25%) occurring in one patient. Of those treated between one to three days post-op, 25% (one of four) were salvaged with the remaining three undergoing partial necrosis. All three patients treated after three days post-op resulted in complete loss. Necrosis of a free tissue transfer is a significant loss because the defect, which the free flap was used to close, is recreated along with the donor site morbidity. This study also underscored the rationale of initiating HBO$_2$ therapy as soon as signs of flap compromise appear, particularly in free flaps and replantations where the time to restoration of perfusion is even more critical, as the cutoff for salvage was much shorter in this study compared to the Bowersox et al. study evaluating skin flaps.

A more recent case series by Larson et al.[69] retrospectively reviewed 15 patients being treated with HBO$_2$ therapy for failing or threatened post-reconstructive flaps. Eleven of the fifteen (73.3%) flaps survived with four healing completely, and seven with substantial improvement. Average area of improvement was 68.3% of flap area. The authors noted that successful outcomes were associated with patient compliance with the treatment regimen and high pretreatment transcutaneous oxygen levels. Another case series from 2015 noted a 75.7% success rate when treating compromised free flaps with HBO$_2$ therapy for a median of 30 days.[70]

There have been several favorable case reports[71-74] on the use of HBO$_2$ therapy in compromised composite grafts consisting of skin, subcutaneous tissue, and cartilage for nasal reconstruction after traumatic injuries. In addition, there have been reported cases[75-76] of successful salvage of compromised flaps following trauma including a compromised facial flap avulsion from a severe dog bite and a complete scalp degloving injury both treated with adjunctive HBO$_2$ therapy. Several case reports have demonstrated the successful salvage of compromised mastectomy skin flaps.[77-79] Most recently, a 2016 case report by Copeland-Halperin et al.[79] described a patient with a history of breast irradiation who suffered mastectomy skin flap ischemia after nipple-sparing mastectomies and immediate reconstruction with tissue expanders. The patient received 15 treatments of HBO$_2$ therapy which resulted in complete mastectomy flap salvage and completion of her reconstruction.

Zhou et al.[80] performed the largest review of randomized controlled studies on the use of HBO$_2$ therapy in flaps and grafts to date. Twenty years of data from China were reviewed including 957 HBO$_2$ therapy patients with 583 control patients from a total of 23 clinical trials. A survival rate of 62.5-100% was reported for HBO$_2$ therapy patients compared to a 35.0-86.5% rate reported in controls. There was heterogeneity in treatment time and regimen, and most studies had small sample sizes.

Summary

It can be noted that a variety of types of grafts and flaps have been investigated in animal and human studies. Baynosa and Zamboni provide a critical review of HBO_2 therapy and its applications to different types of compromised flaps and grafts in a recent book chapter.[81] Friedman et al.[82] has also presented an evidence-based appraisal of the use of HBO_2 therapy on compromised flaps and grafts. Results of the preponderance of work in the literature clearly show the efficacy of HBO_2 therapy with respect to enhancement of skin graft and flap survival. Of importance is that different types of flaps have been analyzed in these studies, including free skin grafts, pedicle flaps, random flaps, irradiated wounds and flaps, composite grafts, as well as free flaps. Although each flap problem is unique, a key factor to flap necrosis is tissue hypoxia. The results indicate that viability of flaps can be enhanced by HBO_2 therapy through a reduction of the hypoxic insult. Other mechanisms of action whereby HBO_2 therapy enhances flap survival include the enhancement of fibroblasts and collagen synthesis, creation of neovascularity,[40,83] the possibility of closing off arteriovenous shunts,[84-85] and the favorable effects on the microcirculation.[48]

A summary of the available clinical evidence is provided in Figure 2. The prospective randomized controlled trial evaluating 48 patients with compromised grafts by Perrins et al.[58] provides the best level I evidence. Level II evidence is provided by Roje et al.[59] in a retrospective, controlled cohort evaluating 388 patients with compromised grafts and flaps used in the reconstruction of traumatic extremity war injuries. A second level II study by Zhou et al.[80] reviewed 23 randomized controlled and controlled trials on HBO_2 therapy in grafts and flaps, encompassing a total of 957 HBO_2 therapy patients and 583 controls. A total of 1928 patients provide level II evidence to support the use of HBO_2 therapy for compromised grafts and flaps. Level IV evidence is represented by 11 case series[60-70] encompassing 109 skin grafts, 53 composite grafts, and 139 flaps as well as nine case studies[71-79] involving four composite grafts and five flaps. Given this available data, the use of HBO_2 therapy for the salvage of compromised grafts and flaps should be considered as a class 1B intervention according to the American Heart Association (AHA) Evidence Based Guidelines as it is both useful and effective based on evidence from a single, randomized trial and non-randomized studies with the potential benefit far outweighing the risks.

Figure 2. Summary of the Available Clinical Evidence Evaluating HBO_2 Therapy for Compromised Grafts and Flaps

SUMMARY OF THE EVIDENCE	
Level I Evidence	One Study – 48 patients (Compromised grafts)
Level II Evidence	Two Studies – 1928 patients (Compromised grafts and flaps)
Level IV Evidence	Eleven Case Series – 109 skin grafts, 53 composite grafts, 139 flaps
	Nine Case Studies – 4 composite grafts, 5 flaps

Clinical Management

The hyperbaric oxygen treatments are given at a pressure of 2.0-2.5 ATA and range from 90 to 120 minutes (depending on the type of HBO_2 therapy facility available, patient status, etc.). Mechanical causes of flap compromise that can be treated surgically should be addressed prior to initiation of HBO_2 therapy. Currently, there is no consensus as to the optimal HBO_2 therapy treatment regimen for compromised flaps and grafts. Weber et al.[86] *used the rat random flap model to compare the efficacy of daily to twice daily (BID) HBO_2 therapy.* Results of this study suggest no additional benefit when performing BID HBO_2 therapy. Should the compromised graft of flap fail, daily HBO_2 therapy treatments may be continued to prepare the compromised wound bed for a salvage graft or flap reconstruction.

To be maximally effective, HBO_2 therapy should be started as soon as signs of flap or graft compromise appear. Flap viability can be assessed by clinical judgment as well as by a variety of non-invasive and invasive techniques, including transcutaneous oximetry and laser Doppler studies. The diagnosis of graft/flap compromise and evaluation of the subsequent response to HBO_2 therapy treatment should be a multidisciplinary effort between the hyperbaric physician and plastic surgeon. Objective measures should be used to assess and monitor the compromised flap or graft whenever possible.

Utilization Review

Utilization review is required after 20 treatments when preparing a recipient site (such as a radiated tissue bed) for a flap or graft, although the indication for HBO_2 therapy may be better classified by the underlying cause of wound healing compromise (i.e., soft tissue radionecrosis, osteoradionecrosis, chronic osteomyelitis, diabetic foot ulcer) unless treatments are continued immediately following compromised graft or flap failure. Utilization review should also be employed following 20 treatments after a flap or graft has been placed into its recipient site.

Cost Impact

Failed flaps are extremely expensive and result in significant morbidity and distress for both the patient and the surgeon. Adjunctive HBO_2 therapy can reduce these financial, physical, and mental costs by salvaging skin grafts, pedicle flaps, random flaps, composite grafts, as well as free flaps and thus eliminating or minimizing the need for secondary surgeries and alternate donor sites.

Acknowledgment

William A. Zamboni MD, FACS contributed to the earlier editions of this review.

Figure 3. Flowchart for Compromised Grafts and Flaps
Details of management are described in the text.

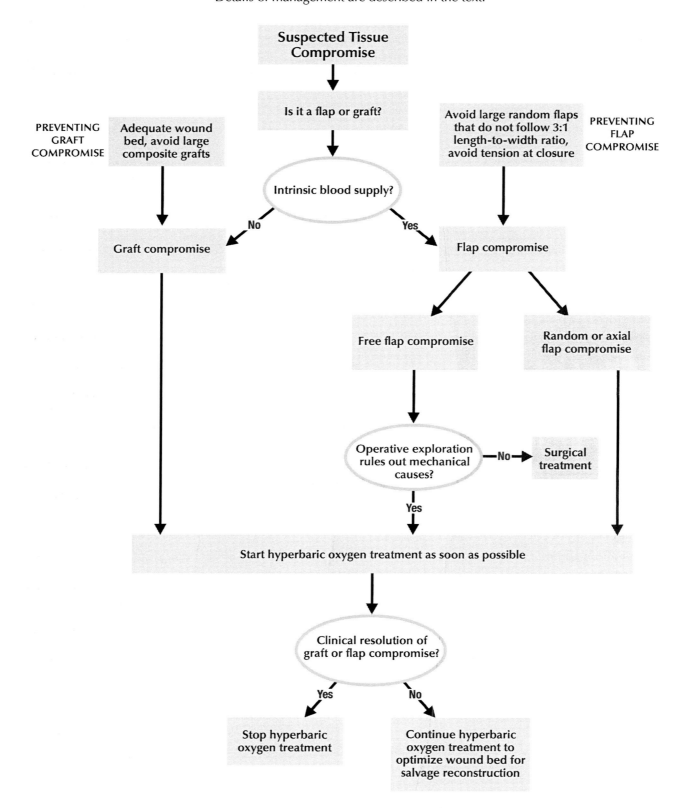

References

1. Francis A, Baynosa RC. Hyperbaric Oxygen Therapy for the Compromised Graft or Flap. Adv Wound Care (New Rochelle). 2017 Jan 1;6(1):23-32.
2. Francis A, Baynosa RC. Ischaemia-reperfusion injury and hyperbaric oxygen pathways: a review of cellular mechanisms. Diving Hyperb Med. 2017 Jun;47(2):110-117.
3. Kivisaari J, Niinikoski J. Effects of hyperbaric oxygen and prolonged hypoxia on the healing of open wounds. Acta Chir Scand. 1975;141:14-19.
4. Shulman AG, Krohn HL. Influence of hyperbaric oxygen and multiple skin allografts on the healing of skin wounds. Surgery. 1967;62:1051-1058.
5. Erdmann D, Roth AC, Hussmann J, et al. Skin allograft rejection and hyperbaric oxygen treatment in immunohistocompatible mice. Undersea Hyperbaric Med. 1995;22: 395-399.
6. Erdmann D, Roth AC, Hussman J, et al. Hyperbaric oxygen and cyclosporine as a combined treatment regimen to prevent skin allograft rejection in immunohistocompatible mice. Ann Plast Surg. 1996;36:304-308.
7. Renner G, McClane SD, Early E, et al. Enhancement of auricular composite graft survival with hyperbaric oxygen therapy. Arch Facial Plast Surg. 2002;4:102-104.
8. Rubin JS, Marzella L, Myers RA, et al. Effects of hyperbaric oxygen on the take of composite skin grafts in rabbit ears. J Hyperbaric Med. 1988;3:79-88.
9. Zhang F, Cheng C, Gerlach T, et al. Effect of hyperbaric oxygen on survival of the composite ear graft in rats. Ann Plast Surg. 1998;41:530-534.
10. Li EN, Menon NG, Rodriguez ED, et al. The effect of hyperbaric oxygen therapy on composite graft survival. Ann Plast Surg. 2004; 53:141-145.
11. Fodor L, Ramon Y, Meilik B, et al. Effect of hyperbaric oxygen on survival of composite grafts in rats. Scand J Plast Reconstr Surg Hand Surg. 2006;40:257-260.
12. Kernahan KA, Zingg W, Kay CW. The effect of hyperbaric oxygen on the survival of experimental skin flaps. Plast Reconstr Surg. 1965;36:19-25.
13. McFarlane RM, DeYoung G, Henry RA. Prevention of necrosis in experimental pedicle flaps with hyperbaric oxygen. Surg Forum. 1965;6:481-482.
14. Wald HI, Georgiade NG, Angelillo J, et al. Effect of intensive hyperbaric oxygen therapy on the survival of experimental skin flaps in rats. Surg Forum. 1968;19:497-499.
15. Niinikoski J. Viability of ischemic skin in hyperbaric oxygen. Acta Chir Scand. 1970: 136: 567-568.
16. Gruber RP, Heitkamp DH, Lawrence JB. Skin permeability to oxygen and hyperbaric oxygen. Arch Surg. 1970;101:69-70.
17. Pellitteri PK, Kennedy TL, Youn BA. The influence of intensive hyperbaric oxygen therapy on skin flap survival in a swine model. Arch Otolaryngol Head Neck Surg. 1992;118:1050-1054.
18. Arturson GG, Khanna NN. The effects of hyperbaric oxygen, dimethyl sulfoxide and complamin on survival of experimental skin flaps. Scand J Plast Reconstr Surg. 1970;4:8-10.
19. Esclamado RM, Larrabee WF Jr, Zel GE. Efficacy of steroids and hyperbaric oxygen on survival of dorsal skin flaps in rats. Otolaryngol Head Neck Surg. 1990;102:41-44.
20. Stewart RJ, Moore T, Bennett B, et al. Effect of free-radical scavengers and hyperbaric oxygen on random-pattern skin flaps. Arch Surg. 1994;129:982-987.
21. Da Rocha FP, Fagundes DJ, Rivoire HC, et al. Immunohistochemical expression of apoptosis and VEGF expression on random skin flaps in rats treated with hyperbaric oxygen and N-acetylcysteine. Undersea Hyperbaric Med. 2011;38:167-174.
22. Da Rocha FP, Fagundes DJ, Pires JA, et al. Effects of hyperbaric oxygen and N-acetylcysteine in survival of random pattern skin flaps in rats. Indian J Plast Surg. 2012;45:453-458.
23. Greenwood TW, Gilchrist AG. The effect of HBO on wound healing following ionizing radiation. In: Trapp WC, et al., Eds. Proceedings of the fifth international congress on hyperbaric medicine, Vol I. Barnaby, Canada: Simon Fraser University. 1973;253-263.
24. Nemiroff PM, Merwin GE, Brant T, et al. HBO and irradiation on experimental skin flaps in rats. Surg Forum. 1984;35:549-550.
25. Nemiroff PM, Merwin GE, Brant, et al. Effects of hyperbaric oxygen and irradiation on experimental flaps in rats. Otolaryngol Head Neck Surg. 1985;93: 485-491.
26. Zhang T, Gong W, Li Z, et al. Efficacy of hyperbaric oxygen on survival of random pattern skin flap in diabetic rats. Undersea Hyperbaric Med. 2007;335-339.

27. Selcuk CT, Kuvat SV, Bozkurt M, et al. The effect of hyperbaric oxygen therapy on the survival of random pattern skin flaps in nicotine-treated rats. J Plast Reconstr Aesthet Surg. 2012;65:489-493.

28. Demirtas A, Azbo I, Bulut M, et al. Effect of hyperbaric oxygen therapy on healing in an experimental model of degloving injury in tails of nicotine-treated rats. J Hand Surg Eur Vol. Epub ahead of print. 2012 Dec 7.

29. Nemiroff PM, Lungu AL. The influence of hyperbaric oxygen and irradiation on vascularity in skin flaps: a controlled study. Surg Forum. 1987;38:565-567.

30. Manson PN, Im MJ, Myers RA, et al. Improved capillaries by hyperbaric oxygen in skin flaps. Surg Forum. 1980;31:564-566.

31. Hartwig J, Kohnlein HE. The influence of hyperbaric oxygen therapy and Dextran 40 on wound healing. Eur Surg Res. 5(Suppl). 1973:109.

32. Meltzer T, Myers B. The effect of hyperbaric oxygen on the bursting strength and rate of vascularization of skin wounds in rats. Am Surg. 1986;52: 659-662.

33. Marx RE and Ames JR. The use of hyperbaric oxygen therapy in bony reconstruction of the irradiated and tissue deficient patient. J Oral Maxillofac Surg. 1982;40: 412-420.

34. Champion WM, McSherry CK, Goulian D. Effect of hyperbaric oxygen on survival of pedicled skin flaps. J Surg Res. 1967;7:583-586.

35. McFarlane RM, Wermuth RE. The use of hyperbaric oxygen to prevent necrosis in experimental pedicle flaps and composite skin grafts. Plast Reconstr Surg. 1966;37:422-430.

36. Jurell G, Kaijser L. The influence of varying pressure and duration of treatment with hyperbaric oxygen on the survival of skin flaps: an experimental study. Scand J Plast Reconstr Surg. 1973;7:25-28.

37. Tan CM, Im MJ, Myers RA, et al. Effect of hyperbaric oxygen and hyperbaric air on survival of island skin flaps. Plast Reconstr Surg. 1974;73:27-30.

38. Ramon Y, Abramovich A, Shupak A, et al. Effect of hyperbaric oxygen on a rat transverse rectus abdominis myocutaneous flap model. Plast Reconstr Surg. 1998;102;416-422.

39. Prada FS, Arrunategui G, Alves MC, et al. Effect of allopurinol, superoxide-dismutase, and hyperbaric oxygen on flap survival. Microsurg. 2002;22;352-360.

40. Nemiroff PM. Synergistic effects of pentoxifylline and hyperbaric oxygen on skin flaps. Arch Otolaryngol Head Neck Surg. 1988;114:977-981.

41. Collins TM, Caimi R, Lynch PR, et al. The effects of nicotinamide and hyperbaric oxygen on skin flap survival. Scand J Plast Reconstr Surg Hand Surg. 1991;25:5-7.

42. Lozano DD, Stephenson LL, Zamboni WA. Effect of hyperbaric oxygen and medicinal leeching on survival of axial skin flaps subjected to total venous occlusion. Plast Reconstr Surg. 1999;104:1029-1032.

43. Yucel A, Bayramicli. Effects of hyperbaric oxygen treatment and heparin on the survival of unipedicled venous flaps: and experimental study in rats. Ann Plast Surg. 2000;295-303.

44. Ulkur E, Yuksel F, Acikel C, et al. Effect of hyperbaric oxygen on pedicle flaps with compromised circulation. Microsurg. 2002;22:; 16-20.

45. Zamboni WA, Roth AC, Russell RC, et al. The effect of acute hyperbaric oxygen therapy on axial pattern skin flap survival when administered during and after total ischemia. J Reconstr Microsurg. 1989;5:343-347.

46. Zamboni WA, Roth AC, Russell RC, et al. The effect of hyperbaric oxygen on reperfusion of ischemic axial skin flaps: a laser Doppler analysis. Ann Plast Surg. 1992;28:339-341.

47. Kaelin CM, Im MJ, Myers RA, et al. The effects of hyperbaric oxygen on free flaps in rats. Arch Surg. 1990;125:607-609.

48. Zamboni WA, Roth AC, Russell RC, et al. Morphological analysis of the microcirculation during reperfusion of ischemic skeletal muscle and the effect of hyperbaric oxygen. Plast Reconstr Surg. 91. 1993;1110-1123.

49. Jones SR, Carpin KM, Woodward SM, et al. Hyperbaric oxygen inhibits ischemia-reperfusion-induced CD18 neutrophil polarization by a nitric oxide mechanism. Plast Reconstr Surg. 2010:126:403-411.

50. Baynosa RC, Naig AL, Murphy PS, et al. The effect of hyperbaric oxygen on nitric oxide synthase activity and expression in ischemia-reperfusion injury. J Surg Res. Epub ahead of print. 2013 Feb 1.

51. Francis A, Kleban SR, Stephenson LL, et al. Hyperbaric Oxygen Inhibits Reperfusion-Induced Neutrophil Polarization and Adhesion Via Plasmin-Mediated VEGF Release. Plast Reconstr Surg Glob Open. 2017 Sep 25;5(9):e1497.

52. Hong JP, Kwon H, Chung YK, et al. The effect of hyperbaric oxygen on ischemia-reperfusion injury: an experimental study in a rat musculocutaneous flap. Ann Plast Surg. 2003;51:478-487.

53. Tomur A, Etlik O, Gundogan NU. Hyperbaric oxygenation and antioxidant vitamin combination reduces ischemia-reperfusion injury in a rat epigastric island skin-flap model. J Basic Clin Physiol Pharmacol. 2005;16: 275-285.

54. Stevens DM, Weiss DD, Koller WA, et al. Survival of normothermic microvascular flaps after prolonged secondary ischemia: Effects of hyperbaric oxygen. Otolaryngol Head Neck Surg. 115: 360-364, 1996.

55. Wong HP, Zamboni WA, Stephenson LL. Effect of hyperbaric oxygen on skeletal muscle necrosis following primary and secondary ischemia in a rat model. Surg Forum. 1996;47:705-707.

56. Gampper TJ, Zhang F, Mofakhami NF, et al. Beneficial effect of hyperbaric oxygen on island flaps subjected to secondary venous ischemia. Microsurg. 2002;22:49-52.

57. Perrins DJD. Hyperbaric oxygenation of skin flaps. Br J Plast Surg. 1966;19:110-112.

58. Perrins DJD, Cantab MB. Influence of hyperbaric oxygen on the survival of split skin grafts. Lancet. 1967;1: 868-871.

59. Roje Z, Roje Z, Eterovic D et al. Influence of adjuvant hyperbaric oxygen therapy on short-term complications during surgical reconstruction of upper and lower extremity war injuries: retrospective cohort study. Croat Med J. 2008;49:224-232.

60. Gonnering RS, Kindwall EP, Goldmann RW. Adjunct hyperbaric oxygen therapy in periorbital reconstruction. Arch Opthalmol. 1986;104: 439-443.

61. Bowersox JC, Strauss MB, Hart GB. Clinical experience with hyperbaric oxygen therapy in salvage of ischemic skin flaps and grafts. J Hyperbaric Med. 1986; 141-149.

62. Friedman HI, Stonerock C, Brill A. Composite earlobe grafts to reconstruct the lateral nasal ala and sill. Ann Plast Surg. 2003;3:275-281.

63. Qing Y, Cen Y, Chen J, Ke S. Reconstruction of a large through-and-through defect of the nasal tip using a modified auricular composite graft. J Craniofac Surg. 2015;26:382-383.

64. Saber AA, Yahya KZ, Rao A, et al. A new approach in the management of chronic nonhealing leg ulcers. J Invest Surg. 2005;18: 321-323.

65. Assaad NN, Chong R, Tat LT, et al. Adjuvant hyperbaric oxygen therapy to support limbal conjunctival graft in the management of recurrent pterygium. Cornea. 2011;30:7-10.

66. Ueda M, Kaneda T, Takahashi H, et al. Hyperbaric oxygen therapy of ischemic skin flaps: clinical and experimental study. Proceedings of 9th International Symposium on Underwater Hyperbaric Physiology. Undersea & Hyperbaric Medical Society. 1987;823.

67. Mathieu D, Neviere R, Pellerin P, et al. Pedicle musculocutaneous flap transplantation: Prediction of final outcome by transcutaneous oxygen measurements in hyperbaric oxygen. Plast Reconstr Surg. 1993;91: 329-334.

68. Waterhouse MA, Zamboni WA, Brown RE, et al. The use of HBO in compromised free tissue transfer and replantation, a clinical review. Undersea Hyperbaric Med.1993; 20(Suppl):64.

69. Larson JV, Steensma EA, Flikkema RM, Norman EM. The application of hyperbaric oxygen therapy in the management of compromised flaps. Undersea Hyperb Med. 2013;40:499-504.

70. Skeik N, Porten BR, Isaacson E, et al. Hyperbaric oxygen treatment outcome for different indications from a single center. Ann Vasc Surg 2015; 29:206-214.

71. Nichter LS, Morwood DT, Williams GS, et al. Expanding the limits of composite grafting: a case report of successful nose replantation assisted by hyperbaric oxygen therapy. Plast Reconstr Surg. 1991;87: 337-340.

72. Rapley JH, Lawrence WT, Witt PD. Composite grafting and hyperbaric oxygen therapy in pediatric nasal tip reconstruction after avulsive dog-bite injury. Ann Plast Surg. 2001;46: 434-438.

73. Cantarella G, Mazzola RF and Pagani D. The fate of an amputated nose after replantation. Am J Otolaryngol. 2005;26: 344-347.

74. Pou JD, Graham HD. Pediatric Nasal Tip Amputation Successfully Treated with Nonmicrovascular Replantation and Hyperbaric Oxygen Therapy. Ochsner J. 2017 Summer;17(2):204-207.

75. McCrary BF. Hyperbaric oxygen treatment for a failing facial flap. Postgrad Med J. 2007;83: e1-e3.

76. Khandelwal S, Wall J, Kaide C, et al. Case report: successful use of hyperbaric oxygen therapy for a complete scalp degloving injury. Undersea Hyperbaric Med. 2008;35: 441-445.

77. Mermans JF, Tuinder S, von Meyenfeldt MF, et al. Hyperbaric oxygen treatment for skin flap necrosis after a mastectomy: a case study. Undersea Hyperbaric Med. 2012;39:719-723.

78. Fredman R, Wise I, Friedman T, Heller L, Kami T. Skin-sparing mastectomy flap ischemia salvage using urgent hyperbaric chamber oxygen therapy: a case report. Undersea Hyperb Med 2014;41:145-147.

79. Copeland-Halperin LR, Bruce SR, Mesbahi AN. Hyperbaric oxygen following bilateral skin-sparing mastectomies: a case report. Plast Reconstr Surg Glob Open. 2016;4:e680.

80. Zhou YY, Liu W, Yang YJ, Lu GD. Use of hyperbaric oxygen on flaps and grafts in China: analysis of studies in the past 20 years. Undersea Hyperb Med. 2014;41:209-216.

81. Baynosa RC and Zamboni WA. Compromised grafts and flaps. In: TS Neuman & SR Thom, Eds. Physiology and Medicine of Hyperbaric Oxygen Therapy. Philadelphia, PA: Saunders/Elsevier. 2008; 373-395.

82. Friedman HI, Fitzmaurice M, Lefaivre JF, et al. An evidence-based appraisal of the use of hyperbaric oxygen on flaps and grafts. Plast Reconstr Surg. 2006;117 (Suppl):175S-190S.

83. Nemiroff PM, Rybak LP. Applications of hyperbaric oxygen for the otolaryngologist-head and neck surgeon. Am J Otolaryngol. 1988;9:52-57.

84. Reinisch JF. Pathophysiology of skin flap circulation: The delay phenomenon. Plast Reconstr Surg. 1974;54:585-598.

85. Reinisch JF. The role of arteriovenous anastomosis in skin flaps. In: Grabb WC, Myers MBG, Eds. Skin Flaps. Boston, MA: Little Brown & Co. 1975;81-92.

86. Weber R, Silver A, Williams SJ, et al. Random flap survival with hyperbaric oxygen: daily versus twice-daily treatments. Undersea Hyperb Med. 2018 Mar-Apr;45(2):157-164.

CHAPTER 6

The Role of Hyperbaric Oxygen for Acute Traumatic Ischemias

Michael B. Strauss MD

Abstract

Acute traumatic ischemias are an array of disorders that range from crush injuries to compartment syndromes, from burns to frostbite and from threatened flaps to compromised re-implantations. Two unifying components common to these conditions are a history of trauma be it physical, thermal, or surgical coupled with ischemia to the traumatized tissues. Their pathophysiology resolves around the self-perpetuating cycle of edema and ischemia and their severity represents a spectrum from mild, almost nonexistent, to tissue death.

Since ischemia is a fundamental component of the traumatic ischemias and hypoxia is a consequence of ischemia, hyperbaric oxygen is a logical intervention for those conditions where tissue survival, infection control and healing is at risk. Unfortunately, even with mechanisms of hyperbaric oxygen that strongly support its usefulness in traumatic ischemias coupled with supportive clinical data, clinicians are disinclined to utilize it for these conditions. This section will focus on the orthopedic aspects of the traumatic ischemias, namely crush injury and compartment syndrome and show how hyperbaric oxygen treatments can mitigate their severity. Other sections in this committee report will discuss the thermal and threatened flaps/re-implantation conditions.

Introduction

Crush injuries of the extremities involve multiple tissue levels. These range from skin and subcutaneous tissues to muscle and tendons to bone and joints and often include nerves and arteries. In their most severe presentations, predictable complications including failed flaps, nonunions of fractures, osteomyelitis, and amputations approach 50% of the cases with standard of practice surgical and medical interventions.[1-3]

Skeletal muscle-compartment syndrome (SMCS) is another consequence of trauma, but in this situation the target tissues are muscles and nerves. Edema and/or bleeding within the confines of the fascial envelope increase the pressure within the skeletal muscle-compartment. When the tissue fluid pressure within the compartment exceeds the capillary perfusion pressure to the muscles and nerves in the compartment, these tissues become ischemic and manifest the signs and symptoms of SMCS. The SMCS, especially in its **Impending Stage** before a fasciotomy is required, is a therapeutic challenge since no means to arrest its progression exist other than hyperbaric oxygen.

Unfortunately, despite endorsement by professional societies[4] hyperbaric oxygen is woefully neglected as an adjunct for managing crush injuries and SMCS. The neglect is threefold: 1) A dearth of hyperbaric facilities at major trauma centers; 2) Failure of insurance carriers (especially CMS/Medicare) to reimburse hyperbaric oxygen treatments for hospitalized patients; and 3) Apparent lack of clinicians familiar with the benefits of this intervention for mitigating the complications of traumatic ischemias.

This section on the crush injuries and skeletal muscle compartment syndromes components of the traumatic ischemias will explain the pathophysiology of these problems, show the roles hyperbaric oxygen have in managing them and provide answers on how to improve awareness of its benefits and consequent use for these conditions.

Pathophysiology

Trauma plus tissue hypoxia are the common denominators of crush injuries and SMCS. This leads to two consequences: a continuum of injury from normal to irreversibly damaged and a self-perpetuating (i.e., vicious cycle) progression of edema contributing to tissue ischemia and vice versa (Figure 1). Consequences of trauma include damage to tissues, impairment of perfusion, and biochemical alterations. If the trauma and consequent energy transfer to the tissues is great enough, the tissues will immediately die. The only options in these circumstances are debridement if the site of involvement is contained or major limb amputation, if not.

Figure 1. Unifying Features of Crush Injuries & Compartment Syndromes

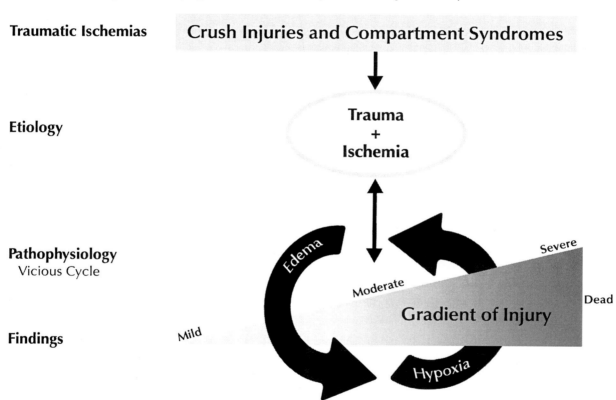

Legend: The unifying features of crush injuries and compartment syndromes are 4-fold and apply equally to the other traumatic ischemias such as burns, frostbites and threatened flaps/replantations.

From the perfusion perspective the traumatic ischemias manifest themselves as trauma to blood vessels, especially at the microcirculation level (Figure 1). This leads to leakage and transudation of fluid (i.e., edema formation), swelling, interstitial bleeding (ecchymoses and hematomas), sluggish flow in the microcirculation, stasis, slugging of cellular elements, Rouleau formation of red blood cells and obstruction. The consequences are ischemia and hypoxia to the tissues perfused by the damaged vasculature. With the hypoxic insult, cells are no longer able to maintain their metabolic functions including ability to retain their intracellular water. This further contributes to edema and third spacing of fluid. If the edema occurs in a closed space, the increased pressure will collapse the microcirculation, eliminate oxygen transfer across the capillary endothelium and further contribute to the hypoxic insult. This information accounts for the pathophysiology of the skeletal muscle-compartment syndrome.

Events at the biochemical level, the ultimate determinants of outcome, are manifested in two ways. First, oxygen is required for all cellular metabolic functions. If oxygen tensions are insufficient, cell signaling factors, wound healing and angiogenesis responses as elaborated through the fibroblast and bacterial killing by the neutrophil are thwarted.[5-7] Oxygen tensions in the tissue fluids greater than 30 mmHg are required for these responses to occur.[8]

The second biochemical event is that of reperfusion injury.[9] Once perfusion is temporarily interrupted, occurring in varying degrees with crush injuries and compartment syndromes, the endothelium becomes sensitized to the hypoxic insult. This results in activation of adhesion molecules leading to the attachment of neutrophils to the endothelium and their release of reactive oxygen species. The consequence is a cascade of biochemical events. The oxygen radicals damage tissue often beyond repair and cause severe vasoconstriction which defines the reperfusion injury and the no-reflow phenomenon associated with it.

Mechanisms of HBO$_2$

The justifications for using hyperbaric oxygen acutely in crush injuries and compartment syndromes are twofold: First, hyperbaric oxygen supplements oxygen availability to hypoxic tissues during the immediate post-injury period when perfusion is most likely to be inadequate and the oxygen needs are the greatest.[10] Second, HBO$_2$ increases tissue oxygen tensions to sufficient levels for the host responses mentioned above to function. Hyperbaric oxygen exposures at two atmospheres absolute (ATA) increase the blood oxygen content (the combination of hemoglobin and plasma carried oxygen) by 125%. The oxygen tensions in plasma as well as tissue fluids is increased tenfold (1000%).[10-12] Sufficient oxygen can be physically dissolved in plasma under HBO$_2$ conditions to keep tissues alive without hemoglobin-borne oxygen.[13] Increased tissue oxygen tensions result in a threefold driving force (mass effect) for oxygen to diffuse through tissue fluids.[14] This helps to compensate for the hypoxia (at normoxic tensions) that results from the increased oxygen diffusion distance from the capillary to the cell through edema fluid.

Edema reduction is a secondary effect of tissue hyperoxygenation. The hyperoxygenation effect of hyperbaric oxygen triggers vasoconstriction. In healthy vasculature (i.e., not affected by atherosclerosis), blood flow is reduced by 20%.[15-16] Since inflow is decreased by 20% through vasoconstriction while outflow is maintained, the net effect is edema reduction of 20%.[16-20] Edema reduction occurs because of decreased filtration of fluid from the capillary to the extracellular space as a consequence of vasoconstriction (resulting in decreased perfusion pressure in the capillary bed), while resorption of fluid at the capillary level is maintained by the oncotic pressure within the capillary. Hyperoxygenation of the plasma maintains oxygen delivery to tissues in the presence of HBO$_2$-induced vasoconstriction.[15,21-22]

Another consequence of decreasing the interstitial fluid pressure through edema reduction is improved blood flow through the microcirculation. The explanation for this is that once the interstitial fluid pressure is reduced below the capillary perfusion pressure, the collapsed microcirculation can reopen and allow perfusion to resume. By reducing edema while supplementing tissue oxygenation, hyperbaric oxygen interrupts the self-perpetuating, edema-ischemia cycle to prevent progression of the injury. The decreased interstitial fluid pressure is especially applicable to mitigating the effects of the skeletal muscle-compartment syndrome.

Mitigation of the reperfusion injury is another effect of hyperbaric oxygen for traumatic ischemias.[23-25] It interrupts the interactions between toxic oxygen radicals and cell membrane lipids by perturbing lipid peroxidation of the cell membrane and by inhibiting the sequestration of neutrophils on post-capillary venules.[26-28] The biochemical mechanism that explains this latter effect is that HBO_2 perturbs the adherence of neutrophils elaborated through the Beta$_2$ integrin (Cluster of designation-11 cell surface protein) on the sensitized capillary endothelium.[25] This reduces/eliminates the release of toxic oxygen radicals and their resultant damage to tissues. The problem is compounded by a hypoxic environment where toxic oxygen species react with reactive nitrogen oxide species to produce peroxynitrite radicals, the most toxic of all the reactive species generated by the human body.[29] Oxygen radical scavengers (such as superoxide dismutase, catalase, peroxidase and glutathione reductase) that normally detoxify reactive oxygen species are generated in a normoxic environment.[30-31] Hyperbaric oxygen can facilitate this process when the injury site is hypoxic when breathing room air.

Patient Selection Criteria for Crush Injuries

Clinical findings coupled with accepted grading systems should be used to make decisions to use HBO_2 for crush injuries. Not only must the seriousness of the injury be considered, but the ability of the host to respond to the injury needs to be factored into the decision-making process. Obviously, better criteria for using HBO_2 in crush injuries must be employed than saying the injury is very severe or limb threatening. The indication for using HBO_2 for crush injuries is the injury severity is so great that the survival of deep tissues and/or skin flaps is threatened. Consequently, trauma surgeons, reconstructive plastic surgeons, orthopedic surgeons and podiatrists are the specialists who need to make the decisions whether or not HBO_2 is needed for the traumatic ischemias.

The widely used Gustilo Open-Fracture Crush-Injury Grading System coupled with an intuitive 5-criteria 0-to-10 point objective Wellness Score is useful for making decisions if hyperbaric oxygen is needed for the traumatic ischemia injury (Tables 1 and 2).[1-2,32] The Wellness Score utilizes 5 assessments considered most useful for making decisions as to whether the patient's health warrants using interventions to avoid amputation or hold treatments in favor of comfort care measures only. Each assessment is graded on a 2 (best) to 0 (worst) analogue scale. High Wellness Score (coupled with the severity of the injury) justify doing everything possible including hyperbaric oxygen to salvage the extremity; low scores favor amputation.[32-33]

Unfortunately, too often, hyperbaric oxygen treatments are requested only after complications from a crush injury have arisen, such as slough of a flap, wound dehiscence, threatened flap after delayed coverage and/or closure, muscle necrosis from residuals of a skeletal muscle-compartment syndrome and/or osteomyelitis. The time to start hyperbaric oxygen is with the initial management in those crush injuries where complications are predictable, such as the Gustilo III-B and C fractures and in lesser Gustilo grades in impaired and decompensated patients as quantified by the Wellness Score (Table 2).

Compartment Syndromes: The skeletal muscle-compartment syndrome, like the crush injury, represents a continuum of severities divided into **Suspected**, **Impending** and **Established Stages**. The unifying pathophysiological feature of compartment syndromes is the self-perpetuating edema-ischemia cycle. In the **Suspected Stage**, the compartment syndrome is not actually present (i.e., an emergency fasciotomy is not indicated), but the severity of the injury or the circumstances (i.e., prolonged ischemia time) raises suspicions that a compartment syndrome could develop. In the **Suspected Stage** hyperbaric oxygen is not indicated, but frequent neurocirculatory checks of the injured extremity are required to recognize the earliest possible progression to the **Impending Stage.**

If the edema-ischemia cycle perpetuates itself, the condition may evolve into the **Impending Stage**. In this stage, signs include the following: 1) increasing pain; 2) hypesthesia; 3) muscle weakness; 4) discomfort with passive stretch of the toes/fingers; and /or 5) tautness of the contents of the compartment. If any of these signs exist, muscle compartment tissue pressure measurements should be made. If the compartment pressure(s) and clinical

Table 1. The Health Status Score—Quantifying Health and Function

Assessment	2 Points	1 Point	0 Points
	Use half points if mixed or intermediate between 2 grades		
Activities of daily living	Full	Some	None
Ambulation	Community	Household	None
	Subtract ½ point if aids are used.		
Comorbidities	No significant	Impaired	Decompensated
	Omit neurological deficits which is separate assessment below.		
Inhibitors smoking, collagen vascular diseases, and immunosuppressors	None	Past	Current
Neurological deficits	None	Some/Minor Sensation, imbalances	Major Cognitive, paralysis

Notes: Five assessments (considered to be the most important to determine how healthy and functional the patient is) are each graded from 2 points (best) to 0 points (worst) and summated to generate a 0 to 10 score. "Healthy" patients generate scores in the 7½ -10 range, "impaired" patients in the 3½-7 range and decompensated patients in the 0-3 range.

Table 2. Guidelines for using Hyperbaric Oxygen in Crush Injuries using the Gustilo Classification Paired with the Patient's Wellness Score[30]

Gustilo Type	Findings Soft tissue injury with the fracture	Outcomes in Healthy Hosts	HBO$_2$ Indications paired with Wellness Score[1]		
			Healthy	Impaired	Decompensated
I	Minimal (<1 cm wide) puncture wound from inside to out	Usually no different from a closed fracture of the same severity			Yes
II	Laceration with minimal deep soft tissue damage	Same as above			Yes
III	Crush Injuries	Depend on Subtypes A, B, and C			
A	Sufficient soft tissue to close the wound (after debridement)	~10% completion rate[2]		Yes	Yes
B	Flaps and/or grafts needed for bone coverage	≥50% incidence of complications[2]	Yes	Yes	Yes/No[3]
C	III-B injuries with major vascular damage		Yes	Yes/No[3]	Yes/No[3]

Notes: Table 2 shows how the Wellness Score is combined with the Gustilo open fracture grading system to add objectivity to the indications for using hyperbaric oxygen in crush injuries.

Scores greater than 4 points support the decision for doing everything possible to salvage the injured tissue including the adjunctive use of hyperbaric oxygen.

Figure 2-a. Indications for HBO$_2$ in the Skeletal Muscle-Compartment Syndrome

Clinical Findings
1. Post-traumatic edema
2. Infiltrations
3. Venous outflow obstruction
4. Prolonged ischemia
5. Comatose posturing; "crunch" syndrome
6. Snake bites (unusual)
7. Shock (hypoperfusion) plus injury to soft tissues

Suspected Stage
(HBO$_2$ not indicated)

Edema

Ischemia

Management
A. High "index of suspicion" for a SMCS
B. Frequent neurocirculatory checks (The "5 P's)
  --Pain
  --Paresthesia
  --Paralysis
  --Pallor
  --Pulselessness
C. Treat primary injuries

Impending Stage

3 or more clinical findings

1 or more manometric findings

Clinical Findings
1. Increasing pain
2. Anesthesia
3. Muscle weakness
4. Discomfort with passive stretch
5. Tenseness of muscle compartment

Hyperbaric Oxygen Indications

Pressure Measurements
(manometrics) when available
Increasing serial measurements
AND/OR
Paired with Wellness Score
(refer to Table 1)

$\leq$45 mmHg "healthy" patient
$\leq$35 mmHg "impaired" patient
$\leq$25 mmHg "decompensated" patient and/or in shock

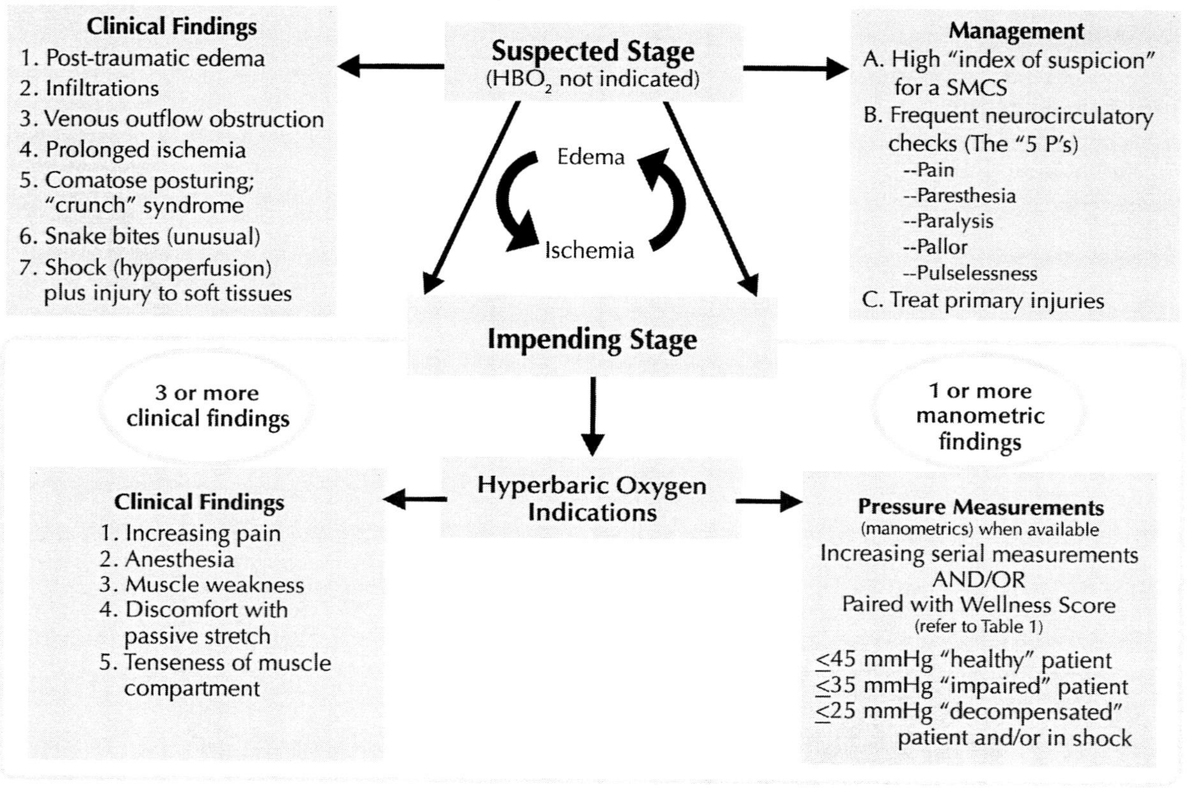

Legend: The skeletal muscle-compartment syndrome starts with an injury or an insult (see findings in **Suspected Stage** above). If the edema-ischemia "vicious cycle" progresses, the **Suspected Stage** evolves into the **Impending Stage**. Hyperbaric oxygen is the only known intervention that will mitigate the edema-ischemia "vicious cycle" during the **Impending Stage**.

finding are such that fasciotomy is not required at this time, hyperbaric oxygen should be started to prevent progression from the **Impending Stage** to the **Established Stage**. If pressure testing is not available and the compartment syndrome is not in the **Established Stage**, three or more clinical findings are sufficient justification to initiate hyperbaric oxygen treatments in the **Impending Stage** (Figure 2-a).

A second indication for hyperbaric oxygen in the **Impending Stage** (if pressure testing is available) is increasing compartment pressures with serial measurements even if the threshhold for fasciotomy has not been reached. The increasing pressures indicate that the edema-ischemia cycle is continuing and without hyperbaric oxygen, will reach a level where fasciotomy is required. As in crush injuries, the patient's Wellness Score needs to paired with compartment pressure measurements when making decisions when to use hyperbaric oxygen for the **Impending Stage** of the SMCS (Figure 2-a).

In the **Established Stage** of the SMCS, symptoms, signs, pressure measurements or combinations of these confirm the diagnosis and dictate that immediate fasciotomy be done (Figure 2-b). Hyperbaric oxygen must not be used as reason to defer surgery in the above situations. However, after fasciotomy, hyperbaric oxygen should be used as an adjunct to wound management if significant residual problems remain, such as ischemic muscle, threatened flaps, unclear demarcation between viable and non-viable tissue, residual neuropathy, massive swelling, prolonged (more than six hours) ischemia time and/or significant comorbidities as determined by the Wellness Score.

Figure 2-b. Requirements for Fasciotomy in the Skeletal Muscle-Compartment Syndrome and Indications for Hyperbaric Oxygen Post-Fasciotomy

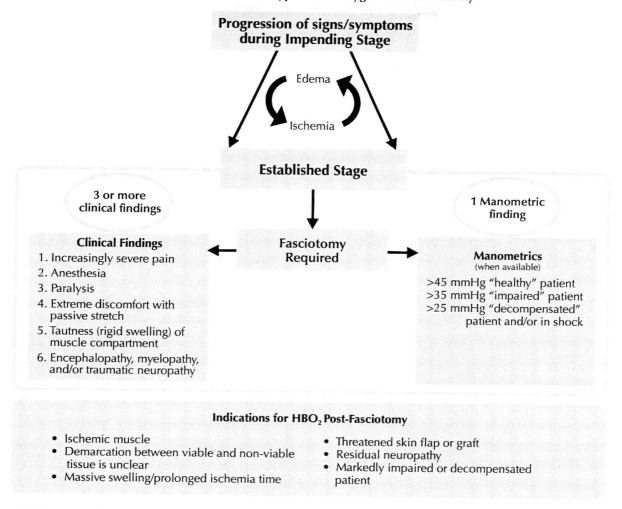

Legend: If the Impending Stage progresses to the Established Stage, HBO$_2$ must not be used as a substitute for fasciotomy. HBO$_2$ should be used post-fasciotomy if 1 or more findings as listed above are present.

The term "lag phase" refers to the time interval from the injury or insult to the time symptoms of SMCS are severe enough to make the diagnosis. It may vary from an hour or two, with bleeding into the compartment, to 24 hours or more with blunt trauma. The lag phase reflects the self-perpetuating edema-ischemia "vicious" circle that precedes the impending and established phases of the SMCS.

Clinical Management

Crush Injuries

Early application of HBO$_2$, preferably within four to six hours of the injury, is recommended. Treatment schedules for crush injuries should be tailored to mitigate the suspected pathophysiology; for example, three or more treatments in the first 24-hour period for critical ischemias; twice a day for threatened flaps and oxygenating an environment so host factors can function; and once a day for dealing with infections, remodeling or resorption of calcified tissues (Table 3). For the isolated reperfusion injury after revascularization or thrombectomy of an extremity that otherwise has sustained minimal physical trauma, a single hyperbaric oxygen treatment, based on animal studies and limited clinical observations, is probably adequate.[25,27] Typically, treatment pressures range from 2 ATA in monoplace chambers to 2.4 ATA in multiplace chambers, with oxygen breathing periods of 90 minutes for two or more treatments a day to 120 minutes for single daily treatments.

Injury and Compartment Syndrome

Compartment Syndromes

For the **Impending Stage** of the SMCS, hyperbaric oxygen treatments should be given twice a day for 24 to 36 hours, the time that the self-perpetuating edema-ischemia cycle would be expected to end. Symptoms and signs of pain reduction, absence of neurological abnormalities, and less tautness in the compartment should be used in deciding when to stop hyperbaric oxygen treatments.

For residual complications after fasciotomy has been performed for the **Established Stage** compartment syndrome, hyperbaric oxygen treatments should be done twice a day for a 7- to 10-day period or when the problems have stabilized enough that no additional improvement is observed from the treatments. Treatment durations and pressures are the same for crush injuries: that is, 90 to 120-minute durations at 2.0 to 2.4 ATA.

Table 3. Treatment Recommendations and Peer Review when using Hyperbaric Oxygen for Crush

Conditions	Peer Review[1] Obtain after # of Rxs	Comments
Primary Conditions		
1. Reperfusion injury	1-2 treatments	Minimal tissue trauma, e.g. after free flaps, revascularizations, and transient edema
2. Crush injury	9 (TID 1st 24 hours; BID 2 days and daily 2 days)	If deterioration noted when HBO_2 treatments are decreased, resume the previous schedule
3. Compartment Syndromes	3 (BID day 1 and single treatment day 2)	HBO_2 is not a substitute for fasciotomy; use it for the impending stage of the SMCS
Residual Problems and/or Complications		
1. Threatened flaps and grafts	14 (BID for 7 days)	If site remains tenuous, consider an additional week of twice a day treatments
2. Problem wounds/infected wounds	21 (BID for 7 days, daily for 7 days)	Refer to Problem Wounds section of this Hyperbaric Oxygen Committee Report
3. Refractory osteomyelitis	30 (Daily for 21 days; possible extension to 40 treatments)	HBO_2 must be integrated with a combined antibiotic and surgical strategy
4. Post-fasciotomy concerns after SMCS	14 (BID for 7 days)	Concerns include massive swelling, threatened flaps, unclear demarcation, neuropathy, etc.

Notes: [1]Peer review should be done by two or more of the following: 1) Hyperbaric medicine physician; 2) Trauma/orthopedic/plastic surgeon requesting HBO_2 and/or patient's primary care physician to decide whether to continue or stop hyperbaric oxygen treatments.

Abbreviations: BID = Twice a day, HBO_2 = Hyperbaric oxygen, # = Number, Rxs = Treatments, SMCS = Skeletal muscle-compartment syndrome, TID = Three times a day.

Supporting Literature and Evidence-Based Indications

Crush Injury Literature Review

More than 600 clinical cases reported in over 20 publications attest to the usefulness of hyperbaric oxygen in crush injuries.[34-36] Although most of the reports describe its benefits in subjective terms such as hyperbaric oxygen treatments were helpful, good results were achieved, or from past experiences problems of similar magnitude would have resulted in amputations, overall outcomes were positive in about 80% of the reports in a historical review.[34]

The most important observation from the historical review was that, as the frequency of treatments increased, the outcomes improved.[34,37-39] Specifically, in traumatic ischemias, Schramek reported 100% salvage rates with six hyperbaric oxygen treatments a day, Loder reported 80% complete or partial recoveries with three treatments a day and Slack reported that 59% responded well with a single treatment daily. In 2005 Garcia-Covarubias, et al. published an evidenced-based approach regarding the use of hyperbaric oxygen in the management of crush injuries and traumatic ischemias.[40] They found nine reports comprising approximately 150 patients that met their inclusion criteria. Eight of nine studies showed a beneficial effect of hyperbaric oxygen treatments with only one reported major complication. They concluded that hyperbaric oxygen as an adjunct to managing crush injuries and traumatic ischemias is not likely to be harmful and could be beneficial if administered early.

The one randomized controlled trial in their report was that of Bouachour's crush injury-fracture study.[41] Bouachour and his co-authors reported complete healing in 94% of the hyperbaric oxygen treated group versus 33% in the controls ($p<0.01$) while the need for additional surgeries was 6% in the hyperbaric oxygen leg compared to 33% in the controls ($p<0.05$). The hyperbaric oxygen patients also demonstrated benefits when age was used as a marker of wellness.

Compartment Syndromes Literature Review

In the 1980s the effects of hyperbaric oxygen on the SMCS were reported in a series of articles using a canine model.[18-20,40,42] The hyperbaric oxygen treated group had significantly less skeletal muscle necrosis than the controls when radiopharmaceutical and histological methods were used to study outcomes. When hyperbaric oxygen treatments were delayed, more injury was observed in the treated canines but was still significantly less than in the controls. In animals rendered shocky by exsanguination, hyperbaric oxygen treatments minimized injury as confirmed by absence of muscle necrosis and more edema reduction as compared to the controls. Nylander's studies with tourniquet ischemia showed similar benefits in the hyperbaric oxygen treated animals.[16] Bartlett, et al. reported significantly improved muscle function confirmed by electrophysiological monitoring in a canine SMCS with a combination of fasciotomy and hyperbaric oxygen versus the fasciotomy group alone.[43] These findings are consistent with several hundred reported clinical experiences using hyperbaric oxygen for SMCS.[44-46]

American Heart Association Level of Classification

Using the American Heart Association (AHA) criteria,[47] hyperbaric oxygen meets the criteria for Class-I, Level-R evidence for treatment of crush injuries. This is based on the findings that hyperbaric oxygen treatments are useful and/or effective, a single randomized control trial exists and the benefits outweigh the risks. In terms of comparative effectiveness research, hyperbaric oxygen is an adjunct to other interventions and should be used for the indications previously stated, rather than in place of another intervention. There are no other comparable interventions to use as an adjunct to managing crush injuries.

For the SMCS, the AHA criteria fits into the Class-I, Level-C category with the benefits outweighing the risks, the treatments are useful/effective based on expert opinion (including laboratory data) and case studies support its use, but no randomized control trials exist. Again, comparative effectiveness research studies are not appropriate for using hyperbaric oxygen for the SMCS in as much as during the **Impending Stage** of the SMCS, no other treatments are beneficial. Consequently, hyperbaric oxygen is the only possible intervention to prevent the progression of the SMCS from the **Impending** to the **Established Stage**. After fasciotomy for the **Established Stage** of the SMCS, hyperbaric oxygen is indicated for reasons of mitigating wound healing complications and promoting recovery.

Effectiveness-Based Indications

With less than 20% of the decisions made in clinical medicine meeting the criteria of evidenced-based indications, a more pragmatic system is needed for making decisions for using hyperbaric oxygen in crush injuries and compartment syndromes as well as for the other traumatic ischemias.[48] Consequently, I propose using an effectiveness-based indications (EBI) evaluation system[49] (Table 4). Five assessments considered most useful for making EBI decisions each graded on a 2 (best) to 0 (worst) analogue scale are summated. This generates a 0 to 10 score. Scores greater than 4 points are considered justification for using the intervention. For crush injuries the EBI score is 7 and for compartment syndrome it is 6 using this system.

Table 4. Effectiveness-Based Indications (EBI) to Justify Hyperbaric Oxygen for Crush Injury and Compartment Syndrome

Assessments	Scoring Criteria[1] For each assessment	EBI Grading (points) for Using Hyperbaric Oxygen	
		Crush Injury	**Compartment Syndrome**
1. Treating physician's experiences	**2 POINTS** Strong evidence to support the intervention	1	1
2. Mechanisms (of HBO$_2$) and lab studies support the intervention		2	2
3. Publications and supporting literature	**1 POINT** Evidence is consistent with supporting the intervention	1½	1
4. No other treatments available (Failure and/or poor outcomes with current management)		1	2 (Impending Stage)
5. Randomized control trials and/or head-to-head studies (2 or more)	**0 POINTS** No benefit, no information or possible harm with the intervention	1½	0
		7 Points[2]	**6 points[2]**

Notes: [1]Use half points if the information is between two scoring criteria.
[2]Greater than 4 points qualifies the interventions as an Effective-Based Indication.

Utilization Review

Crush Injuries

Recommendations for utilization review for crush injuries have been listed previously (Table 3). Before making a decision whether to continue or stop hyperbaric oxygen treatments for crush injuries, the conditions for which the treatments were started must be carefully assessed. If the injury process has not stabilized, that is there is still a risk for further progression, hyperbaric oxygen treatments should be continued until the injury pathology has stabilized and improvement is occurring. A secondary consideration for continuing hyperbaric oxygen treatments is appreciation that the indications for treatments change as recovery is continuing. Initially, hyperbaric oxygen may be indicated for mitigating the reperfusion injury (two or three treatments), then for survival of threatened flaps (7-15 treatments), then for wound healing (14-21 treatments) and finally for managing osteomyelitis and fracture union (21-40 treatments). Utilization review should be initiated by the hyperbaric medicine physician and the decision whether to extend the treatments or stop them should be the consensus of the hyperbaric physician, the trauma/orthopedic surgeon, the plastic/reconstructive surgeon and/or the primary care physician attending the patient.

Compartment Syndromes

For the **Impending Stage** of the skeletal muscle-compartment syndrome when findings do not require a fasciotomy, utilization review is recommended after three hyperbaric oxygen treatments. For managing complications post-fasciotomy, utilization review should be done after seven days or 14 treatments using the same approach as described for the crush injuries.

Cost Impact

Crush Injuries

The additional expenses associated with hyperbaric oxygen treatments when used in crush injuries weigh favorably against the costs of dealing with 50% complication rates associated with Gustilo Type III-B and C open-fracture crush injuries.[1-3] From a historical perspective, Brighton in 1977 estimated that in the United States, $140,000 was the average cost per patient required to resolve the 100,000 open fracture-crush injuries that failed to heal primarily each year.[50] Costs would be many-fold higher today. Hyperbaric oxygen in general and oxygen in particular have defined roles in fracture healing especially in those fractures were healing challenges are anticipated.[51]

Even with state of the art technologies, complication rates are predictable for the most severe open-fracture crush injuries (Gustilo II-B and C).[1-2] Because of the large number of open-fracture crush injuries that occur in the United States each year, a reduction in complications and the morbidity associated with them could have a substantial impact on health care costs and far outweigh additional expenses associated with hyperbaric oxygen treatments.[51] Not to be dismissed are the intangible benefits that primary healing and avoidance of limb amputations have for the patient's mental outlook, ability to function independently and return to gainful employment.[52] Experiences from the literature with hyperbaric used as an adjunct for managing open-fracture crush injuries, report healing complication rates of approximately 20%.[53] This compares favorably to the 50% complication rates reported in the literature when hyperbaric oxygen was not used.[1-3] An editorial in *Undersea and Hyperbaric Medicine* further substantiated the predictable high complication rates, primarily in war related extremity injuries, that have been reported in current literature and for which hyperbaric oxygen treatments were not used.[53]

Compartment Syndromes

In a review, total costs were reported to be 75% less when hyperbaric oxygen was initiated in the **Impending Stage** of the SMCS to prevent its progression to the **Established Stage** (and the need for fasciotomy) than for managing complications using hyperbaric oxygen as an adjunct after a fasciotomy had been done.[54] The cost savings of one patient not progressing from the **Impending Stage** to the **Established Stage** of the SMCS and requiring fasciotomy would be about equivalent to the costs to arrest progression of 10 patients in the **Impending Stage** using hyperbaric oxygen. The cost benefits for preventing fasciotomy in the **Impending Stage** include elimination of the extended hospitalizations for wound care and closure/coverage of the fasciotomy site.

The New Reality

Previously, the orthopedic surgeon was the primary referral consideration for hyperbaric oxygen as an adjunct to manage crush injuries and compartment syndromes. Now the orthopaedic trauma surgeons are so skilled and the hardware, bone grafting materials and healing adjuncts so refined, that fracture healing of the crush injury is often the least concern. Soft tissue survival and recovery of function become the major outcome determinants. These are what the major benefits of hyperbaric oxygen address. This places the reconstructive plastic surgeon and the trauma surgeon as the primary decision makers for using hyperbaric oxygen for the traumatic ischemias.

It behooves our committee and our society to inform the "new" referral sources the roles hyperbaric oxygen has for traumatic ischemias, encourage hyperbaric medicine programs to accept treat patients with these diagnoses and have payers reimburse for these specialized services which can reduce complications, shorten hospitalizations, prevent limb loss and enhance recovery.

49. Strauss MB. The role of hyperbaric oxygen in the surgical management of chronic refractory osteomyelitis. In: Bakker DJ, Cramer FS, editors. Hyperbaric Surgery Perioperative Care. Flagstaff, AZ: Best Publishing; 2002. Pp. 37-62.

50. Brighton CT. Hospital Tribune. May 9, 1977.

51. Strauss MB, Tan AM, Lu LQ. Fracture healing and the roles of hyperbaric oxygen. In: Whelan HT, Kindwall EP, editors. Hyperbaric Medicine Practice. North Palm Beach, FL: Best Publishing Company; 2017. Pp. 623-40.

52. MacKenzie EJ, Bosse MJ, Pollak AN, Webb LX, Swiontkowski MF, Kellam JF, Smith DG, Sanders RW, Jones AL, Starr AJ, McAndrew MP, Patterson BM, Burgess AR, Castillo RC. Long-term persistence of disability following severe lower-limb trauma. Results of a seven-year follow-up. J Bone Joint Surg Am. 2005;87(8):1801-9.

53. Strauss MB. Cost-effective issues in hyperbaric oxygen therapy: complicated fractures [Editorial]. J Hyperbaric Med. 1988;3(4):199-205.

54. Strauss MB. Why hyperbaric oxygen therapy may be useful in treating crush injuries and skeletal muscle-compartment syndrome [Editorial]. Undersea Hyperb Med. 2012;39(4):799-800.

CHAPTER 7

Decompression Sickness

Richard E. Moon MD, Simon J. Mitchell MD, MBChB, PhD

Rationale

Decompression sickness (DCS, "bends") is caused by formation of bubbles in tissues and/or blood when the sum of dissolved gas pressures exceeds ambient pressure (supersaturation).[1] This may occur when ambient pressure is reduced during any of the following: ascent from a dive; depressurization of a hyperbaric chamber; rapid ascent to altitude in an unpressurised aircraft or hypobaric chamber; loss of cabin pressure in an aircraft;[2] and during space walks. In diving, compressed gas breathing is usually necessary, although rarely DCS has occurred after either repetitive or very deep breath-hold dives.[3-4] Although arterial gas embolism due to pulmonary barotrauma can occur after a dive as shallow as 1 meter, the threshold depth for DCS in compressed gas diving is around 20 feet of sea water (fsw).[5] DCS after a dive can be provoked by mild altitude exposure, such as a commercial aircraft flight,[6-7] but without a preceding dive the threshold altitude for DCS occurrence in unpressurized flight is 18,000-20,000 ft.[8-9]

Several mechanisms have been hypothesized by which bubbles may exert their deleterious effects. These include direct mechanical disruption of tissue,[10] occlusion of blood flow, platelet deposition and activation of the coagulation cascade,[11] endothelial dysfunction,[12-13] capillary leakage,[14-18] endothelial cell death, complement activation,[19-20] inflammation[21] and leukocyte-endothelial interaction.[22] Recent evidence suggests that circulating microparticles may play a pro-inflammatory role in DCS pathophysiology.[23-24]

The diagnosis of DCS is made on the basis of careful evaluation of the circumstances of the dive (or altitude exposure), the presence of known risk factors, and the post-dive latency and nature of the manifestations.[25-28] DCS manifestations most commonly include paresthesias, hypesthesia, musculoskeletal pain, skin rash and malaise.[25-28] Less common but more serious signs and symptoms include motor weakness, ataxia, vertigo, hearing loss, dyspnea, pulmonary edema,[29] bladder and anal sphincter dysfunction, shock and death.[25-28] Severe DCS may be accompanied by hemoconcentration, hypotension and coagulopathy.[17,30] Severe symptoms usually occur within one to three hours of decompression; the vast majority of all symptoms manifest within 24 hours, unless there is an additional decompression (e.g. altitude exposure).[27] Altitude DCS has similar manifestations, although cerebral manifestations seem to occur more frequently.[27]

Investigations have limited value in diagnosis of DCS. Chest radiography prior to hyperbaric oxygen (HBO$_2$) treatment in selected cases may be useful to exclude pneumothorax (which may require tube thoracostomy placement before recompression). If the clinical presentation is not typical of DCS or notably inconsistent with the circumstances of the dive, neural imaging is occasionally useful to exclude causes unrelated to diving for which treatment other than HBO$_2$ would be appropriate (e.g. herniated disc or spinal hemorrhage). However, imaging studies are rarely helpful for the evaluation or management of DCS.[31-32] Magnetic resonance imaging is not sufficiently sensitive to consistently detect early anatomic correlates of neurological DCI.[33-34] Bubbles causing limb pain cannot be detected radiographically. Neither imaging nor neurophysiological studies should be relied upon to confirm the diagnosis of DCS or be used in deciding whether a patient with suspected DCS needs HBO$_2$.

Improvement of decompression sickness symptoms as a result of recompression was first noted in the nineteenth century.[35] Recompression with air was first implemented as a specific treatment for that purpose in 1896.[36] Oxygen breathing was observed by Bert in 1878 to improve the signs of decompression sickness in animals.[37] The use of oxygen with pressure to accelerate gas diffusion and bubble resolution in humans was first suggested in 1897[38] and eventually tested in the 1930s for human DCS and recommended for the treatment of divers.[39] The rationale for treatment with HBO_2 includes immediate reduction in bubble volume, increasing the diffusion gradient for inert gas from the bubble into the surrounding tissue, oxygenation of ischemic tissue and reduction of CNS edema. It is also likely that HBO_2 has other beneficial pharmacological effects, such as a reduction in neutrophil adhesion to the capillary endothelium.[40-41] The efficacy of HBO_2 is now widely accepted, and HBO_2 is the mainstay of treatment for this disease.[27,42-47]

Patient Selection Criteria

Treatment is recommended for patients with a history of a decompression and whose manifestations are consistent with DCS. HBO_2 treatment is recommended for all patients with symptoms of DCS whenever feasible, although normobaric oxygen administration may be sufficient for the treatment of altitude DCS when neurological manifestations are absent, and for mild DCS (as defined below) following diving. For definitive treatment of altitude-induced cases that do not respond to ground level oxygen, and for more serious cases of DCS after diving, HBO_2 remains the standard of care.[44-45,48-49]

At a consensus workshop on remote treatment of mild DCS (limb pain, constitutional symptoms, subjective sensory symptoms or rash, with non-progressive symptoms, clinical stability for 24 hours or more and a normal neurological exam), it was concluded that some patients with mild symptoms and signs after diving can be treated adequately without recompression.[50] Thus, although HBO_2 remains the preferred intervention in all cases of DCS, not least because DCS may recover more slowly without recompression,[50] it is acceptable to treat cases fitting the mild classification with first aid measures (see below) alone if access to HBO_2 is logistically difficult or hazardous. Such decisions should only be made on a case by case basis and must always involve a diving medicine physician.[51]

Clinical Management

First Aid. In addition to general supportive measures, including fluid resuscitation, airway protection and blood pressure maintenance, administration of 100% oxygen at ground level (1 atmosphere absolute [ATA]) is recommended as first aid for all cases of DCS. Normobaric oxygen can be definitive treatment for altitude-induced DCS.[51, 52]

The following consensus guidelines for pre-hospital care have been developed by a group of international physicians organized by the Divers Alert Network.[51]

- Normobaric oxygen (surface oxygen administered as close to 100% as possible) is beneficial in the treatment of DCI. Normobaric oxygen should be administered as soon as possible after onset of symptoms.

- Training of divers in oxygen administration is highly recommended.

- A system capable of administering a high percentage of inspired oxygen (close to 100%) and an oxygen supply sufficient to cover the duration of the most plausible evacuation scenario is highly recommended for all diving activities. In situations where oxygen supplies are limited and where patient oxygenation may be compromised (such as when drowning and DCI coexist), consideration should be given to planning use of available oxygen to ensure that some oxygen supplementation can be maintained until further supplies can be obtained.

- A horizontal position is generally encouraged in early presenting DCI and should be maintained during evacuation if practicable. The recovery position is recommended in unconscious patients. The useful duration of attention to positioning in DCI is unknown. The head-down (Trendelenburg) position is no longer recommended in management of DCI.

- Oral hydration is recommended but should be avoided if the patient is not fully conscious. Fluids should be noncarbonated, noncaffeinated, nonalcoholic and ideally an electrolyte-containing oral resuscitation fluid such as WHO oral rehydration solution or Pedialyte™ (but drinking water is acceptable).

- If suitably qualified and skilled responders are present, particularly in severe cases, intravascular rehydration (intravenous or intraosseous access) with non-glucose containing isotonic crystalloid is preferred. Intravenous glucose-containing solutions should not be given.

- Treatment with a nonsteroidal anti-inflammatory drug (NSAID) is appropriate if there are no contraindications.

- Other agents such as corticosteroids, pentoxifylline, aspirin, lidocaine and nitroglycerine have been utilized by suitably qualified responders in early management of DCI, but there is insufficient evidence to support or refute their application.

- Divers should be kept thermally comfortable (warm but not hyperthermic). Hyperthermia should be avoided especially in cases with severe neurological signs and symptoms. For example, avoid exposure to the sun, unnecessary activity or excess clothing.

Hyperbaric Oxygen. Recommended treatment of DCS is administration of oxygen at suitable pressures greater than sea level (hyperbaric oxygen). The choice of treatment table and the number of treatments required will depend upon the following: (a) the clinical severity of the illness; (b) the clinical response to treatment; and (c) residual symptoms after the initial recompression. A wide variety of initial hyperbaric regimens have been described, differing in treatment pressure and time, partial pressure of oxygen and diluent gas. Although there are no human outcome data obtained in prospective, randomized studies for the treatment of diving related decompression sickness, broad principles that are generally agreed upon include the following: (a) complete resolution is more likely to result from early hyperbaric treatment;[27,44] (b) the U.S. Navy oxygen treatment tables[49] (and the similar RN and Comex tables), with initial recompression to 60 fsw (18 msw, 2.82 ATA) have been the most widely used recompression procedures for DCS treatment beginning at the surface, and have achieved a high degree of success in resolving symptoms.[27,43,46-47,52-53] Treatment at shallower depths (e.g. 33 fsw, 10 msw, 2 ATA) can also be effective, although published case series suggest that the success rate may be lower at treatment depths less than 60 fsw.[46,54]

Treatment Depth Exceeding 60 fsw (18 msw). For the vast majority of cases of DCS, superiority of treatments at pressure exceeding 2.82 ATA or using helium as the diluent gas has not been demonstrated.[55] The speculative use of treatment schedules that deviate from the U.S. Navy oxygen treatment tables or published monoplace tables are best reserved for facilities and personnel with the experience, expertise and hardware necessary to deal with untoward responses.

Number of Treatments. Most cases of DCS respond satisfactorily to a single hyperbaric treatment, although repetitive treatments (typically once daily) may be required depending on the patient's initial response. For patients with residual deficits following the initial recompression, repetitive treatments are recommended until clinical stability has been achieved. HBO_2 should be administered repetitively as long as stepwise improvement occurs, based upon clearly documented symptoms and physical findings. The need for such follow-up "tailing" treatments should be supported by documentation of the clinical evaluation before and after each treatment. Complete resolution of symptoms or lack of improvement on two consecutive treatments establishes the endpoint of treatment; typically no more than one to two treatments.[27] The optimal choice of recompression table for repetitive treatments has not been established. It is generally agreed that for tailing treatments, repetitive long treatment tables (such as the U.S. Navy Table 6)[49] are not justified, and it is typical to utilize shorter treatments (such as the U.S. Navy Table 5)[49] or even wound treatment tables conducted at 2-2.4 ATA for this purpose. Although a small minority of divers with severe neurological injury may not reach a clinical plateau until 15-20 repetitive treatments have been administered, formal statistical analysis of approximately 3,000 DCI cases supports the efficacy of no more than 5-10 repetitive treatments for most individuals.[56]

Time from Symptom Onset to Hyperbaric Treatment. Available data do not convincingly demonstrate superior outcomes in "rapid" vs. delayed treatment.[53,57] For example, in two published series, time to treatment greater than 24[47] or 48[46] hours was as effective as earlier treatment. However, most series in recreational diving lack cases with extremely short symptom-to-recompression latency as comparators. In contrast, there are data from military experimental diving, which suggest immediate recompression is extremely effective in controlling symptoms.[43,58-59] As a general principle, timely treatment is preferred. Currently available data have not established a maximum time (hours or days) after which recompression is ineffective.[59-65]

Monoplace Chamber Treatment. Monoplace chambers were originally designed for the continuous administration of 100% oxygen and were not equipped to administer air for "air breaks," which are incorporated in U.S. Navy treatment tables for DCS. For monoplace chambers of this type, tables are available for treatment of decompression sickness that are shorter than standard USN treatment tables.[66-68] Retrospective evidence, using telephone follow-up, suggests that such tables may be as effective as standard USN tables for the treatment of mildly or moderately affected patients.[42,69-70] However, many monoplace chambers are now fitted with the means to deliver air to the patient, and thus can be used to administer standard 2.82 ATA USN treatment tables.[71]

Saturation Treatment. For severe DCS in which gradual but incomplete improvement occurs during hyperbaric treatment at 60 fsw, saturation treatment may be considered if the hyperbaric facility has the capability. There is, however, no convincing evidence that such interventions are associated with a better outcome than other approaches.

In-Water Recompression. In-water recompression (IWR) of injured divers has been proposed as an emergency treatment modality if evacuation of a symptomatic diver to a hyperbaric facility cannot be performed in a timely manner. The advantage of IWR is that it can be initiated within a very short time after symptom onset. IWR breathing air has been used by indigenous divers with a high reported success rate, although clinical details are scant.[72] There is anecdotal evidence that IWR using oxygen is more effective.[73] However, a major risk is an oxygen convulsion resulting in fatal drowning. IWR using oxygen has been discussed in the literature[51,73-74] and is described in the *U.S. Navy Diving Manual*.[49] Typical IWR oxygen-breathing protocols recommend depths no greater than 30 fsw (USN) or shallower.[73] Recommendations include a requirement that the diver not use a regular scuba mouthpiece but rather a full face mask, surface-supplied helmet breathing apparatus or regulator retention strap ("gag strap").[75] Other requirements include the need for a tender in the water and the symptomatic diver to be tethered.[73] IWR is not recommended or may cause harm in the setting of isolated hearing loss, vertigo, respiratory distress, airway compromise, altered consciousness, extreme anxiety, hypothermia and hemodynamic instability.

In the absence of a sufficiently detailed case series from which risks and benefits can be assessed, IWR is not presently endorsed by the UHMS but was cautiously endorsed in a recent expert consensus for use by properly trained and equipped divers.[51] It should not be attempted without the necessary equipment, training and a full understanding of the necessary procedures.

Altitude DCS. The following algorithm has been used effectively by the U.S. Air Force.[44,76]

- Mild symptoms that clear on descent to ground level with normal neurological exam: 100% oxygen by tightly fitted mask for a two-hour minimum; aggressive oral hydration; observe 24 hours.

- Symptoms that persist after return to ground level or occur at ground level: 100% oxygen; aggressive hydration; hyperbaric treatment using U.S. Navy (USN) Treatment Tables 5 or 6, as appropriate. For individuals with symptoms consisting only of limb pain, which resolves during oxygen breathing while preparing for hyperbaric treatment, a 24-hour period of observation should be initiated; hyperbaric therapy may not be required.

- Severe manifestations of DCS (neurological, "chokes", hypotension or manifestations that progress in intensity despite oxygen therapy): continue 100% oxygen; administer intravenous hydration; initiate immediate hyperbaric therapy using USN Treatment Table 6. Recompression to 2 ATA (USAF Table 8) has also been used effectively for altitude DCS.[77]

Adjunctive Therapy. Adjunctive treatments such as first-aid oxygen administration, fluid resuscitation and for patients with leg immobility, venous thromboembolism prophylaxis, are indicated. These are discussed in detail in a separate monograph,[78] which is available on the Undersea and Hyperbaric Society website (www.uhms.org/images/Publications/ADJUNCTIVE_THERAPY_FOR_DCI.pdf).

Evidence-Based Review

The use of HBO_2 for decompression sickness is an AHA level I recommendation (level of evidence C). A number of adjunctive therapies have been used for the treatment of DCS (see Table 1) and discussed in the Report of the Decompression Illness Adjunctive Therapy Committee of the Undersea and Hyperbaric Medical Society.[78] These guidelines can be accessed via the internet at www.uhms.org/images/Publications/ADJUNCTIVE_THERAPY_FOR_DCI.pdf.

Utilization Review

Utilization review should occur after 10 treatments.

Cost Impact

Only those people exposed to increased ambient pressure (divers or compressed air workers) or who suffer decompression sickness at altitude are affected. Because there are relatively few individuals who develop this condition, the application of HBO_2 will be limited. HBO_2 is a treatment that usually provides resolution or significant improvement of this disorder that can otherwise result in permanent spinal cord, brain or peripheral nerve damage or death, and is therefore an exceptionally cost-effective treatment.

Table 1. Evidence-based Review of Adjunctive Therapies for DCS
(from Moon:[78] www.uhms.org/images/Publications/ADJUNCTIVE_THERAPY_FOR_DCI.pdf)

	Condition							
	AGE (no significant inert gas load)		**DCS: pain only/mild**		**DCS: neurological**		**DCS: chokes (cardiorespiratory)**	
	Class	Level	Class	Level	Class	Level	Class	Level
Surface O$_2$ (1 ATA)	I	C	I	C	I	C	I	C
Intravenous Fluid Therapy	D5W[†] III LR/crystalloid[‡] IIb Colloid[‖] IIb	C	D5W[†] III LR/crystalloid[‡] I Colloid[‖] I	C	D5W[†] III LR/crystalloid[‡] I Colloid[‖] I	C	D5W[†] III LR/crystalloid[‡] IIb Colloid[‖] IIb	C
Aspirin	IIb	C	IIb	C	IIb	C	IIb	C
NSAIDs	IIb	C	IIb	B	IIb	B	IIb	C
Anti-coagulants*	IIb	C	III	C	IIb[§]	C	IIb	C
Cortico-steroids	III	C	III	C	III	C	III	C
Lidocaine	IIa	B	III	C	IIb	C	III	C

[§]For decompression illness with leg immobility, low molecular weight heparin is recommended as soon as possible after injury (enoxaparin 30 mg or equivalent, subcutaneously every 12 hours).
[†]5% dextrose in water.
[‡]Lactated Ringer's solution, normal saline or other isotonic intravenous fluid not containing glucose.
[‖]Starch, gelatin or protein fraction with isotonic electrolyte concentration.
*Full dose heparin, warfarin, thrombin inhibitors, thrombolytics, IIB/IIIA antiplatelet agents.

Figure 1. Flowchart for DCS Symptoms
Details of management are described in the text.

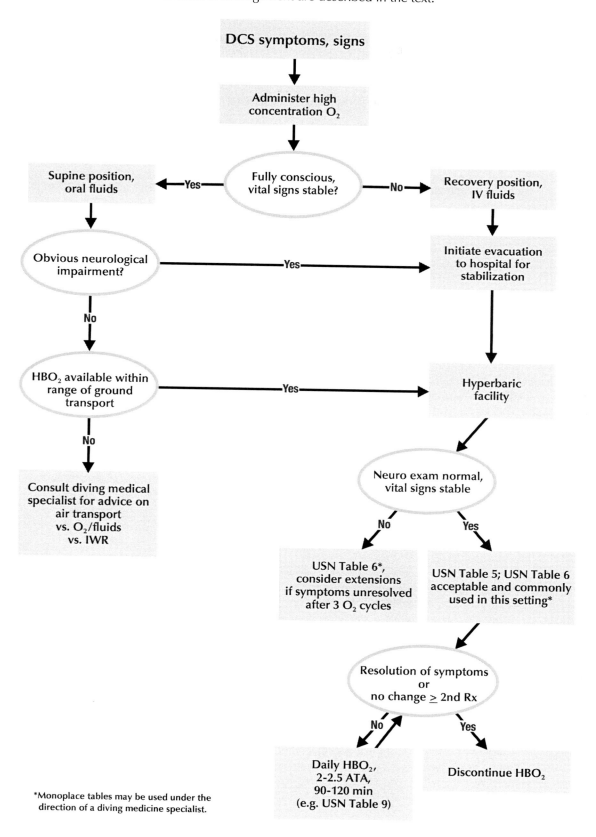

DCS symptoms, signs

Administer high concentration O_2

Fully conscious, vital signs stable?

Yes → Supine position, oral fluids

No → Recovery position, IV fluids

Obvious neurological impairment?

Yes → Initiate evacuation to hospital for stabilization

No → HBO$_2$ available within range of ground transport

Yes → Hyperbaric facility

No → Consult diving medical specialist for advice on air transport vs. O$_2$/fluids vs. IWR

Neuro exam normal, vital signs stable

No → USN Table 6*, consider extensions if symptoms unresolved after 3 O$_2$ cycles

Yes → USN Table 5; USN Table 6 acceptable and commonly used in this setting*

Resolution of symptoms or no change ≥ 2nd Rx

No → Daily HBO$_2$, 2-2.5 ATA, 90-120 min (e.g. USN Table 9)

Yes → Discontinue HBO$_2$

*Monoplace tables may be used under the direction of a diving medicine specialist.

References

1. Mitchell SJ. Decompression sickness: pathophysiology. In: Edmonds C, Bennett MH, editors. Diving and Subaquatic Medicine. 5 ed. Boca Raton, FL: Taylor and Francis; 2015. p. 125-40.

2. Hundemer GL, Jersey SL, Stuart RP, Butler WP, Pilmanis AA. Altitude decompression sickness incidence among U-2 pilots: 1994-2010. Aviat Space Environ Med. 2012;83(10):968-74.

3. Kohshi K, Wong RM, Abe H, Katoh T, Okudera T, Mano Y. Neurological manifestations in Japanese Ama divers. Undersea Hyperb Med. 2005;32(1):11-20.

4. Schipke JD, Gams E, Kallweit O. Decompression sickness following breath-hold diving. Res Sports Med. 2006;14(3):163-78.

5. Van Liew HD, Flynn ET. Direct ascent from air and N_2-O_2 saturation dives in humans: DCS risk and evidence of a threshold. Undersea Hyperb Med. 2005;32(6):409-19.

6. Freiberger JJ, Denoble PJ, Pieper CF, Uguccioni DM, Pollock NW, Vann RD. The relative risk of decompression sickness during and after air travel following diving. Aviat Space Environ Med. 2002;73:980-4.

7. Vann RD, Pollock NW, Freiberger JJ, Natoli MJ, Denoble PJ, Pieper CF. Influence of bottom time on preflight surface intervals before flying after diving. Undersea Hyperb Med. 2007;34(3):211-20.

8. Webb JT, Pilmanis AA, O'Connor RB. An abrupt zero-preoxygenation altitude threshold for decompression sickness symptoms. Aviat Space Environ Med. 1998;69(4):335-40.

9. Webb JT, Kannan N, Pilmanis AA. Gender not a factor for altitude decompression sickness risk. Aviat Space Environ Med. 2003;74(1):2-10.

10. Francis TJ, Griffin JL, Homer LD, Pezeshkpour GH, Dutka AJ, Flynn ET. Bubble-induced dysfunction in acute spinal cord decompression sickness. J Appl Physiol (1985). 1990;68:1368-75.

11. Philp RB, Schacham P, Gowdey CW. Involvement of platelets and microthrombi in experimental decompression sickness: similarities with disseminated intravascular coagulation. Aerosp Med. 1971;42(5):494-502.

12. Nossum V, Koteng S, Brubakk AO. Endothelial damage by bubbles in the pulmonary artery of the pig. Undersea Hyperb Med. 1999;26(1):1-8.

13. Nossum V, Hjelde A, Brubakk AO. Small amounts of venous gas embolism cause delayed impairment of endothelial function and increase polymorphonuclear neutrophil infiltration. Eur J Appl Physiol. 2002;86:209-14.

14. Berry CA, King AH. Severe dysbarism in actual and simulated flight; a follow-up study of five cases. U S Armed Forces Med J. 1959;10(1):1-15.

15. Malette WG, Fitzgerald JB, Cockett AT. Dysbarism. A review of thirty-five cases with suggestion for therapy. Aerosp Med. 1962;33:1132-9.

16. Brunner F, Frick P, Bühlmann A. Post-decompression shock due to extravasation of plasma. Lancet. 1964;1:1071-3.

17. Boussuges A, Blanc P, Molenat F, Bergmann E, Sainty JM. Haemoconcentration in neurological decompression illness. Int J Sports Med. 1996;17:351-5.

18. Levin LL, Stewart GJ, Lynch PR, Bove AA. Blood and blood vessel wall changes induced by decompression sickness in dogs. J Appl Physiol (1985). 1981;50:944-9.

19. Ward CA, Koheil A, McCullough D, Johnson WR, Fraser WD. Activation of complement at plasma-air or serum-air interface of rabbits. J Appl Physiol (1985). 1986;60:1651-8.

20. Ward CA, McCullough D, Yee D, Stanga D, Fraser WD. Complement activation involvement in decompression sickness of rabbits. Undersea Biomed Res. 1990;17:51-66.

21. Little T, Butler BD. Pharmacological intervention to the inflammatory response from decompression sickness in rats. Aviat Space Environ Med. 2008;79(2):87-93.

22. Helps SC, Gorman DF. Air embolism of the brain in rabbits pre-treated with mechlorethamine. Stroke. 1991;22:351-4.

23. Thom SR, Yang M, Bhopale VM, Huang S, Milovanova TN. Microparticles initiate decompression-induced neutrophil activation and subsequent vascular injuries. J Appl Physiol (1985). 2011;110(2):340-51.

24. Yang M, Kosterin P, Salzberg BM, Milovanova TN, Bhopale VM, Thom SR. Microparticles generated by decompression stress cause central nervous system injury manifested as neurohypophisial terminal action potential broadening. J Appl Physiol (1985). 2013.

25. Elliott DH, Moon RE. Manifestations of the decompression disorders. In: Bennett PB, Elliott DH, editors. The Physiology and Medicine of Diving. Philadelphia, PA: WB Saunders; 1993. p. 481-505.

26. Francis TJR, Mitchell SJ. Manifestations of decompression disorders. In: Brubakk AO, Neuman TS, editors. Bennett & Elliott's Physiology and Medicine of Diving. New York, NY: Elsevier Science; 2003. Pp. 578-99.

27. Vann RD, Butler FK, Mitchell SJ, Moon RE. Decompression illness. Lancet. 2011;377(9760):153-64.

28. Mitchell SJ. Decompression sickness: manifestations. In: Edmonds C, Bennett MH, editors. Diving and Subaquatic Medicine. 5 ed. Boca Raton, FL: Taylor and Francis; 2015. Pp. 141-51.

29. Zwirewich CV, Müller NL, Abboud RT, Lepawsky M. Noncardiogenic pulmonary edema caused by decompression sickness: rapid resolution following hyperbaric therapy. Radiology. 1987;163:81-2.

30. Trytko B, Mitchell SJ. Extreme survival: a deep technical diving accident. SPUMS J. 2005;35:23-7.

31. Warren LP, Djang WT, Moon RE, Camporesi EM, Sallee DS, Anthony DC. Neuroimaging of scuba diving injuries to the CNS. AJNR Am J Neuroradiol. 1988;9:933-8.

32. Reuter M, Tetzlaff K, Hutzelmann A, Fritsch G, Steffens JC, Bettinghausen E, Heller M. MR imaging of the central nervous system in diving-related decompression illness. Acta Radiol. 1997;38(6):940-4.

33. Gempp E, Blatteau JE, Stephant E, Pontier JM, Constantin P, Peny C. MRI findings and clinical outcome in 45 divers with spinal cord decompression sickness. Aviat Space Environ Med. 2008;79(12):1112-6.

34. Chung JM, Ahn JY. Relationship between clinical and radiologic findings of spinal cord injury in decompression sickness. Undersea Hyperb Med. 2017;44(1):57-62.

35. Pol B, Wattelle TJJ. Mémoire sur les effets de la compression de l'air appliquée au creusement des puits à houille. Ann Hyg Pub Med Leg. 1854;2:241-79.

36. Moir EW. Tunnelling by compressed air. J Soc Arts. 1896;44(May 15):567-85.

37. Bert P. Barometric Pressure (La Pression Barométrique). Bethesda, MD: Undersea Medical Society; 1978.

38. Zuntz N. Zur Pathogenese und Therapie der durch rasche Luftdruckänderungen erzeugten Krankheiten. Fortschr Med. 1897;15:632-9.

39. Yarbrough OD, Behnke AR. The treatment of compressed air illness using oxygen. J Ind Hyg Toxicol. 1939;21:213-8.

40. Zamboni WA, Roth AC, Russell RC, Graham B, Suchy H, Kucan JO. Morphological analysis of the microcirculation during reperfusion of ischemic skeletal muscle and the effect of hyperbaric oxygen. Plast Reconstr Surg. 1993;91:1110-23.

41. Martin JD, Thom SR. Vascular leukocyte sequestration in decompression sickness and prophylactic hyperbaric oxygen therapy in rats. Aviat Space Environ Med. 2002;73(6):565-9.

42. Kindwall EP. Use of short *versus* long tables in the treatment of decompression sickness and arterial gas embolism. In: Moon RE, Sheffield PJ, editors. Treatment of Decompression Illness. Kensington, MD: Undersea and Hyperbaric Medical Society; 1996. Pp. 122-6.

43. Thalmann ED. Principles of US Navy recompression treatments for decompression sickness. In: Moon RE, Sheffield PJ, editors. Treatment of Decompression Illness. Kensington, MD: Undersea and Hyperbaric Medical Society; 1996. Pp. 75-95.

44. Moon RE, Sheffield PJ. Guidelines for treatment of decompression illness. Aviat Space Environ Med. 1997;68:234-43.

45. Moon RE, Gorman DF. Treatment of the decompression disorders. In: Neuman TS, Brubakk AO, editors. Bennett & Elliott's Physiology and Medicine of Diving. New York, NY: Elsevier Science; 2003. Pp. 600-50.

46. Hadanny A, Fishlev G, Bechor Y, Bergan J, Friedman M, Maliar A, Efrati S. Delayed recompression for decompression sickness: retrospective analysis. PLoS ONE. 2015;10(4):e0124919.

47. Chin W, Joo E, Ninokawa S, Popa DA, Covington DB. Efficacy of the U.S. Navy Treatment Tables in treating DCS in 103 recreational scuba divers. Undersea Hyperb Med. 2017;44(5):399-405.

48. Moon RE, Gorman DF. Decompression sickness. In: Neuman TS, Thom SR, editors. The Physiology and Medicine of Hyperbaric Oxygen Therapy. Philadelphia, PA: Saunders Elsevier; 2008. Pp. 283-319.

49. Navy Department. US Navy Diving Manual. Revision 7. Vol 5 : Diving Medicine and Recompression Chamber Operations. NAVSEA 0910-LP-115-1921. Washington, DC: Naval Sea Systems Command; 2016.

50. Mitchell SJ, Doolette DJ, Wachholz CJ, Vann RD, editors. Management of Mild or Marginal Decompression Illness in Remote Locations. Durham, NC: Divers Alert Network; 2005.

51. Mitchell SJ, Bennett MH, Bryson P, Butler FK, Doolette DJ, Holm JR, Kot J, Lafere P. Pre-hospital management of decompression illness: expert review of key principles and controversies. Diving Hyperb Med. 2018;48(1):45-55.

52. Ball R. Effect of severity, time to recompression with oxygen, and retreatment on outcome in forty-nine cases of spinal cord decompression sickness. Undersea Hyperb Med. 1993;20:133-45.

53. Ross JAS. Clinical Audit and Outcome Measures in the Treatment of Decompression Illness in Scotland. A report to the National Health Service in Scotland Common Services Agency, National Services Division on the conduct and outcome of treatment for decompression illness in Scotland from 1991-1999. Aberdeen, UK: Department of Environmental and Occupational Medicine, University of Aberdeen Medical School; 2000 27 April 2000.

54. Goodman MW, Workman RD. Minimal recompression oxygen-breathing approach to treatment of decompression sickness in divers and aviators. Washington, DC: US Navy Experimental Diving Unit Report #5-65; 1965.

55. Bennett MH, Mitchell SJ, Young D, King D. The use of deep tables in the treatment of decompression illness: the Hyperbaric Technicians and Nurses Association 2011 Workshop. Diving Hyperb Med. 2012;42(3):171-80.

56. Vann RD, Bute BP, Uguccioni DM, Smith LR. Prognostic factors in DCI in recreational divers. In: Moon RE, Sheffield PJ, editors. Treatment of Decompression Illness. Kensington, MD: Undersea and Hyperbaric Medical Society; 1996. Pp. 352-63.

57. Gempp E, Blatteau JE. Risk factors and treatment outcome in scuba divers with spinal cord decompression sickness. J Crit Care. 2010;25:236-42.

58. Rivera JC. Decompression sickness among divers: an analysis of 935 cases. Mil Med. 1964;129:314-34.

59. Workman RD. Treatment of bends with oxygen at high pressure. Aerosp Med. 1968;39:1076-83.

60. How J, Chan G. Management of delayed cases of decompression sickness--3 case reports. Singapore Med J. 1973;14(4):582-5.

61. Erde A, Edmonds C. Decompression sickness: a clinical series. J Occup Med. 1975;17(5):324-8.

62. Kizer KW. Delayed treatment of dysbarism: a retrospective review of 50 cases. JAMA. 1982;247(18):2555-8.

63. Meyers RAM, Bray P. Delayed treatment of serious decompression sickness. Ann Emerg Med. 1985;14:254-7.

64. Curley MD, Schwartz HJC, Zwingelberg KM. Neuropsychologic assessment of cerebral decompression sickness and gas embolism. Undersea Biomed Res. 1988;15:223-36.

65. Rudge FW, Shafer MR. The effect of delay on treatment outcome in altitude-induced decompression sickness. Aviat Space Environ Med. 1991;62:687-90.

66. Kindwall EP. Decompression sickness. In: Davis JC, Hunt TK, editors. Hyperbaric Oxygen Therapy. Bethesda, MD: Undersea Medical Society; 1977. Pp. 125-40.

67. Hart GB, Strauss MB, Lennon PA. The treatment of decompression sickness and air embolism in a monoplace chamber. J Hyperb Med. 1986;1:1-7.

68. Elliott DH, Kindwall EP. Decompression sickness. In: Kindwall EP, Whelan HT, editors. Hyperbaric Medicine Practice. Flagstaff, AZ: Best Publishing Co; 1999. Pp. 433-87.

69. Bond JG, Moon RE, Morris DL. Initial table treatment of decompression sickness and arterial gas embolism. Aviat Space Environ Med. 1990;61:738-43.

70. Cianci P, Slade JB, Jr. Delayed treatment of decompression sickness with short, no-air-break tables: review of 140 cases. Aviat Space Environ Med. 2006;77(10):1003-8.

71. Weaver LK. Monoplace hyperbaric chamber use of U.S. Navy Table 6: a 20-year experience. Undersea Hyperb Med. 2006;33(2):85-8.

72. Farm FP, Jr, Hayashi EM, Beckman EL. Diving and decompression sickness treatment practices among Hawaii's diving fisherman. Sea Grant Technical Paper UNIHI-SEAGRANT-TP-86-01. Sea Grant Technical Paper. Honolulu: University of Hawaii; 1986. Report No.: UNIHI-SEAGRANT-TP-86-01.

73. Doolette DJ, Mitchell SJ. In-water recompression. Diving Hyperb Med. 2018;48(2):84-95.

74. Pyle RL, Youngblood DA. In-water recompression as an emergency field treatment of decompression illness. SPUMS J. 1997;27:154-69.

75. Dituri J, Sadler R, Siddiqi F, Sadler C, Javeed N, Annis H, Whelan H. Echocardiographic evaluation of intracardiac venous gas emboli following in-water recompression. Undersea Hyperb Med. 2016;43(2):103-12.

76. Dart TS, Butler W. Towards new paradigms for the treatment of hypobaric decompression sickness. Aviat Space Environ Med. 1998;69(4):403-9.

77. Butler WP, Topper SM, Dart TS. USAF treatment table 8: Treatment for altitude decompression sickness. Aviat Space Environ Med. 2002;73(1):46-9.

78. Moon RE, editor. Adjunctive Therapy for Decompression Illness. Kensington, MD: Undersea and Hyperbaric Medical Society; 2003.

CHAPTER 8

Delayed Radiation Injuries (Soft Tissue and Bony Necrosis) and Potential for Future Research

John J. Feldmeier DO, FACRO, FUHM, Laurie B. Gesell MD, FACEP, FUHM

Introduction

The application of hyperbaric oxygen to the treatment and prevention of delayed radiation injury is the core topic for this chapter. A few miscellaneous topics will also be discussed, including areas of interest for research. We will also discuss some of the pertinent literature demonstrating the safety of HBO_2 for the cancer patient. The latest information available from the UHMS in 2019 indicates that delayed radiation injuries are now the most frequent indication for hyperbaric treatments in the United States. The management of delayed radiation injury, especially when bone is involved, requires a multi-disciplinary approach. Importantly, each aspect of treatment, including technique when surgery is needed, must be optimized to give the best chance for a successful therapeutic effort. In the pages that follow, the nature of delayed radiation injury, the mechanisms whereby hyperbaric oxygen is effective, clinical results, the effects of hyperbaric oxygen on cancer growth and future areas for research will be discussed. Recently, there have been several negative articles for hyperbaric oxygen in the management or prevention of mandibular necrosis. Many of these articles are limited in value since they either include patients who are at low risk for ORN after extractions because of any of the following: they were treated only to moderate doses of radiation; or the teeth extracted were outside the region of high radiation dose deposition; or they were maxillary teeth. With previous radiation techniques we would say outside the radiation field, but given the complexity of modern radiation planning, these areas might not be totally outside a combination of many beamlets that are employed in intensity modulated radiation therapy (IMRT), the common standard targeted therapy for head and neck cancers. Many in the radiation oncology community have predicted much lower incidence of radiation injury as the consequence of image-guided targeted techniques including IMRT.[1] It has not yet been firmly established that IMRT will deliver a lower incidence of ORN and other serious radiation complications at various sites.

In the treatment of osteoradionecrosis (ORN), other recent papers question the need for HBO_2 and instead advocate for microvascular surgery and free flaps when treating a Marx Stage III ORN patient who requires a segmental resection and reconstruction. See below for a more extensive discussion of these topics within the specific sections dedicated to them.

The Nature of Radiation Injury

Radiation injuries should be classified as acute, subacute or delayed complications.[2] Acute injuries are due to direct and essentially immediate cellular toxicity caused by free radical-mediated damage to DNA in normal cells surrounding the tumor. Many cells suffer a mitotic or reproductive death, i.e., enough damage has been rendered to the DNA that successful subsequent cell division and reproduction are prevented. This mechanism is felt to be the primary method by which most cancer cells are destroyed.[3] In normal tissues, these acute injuries occur most notably in rapidly dividing cells such as those lining the GI tract from mouth to anus.[4] These injuries are seen frequently in the oral and pharyngeal mucosa. Acute injuries to normal tissues are typically self-limited and almost invariably resolve within a few weeks of completing the course of radiation. They rarely persist beyond two months. Treatment is generally symptomatic providing nutritional support and pain control. Though self-limited, the acute injuries can be very debilitating throughout their duration and must not be neglected. Subacute injuries are typically identifiable in only a few organ systems. Subacute injuries have been shown to occur in the lung with a clinical syndrome mimicking bronchitis with onset between 8 to 12 weeks post radiation. When this syndrome occurs, it is termed radiation pneumonitis. Subacute injuries also occur in the spinal cord as the result of temporary demyelinization. The so-called Lhermitte's sign is caused by this damage.[5] In this syndrome, patients experience electric-like shocks (paresthesias) down their legs with spinal extension (forward bending). Subacute effects, too, are most often self-limited but on a rare occasion evolve to become delayed injuries. Some subacute injuries may persist for several months. Treatment is symptomatic. No specific treatment is especially effective although steroids are commonly employed. Supplemental oxygen may be required for patients with radiation pneumonitis. Delayed radiation complications are typically seen after a latent period of six months or more and may rarely develop many years after the radiation exposure.[4,6] Sometimes, especially when chemotherapy and radiation are given as combined modality treatment, acute injuries are so severe that they never resolve and evolve to become chronic injuries indistinguishable from other delayed radiation injuries.[7] Harmful effects evolving in this fashion are termed "consequential effects" and are not characterized by a symptom-free latent period. Often, delayed injuries are precipitated by an additional tissue insult such as trauma or surgery within the radiation field. On the other hand, frequently late radiation injuries are spontaneous, and no immediate precipitating insult or injury can be identified.

A role for hyperbaric oxygen in acute and subacute radiation injuries has not been well-studied or established, although there is some interest in pursuing this application.[8] Considerations of cost (both direct and indirect) would have to be considered along with efficacy in any hyperbaric intervention for these injuries because they almost always resolve with supportive care.

The Etiology of Delayed Radiation Injury

The exact causes and physical and biochemical processes leading to delayed radiation injury are complex and still only partially understood.[9] They continue to be studied.[4] In virtually all instances which demonstrate late radiation damage, we observe vascular changes characterized by obliterative endarteritis.[6,10-11] Because hyperbaric oxygen has been shown to enhance angiogenesis in hypoxic tissues, the hyperbaric oxygen community has traditionally postulated that the enhancement of angiogenesis is the primary therapeutic effect of hyperbaric oxygen in radiated tissues. Some radiation scientists are now convinced that at least in some organ systems, vascular changes play only a minor role in the evolution of delayed radiation injury and instead radiation-induced apoptosis and exuberant fibrosis are the predominant causes of delayed radiation injuries.[12]

Therefore, a more complex model of radiation damage continues to evolve in the radiation oncology community. In the past, radiation oncologists had made a distinction between the causes of acute and delayed injuries, suggesting that the mechanisms of injury were unrelated. Indeed, it is not uncommon to find a patient with serious acute reactions who does not suffer late complications or someone with severe delayed complications who had experienced no worse than minor acute radiation reactions. Radiation researchers now appreciate that the process of radiation injury is initiated at the time of radiation treatment and involves the elaboration and release of many bioactive substances prominently including fibrogenic cytokines.[13] The process whereby therapeutic radiation inflicts delayed damage on normal tissues has been recently described as the fibroatrophic effect by Delainian and associates.[12] This model emphasizes the consequences of the observed depletion of stem cells and subsequently parenchymal cells. It also highlights the exuberant fibrosis found in severely damaged irradiated tissues. In this model, vascular damage and stenosis continue to be recognized as a consistent finding in tissues exhibiting radiation damage including frank necrosis; however, endarteritis as a causative factor for delayed radiation injuries is not felt by this group to contribute significantly to delayed radiation injury, at least as a primary cause.

It has been demonstrated that chronically hypoxic tissues are subject to exuberant fibrosis mediated by HIF-1.[14] It is very likely that the fibrosis that is generated in radiated tissues is at least a partial consequence of radiation-induced vascular damage and consequent tissue hypoxia.[15] It is also likely that exuberant fibrosis seen in radiated tissues also is at least a partial causative factor of subsequent vascular damage by "squeezing out" or compressing small vessels.

A recent review of the mechanism of delayed effects of radiation has been accomplished by Fleckenstein et al.[13] The author of this paper focuses on delayed radiation injuries of the lung. This paper identifies TGF-beta as the most frequently studied cytokine associated with radiation injury. Additional cytokines associated with radiation injury include IL-1 (Interleukin-1), IL-2, IL- 4, IL-5, IL-6, IL-7, IL-8, IL-10, IL-12, IL-13, IL-17, TNF-alpha and GMCSF. The increase in these cytokines begins at the time of radiation, but the damage caused may take months or even years to be clinically expressed.

Many studies of cytokines and radiation injuries have been accomplished in animal models of radiation-induced pneumonitis.[16] To date, we have not been able to make practical clinical application of these observed associations, either as a predictor of or therapy for radiation injury. No single marker is likely to provide us with a reliable estimate of future radiation damage.[13] Similarly, no practical strategies have yet been developed to prevent or reduce the production of these cytokines or reduce their impact in a preventive fashion. We know that there is a very wide range of tolerance to radiation by individual patients based on heterogenous genetic makeup and that some patients are much more sensitive to radiation injury.[17] If reliable predictors of delayed radiation injury were available during or before treatment, adjustments to the radiation dosing and targeting scheme could be made for the radio-sensitive patient. Some exquisitely sensitive patients might be advised to seek alternative therapies (if available) instead of radiation if indeed these determinants reliably predict severe complications. Moreover, prophylactic interventions such as hyperbaric oxygen or other yet-to-be studied or applied pharmacologic interventions could be given before or during the latent period, i.e., before the manifestation of the chronic injury. Drugs that have shown promise to mitigate radiation injuries include antioxidants, free radical scavengers, inhibitors of apoptosis, anti-inflammatory drugs, angiotensin-converting enzyme inhibitors, growth factors, and cytokines.[9,18] The hope and expectation would be that, by identifying a group at risk and intervening in this group before manifestation of the injury, delayed radiation injury could be prevented or at least reduced in severity. Obviously, this premise will have to be subjected to clinical trials, and the most important consideration would be to do nothing that jeopardizes tumor control, i.e., do nothing that protects the tumor as well as normal tissues from radiation damage.

A similar intent (the prevention of radiation damage) led to the development of the Marx 20/10[19] protocol prior to dental extractions in heavily radiated patients (doses over 6000cGy) to prevent the clinical expression of mandibular necrosis, when not only the mandible itself but also the surrounding soft tissues suffer damage. This damage might be subclinical at that time. This group of patients will also have had significant compromise in the soft tissue of the head and neck surrounding the mandible that can be mitigated by HBO_2.

The Effects of Hyperbaric Oxygen on Irradiated Tissues

The impact of hyperbaric oxygen in terms of its beneficial effects is likely to involve at least three mechanisms in radiation damaged tissues:

1. Hyperbaric oxygen stimulates angiogenesis and secondarily improves tissue oxygenation.
2. Hyperbaric oxygen reduces fibrosis.
3. Hyperbaric oxygen mobilizes and induces an increase of stem cells within irradiated tissues that can differentiate, as needed, by that tissue.

Because a consistent manifestation of radiation injury is vascular damage and resultant hypoxia, the known impact of hyperbaric oxygen in stimulating angiogenesis continues to be an obvious and important mechanism, whereby hyperbaric oxygen is effective in radiation injury. HBO_2 induces neovascularization in hypoxic tissues. A recent animal study by Deschpande and colleagues[20] demonstrates a significant and quantifiable reduction in irradiated vasculature in rat mandible following irradiation. Marx[21] has demonstrated both the prehyperbaric oxygen vascular damage and the enhanced vascularity and cellularity in heavily irradiated tissues after hyperbaric oxygen therapy by comparing histologic specimens from patients pre- and posthyperbaric oxygen. Marx[21] has also demonstrated the serial improvement in transcutaneous oxygen measurements of patients receiving hyperbaric oxygen as an indirect measure of increased vascular density. Marx et al[21] in an animal model of irradiated rabbit mandibles with angiography have shown increased vascularity in mandibles after exposure to hyperbaric oxygen. Svalestad and associates[22] demonstrated in a controlled human study of irradiated patients employing Doppler flow studies and transcutaneous oxygen measurements that patients after HBO_2 had improved blood flow and improved tissue oxygen content as measured by serial transcutaneous measurements. Johnson-Arbor and her associates[23] have published a case report employing indocyanine green fluorescent angiography in a patient treated for breast necrosis and was shown to have a region of poor vascularity at the site of the injury that showed improved vascularity with HBO_2.

In fibrosis as one of the elements of radiation, Feldmeier and his colleagues[24-25] in a murine model of radiation damage to the small bowel have shown that hyperbaric oxygen given seven weeks after radiation can reduce the degree and mechanical effects of fibrosis by being applied prior to the manifestation of radiation injury. Assays of the murine bowel for collagen content included a mechanical stretch assay of compliance as well as quantitative histologic morphometric assays of fibrosis in the tunica media of the animal bowel utilizing Mason's trichrome staining, which stains collagenous materials blue.

Many head and neck cancer patients sustain woody fibrosis of the soft tissues of the neck after a full course of radiation.[26] The authors have personally observed and other clinicians have noted significant reduction in this woody fibrosis of soft tissues of the neck following a course of hyperbaric oxygen intended to treat mandibular necrosis. To our knowledge, this effect has not yet been systematically studied, and it is not readily apparent in all patients but is a frequent finding.

The hyperbaric study group headed up by Dr. Thom[27-28] while at the University of Pennsylvania has published studies demonstrating the mobilization of stem cells mediated through nitric oxide with HBO_2. These papers include an animal model as well as a group of head and neck cancer patients who had received radiation treatments. A putative effect on increasing stem cells at the site of radiation injury is confirmed to some extent by Marx's demonstration of increased cellular density in histologic preparations from patients initially demonstrating hypocellularity after hyperbaric oxygen for mandibular osteoradionecrosis.[21]

Hyperbaric oxygen has been applied as a therapy for delayed radiation injury for more than 40 years.[29-30] Hyperbaric oxygen as a neoadjuvant treatment prior to dental extractions is also supported by a randomized controlled trial and several other case series. The following sections will discuss the application of hyperbaric oxygen to radiation complications on an anatomic basis beginning with mandibular osteoradionecrosis.

Hyperbaric Oxygen as Treatment for Mandibular Radiation Necrosis (ORN)

One of the earliest and most frequently applied applications for hyperbaric oxygen in late and chronic radiation injury is its utilization in the treatment and prevention of radiation necrosis of the mandible. Multiple publications describing the use of hyperbaric oxygen in the treatment of mandibular necrosis have appeared in the medical literature since the 1970s.[29-30]

The likelihood of mandibular necrosis as a result of therapeutic radiation varies widely among several reports. During the era of mostly cobalt therapy and before IMRT, Bedwinek[31] reported a 0% incidence below doses of 6,000 cGy increasing to 1.8% at doses from 6,000 to 7,000 cGy and to 9% at doses greater than 7,000 cGy. In his comprehensive review of radiation tolerance, Emami[32] estimated a 5% incidence when a small portion of the mandible (less than one-third) is irradiated to 6500 cGy or higher and a 5% incidence at 6000 cGy or higher when a larger volume of the mandible is irradiated. Reuther and associates[33] at the University of Heidelberg in a 30-year review of 830 patients reported an 8.2% incidence of ORN and interestingly also reported resolution in only 40% of their patients of which the vast majority were managed conservatively. The current application of IMRT has been predicted to reduce mandibular radiation necrosis compared to older radiation techniques.[1,34] These referenced studies show that the volume of mandible included within the high dose volume is an important determinant of the occurrence of ORN. Recent publications of a now mature experience with IMRT are demonstrating an incidence of 7 to 10% of ORN in the IMRT era.[35-36] Besides the wide adoption of IMRT for head and neck cancers, an even more drastic change has been the adoption of primary radiation with chemotherapy sensitization as initial treatment for most head and neck cancers. Radical surgery is saved as an option for salvage of persistent or recurrent tumor.[37] This change in philosophy has increased radiation doses from 5,000 to 6,000 cGy as an adjuvant treatment to doses of 7,000 cGy or higher as curative primary doses. Chemotherapy, given often to act as a radiosensitizer, would be expected to increase normal tissue damage as well as enhance control of the malignancy.

Not all cases of exposed mandibular bone after radiation are ORN. It has been reported that 85% or more of cases resulting in initially exposed mandibular bone will resolve spontaneously with conservative management.[38] Unfortunately, when the exposed bone persists, the remaining cases generally become chronic and progressive. When ORN develops, it is typically accompanied by considerable insult to the surrounding soft tissues as well as bone. A useful impact of HBO$_2$ is to enhance the quality of soft tissues that surround the necrotic bone and, in this way, indirectly support its resolution.

Much of the early work in this area considered radiation-induced mandibular necrosis to be a subset of mandibular osteomyelitis. At the USAF Hyperbaric Medicine Center in San Antonio, there was an initial experience in delivering HBO$_2$ often along with antibiotics as treatment for mandibular necrosis without surgical management and after failure of more conservative therapy.[39] Although most cases would show temporary improvement including alleviation of the characteristic pain of ORN with HBO$_2$ as monotherapy, virtually all cases of moderate to severe ORN would recur if hyperbaric oxygen was administered without appropriate surgical debridement or resection.

Dr. Robert Marx, DDS. and his colleagues[21,39-40] elucidated many fundamental principles in the etiology and management of mandibular ORN which have led to a rationale approach to its management. Dr. Marx has provided several key principles in the understanding of the pathophysiology of mandibular necrosis. He has demonstrated that infection is not the primary etiology of mandibular necrosis by obtaining deep cultures of affected bone and showing the absence of bacteria.[39] Consistent with Marx's elucidation of the pathophysiology of mandibular ORN, it is appropriate to think of ORN as an avascular necrosis.[39] Since a major goal in applying hyperbaric oxygen is to enhance the vascular milieu, the bulk of the hyperbaric oxygen in his protocols is given prior to surgical wounding including dental extractions.[21] In this fashion, the normal soft tissues are conditioned to better deal with the stress and increased metabolic demand of surgical wounding. Marx has also shown that for hyperbaric oxygen to be consistently successful, it must be combined with surgery in an optimal fashion. The surgical procedures have evolved over the years with the advent of microvascular free flaps and other technical improvements including the use of adjuncts in bony reconstruction, but the importance of adjunctive HBO$_2$ has not changed and is still essential in Dr. Marx's experience.[21]

Marx has developed a staging system for classifying mandibular necrosis. This staging system is applied to determine the severity of mandibular necrosis. In addition, it permits a plan of therapeutic intervention, which is a logical outgrowth of the stage/severity of necrosis.[21] Note: There are other staging systems, but none has shown any clear superiority to the Marx system.[21,41]

Marx Stage I ORN: This stage includes those patients with persistently devitalized exposed bone who have none of the serious manifestations found in Stage III as described below. Generally, before hyperbaric oxygen, these patients have had chronically exposed bone for months or they have rapidly progressive ORN. These patients begin treatment with 30 HBO$_2$ sessions followed by relatively minor bony debridement. If these patients' response is adequate, an additional 10 daily treatments are given, and the patients are followed to complete clinical resolution.

Marx Stage II ORN: If patients are not progressing appropriately at 30 daily treatments or if a more major debridement is needed, they are advanced to Stage II and they receive a more radical surgical debridement or resection in the operating room followed by 10 postoperative treatments. This surgery is often an en bloc resection of the alveolar ridge. Surgery for Stage II patients must maintain mandibular continuity. If mandibular segmental resection is required, patients are advanced to Stage III and require reconstruction.

Marx Stage III ORN: In addition to those failing treatment in Stage I or II, patients who present initially with grave prognostic signs such as pathologic fracture, orocutaneous fistulae or evidence of lytic involvement extending to the inferior mandibular border are treated in Stage III from the outset. When a patient is assessed to be at Stage III, mandibular segmental resection is a planned part of the treatment from its initiation. In Stage III patients are entered into a reconstructive protocol after mandibular resection. Marx has established the principle that all necrotic bone must be surgically eradicated here just as in Stages I and II. Stage III patients receive 30 daily hyperbaric treatments prior to mandibular resection followed by 10 postresection treatments. At this surgery, this group of patients may require soft tissue enhancing procedures including free flaps or myocutaneous flaps.[21] Typically, after a period of about three months, the patients complete a reconstruction, which may involve various surgical techniques. In the original reports, the reconstruction made use of freeze-dried cadaveric bone trays from a split rib or iliac crest combined with autologous corticocancellous bone grafting. In 2019, microvascular free flaps are frequently used, most often employing an autologous fibula. In his original work at Wilford Hall USAF Medical Center, Marx had reconstruction patients complete a full additional course of hyperbaric treatments in support of the reconstruction. Marx has subsequently found that the vascular improvements accomplished during the initial 40 hyperbaric exposures are maintained over time and patients can undergo reconstruction without a second full course of HBO$_2$. Also, typically in the current version of the protocol, at the time of the resection a customized titanium tray is placed internally to maintain the anatomic and functional relationships of the mandible until the formal reconstruction is accomplished. In Marx's hands currently, cancellous bone is obtained by aspiration with a trocar from the ilium and that bone along with several adjuvants including growth factors, bone morphogenic protein and platelet rich plasma are combined in a cocktail and inserted into the mandibular deficit to complete the bony reconstruction.[21]

Marx[21] has recently reported his updated results in 914 patients treated according to the above protocol. In his hands with this technique, successful resolution has been achieved in 100% of patients. Unfortunately, the vast majority of patients require treatment as Stage III patients necessitating mandibular resection and reconstruction.[42] Dr. Marx has always sought cosmetic restoration as well as the success in supporting a denture. These two issues, cosmesis and restoration of dentition for mastication, are necessary components in improving quality of life in this group of patients.[43] In fact, Dr. Marx[21] has established six criteria for a successful mandibular reconstruction in an ORN patient requiring mandibular segmental resection:

1. Restoration of Jaw Continuity
2. Restoration of Alveolar Height
3. Restoration of Alveolar Width Suitable for Dental Implants
4. Restoration of Arch Form
5. Maintenance of Bone
6. Restoration of Facial Contours

Feldmeier and Hampson[44] published a review of hyperbaric oxygen in the treatment of radiation injury in 2002. A total of 14 papers reporting the results in the treatment of mandibular necrosis were included. All but one of these was a case series. A single study by Tobey et al.[22] was a positive randomized controlled trial. It was a very small study with only 12 patients enrolled; however, it was double-blinded and reported to be a positive trial by the authors. Details of randomization and outcome determinants were not clearly stated. Patients received either 100% oxygen at 1.2 atmospheres absolute (ATA) or 2.0 ATA. The paper states that those treated at 2.0 ATA "experienced significant improvement" compared to the control group.

Of the reports included in this review paper of 2002, only one report, the publication by Maier et al.,[45] failed to report a positive outcome in applying hyperbaric oxygen to the treatment of mandibular ORN. In this paper, Maier and colleagues added hyperbaric oxygen to their management only after the definitive surgery was done. They failed to heed Marx's guidance that the optimal management of mandibular ORN requires that the majority of HBO$_2$ be given prior to surgical debridement, resection or reconstruction in order to improve the quality of tissues prior to surgical wounding. Of note was how readily the Marx protocol was adopted and transferred successfully in both the academic and private practice setting as employed by those authors reviewed in this section of the Feldmeier-Hampson paper.[44]

Since that review, several additional papers have been added to the literature. A paper not included in the 2002 systemic review by Feldmeier and Hampson comes from Freiberger[46] and associates at Duke University. The authors of this publication report a high resolution or response rate of 88% with mean duration of 86.1 months of follow-up in their patients in non-smokers. Nine of their 57 patients receiving HBO$_2$ had recurrent malignancy. Forty-one of this group of 57 had ultimately failed previous treatment.

A multi-institutional randomized controlled trial by Annane et al.[47] reported negative results in their study applying hyperbaric oxygen to Marx Stage I ORN. These results have created a stir in the hyperbaric oxygen community. Patients were randomized to receive either 90 minutes of 100% O$_2$ at 2.4 ATA or a breathing gas mix delivering an equivalent partial pressure of oxygen to air at sea level for 30 daily treatments. The study design has received criticism from several circles. The most serious flaw in the study design was its failure to adhere to Marx's guidance and to integrate hyperbaric oxygen into a multi-disciplinary approach to ORN treatment. The study's apparent intent was to investigate whether the application of hyperbaric oxygen could obviate the need for surgery in early mandibular ORN. It is not surprising that the study had negative results because more than three decades earlier, Marx[40] had shown an absolute necessity of surgically eradicating all necrotic bone. The need to remove all necrotic bone to achieve resolution was also confirmed by Feldmeier et al.[48] in their earlier report of chest wall necrosis including some cases with ORN of the ribs and sternum.

Additional criticisms of this study by Annane have been made. Moon et al.[49] have shown that nearly two-thirds of the hyperbaric group received fewer than 22 hyperbaric treatments. Laden[50] points out that the patients assigned to the control group had a risk for developing decompression sickness with the gas mix they breathed (9% oxygen and 91% nitrogen) at 2.4 ATA. Mendenhall,[51] a prominent radiation oncologist from the University of Florida, in an editorial accompanying the Annane paper in the *Journal of Clinical Oncology* points out that the Annane paper was underpowered and therefore subject to question. He goes on, however, to state his belief that hyperbaric oxygen is not indicated for mandibular ORN. Interestingly, he also remarks that it is hard to understand why the HBO_2 group in the Annane study did worse than control.

In another paper subsequent to the Feldmeier and Hampson[44] review paper, Gal and associates[52] have published their results in treating a series of 30 patients with Marx Stage III mandibular ORN with debridement and often segmental resection and reconstruction employing microvascular anastomosis for free flaps. Twenty-one of these patients had previously been treated with hyperbaric oxygen without resolution. The specific number and profile of hyperbaric treatments was not described for any of these patients. At least some had undergone some debridement prior to coming to Gal. Once in the author's hands, they all had appropriate debridement or resection of all necrotic bone and reconstruction with free flaps. Those patients who had not seen hyperbaric oxygen previously had a complication rate of 22%, while the group who had received at least some hyperbaric oxygen had a much higher rate of complications of 52%. Of course, this was not a randomized trial, and even the authors suggest that the hyperbaric group may have represented a group with more refractory mandibular ORN. Obviously, in these patients those principles previously established by Marx, i.e., an emphasis on presurgical hyperbaric oxygen and debridement of all necrotic bone followed by reconstruction with postoperative hyperbaric oxygen, were not adhered to. The authors of this paper also discuss that Marx Stage III ORN patients represent a heterogeneous group with a broad range of injuries, severity of injuries, and a subsequent broad range of outcomes.

In a 2017 publication by Dielman et al.,[53] the authors present their recommendations for treatment of ORN based on experience with 27 patients with ORN out of 509 evaluated (5.3%) radiated patients in a retrospective review. They continue to recommend hyperbaric oxygen for Stage I and II ORN, but recommend primary surgical intervention for Stage III consisting of segmental resection and a free flap reconstruction without HBO_2. Hyperbaric oxygen is recommended in Stage III when there is extensive soft tissue damage or other complications which are not well delineated by the authors.

A series of papers from several centers beginning in 2008 and extending to 2018 recommend free flap reconstructions after resection of necrotic bone, including segmental resection of the mandible without hyperbaric oxygen for Stage III mandibular necrosis.[54-56] Their success rate in re-establishing mandibular continuity was on average approximately 85%. However, serious complication rates are on the order of 50%. In one report, re-operation is required in about 60% of patients. In these papers, dental rehabilitation with implants when reported was only accomplished on the order of 7 to 10%. Free flap patients characteristically require one or two days' care in an ICU and continued hospital-care thereafter for a week or more.

Teng and Futran[57] have also published their opinion that hyperbaric oxygen has no role in treating ORN. Their article presents no new clinical data and is a review article. The authors base their conclusions on the Annane study and the advancement of the fibro-atrophic model of radiation injury as now dominant in the opinion of many experts of radiation pathology.

Dr Sylvie Delainian,[58] a French radiation oncologist who has been the major proponent of the fibro-atrophic model of delayed radiation injury, has published several papers advocating a medical treatment for late radiation injuries including ORN. The protocol consists of pentoxifylline (800mg), Vitamin E 1000 IU) and clodronate (a bisphosphonate) (1600mg) daily Monday through Friday. On Saturday and Sunday, the patients receive prednisone (20mg) and ciprofloxacin (1000mg). Most notably she and her colleagues have completed and published a Phase II trial applying this treatment to 54 patients.[58] Thirteen of these patients are said to have failed HBO$_2$. Twenty-five patients had undergone surgical intervention previously. These patients were treated for 16±9 months. She reports complete response in all patients in a median time of nine months. She also reports that two-thirds of her patients were Stage III disease by the Epstein scale with fistula, fracture or "osteitis." Nearly one half (24) of these patients had only 1mm of exposed bone. The authors do state that the lesions were fairly minimal in extent with the average length of exposed bone 17±8mm. Thirty-six of these patients required "iterative sequestrectomies." Eight patients are reported to have nondisplaced fractures. Fifteen of 54 patients stopped their medical therapy early, and six of 54 or 11% of patients died of sepsis attributed to local severe infection, fistula or mandibular fracture progressing to cellulitis and sepsis. The authors considered even those patients who had exposed bone of up to 5 mm length at the completion of PENTOCLO treatment as "complete responders!"

These results are quite interesting and need to be confirmed in a randomized trial. Dr. Delianian[59] suggests that the medical combination therapy she advocates for ORN may have broad applicability to delayed radiation injuries of many organs and tissue types. She does advocate randomized controlled trials to confirm its routine use.

Hampson et al.[60] have recently reported a series of 411 patients treated for radiation injury involving multiple anatomic sites at the Virginia Mason Hyperbaric Center since 2002. The outcome of many of these patients has been previously reported in earlier publications. Among these patients, 62 patients were treated for mandibular necrosis. Forty-three were available for analysis and among these 73% showed resolution, 21% had 50-90% improvement, and the other 5% were unchanged.

Suffice it to say that recent papers addressing the efficacy of hyperbaric oxygen in the treatment of ORN have expressed divergent opinions. Several publications advocate no hyperbaric oxygen and instead fibular free flaps for mandibular reconstruction following segmental resection of Stage III ORN of the mandible. [53-55] As previously noted, these procedures have a high complication rate and rarely allow for dental rehabilitation with dental implants.

Advocates of this technique point out that patients are planned for a single surgery to resect the necrotic bone and accomplish the reconstruction. In part, they argue that patients are eager to have the surgery done in a single stage because they are impatient. Yet, these patients have been dealing with a chronic problem typically at least for several months, and are not likely to be too impatient at this point as long as they are seeing progress toward resolution. The free flap procedures typically require a hospital stay of several days or a week, and for the first day or two require intensive care. The procedure is quite expensive, especially when the required in-patient stay is considered. Per Dr. Marx, the cost is more than $90,000 per patient and increases even more if the patient must be returned to the operating room to relieve flap congestion, remove a venous clot or repair the anastomosis. These needed returns to the operating room occur from 5%-25% of patient reconstructions.

Only one of these recent publications (The Annane Study) was a randomized controlled trial, and it is subject to the criticisms in design as discussed above. If we look at the total body of literature reporting the impact of hyperbaric oxygen on mandibular ORN, we find that the publications reviewed in the Feldmeier/Hampson analysis,[21] a total of 371 cases of mandibular ORN are reported with a positive outcome in 310 or 83.6%. Unfortunately, some of the papers report improvement rather than resolution as their outcome determinate. Of course, a better determination of outcome would be resolution. In Marx's[21] studies, resolution is noted in 100% of cases and he has now reported on the treatment of 914 patients. Marx also indicates that success in Stage III patients requires not only re-establishment of mandibular continuity but also rehabilitation including the six criteria listed in the text above. The Freiberger[46] paper demonstrates a positive durable outcome in 86% of their 65 patients. By contrast, if we look at the recent trials not employing HBO$_2$, only 22 patients are included in the Gal report[28] and 31 patients randomized to hyperbaric oxygen in the Annane study.[47] The Delainian[58] Phase II study reported results in 54 patients.[57] Those papers reported above by Hirsch, Nolen and van Gemert employing free flap reconstruction for ORN, the numbers of patients studied in the respective publications were 21, 89 and 79 respectively. Practitioners of hyperbaric oxygen who treat mandibular ORN must do so in a multidisciplinary manner and ensure that treatment includes a reconstructive surgeon who can and will accomplish the needed extirpation of all necrotic bone. For Stage III patients, after resection and resultant discontinuity, patients must have the advantage of skilled reconstructive surgeons and the best modern surgical techniques.

Neoadjuvant HBO$_2$ Prior to Dental Extractions

Extraction of teeth from heavily irradiated jaws is a common precipitating factor for mandibular necrosis. In roughly one half of cases of ORN of the mandible, extractions or some other surgery is the precipitating event. The rest are spontaneous and may develop several to many years after the radiation.[33] Marx[19] has published the results of a randomized prospective trial wherein patients who had received a radiation dose of at least 6,800 cGy were randomly assigned to pre-extraction HBO$_2$ versus penicillin prophylaxis. Those patients assigned to the hyperbaric group completed 20 pre-extraction daily HBO$_2$ treatments with ten additional postextraction daily hyperbaric treatments. Thirty-seven patients were treated in each group. In the penicillin group, a total of 29.9% of patients developed ORN while only 5.4% of patients in the hyperbaric group developed necrosis. Also, the severity of ORN was more pronounced in the penicillin group with nearly three-quarters (8/11) requiring treatment as Stage III patients. Neither patient with ORN from the hyperbaric group required a resection with reconstruction and both resolved with treatment as Stage II ORN patients with additional hyperbaric oxygen and appropriate debridement.

The important principles advocated by Marx in the treatment as well as prevention of ORN include an emphasis on presurgical/pre-extraction hyperbaric oxygen to improve tolerance to surgical wounding including the soft tissues surrounding the mandible. Extraction technique is also very important in radiated patients. Many recommend that extraction sockets be closed, and a careful alveoloplasty should be accomplished to prevent any prominent or sharp bony prominences. Several reports recommend against elevation of the mucoperiosteum unless absolutely required. Other practitioners have applied these principles established by Marx and his colleagues and have had similar success in the prevention and treatment of mandibular necrosis. There are several additional positive case series reporting outcome in applying hyperbaric oxygen prior to dental extractions. Dr. Paul Lambert and associates[61] from Dayton, OH, VA Medical Center report their series of 47 evaluable patients who underwent HBO$_2$ in support of dental extractions following the Marx protocol. No ORN occurred following these extractions. In the publication of Vudiniabola et al.[62] following the Marx protocol in ORN prophylaxis, one of 29 patients experienced ORN while in a similar case series from David et al.,[63] one of 24 patients experienced mandibular ORN after extractions from a radiated mandible following the prophylactic application of hyperbaric oxygen. Another publication is the report of 40 patients by Chavez and Atkinson[64] in whom hyperbaric oxygen was applied in the manner prescribed by Marx (20 pre-extraction hyperbaric treatments followed by 10 postextraction). The authors report that uncomplicated healing of tooth sockets was observed in 98.5% of extractions. In the recent review by Hampson et al.,[60] a total of 210 patients were treated prior to dental extractions to prevent frank ORN. One hundred sixty-six patients were available for evaluation, and among this group, 100% were felt to have a major response and 92% had no evidence of ORN.

An even larger experience comes from the latest update of Marx's[21] results in extracting teeth in high risk patients. In this update applying the 20/10 protocol for over 30 years in high-risk patients, he reports a 0.75% incidence of ORN in 936 patients involving the extraction of 2,019 teeth.

Sulaiman et al.[65] from Sloan-Kettering report their results in dental extractions in a series of 187 previously irradiated patients. Only three patients in this group received hyperbaric oxygen, and the authors report that most received radiation doses between 6000 and 7000 cGy. Mandibular ORN developed in only four of the 180 cases (2.2%). The authors attribute this excellent result to their "atraumatic" technique in extracting the teeth. They question the need for hyperbaric oxygen if their surgical techniques are emulated. In this group of patients one half of the teeth extracted were outside the radiation field. Marx's patients in his prophylactic study all had teeth extracted from within the radiation fields and had doses of 6800cGy or greater while in the Sulaiman report 68% received doses lower than 6900 cGy. Twenty-one percent received doses less than or equal to 5900 cGy. Twenty percent of patients had extractions of anterior teeth, likely outside the radiation treatment ports.

Other authors have likewise presented series of patients in whom hyperbaric oxygen was not used pre-extractions and ORN incidence was low. In all these papers, groups of low-risk patients were included, including extractions of maxillary teeth, anterior mandibular teeth outside the radiation field and patients who received low total radiation doses. In the paper by Makkonen et al.[66] from 1986, i.e., before the IMRT era, the authors report the results in 25 patients who had a total of 94 teeth extracted after radiation and found no cases of ORN. However, this group included many low-risk patients. Six patients had maxillary tooth extractions. Eleven were lymphomas, and the median radiation dose for this group was only 4,100 cGy. Of the 66 mandibular extractions, 47 were either incisors or canine teeth, i.e., anterior teeth outside the typical radiation fields.

In another paper from 1991, Maxymiw et al.[67] from Princess Margaret, the group reported 72 patients with 449 teeth extracted. This group of patients was largely a low-risk group: median radiation dose less than 5,000 cGy, only 44% of teeth were within the radiation field and 44% of the teeth were in the maxilla.

In 2007 Lye and co-authors[68] reported another series of 40 patients undergoing a total of 155 extractions without HBO$_2$ and prospectively followed and evaluated for delayed healing and ORN after radiation. Patients were classified as demonstrating normal healing, delayed healing or ORN. Those patients exhibiting delayed healing were 5.8% of the total and those developing ORN was 1.9%. This report also included a sizeable number of low-risk patients. Forty-one percent were maxillary teeth, and another 23% were anterior mandibular teeth likely outside the radiation field.

Dr. Lewis Clayman[69] published a review paper in 1997 stating the data didn't support mandatory use of HBO$_2$ before removing teeth in irradiated mandibles." As a review paper, the publication included no original data. Dr. Clayman presents a series of articles in which patients with low risk for ORN are key to his conclusions. These include the papers by Makkonen[66] and Maximiw,[67] which are discussed above pointing out their inclusion of low-risk patients, including those with low doses, teeth outside the radiation portals and maxillary teeth. Dr. Clayman recommends that extractions be done by dentists experienced in dealing with irradiated patients and that they utilize careful technique.

Michael Wahl,[70] a dentist in private practice, published a review article in 2006 in the most prominent radiation oncology journal. Many of the papers included in his review are subject to the same criticisms applied to the Clayman paper. No new data were presented in this paper. In this review, he concluded there was not sufficient evidence to support the use of prophylactic HBO_2 treatments before extractions or other oral surgical procedures in radiation patients.

Again, in evaluating the literature both positive and negative for peri-extraction HBO_2 in support of dental extractions, we must look carefully to the details of the publication. When high-risk patients are included, the publications recorded above do indeed support HBO_2 with the intent of extracting teeth without triggering the onset of ORN; whereas, patients in a low-risk status do not benefit from HBO_2 to support their dental extractions. In order to sort out which patients are in the high- versus low-risk categories, the hyperbaric physician must obtain the radiation records and ideally discuss the case with the treating radiation oncologist given the complexity of modern IMRT-based radiation treatment planning.

Laryngeal Necrosis and Other Soft Tissue Necroses of the Head and Neck

Laryngeal necrosis is an uncommon complication of radiation therapy for head and neck cancer. In well designed and appropriately fractionated radiation treatments, its incidence should be less than 1%. [71-72] However, when persistent edema, fetid breath or visible necrosis persist for more than six months after completion of irradiation, the standard recommendation has been to accomplish a laryngectomy because the likelihood of persistent tumor is very high and even if there is no recurrent or persistent malignancy, there are no effective therapies to reverse necrosis.[73] Biopsy in order to eliminate the presence of cancer may be necessary. Biopsies, however, must be done with caution and are subject to sampling error. Often, the residual cancer is not readily visible on endoscopy and may be submucosal, thus requiring several random biopsies. Aggressive biopsies and the resultant surgical wounding of already injured tissues may further exacerbate tissue damage.

Chandler[74] has established a system to grade the severity of laryngeal necrosis. Most with Grade 1 and 2 levels of necrosis will resolve with conservative treatment. Patients suffering from Grade 3 or 4 necrosis are very likely to require laryngectomy. Five institutions have now published case series in applying hyperbaric oxygen to the treatment of radiation laryngeal necrosis.[60,75-78] Additionally, a new single case report has also been published.[79] In the earlier reports, most patients were treated for severe laryngeal necrosis (Chandler Grade 3 or 4). The outcome in a total of 44 cases is reported and only six patients were failures to treatment and required total laryngectomy.[75-79] The other 38 patients maintained their voice box and most ultimately had good voice quality.

In the recent very large case series of multiple different sites of radiation injury assessed prospectively and reported by Hampson et al.,[60] there were 27 patients treated and evaluable for soft tissue necrosis of the larynx. Improvement by at least 50% was seen in 82% of these patients. Twenty patients were retrospectively graded by the Chandler's system described above, and 18 of 20 were advanced Grade (Chandler's Grade 3 or 4). All but one of these patients improved by at least one Chandler's grade and 11 improved by two or more Chandler's grades. Two patients completed HBO_2 at a Grade 3 or 4 and likely progressed to laryngectomy although that information was not provided in the manuscript. In the case report by Hsu et al.,[79] their patient with Chandler's Grade 4 had complete resolution after 40 hyperbaric oxygen treatments.

In addition to laryngeal necrosis, there are several published reports addressing the results of hyperbaric oxygen treatment in other soft tissue injuries of the head and neck. Many of these deal with soft tissue necrosis of the neck and failing flaps within irradiated fields. In the Whelan-Kindwall *Hyperbaric Medicine Practice 4th Edition* textbook, Dr. Marx[21] has reported extensive experience in treating soft tissue radiation injuries of the head and neck. In a controlled, randomized report of 240 patients requiring flaps (pedicled or free flaps) to repair soft tissue damage or replace surgically removed or damaged soft tissues, he has compared wound infection, dehiscence and delayed healing in a hyperbaric group receiving the 20/10 protocol versus a control group. He found that HBO_2 patients experienced 11% wound infection versus 37% control; 6% dehiscence versus 26% control; and 14% delayed wound healing versus 46% control respectively in HBO_2 vs non-HBO_2 patients. All differences are statistically significant with a P value equal to 0.005.

Like results have also been reported by other authors. Davis and his colleagues[80] have reported successful treatment in 15 of 16 patients with soft tissue necrosis of the head and neck including many with extensive necrotic wounds.

In 1997, Neovius and colleagues[81] reported a series of 15 patients treated with hyperbaric oxygen for wound complications after surgery within an irradiated field. They compared this group to a carefully matched historical control group from the same institution. Twelve of the 15 patients in the hyperbaric group healed completely with improvement in two and only one without benefit. In the control group only seven of 15 patients healed. Two patients in the control group also developed life-threatening hemorrhage and one of these did indeed exsanguinate. Any practitioner experienced in the management of head and neck cancer patients has experienced at least one patient in his or her career who has died from exsanguination as the result of a soft tissue necrosis of the neck, which progressed to erode into the carotid artery or other major vessel. No serious bleeds occurred in the hyperbaric group.

In another group of patients, Feldmeier and colleagues[82] have reported in abstract form the successful adjuvant treatment of patients undergoing radical surgical resection for salvage of recurrent or persistent head and neck cancer following full course prior irradiation. Serious surgical complications, including occasional fatalities, have been reported to occur in over 60% of patients undergoing radical cancer salvage surgery within a previously irradiated field without the benefit of HBO_2.[83-84] With a short course of HBO_2 initiated immediately after surgery (median number of treatments 12), 87.5% of patients healed their surgical wounds with no serious complications. In this group, no deaths occurred in the immediate postoperative period.

Miscellaneous Soft Tissue Injuries of Head and Neck Cancer Patients: A Potential as Preventive Treatment and to Enhance Quality of Life (QoL)

Head and neck cancer patients are now being cured in about two-thirds of cases. Radiation therapy is a mainstay of this curative treatment. An interesting new promising application for hyperbaric oxygen is an application to head and neck cancer patients soon after radiation to ameliorate acute radiation injuries and improve quality of life.

Gerlach and associates[85] accomplished a quality of life prospective study on a group of 21 head and neck patients receiving hyperbaric oxygen for either prevention or treatment of ORN. The patients received hyperbaric oxygen between four months and five years after completion of their radiation. The hyperbaric exposure was 85 minutes of 100% oxygen at 2.5 ATA for a total of 30 to 40 treatments with the majority given before any surgical procedures much like the Marx 20/10 and 30/10 protocols. Radiation doses varied from 5,000 to 7,000 cGy. The patients completed a subjective questionnaire before HBO_2 and at one and two years post-HBO_2. A European

Organization for Research and Treatment of Cancer questionnaire was employed to compare several parameters of quality of life (QoL). The questionnaire was completed before HBO_2 and at 12 and 24 months post-HBO_2. The authors report improvement in swallowing, subjective improvement in volume of saliva and improvement in taste at both follow-up time intervals. At 24 months, swallowing problems had decreased by 23%, the subjective perception of saliva had improved by 13%, and subjective improvement in taste had improved by 22%. Subsequent to this study, Teguh and colleagues[9] have conducted a small randomized trial of 19 patients where the study group of patients immediately following a full course of radiation received 30 hyperbaric treatments at 2.5 ATA for 90 minutes. These investigators also employed a quality of life questionnaire from the European Organization for Research and Treatment of Cancer. Improved outcomes for these patients compared to control included improved swallowing, improved quality and quantity of saliva and decreased oral pain.

These reports are certainly promising and warrant further investigation. While we make progress in the control of cancer, QoL issues have become all the more important and are rightfully the topic of frequent study in the oncology community. The discussion above in developing biochemical predictors of the severity of effects of treatment on the individual cancer patient might allow us to intervene early in a group of patients found to have a high likelihood of significant diminishment in QoL based on a reliable predictor or group of predictors or clinical considerations such as re-irradiation after an initial failure. While it is probably not fiscally possible to offer all cancer patients a course of HBO_2 to result in an improved QoL and it is unlikely that this entire group would be willing to subject themselves to HBO_2 after a long and rigorous course of oncologic treatment, it may be possible and appropriate to offer this therapy to a subset of patients at high risk for these long-term effects of treatment that will decrease their enjoyment of the years of life provided by modern aggressive oncologic treatments. Here, too, the promise of this type of treatment must be established by additional quality research.

Chest Wall Necrosis

Radiation therapy after lumpectomy has become the preferred treatment for most early breast cancers.[86] After this treatment, fat necrosis of the intact breast has been reported but is an uncommon clinical problem. Radiation therapy is frequently used as an adjuvant treatment following mastectomy in more advanced cancers for large tumors, when axillary metastases are present or if it is the patient's preference. When a patient is irradiated after mastectomy, the radiation dose to the skin is not designed to provide a skin dose sparring effect because the treatment is designed to cover the dermal lymphatic vessels which may harbor microscopic metastases. As a result of this standard radiation technique, most women irradiated after mastectomy are subject to brisk acute radiation reactions including inflammation, brisk dermatitis, sometimes ulceration and accompanying pain. Some patients experience large areas of moist desquamation accompanied by superficial ulceration during and just after radiation treatments. Frank necrosis of the chest wall is fairly uncommon but is very difficult to manage when it does occur. Traditional treatment for chest wall necrosis has required extensive surgical debridement and frequently closure with omental or myocutaneous flaps originating outside the radiation field to ensure a vascular supply which is unimpaired by radiation vascular injury.

As early as 1976, Hart and Mainous[29] reported the successful application of hyperbaric oxygen as an adjunct to skin grafting in women treated for necrosis of the chest wall after mastectomy. Feldmeier and colleagues[87] in 1995 reported the outcome in applying hyperbaric oxygen as treatment of both soft tissue and bony necrosis of the chest wall. In this report, all patients who were cancer-free and suffered only soft tissue necrosis were treated successfully. However, only eight of 15 patients who also had ORN of the ribs or sternum achieved resolution. The common characteristic in these failed cases was the failure to surgically eliminate all necrotic bone. As discussed above, Marx had previously demonstrated the necessity of total extirpation of necrotic bone for the treatment of mandibular necrosis. This general principle should apply to osteoradionecrosis at any site.

Carl and Hartmann,[88] then from the University of Düsseldorf in 1998, reported a single case of a patient who had experienced long-standing, painful breast edema following lumpectomy and postoperative radiation. After 15 daily hyperbaric treatments of 90 minutes of 100% hyperbaric oxygen at 2.4 ATA, the patient experienced complete resolution of pain and edema.

In a second publication, Carl and his associates[89] in 2001 reported the outcome of 44 patients who experienced complications following lumpectomy and irradiation for early breast cancers. These patients were found to have pain, edema, fibrosis and telengectasias as a consequence of their irradiation. Each patient experienced these complications in various combinations and to varying degrees of severity. The severity of symptoms was assessed with a score for each patient based on a modified LENT-SOMA score, (Late Effects Normal Tissue Task Force-Subjective, Objective, Management, Analytic), a validated and often applied system for grading radiation damage.[90] Each patient was assessed a score from 1 to 4 in the severity of symptoms in the categories of pain, edema, fibrosis/ fat necrosis and telangectasia/erythema. Only patients with at least grade 3 pain (persistent and intense) or a summed LENT-SOMA score of at least 8 were studied. Thirty-two patients agreed to undergo hyperbaric oxygen treatment while 12 women refused HBO$_2$ and constituted the control group. Hyperbaric oxygen treatments resulted in a statistically significant reduction in the post-treatment LENT-SOMA scores in women receiving treatment compared to those who did not; however, in this study fibrosis and telangiectasia were not reduced. All women in the control group continued to demonstrate symptoms at the completion of the trial with no improvement in pain or edema. Seven women in the hyperbaric group had complete resolution of their symptoms.

Teguh and associates[91] reported a group of 57 prospectively followed women who suffered late radiation damage and symptoms after breast conserving treatment. Their symptoms and response are as follows: For severe pain in the arm and shoulder prior to HBO$_2$ 46%, post-HBO$_2$ 17%; for swollen arm and hand prior to HBO$_2$ 14%, after 7%; for difficulty in lifting arm or moving it sideways before HBO$_2$ 45%, after 22%; for pain in the breast before HBO$_2$ 67%, after 15%; for swelling in breast 45% before HBO$_2$, after 13%; for hypersensitivity of the breast before HBO$_2$ 54%, and after 15%; for abnormal skin changes in the breast before HBO$_2$ 32% and after 11%. Symptoms were reduced by two-thirds in most categories and at least one-half in the rest.

Enomoto and colleagues[92] reported in 2017 a case of a 74-year-old woman who 25 years after adjuvant radiation following mastectomy to her chest wall and lymphatics developed a chronic draining skin ulcer with undermining and a fistulous tract. She was reported to also have "osteomyelitis" of the ribs. More likely this was ORN. She completed 101 HBO$_2$ treatments consisting of 100% oxygen at 2.5 ATA with complete resolution.

Radiation Cystitis

Radiation therapy is commonly delivered to tumors of the pelvis including rectal cancers, gynecologic malignancies and prostate cancer. Radiation cystitis is not a common complication but can be very difficult to manage when it does occur. In its most serious manifestations, it may even require cystectomy and diversion of the urinary stream. Conservative measures include the installation of formalin or alum as chemical cautery agents into the bladder lumen. Feldmeier and Hampson[44] in a review article discuss 17 papers wherein hyperbaric oxygen has been delivered for this indication. At the time of this review, the paper by Bevers et al.[93] was the largest series. It was a prospective but nonrandomized and noncontrolled trial. All the other reports were case series. Many, if not most, of the patients reported in these series and subsequent series had already failed other conservative measures. When we combine all of the patients from these 17 papers, we find that 76.3% of 145 patients resolved with HBO$_2$.

Since this review article, there have been additional reports of hyperbaric oxygen for radiation cystitis. Neheman et al.[94] from Israel have published their results in a case series of seven patients. These patients received a mean number of 30 daily hyperbaric oxygen treatments. Patients were treated at 2.0 ATA for 90 minutes of 100% oxygen exposure. All seven patients had initial resolution of their hematuria. Two recurred and again received hyperbaric oxygen, with an additional 30 and 37 treatments respectively, the recurrent hematuria again resolved. Another patient had resolution of hematuria after 20 hyperbaric oxygen treatments but had progressive tumor (a primitive neuroectodermal tumor) and died as a result of the malignancy.

In a publication from 2003 Corman et al.,[95] the authors report a series from Virginia Mason of 57 patients in 2003 treated for radiation cystitis with HBO_2. Chong et al.[96] have updated this series in 2005 with an additional three patients. In this report, the average number of treatments was 33 at 2.36 ATA for 90 minutes of 100% oxygen. In the first paper, 80% of those treated had either complete or partial resolution. For those experiencing clot retention, six had complete resolution and 26 partial resolution. Eight had no change and two worsened.

In the publication by Chong et al.[96] discussed above, the authors report the importance of early intervention. In their analysis, they have found that the rate of improvement increases from 80 to 96% when HBO_2 begins within six months of onset of hematuria. Improvement in clot retention was seen in 100% of those who began treatment within six months. Another notable advantage of this trial is that outcomes were reported at least 12 months after completion of HBO_2 treatment. The evaluation at this point is indicative of a durable response and does not include that group which may see early response but then experience recurrence in a relatively short time period.

In a third publication from this group, results in the hyperbaric treatment of 411 patients with various radiation injuries treated at the Virginia Mason Hyperbaric Medicine Section between 2002 and 2010 are reported. Hampson et al.[60] report 44 evaluable cases treated for radiation cystitis. In this group, the average number of treatments was 42. Fifty-seven percent achieved complete response and another 32% improved from 50 to 90%. No patients receiving HBO_2 demonstrated progression during the period of follow-up.

A very recent review article was accomplished in 2018 by Cardinal et al.[97] The authors selected 16 papers for inclusion. These papers reported the results on 602 patients with radiation-induced cystitis of whom 84% had at a partial or complete response. Recurrences were reported in 10 of the papers included in this review where 12-month follow-up was available. Fourteen percent recurred at time intervals between three and 120 months (median 10 months).

Hemorrhagic cystitis is often a serious and not uncommonly a life-threatening disorder. Cheng and Foo[98] have reported their results in treating nine patients with refractory radiation-induced hemorrhagic cystitis without hyperbaric oxygen. Six of these patients required bilateral percutaneous nephrostomies while three patients required cystectomy and ileal loop diversions of their urinary stream. In spite of aggressive surgical intervention, 44% of the patients in this series died as the result of their cystitis. In another review by Li and colleagues,[99] the authors report a 3.7% mortality rate in their review of 378 patients experiencing hemorrhagic cystitis. All these patients had been irradiated for cervical cancer.

In summary, the vast majority of published series applying hyperbaric oxygen to radiation cystitis are positive reports. This success rate is especially noteworthy when compared to those publications cited above highlighting a poor outcome and significant mortality rate when HBO_2 is not administered, even when radical surgical intervention is employed. Also, many of those reporting HBO_2 for radiation cystitis identify a significant recurrence rate in spite of a good initial response. Hampson has reported an average of 40 or more treatments in the treatment of radiation cystitis and has also noted the importance of early intervention. Several authors report a second course of HBO_2 for those with recurrence and that in most cases they also report a positive response. The authors of this chapter have experienced a group of patients who may require 60 or more treatments to achieve durable resolution and believe that it is reasonable to offer patients more than the typical number of 40 HBO$_2$ treatments recommended in radiation injury elsewhere as long as these patients continue to demonstrate response but still have significant evidence of ongoing radiation damage. It is also reasonable to offer patients a second course of hyperbaric oxygen therapy if they recur after a positive response to an initial course of therapy.

Radiation Proctitis and Enteritis

For the most part, radiation enteritis and proctitis have been addressed together in previous publications. In regard to their incidence, a paradox exists. The small intestine is known to be more sensitive, i.e., subject to damage at lower radiation doses, but the colon and especially the rectum are more frequently injured in clinical practice. This seeming contradiction occurs because modern targeted radiation techniques are much more successful in avoiding the small bowel. Whereas, the large bowel, because much of it is in a fixed position in the retroperitoneum and because it is usually in much closer proximity to tumor sites in the prostate, uterus, uterine cervix or even the rectum itself, more commonly receives a potentially damaging radiation dose.

An animal study has been reported by Feldmeier and associates[24-25] wherein HBO$_2$ was shown to be highly successful in preventing radiation-induced enteritis. In this study, experimental animals received HBO$_2$ in a prophylactic setting seven weeks after radiation exposure. Animals were euthanized seven months after the radiation exposure. Both gross and histologic morphometry were accomplished and demonstrated a statistically significant reduction in signs of enteritis in the experimental group compared to the radiation only control group. Additionally, both quantitative histologic morphometry and a mechanical stretch test demonstrated significant reduction in submucosal fibrosis and an increase in mechanical compliance for hyperbaric treated animals.

In the review by Feldmeier and Hampson from 2002,[44] nine clinical papers reporting the results of hyperbaric oxygen in the treatment of enteritis or proctitis had been identified. These publications present a total of 114 cases. Forty-one (36%) of these patients were treated with complete resolution while another 68 (60%) had improved symptoms. Four percent of patients had no benefit from treatment.

A case report by Neurath and colleagues[100] documents the successful resolution of severe malabsorption due to established radiation enteritis in a 53-year-old female following 20 hyperbaric treatments at 3.0 ATA for 90 minutes.

Since the systematic review of 2002, additional papers on this topic have been published. Jones et al.[101] have reported their experience in treating 10 patients with HBO$_2$ for radiation-induced proctitis. Three of their patients had grade 3 toxicity (bleeding necessitating transfusion). The seven remaining patients had grade 2 toxicity, due to rectal pain and/or diarrhea. Six of these had rectal bleeding but had not required transfusion. Nine of these 10 patients completed treatment without complications. Rectal bleeding resolved in four patients while improvement was seen in three others. One patient discontinued treatment after the chamber facility at which he was being treated had been closed for an extended time due to concerns related to potential SARS exposure. Two patients failed to respond. Rectal pain resolved in three of five patients affected. In those suffering chronic diarrhea, one of five resolved and three improved. Of the 10 patients in this series, only two failed to experience demonstrable improvement. In this study, median follow-up was 25 months showing durability.

In another series from Girnius et al.[102] from Cincinnati, nine patients with hemorrhagic proctitis were treated with hyperbaric oxygen. Five patients had previously required transfusion, and three had been unsuccessfully treated with argon plasma coagulation or electrocautery. The authors report with median follow-up of 17 months, complete resolution in seven of the nine. The remaining two had improvement but still had some bleeding.

The Virginia Mason group has published their previous experience with radiation-induced proctitis and enteritis in two publications.[103-104] A total of 65 patients are reported, 37 male and 28 female. All had endoscopic documentation of their injury. The injuries included 54 rectal injuries with 15 in the more proximal GI tract (4 stomach, 7 small bowel, 6 colon and 6 duodenum). More than 65 injuries are reported because some patients had multiple injuries. These patients had an initial 30 HBO_2 treatments at 2.36 ATA for 90 minutes of 100% O_2. In those patients demonstrating a partial response at this point, additional treatments were delivered (6 to 30 treatments). Complete overall response rate was 43% (28 patients), and partial response 25% (16 patients). The results were somewhat worse for rectal cancer with a response rate of 65% compared to 73% for more proximal lesions.

In a randomized, controlled, double-blinded trial sponsored by the Baromedical Research Foundation, Clarke et al.[105] have reported their results in applying hyperbaric oxygen to patients with refractory chronic radiation-induced proctitis. One hundred fifty patients were enrolled in the trial, and 120 were evaluable. Patients were assessed utilizing the LENT-SOMA scoring systems which have become standard in studies of radiation injuries/complications. Patients in the active arm were treated on 100% at 2.0 ATA. Sham patients were exposed to very slightly elevated pressures (1.1 ATA) breathing air. The intent was to accomplish blinding of the control patients by giving them a sense of pressurization without enhanced oxygenation. After 30 treatments, reassessment was made by the referring physician who was blinded, and, in select patients who had shown partial response, an additional 10 treatments were accomplished. Ultimately, control patients were offered the opportunity to cross over to hyperbaric oxygen and all but three agreed to do so. With an average follow-up of two years (minimum one1 year), those patients in the active arm showed a statistically increased improvement in their LENT-SOMA scores (5.00 vs 2.61) with a p value of 0.0019. Responders in the active arm were 88.9% vs. 62.5% in the control arm (p = 0.00009). The absolute risk reduction was 32% and the number needed to treat was three. These results are impressive. The researchers are to be commended in the rigorous design and conduct of the trial. This report adds an important contribution of Level 1 evidence to the case series and reports discussed above.

An updated experience in treating radiation-induced proctitis and enteritis from the Virginia Mason group is included in their general review of the treatment of radiation injuries from 2002 to 2010. For enteritis and proctitis, this group reports a resolution rate of 25%; an improvement of 50-90% in 38%; an improvement of less than 50% in 25%; and an unchanged status in 12%.[60] It is likely that some patients had been reported in earlier papers from this same group.

Glover and co-investigators[106] in 2015 reported the results of a randomized, double-blinded controlled trial investigating HBO_2 for radiation proctitis. Eighty-four patients were randomized (55 to hyperbaric treatment and 29 to a sham control). The hyperbaric profile consisted of a total of 40 exposures at 2.4 ATA, five days per week, for 90 minutes of 100% oxygen at pressure over eight weeks' time. The investigators had two major endpoints for the study: change in the inflammatory bowel disease questionnaire (IBDQ) and change in rectal bleeding score. These metrics were determined for each patient at initiation of treatment, at two weeks post-treatment and 12 months post-treatment. No significant changes were detected in either measure at these follow-up points.

Several criticisms have appeared in print relative to this study. These include their reports of some patients with minimal symptoms, the employment of the IBDQ which was designed to follow patients with inflammatory bowel problems not radiation injury, and the long duration of proctitis before entering into the trial (a median of 43 months).

The American Society of Colon and Rectal Surgeons published their clinical practice guidelines for the treatment of chronic radiation proctitis in 2018.[107] In this paper, they define the problem of chronic radiation proctitis, discuss systemic and topical chemical and pharmacologic interventions, including oral mesalamine, formalin instillation and sucralfate enemas, as well as review physical measures such as argon plasma coagulation, electrocoagulation and radiofrequency ablation. They also discuss hyperbaric oxygen and reference several publications. In this review and in the formulation of their guidelines, they determine that HBO_2 is a class 1B indication, i.e., it is strongly indicated based on moderate quality evidence.

Other Abdominal and Pelvic Injuries

In 1978 Farmer and associates[108] reported a single case of vaginal necrosis, which resolved with hyperbaric oxygen. In 1992, Williams and colleagues[109] reported their results in treating 14 patients with vaginal necrosis. Thirteen of 14 patients had complete resolution, although one responding patient required a second course of hyperbaric oxygen. In 1997 Feldmeier and his co-authors[110] published their results in a review of 44 patients treated with HBO_2 at 2.4 ATA for 90 minutes for a variety of pelvic and abdominal injuries. Forty-one were available for follow-up. Six patients had necrotic wounds in the groin. Four of these healed and two were not available for follow-up. Two patients were treated for pelvic bone necrosis. One healed after 48 treatments. The other refused additional treatments after just five treatments and did not respond. Seven had perineal wounds. Three of these had complete healing. Two had inadequate treatment. One was lost to follow-up, and one did not heal. Five had vaginal necrosis and all healed. Another 16 had cutaneous nonhealing wounds of the abdominal wall and will be discussed in the section on skin injury below. Eight had bowel injuries and were already included in the section above on bowel injury.[44] Thirty-one of these patients in all categories received at least 20 hyperbaric treatments for radiation injuries to the perineum, groin, vagina and pelvic bone. Twenty-six (84%) of these patients had complete resolution of their radiation injury. Of note was the subset of eight patients with rectovaginal or rectovesical fistulae. In this group, six resolved and three of these did not require surgical intervention. Two did not resolve. Closure of fistulae after radiation is an especially difficult problem generally requiring major surgical excisions and reconstructions employing omental flaps, and even with these interventions, the failure rate is high.

In a more recent publication by Fink et al.,[111] a series of 14 patients treated with HBO_2 for a variety of pelvic injuries is reported. Six of these patients had vaginal injuries (four with ulcers, one with stenosis and one characterized only as vaginitis). Several of these patients had injuries to more than one organ simultaneously. In those treated for vaginal injury either alone or in combination with other injuries, the outcome was complete resolution in one, four with greater than 50% response and one with less than 50% improvement. In the entire group including the vaginal injuries and other sites within the pelvis, the authors report that 71% had greater than 50% improvement. Most patients received only 30 hyperbaric treatments at 2.4 ATA.

In a review article, Craighead and colleagues[112] along with authors from several Canadian cancer centers and several hyperbaric centers reported their conclusions after conducting a literature search and analysis of two randomized trials and 11 nonrandomized trials. In these publications, hyperbaric oxygen was delivered for late radiation injuries after pelvic irradiation for gynecologic malignancies. These injuries included radiation-induced cystitis, proctitis and enteritis as well as bone necrosis and quality of life assessments. The authors conclude that HBO_2 is effective for delayed radiation injury, especially in the treatment of anal and rectal injuries. The authors further conclude that there is limited but consistent evidence that HBO_2 has utility in reducing complications in women undergoing surgery within a radiated area to surgically address the radiation-induced necrosis.

Miscellaneous Cutaneous Radiation Injuries

In the review by Feldmeier and Hampson,[44] only two publications were discovered which report the results of hyperbaric treatment in radiation injuries of the skin, mostly in the lower extremities. Farmer and associates[108] in 1978 reported a single patient treated for radiation necrosis of the foot without improvement. Feldmeier et al.[113] in 2000 reported a series of 17 patients treated for radiation necrosis involving the lower extremity. One lesion was a combination of bone and soft tissue necrosis. The rest were cutaneous lesions, i.e., skin necrosis. Five of these were at least 10 cm in the greatest dimension. Eleven of 17 patients had complete resolution of their injury with treatment. If we restrict our review to patients in whom follow-up is available and who were not found to have recurrent malignancy, eleven of 13 or 85% resolved.

In the paper by Feldmeier et al.[110] previously described in the section above discussing miscellaneous pelvic and abdominal injuries, 15 lesions involved skin of the anterior abdominal wall. With adjuvant hyperbaric oxygen, eight healed, four did not heal and three had an inadequate course of HBO_2. A course of therapy was considered inadequate when the patient had fewer than 20 hyperbaric treatments.

In the paper from Virginia Mason reporting 411 radiation injuries at multiple sites, fifty-eight patients who were available for follow-up had skin lesions.[60] The authors report 26% complete response and another 50% who had between 50 to 90% response.

In those anatomic sites mentioned above, especially the patients with breast or chest wall damage, much of the radiation damage involved skin and the discussion for these sites as well as the publications discussed in this section are pertinent to the application of HBO_2 to radiation skin damage including necrosis and ulceration.

Neurologic Injuries Secondary to Radiation

In the review article previously cited, Feldmeier and Hampson[44] have identified 14 publications that report hyperbaric oxygen treatment for a variety of neurologic injuries. These include radiation-induced transverse myelitis (spinal cord injury), brain necrosis, optic nerve injury and brachial plexopathy. Since this review article, additional papers on this topic have been published.

Radiation Myelitis

Radiation myelitis is a very serious but fortunately very rare consequence of radiation. It results in paralysis and is essentially a functional cord transection caused by radiation. Marcus and Million[114] reviewed their experience in the incidence of cervical spinal myelitis in 23 years of treatment of head and neck cancers. They reported an incidence of two patients in a total of 1,112 treated (0.2%). In 1976, Hart and Mainous[29] published their results in the hyperbaric treatment of five cases of transverse myelitis. Glassburn and Brady[116] reported nine cases of transverse myelitis in 1977 treated with HBO_2. In the report by Hart, no improvement in motor function was demonstrated while in Glassburn's report six of nine patients had improvement including some improvement in motor function. Calabro and Jinkins[117] in 2000 reported one case of transverse myelitis treated with hyperbaric oxygen who experienced both clinical and MRI imaging evidence of improvement. In a murine study by Feldmeier et al.,[118] delay but no permanent prevention of myelitis was seen for HBO_2 treated animals administered before objective signs of myelitis at seven weeks after a fairly extreme radiation exposure. In fact, the authors discuss that in the study design, the radiation exposure created a 100% incidence of myelitis where an incidence of 50% had been predicted for the control group. Sminia et al.[119] in another animal model investigated HBO_2 given right after re-irradiation of rat spinal cords or at intervals of 5, 10 or 15 weeks after the first cycle of radiation. Animals had received an initial fractionated dose of 6,500 cGy followed by an additional single dose of

2,000 cGy one year after the first course of radiation. In this study, animals did not demonstrate radioprotection by the hyperbaric oxygen. The HBO_2 regimen consisted of 30 daily treatments at 2.4 ATA, each consisting of 90 minutes of 100% oxygen exposure.

Feldmeier and associates[121] have reported a single case report in 2009 at the UHMS annual meeting. In this case a 51-year-old woman with multiple myeloma after two stem cell transplants and other aggressive chemotherapy along with spinal radiation from vertebral levels T-8 to T-12 developed neurologic deficits consisting of a Brown-Sequard pattern with motor and sensory loss on opposite sides of the body. She had weakness, including foot drop in her right lower extremity with back pain and paresthesias in her left lower extremity. Spinal MRI was consistent with radiation myelitis. She completed 40 hyperbaric treatments at 2.5 ATA for 90 minutes of 100% oxygen at pressure. At the completion of treatment, she had improvement in motor and sensory deficits including resolution of her foot drop and was able to undergo physical therapy for rehabilitation. It should be noted that this successful treatment was offered to a patient who was not suffering from a complete loss of neurologic function in her spinal cord, i.e., the cord had not withstood a complete loss of function due to the radiation. Also, of note is that a post-HBO_2 MRI showed resolution of spinal cord damage when compared to the pre-HBO_2 images which were consistent with radiation myelitis.

Other than HBO_2, no other known successful treatments for radiation-induced myelitis exist, and besides the obvious drastic impact of resultant paralysis, there is a high incidence of mortality in these patients with two-thirds dying within four years as a result of this condition's onset.[122] Although hyperbaric treatment has not been universally successful, because of the severe consequences of progressive transverse myelitis and the total lack of other useful treatments, hyperbaric therapy should be considered on a humanitarian basis for the treatment of radiation-induced transverse myelitis. Treatment should be initiated as soon as possible to enhance the likelihood of a therapeutic response.

Brain Necrosis

In the 1976 paper by Hart and Mainous,[29] a single case of radiation caused brain injury improved with HBO_2. Chuba and co-workers[122] have reported a series of 10 children irradiated for primary brain tumors with radiation-induced brain necrosis who were treated with hyperbaric oxygen. All children in this series improved initially. At the time of their publication, four patients had died due to recurrent/progressive tumor while five of the six remaining patients had maintained their improvement as a result of hyperbaric treatment. Leber and colleagues[123] have reported two cases where patients developed brain necrosis after radiosurgery procedures for arteriovenous malformations. In both of these patients, the authors report clinical improvement and a reduction in the size of necrosis by imaging after hyperbaric oxygen therapy. One had complete resolution by MRI. Neither patient required steroids. Cirafsi and Verderamae[124] have published their experience in the treatment a single case of radiation-induced brain necrosis involving the brainstem. This patient had no clinical improvement with hyperbaric oxygen or steroids or anticoagulants. Interestingly three years after HBO_2, the lesion was not visible by MRI.

In a more recent report, Dear and colleagues[125] report that 9 of 20 patients with radiation brain necrosis improved with hyperbaric oxygen. Eleven of the patients in this group had been irradiated for glioblastoma multiforme and only one patient with this diagnosis showed improvement. Since 7 of the 11 patients with glioblastoma had died by the time of the report, it is likely that some, if not a substantial part of their neurologic deficits and patient deterioration, were the result of tumor as well as radiation injury.

Gesell and her colleagues[126] in the largest series to date have reported the outcome in 29 patients treated with hyperbaric oxygen for radiation-induced brain injury. Objective neurologic exam improved in 58% of these patients and the need for steroids reduced in 69%.

A problem in the study of these patients is the difficulties in distinguishing radiation necrosis from recurrent or persistent tumor. Often, they occur together. Necrosis can cause a mass effect and on anatomic based imaging be indistinguishable from a tumor mass. Metabolic imaging with PET scans and MRI spectroscopy can provide useful information but PET in particular suffers from poor spatial resolution.

In a systematic review of toxicities, Fetcko and colleagues[127] report the pooled results of 29 studies. In this report they discovered a range of radiation necrosis incidence of from 0 to 33% after stereotactic radiosurgery with a pooled average of 6.5% for newly diagnosed high-grade gliomas. For recurrent gliomas treated with radiosurgery, the incidence increases to as high as 44% in one study.

There are few effective treatments for brain necrosis. Surgical resection is an option if the site affected is a "non-eloquent" region of the brain and accessible to surgery. Avastin, which is a VEGF inhibitor, has been found to reduce vascular permeability and in this way reduce perilesional edema.[128] A multi-institutional nonrandomized study employing Avastin (bevacizumab) has been reported to have achieved its primary goal of reducing perilesional edema by at least 30% in 78.9% of patients at three months, but only 42% of patients had an improvement in performance status.[128] In consideration of the dire consequences of radiation necrosis of the brain and the success reported in the case series cited above (60 to 70% improvement), in these instances, based on humanitarian considerations and the absence of other effective options, hyperbaric oxygen should be recommended in these patients on a case by case basis.

Radiation-Induced Optic Neuritis

A total of seven full publications and one letter to the editor addressing the application of hyperbaric oxygen to the treatment of optic neuritis are summarized here.[129-136] Borruat et al.[129] have reported on a single patient with bilateral optic neuritis. After hyperbaric oxygen treatment, this patient had complete resolution of optic neuritis in the eye most recently affected and some but less than total resolution in the first eye affected. This experience supports the need to intervene early with HBO_2. In 1991, Fontanesi et al.[130] have reported a case of a pediatric patient treated for a CNS tumor who sustained complete loss of visual acuity, and these changes were refractory to steroids. Hyperbaric oxygen for 20 treatments at 2.0 ATA each for 90 minutes substantially improved vision in both eyes. Boschetti et al.,[131] in another case study, reported their results in a 41-year-old patient who sustained visual damage after radiosurgery to the pituitary for Cushing disease, consisting of blindness in the left eye and temporal hemianopsia in the right eye refractory to corticosteroid treatment. After hyperbaric oxygen, blindness persisted in the left eye, but the patient had objective improvement in visual fields in the right eye by formal visual field mapping. Hyperbaric oxygen consisted of 41 treatments at 2.2 ATA each delivering 60 minutes of 100% oxygen. Guy et al.,[132] in a series of four patients, report that two who had prompt treatment (within 72 hours of onset) improved, but if treatment was delayed by more than 72 hours, no improvement was detected. These authors contend that unless HBO_2 is initiated early after onset of visual loss, no improvement will be experienced. In the largest series by Roden et al.,[133] no improvement occurred in any of the 13 patients treated in this series. In a letter to the editor commenting on the Roden publication, Guy[134] expresses several criticisms of this paper. Guy points out that none of the patients in Roden's series had HBO_2 treatment within two weeks of onset and sometimes the interval was as long as 12 weeks. He also points out that Roden's patients were treated at 2.0 ATA whereas his patients were treated at 2.8 ATA. Guy also observes that Roden's publication included only central visual acuity and no visual field mapping was done.

Figure 3.

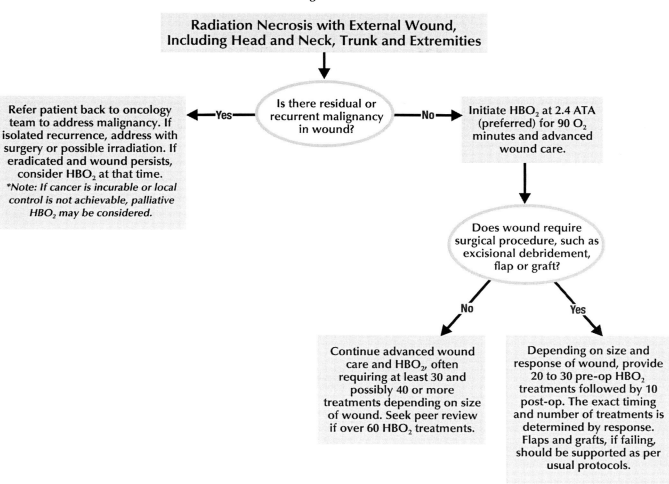

Radiation Necrosis with External Wound, Including Head and Neck, Trunk and Extremities

Is there residual or recurrent malignancy in wound?

Yes → Refer patient back to oncology team to address malignancy. If isolated recurrence, address with surgery or possible irradiation. If eradicated and wound persists, consider HBO$_2$ at that time.
Note: If cancer is incurable or local control is not achievable, palliative HBO$_2$ may be considered.

No → Initiate HBO$_2$ at 2.4 ATA (preferred) for 90 O$_2$ minutes and advanced wound care.

Does wound require surgical procedure, such as excisional debridement, flap or graft?

No → Continue advanced wound care and HBO$_2$, often requiring at least 30 and possibly 40 or more treatments depending on size of wound. Seek peer review if over 60 HBO$_2$ treatments.

Yes → Depending on size and response of wound, provide 20 to 30 pre-op HBO$_2$ treatments followed by 10 post-op. The exact timing and number of treatments is determined by response. Flaps and grafts, if failing, should be supported as per usual protocols.

Figure 4.

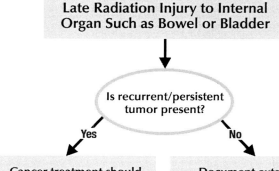

Late Radiation Injury to Internal
Organ Such as Bowel or Bladder

Is recurrent/persistent
tumor present?

Yes

Cancer treatment should
take precedence;
if no effective oncologic
treatment available,
palliative HBO$_2$ should
be considered.

No

Document extent and
severity of radiation injury
by imaging. If accessible
to endoscopy, direct
visualization and/or biopsy
is ideal. Address need for
intervention for anemia or
obstructive symptoms.
Cystitis patients may
require continuous
bladder irrigation.

Initiate HBO$_2$ preferably at 2.4 ATA
for 90 O$_2$ minutes. Recommend
initial 40 treatments unless early
responder. Document response as
patient approaches these 40
treatments. If there is response but
improvement has not yet plateaued,
consider another 10 to 20
treatments. If 60 treatments are to
be exceeded, seek peer review.
*Note: Several cases of radiation cystitis
have recurred but responded to a
second course of treatment.*

Figure 5.

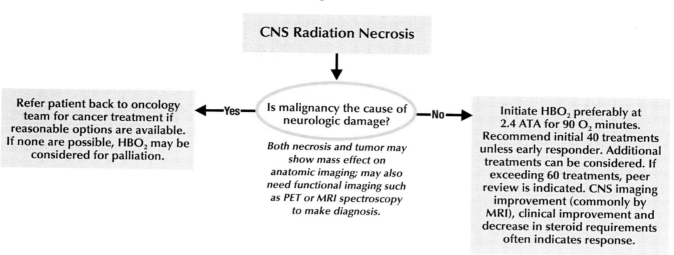

CNS Radiation Necrosis

Is malignancy the cause of neurologic damage?

Both necrosis and tumor may show mass effect on anatomic imaging; may also need functional imaging such as PET or MRI spectroscopy to make diagnosis.

—Yes→ Refer patient back to oncology team for cancer treatment if reasonable options are available. If none are possible, HBO₂ may be considered for palliation.

—No→ Initiate HBO₂ preferably at 2.4 ATA for 90 O₂ minutes. Recommend initial 40 treatments unless early responder. Additional treatments can be considered. If exceeding 60 treatments, peer review is indicated. CNS imaging improvement (commonly by MRI), clinical improvement and decrease in steroid requirements often indicates response.

Figure 6.

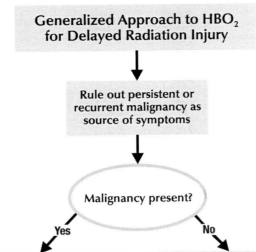

**Generalized Approach to HBO$_2$
for Delayed Radiation Injury**

**Rule out persistent or
recurrent malignancy as
source of symptoms**

Malignancy present?

Yes

No

Patient should be referred back to oncology team for management of malignancy, which will take priority if effective treatment is available. If none available, HBO$_2$ as palliative treatment should be considered since necrosis and tumor may both be present. HBO$_2$ cannot be expected to have benefit for tumor except potentially as adjuvant to concomitant radiation injury.

In most cases HBO$_2$ should be initiated. 2.4 ATA is preferred for 90 minutes of O$_2$ per treatment. Typically, 40 treatments are required. In some instances, up to 60 treatments are appropriate, especially for brain. Rarely, HBO$_2$ may exceed 60 treatments, though peer review should be obtained. If initially responsive but then recurrent symptoms, a repeat course is likely appropriate. HBO$_2$ should be combined with other appropriate medical or surgical interventions. Prior to surgery in a radiated field, 20 to 30 pre-operative treatments should be given. If there is a wound, wound care as in other hypoxic tissues is needed. A team effort including oncologists, surgeons and endoscopists will optimize patient outcome.

References

1. Studer G, Studer SP, Zwahlen RA et al. Osteoradionecrosis of the mandible: minimized risk profile following intensity-modulated radiation therapy (IMRT). Strahlen Onko 2006;182(5):283-8.
2. Rubin P, Casarrett GW. Clinical radiation pathology, vol.1. Philadelphia, PA: WB Saunders; 1968:57-61.
3. Hall EJ, Giaccia A. Radiobiology for the Radiologist.Philadelphia, PA: Lippincot, Williams & Wilkins, and Wolters Kluwer; 2012:9-34.
4. Stone HB,Coleman CN, Anscer MS, McBride WH. Effects of radiation on normal tissues: consequences and mechanisms. Lancet Oncol 2003;4:529-36.
5. Metler FA, Upton AC. Medical effects of ionizing radiation. WB Saunders Company; 1995:230.
6. Hall EJ, Giaccia A. Radiobiology for the radiologist. Lippincot, Williams & Wilkins, and Wolters Kluwer; 2012:327-55.
7. Dorr W, Hendry H. Consequential late effects in normal tissues. Radiotherapy and oncology 2001;61:223-31.
8. Teguh DN, Levendag PC, Noever I. et al. Early hyperbaric oxygen therapy for reducing radiotherapy side effects: early results of a randomized trial in oropharyngeal and nasopharyngeal cancer. Int J Radiation Oncology Biol Phys. 2009;75(3):711-6.
9. Rosenstein BS. Radiogenomics: identification of genomic predictors for radiation toxicity. Semin Radiat Oncol. 2017;27:300-9.
10. Marx RE. Osteoradionecrosis: a new concept of its pathophysiology. J Oral Maxillofac Surg. 1983;41:283-288.
11. Hojan K, Milecki P. Opportunities for rehabilitation of patients with radiation fibrosis syndrome. Reports of Practical Oncology and Radiotherapy. 2014;19:1-6.
12. Delainian S, Lefaix JL. The radiation-induced fibroatrophic process: therapeutic perspective via the antioxidant pathway. Radiother Oncol. 2004;73(2):119-31.
13. Fleckenstein K, Gauter-Fleckenstein B, Jackson IL, Rabbani Z, Anscher M, Vujaskovic Z. Using biological markers to predict risk of radiation injury. Semin Radiat Oncol. 2007;17:89-98.
14. O'Sullivan B, Levin W. Late radiation-related fibrosis:pathogenesis, manifestations, and current management. Seminars in Radiat Oncol. 2003;13(3):274-89.
15. Darby IA, Hewitson TD. Hypoxia in tissue repair and fibrosis. Cell tissue RE. 2016;365:553-62.
16. Hakenjos L, Bamberg M, Rodemann HP. TGF beta-1-mediated alterations of rat lung fibroblast differentiation resulting in the radiation-induced fibrotic phenotype. Int J Radiat Biol. 2000;76:503-9.
17. Andreassen CN, Alsner J, Overgaard J. Does variability in normal tissue reactions after radiotherapy have a genetic basis? Where and how to look for it. Radiotherapy and oncology. 2002;64:131-40.
18. Stewart FA, Akleyev AV, Hauer-Jensen M, et al. ICRP publication 118: ICRP statement on tissue reactions and early and late effects of radiation in normal tissues and organ-threshold doses for tissue reactions in radiation protection context. Ann IRCP. 2012;41(1-20):1-322.
19. Marx RE, Johnson RP, Kline SN. Prevention of osteoradionecrosis: A randomized prospective clinical trial of hyperbaric oxygen versus penicillin. J Am Dent Assoc. 1985;11:49-54.
20. Deschpande SS, Donneys A, Farberg AS et al. Quantification and characterization of radiation-induced changes to mandibular vascularity using micro-computed tomography. Ann Plast Surg. 2014;72(1):100-3.
21. Marx RE. Radiation injury to tissue. In: Kindwall EP, ed. Hyperbaric medicine practice, fourth edition. North Palm Beach, FL: Best Publishing Company; 2017:727- 73.
22. Svalestad J, Thorsen G, VaagboS et al. Effect of hyperbaric oxygen treatment onoxygen tension and vascular capacity in irradiated skin and mucosa. Int J Oral and Maxillofac Surg. 2013;43:107-12.
23. Johnson-Arbor K, Falola R, Kelty J et al. Use of indocyanine green fluorescent angiography in a hyperbaric patient with soft tissue radiation necrosis: a case report. Undersea Hyperb Med. 2017;44(3):273-8.
24. Feldmeier JJ, Davolt DA, Court WS, Onoda JM, Alecu R. Histologic morphometry confirms a prophylactic effect for hyperbaric oxygen in the prevention of delayed radiation enteropathy. Undersea Hyper Med. 1998; 25(2):93-97.
25. Feldmeier JJ, Jelen I, Davolt DA, Valente PT, Meltz ML, Alecu R. Hyperbaric oxygen as a prophylaxis for radiation induced delayed enteropathy. Radiotherapy and Oncology. 1995; 35:138-144.
26. Hamilton SN, Arshad O, Kwok J et al. Documentation and incidence of late effects and screening recommendations for adolescent and young adult patients with head and neck cancer survivors treated with radiotherapy. Support Care Cancer 2018;published online 22 Nov 2018.
27. Milonova TN, Bhopale VM, Sorokino EM et al. Hyperbaric oxygen stimulates vasculogenic stem cell growth and differentiation in vivo. J Appl Physiol. 1985;106(2):711-28.
28. Thom SR, Bhoplae VM, Velazquez OC et al. Stem cell mobilization by hyperbaric oxygen. AJP-Heart. 2005;290:1378-86.

29. Hart GB, Manous EG. The treatment of radiation necrosis with hyperbaric oxygen (OHP). Cancer. 1976;37:2580-5.

30. Tobey RE, Kelly JF. Osteoradionecrosis of the jaws. Otolaryngol Clin North Am. 1979;12(1):183-186.

31. Bedwinek JM, Shukovsky LJ, Fletcher GH, Daly TE. Osteonecrosis in patients treated with definitive radiotherapy for squamous cell cancers of the oral cavity and naso- and oropharynx. Radiology. 1976;119:665-667.

32. Emami B, Lyman J, Brown A, Coia L, Gottein M, Munzenrider JE, Shank B, Solin LJ, Wesson M. Tolerance of normal tissue to therapeutic irradiation. Int J Radiat Oncol Biol Phys. 1991:21:109-122.

33. Reuther T, Schuster T, Mende U, et al. Osteoradionecrosis of the jaws a side effect of radiotherapy of head and neck tumor patients-a report of a thirty-year retrospective review. Int J Oral and Maxillofac Surg. 2003;32:289-295.

34. Gomez DR, Estilo L, Wolden SL, Zelefsky MJ, Kraus DH, Wong RJ, Shaha AR, Jatin JP, Mechalakos JG, Lee NY. Correlation of osteoradionecrosis and dental events with dosimetric parameters in intensity-modulated radiation therapy for head and neck cancer. Int J Radiat Oncol Biol Phys. 2011 Nov 15;81(4):e207-13.

35. Caparrotti F, Huang SH, Bratman SV, et al. Osteoradionecrosis of the mandible in carcinoma treated with intensity-modulated radiotherapy. Cancer. 2017;123(19):369-373.

36. Maesschaick T, Dulguerov N, Caparotti F, et al. Comparison of the incidence of osteoradionecrosis with conventional radiotherapy and intensity-modulated radiotherapy. Head Neck. 2016;38(11):1695-1702.

37. Suntharalingam M. The role of chemotherapy and radiation in the management of patients with squamous cell carciomas of the head and neck. Semin Oncol. 2003:30(4Suppl9):37-45.

38. Parsons JT. The effect of radiation on normal tissues of the head and neck. In: Million RR, Cassisi NJ, eds. Management of head and neck cancer: A multi-disciplinary approach. Philadelphia: JB Lippincott; 1994:245-289.

39. Marx RE.Osteoradionecrosis: a new concept of its pathology. J Oral Maxillofac Surg. 1983;41:351-8.

40. Marx RE. Osteoradionecrosis of the jaws:review and update. HBO Rev. 1984;5:412-9.

41. He Y, Liu Z, Tian Z et al. Retrospective analysis of osteoradionecrosis of the mandible: proposing a novel clinical classification and staging system. Int J Oral Maxillofac Surg. 2015;44:1547-1557.

42. Personal communication with Dr. Robert Marx, January 2019.

43. Lofstrand J, Nyberg M, Karlsson T. Quality of life after fibular free flap reconstryuction of segmental mandibular defects. J Reconstr Microsurg. 2018;34:108-20.

44. Feldmeier JJ, Hampson NB. A systematic review of the literature reporting the application of hyperbaric oxygen prevention and treatment of delayed radiation injuries: an evidence based approach. UHM. 2002;29:4-30.

45. Maier A, Gaggl A, Klemen H, Santler G, Anegg U, Fell B, Karcher H, Smolle-Juttner FM, Friehs GB. Review of severe osteoradionecrosis treated by surgery alone or surgery with postoperative hyperbaric oxygenation. Br J Oral Maxillofac Surg. 2000;38:173-6.

46. Freiberger JJ, Yoo DS, de Lisle Dear G et al. Multimodality surgical and hyperbaric management of mandibular osteoradionecrosis. Int J Radiat Oncol Bio Phys. 2008;75(3):717-24.

47. Annane D, Depondt J, Aubert P et al. Hyperbaric oxygen therapy for radionecrosis of the jaw: a randomized controlled, double-blind trial from ORN96 Study Group. J Clin Oncol. 2004;22:4893-4900.

48. Feldmeier JJ, Heimbach RD, Davolt DA, Court WS, Stegmann BJ, Sheffield PJ. Hyperbaric oxygen as an adjunctive treatment for radiation necrosis of the chest wall. Undersea and Hyperbaric Medicine. 1995:22(4).

49. Moon RE, McGraw TA, Blakey G. Hyperbaric oxygen therapy for radiation necrosis of the jaw: comments on a randomized study. UHM. 2005;32:145-6.

50. Laden G. Hyperbaric oxygen therapy for radionecrosis: clear evidence from confusing data (letter to the editor). J Clin Oncol. 2005;23:4465. Mendenhall WM. Mandibular Osteoradionecrosis (editorial) J Clin Oncol. 2004;22:4867-8.

51. Mendenhall WM. Mandibular osteoradionecrosis (editorial). J Clin Oncol. 2004;22:4867-8.

52. Gal TJ, Yueh B, Futran ND. Influence of prior hyperbaric oxygen therapy in complications following microvascular reconstruction for advanced osteoradionecrosis. Arch Otolaryngol Head Neck Surg. 2003;129:72-76.

53. Dielman FJ, Phan TTT, van den Hoogen FJA et al. The efficacy of hyperbaric oxygen related to clinical stage of osteoradionecrosis of the mandible. Int J Oral and Maxillofac Surg. 2017;46:428-33.

54. Hirsch DL, Bell RB, Dierks EJ, et al. Analysis of microvascular free flaps for reconstruction of advanced mandibular osteoradionecrosis: a retrospective cohort study. J Oral Maxillofac Surg. 2008;66(12):2545-56.

55. Nolen D, Cannady SB, Wax MK, et al. Comparison of complications in free flap reconstruction for osteoradionecrosis in patients with or without hyperbaric oxygen therapy. Head Neck. 2014;36(12):1701-4.

56. Van Gemert JT, Abbink JH, van Es RJ, et al. Early and late complications in the reconstructed mandible with free fibular flaps. J Surg Oncol. 2018;117:773-80.

57. Teng MS, Futran ND. Osteoradionecrosis of the mandible. Cur Opin Otolaryngol Head Neck Surg. 2005;13:217-21.

58. Delainian S, Chatel CC, Porcher R et al. Complete restoration of refractory mandibular osteoradionecrosis by prolonged treatment with a pentoxifylline-tocopherol-clodronate combination (PENTOCLO): a phase II trial. Int J Radiation Oncology Biol Phys. 2011;80(30):832-9.

59. Delainian S, Lefaix JL. The radiation-induced fibroatrophic process: therapeutic perspective via the antioxidant pathway. Radiotherapy and Oncology. 2003;73:119-31.

60. Hampson NB, Holm JR, Wreford-Brown CE, Feldmeier JJ. Prospective assessment of outcomes in 411 patients treated with hyperbaric oxygen for chronic radiation issue injury. Cancer. 2012;118:3860-8.

61. Lambert PM, Intrier N, Eichstaedt R. Management of dental extractions in irradiated jaws: a protocol with hyperbaric oxygen treatment. J Oral Maxillofac Surg. 1997;55:268-74.

62. Vudiniabola S, Pirone C, Williamson J, Goss ANN. Hyperbaric oxygen in the prevention of osteoradionecrosis of the jaws. Australian Dental Journal. 1999; 44:243-247.

63. David LA, Sandor GK, Evans AW, Brown DH. Hyperbaric oxygen therapy and mandibular osteoradionecrosis: a retrospective study and analysis of treatment outcomes. J Can Dent Assoc. 2001; 67:384.

64. Chavez JA, Adkinson CD. Adjunctive hyperbaric oxygen in irradiated patients requiring dental extractions: outcomes and complications. J Oral Maxillofac Surg. 2001; 59:518-22.

65. Sulaiman F, Huryn JM, Ziotolow IM. Dental extractions in the irradiated head and neck patient: a retrospective analysis of Memorial Sloan-Kettering Cancer Center protocols, criteria, and end results. J Oral Maxillofac Surg. 2003;61:1123-31.

66. Makkonen TA, Kiminski A, Makkkonen TK et al. Dental extractions in relation to radiation therapy of 224 patients. Int J Oral Maxillofac Surg.1987; 7;16:56-64.

67. Maxymiw WG, Wood RE. Liu FF. Postradiation dental extractions without hyperbaric oxygen. Oral Surg Oral MedOral Pathol. 1991;72(3):270-4.

68. Lye KW, Wee J Gao F et al. The effect of prior radiation therapy for treatment of nasopharyngeal cancer on wound healing following extractions: incidence of complications and risk factors. Int J Oral Maxillofac Surg. 2007;36:315-20.

69. Clayman L. Management of dental extractions in irradiated jaws: a protocol without hyperbaroc oxygen. J Oral Maxillofac Surg. 1997;55:275-81.

70. Wahl MJ. Osteoradionecrosis prevention myths. Int J Radiation Oncology Biol Phys. 2006;64:661-9.

71. Kim JC, Elkin D, Hendrickson FR. Carcinoma of the vocal cords: results of treatment and time-dose relationships. Cancer. 1978;42:1114-9.

72. Stell PM, Morrison ND. Radiation necrosis of the larynx: etiology and management. Arch Oto Rhin Laryngol. 1973; 98:111-3.

73. Flood LM, brightwell AP. Clinical assessment of the irradiated larynx. J Laryngol Otol.1984;98:493-8.

74. Chandler JR. Radiation fibrosis and necrosis of the larynx. Ann Otol Rhinol & Laryngol. 1979;88:509-14.

75. Ferguson BJ, Hudson WR, Farmer JC. Hyperbaric oxygen for laryngeal radionecrosis. Ann Otol Laryngol. 1987; 96:1-6.

76. Feldmeier JJ, Heimbach RD, Davolt DA, Brakora MJ. Hyperbaric oxygen as an adjunctive treatment for severe laryngeal necrosis: A report of nine consecutive cases. Undersea Hyper Med. 1993;20:329-335.

77. Filintisis GA, Moon RE, Kraft KL, Farmer JC, Scher RL, Piantadosi CA. Laryngeal radionecrosis and hyperbaric oxygen therapy: report of 18 cases and review of the literature. Ann Otol Rhinol Laryngol. 2000;109:554-62.

78. Narzony W, Sicko Z, Kot J et al. Hyperbaric oxygen therapy in the treatment of complications of irradiation in the head and neck area. Undersea Hyperb Med. 2005;32:103-10.

79. HSU YC, Lee KW, Tsai KB et al. Treatment of laryngeal necrosis with hyperbaric oxygen therapy: a case report. Kaohsing Med. 2005;21:88-92.

80. Davis JC, Dunn JM, Gates GA, Heimbach RD. Hyperbaric oxygen: a new adjunct in the management of radiation necrosis. Arch Otolaryngol. 1979;105:58-61.

81. Neovius EB, Lind MG, Lind FG. Hyperbaric oxygen for wound complications after surgery in the irradiated head and neck: a review of the literature and a report of 15 consecutive cases. Head and Neck. 1997;19:315-322.

82. Feldmeier JJ, Newman R, Davolt DA, Heimbach RD, Newman NK, Hernandez LC. Prophylactic hyperbaric oxygen for patients undergoing salvage for recurrent head and neck cancers following full course irradiation (abstract). Undersea Hyper Med. 1998;25(Suppl):10.

83. Sassler AM, Esclamado RM, Wolf GT. Surgery after organ preservation therapy. Analysis of wound complications. Arch Otolaryngol Head Neck Surg. 1995 Feb;121(2):162-5

84. Agra IM, Carvalho AL, Pontes E, Campos OD, Ulbrich FS, Magrin J, Kowalski LP. Postoperative complications after en bloc salvage surgery for head and neck cancer. Arch Otolaryngol Head Neck Surg. 2003 Dec;129(12):1317-21.

85. Gerlach NL, Barkhuysen R, Kaanders JH et al. The effect of hyperbaric oxygen therapy on quality of life in oral and oropharyngeal cancer patients treated with radiotherapy. Int J of Maxillofac Surg. 2008;37:255-9.

86. No authors listed. Breast Cancer Treatment (PDQ®)—Patient Version - National Cancer Institute.

87. Feldmeier JJ, Heimbach RD, Davolt DA, Court WS, Stegmann BJ, Sheffield PJ. Hyperbaric oxygen as an adjunctive treatment for delayed radiation injury of the chest wall: a retrospective review of 23 cases. Undersea Hyperb Med. 1995;22:383-393.

88. Carl UM, Hartmann KA. Hyperbaric oxygen treatment for symptomatic breast edema after radiation therapy. Undersea Hyperb Med. 1998;25;233-234.

89. Carl UM, Feldmeier JJ, Schmitt G et al. Hyperbaric oxygen therapy forn late sequelae in women receiving radiation after breast conservation treatment. Int J Radiat Oncol Bio Phys. 2001;49(4):1029-31.

90. No Authors Listed. LENT SOMA scales for all anatomic sites. Int J Radiat Oncol Biol Phys. 1995;31(5):1049-91.

91. Teguh DN, Bol Raap R, Strikmans H et al. Hyperbaric oxygen therapy for late radiation-induced tissue toxicity: prospectively patient-reported outcome measures in breast cancer patients. Radiat Oncol. 2016;11(1);130.

92. Enomoto M, Yagishita K, Okuma K et al. Hyperbaric oxygen for a refractory skin ulcer after radical mastectomy and radiation therapy: a case report. J Med Case Rep. 2017;11(1):electronically published.

93. Bevers RF, Bakker DJ, Kurth KH. Hyperbaric oxygen treatment for haemorrhagic radiation cystitis. Lancet:1995;346:803-805.

94. Neheman A, Nativ O, Moskovitz B, Melamed Y, Stein A. hyperbaric oxygen therapy for radiation-induced haemorrhagic cystitis. BJU Int. 2005;96:107-9.

95. Corman JM, McClure D, Pritchett R, Kozlowski P, Hampson NB. Treatment of radiation induced hemorrhagic cystitis with hyperbaric oxygen. J Urol. 2003;160:2200-2.

96. Chong KT, Hampson NB, Corman JM. Early hyperbaric oxygen improves outcome for radiation-induced hemorrhagic cystitis. Urology. 2005;65:649-53.

97. Cardinal J, Slade A, McFarland M et al. Scoping review and meta-analysis of hyperbaric oxygen therapy for radiation-induced hemorrhagic cystitis. Current Urology Reports. 2018.;19:38 published on line.

98. Cheng C, Foo KT. Management of severe chronic radiation cystitis. Ann Acad Med. Singapore:1992;21:368-71.

99. Li A, Sun J, Chao H. Late bladder complications following radiotherapy of carcinoma of the uterine cervix. Zhonghua Fu Chan Ke. 1995;30:741-3.

100. Neurath MF, Branbrink A, Meyer zum Buschenfelde KH, Lohse AW. A new treatment for severe malabsorption due to radiation enteritis. Lancet. 1996;347:1302.

101. Jones K, Evans AW, Bristow RG et al. Treatment of radiation proctitis with hyperbaric oxygen. Radiotherapy and Oncology. 2006;78:91-4.

102. Girinius S, Ceronsky N, Gesell L et al. Treatment of refractory radiation-induced hemorrhagic proctitis with hyperbaric oxygen therapy. Am J Clin Oncol. 2006;29:588-92.

103. Dall'Era MA, Hampson NB, His RA et al. Hyperbaric oxygen therapy for radiation induced proctopathy in men treated for prostate cancer. J Urol. 2006;176:87-90.

104. Marshall GT, Thirlby RC, Bredfeldt JE, Hampson NB. Treatment of gastrointestinal radiation injury with hyperbaric oxygen Undersea Hyperb Med. 2007;34:35-42.

105. Clarke RE, Tenorio LMC, Hussey JR et al. Hyperbaric oxygen treatment of chronic refractory radiation proctitis: a randomized and controlled double-blind crossover trial with long term follow-up. Int J Radiat Oncol Biol Phys. 2008;72(1):134.

106. Glover M, Smerdon GR, Andeyev HJ et al. Hyperbaric oxygen for patients with chronic bowel dysfunction after pelvic radiotherapy (HBO$_2$T): a randomized double-blind, sham-controlled phase 3 trial. Lancet Oncol. 2016;17(2):224-33.

107. Paquette IM, Vogel JD, Abbas MA, et al. The American Society of Colon and Rectal Surgeons clinical practice guidelines for the treatment of chronic radiation proctitis. Dis Colon Rectum. 2018;61:1135-40.

108. Farmer JC, Shelton DL, Bennett PD, Angelillo JD, Hudson MD. Treatment of radiation-induced injury by hyperbaric oxygen. Ann Otol. 1978; 87;707-15.

109. Williams JAA, Clarke D, Dennis WAA, Dennis EJJ, Smith STT. Treatment of pelvic soft tissue radiation necrosis with hyperbaric oxygen. Am J Obstet Gynecol. 1992; 167:415-416.

110. Feldmeier JJ, Heimbach RD, Davolt DA, Court WS, Stegmann BJ, Sheffield PJ. Hyperbaric oxygen as an adjunctive treatment for delayed radiation injuries of the abdomen and pelvis. Undersea Hyperb Med. 1997;23(4):205-213.

111. Fink D, Chetty N, Lehm JP, Marsden DE, Hacker NF. Hyperbaric oxygen therapy for delayed radiation injuries in gynecological cancers. Int J Gynecol Cancer. 2006;16:638-42.

112. Craighead P, Shea-Budgell MA,Nation J, Esmail R, Evans AW, Parliament M, Oliver TK, Hagen NA. Hyperbaric oxygen for late radiation tissue injury in gynecologic malignancies. Curr Oncol. 2011;18(5):220-7.

113. Feldmeier JJ, Heimbach RD, Davolt DA, McDonough MJ, Stegmann BJ, Sheffield PJ. Hyperbaric oxygen in the treatment of delayed radiation injuries of the extremities Undersea Hyper Med. 2000;27(1):15-19.

114. Marcus RB Jr, Million RR. The incidence of transverse myelitis after radiation of the cervical spinal cord. Int J Radiat Oncol Biol Phys. 1990;19:3-8.
115. Marcus RB Jr, Million RR. The incidence of transverse myelitis after radiation of the cervical spinal cord. Int J Radiat Oncol Biol Phys 1990;19:3-8.
116. Glassburn JR, Brady LW. Treatment with hyperbaric oxygen for radiation myelitis. Proc. 6th Int Cong on Hyperbaric Medicine. 1977:266-77.
117. Calabro F, Jinkins JR. MRI of radiation myelitis: a report of a case treated with hyperbaric oxygen. Eur Radiol. 2000;10:1079-84.
118. Feldmeier JJ, Lange JD, Cox SD, Chou L, Ciaravino V. Hyperbaric oxygen as a prophylaxis or treatment for radiation myelitis. Undersea Hyper Med. 1993;20(3):249-255.
119. Sminia P, Van der Kleij AJ, Carl UM, Feldmeier JJ, Hartmann KA. Prophylactic hyperbaric oxygen treatment and rat spinal cord re-irradiation. Cancer Lett. 2003 Feb 28;191(1):59-65.
120. Feldmeier J, Borrillo D Siebenhaler G. The benefits of hyperbaric oxygen in the treatment of delayed spinal cord radiation induced injury. Undersea Hyper Med. 2009;36(4).
121. Schulteiss TE, Stephen LC, Peters LJ. Survival in radiation myelopathy. Int J Radiat Oncol Biol Phys. 1986;12:1765-9.
122. Chuba PJ, Aronin P, Bhambhani K, Eichenhorn M, Zamarano L, Cianci P, Muhlbauer M, Porter AT, Fontanesi J. Hyperbaric oxygen therapy for radiation-induced brain injury in children. Cancer. 1997;80:2005-2012.
123. Leber KA, Eder HG, Kovac H, Anegg U, Pendl G. Treatment of cerebral radionecrosis by hyperbaric oxygen therapy. Sterotact Funct Neurosurg. 1998;70(Suppl 1):229-36.
124. Cirafisi C, Verderame F. Radiation-induced rhomboencephalopathy. Ital J Neurol Sci. 1999;20:55-8.
125. Dear GdeL, Rose RE, Dunn R, Piantadosi CA, Stolp BW, Carraway MS, Thalmann ED, Kraft K, Rice JR, Friedman AH, Friedman HS, Moon RE. Treatment of neurological symptoms of radionecrosis of the brain with hyperbaric oxygen: a case series. Presented at the 35th Annual Undersea and Hyperbaric Medical Society Scientific Meeting. San Diego, CA: 28-30 June 2002.
126. Gesell LB, Warnick R, Breneman J, Albright R, Racadio J, Mink, S. Effectiveness of hyperbaric oxygen for the treatment of soft tissue radionecrosis of the brain. Presented at the 35th Annual Undersea and Hyperbaric Medical Society Scientific Meeting. San Diego, CA: 28-30 June, 2002.
127. Fetko K, Lukas RV, Watson L et al. Survival and complications of stereotactic radiosurgery:a systematic review of stereotactic radiosurgery for newly diagnosed and recurrent high-grade gliomas. Medicine (Baltimore). 2017; 96(43):e8293.
128. Furuse M, Nonoguchi N, Kuroiwa T et al. A prospective multi-centre, single-arm clinical trial of bevacizumab for patients with surgically untreatable symptomatic brain radiation necrosis. Neurooncol Pract. 2016;3(4):272-80.
129. Borruat FXX, Schatz NJJ, Glaser JSS, Feun LGG, Matos L. Visual recovery from radiation-induced optic neuropathy. The role of hyperbaric oxygen therapy. J Clin Neuroophthalmol. 1993;13:98-101.
130. Fontanesi J, Golden EB, Cianci PC, Heideman RL. Treatment of radiation-induced optic neuropathy in the pediatric population. Journal of Hyperbaric Medicine. 1991;6(4):245-248.
131. Boschetti M; De Lucchi M; Giusti M; Spena C; Corallo G; Goglia U; Ceresola E; Resmini E; Vera L; Minuto F; Ferone D. Partial visual recovery from radiation-induced optic neuropathy after hyperbaric oxygen therapy in a patient with Cushing disease. Eur J Endocrinol. 01 June 2006;154(6):813-8.
132. Guy J, Schatz NJJ. Hyperbaric oxygen in the treatment of radiation-induced optic neuropathy. Ophthalmology. 1986;93:1083-8.
133. Roden D, Bosley TM, FowbleB, Clark J, Savino PJ, Sergott RC, Schatz NJ. Delayed radiation injury to the retrobulbar optic nerves and chiasm. Clinical syndrome and treatment with hyperbaric oxygen and corticosteroids. Ophthalmolgy. 1990;97:346-51.
134. Guy J. Letter to the Editor. Ophthalmology. 1990;97:1246-7.
135. Malik A, Golnik K. Hyperbaric oxygen in the treatment of radiation optic neuropathy. J Neuroophthalmol. 2012;32(2):128-31.
136. Li CQ, Gerson S, Snyder B. Case report; hyperbaric oxygen and MRI findings in radiation-induced optic neuropathy. Undersea Hyperb Med. 2014;41(1):59-63.
137. Videtic GM, Venkatesan VM. Hyperbaric oxygen corrects sacral plexopathy due to osteoradionecrosis appearing 15 years after pelvic irradiation. Clin Oncol (R Coll Radiol). 1999;11(3):198-9.
138. Pritchard J, Anand P, Broome J,et al. Double-blind randomized phase II study of hyperbaric oxygen in patients with radiation-induced brachial plexopathy. Radiother Oncol. 2001;58:279-86.
139. Granstrom G. Placement of dental implants in irradiated bone: the case for hyperbaric oxygen. Int J Oral Maxillofac. 2006;64:812-8.

140. Ueda M, Kaneda T, Takahashi H. Effect of hyperbaric oxygen therapy on osseointegration of titanium implants in irradiated bone: A preliminary report. Int J Oral Maxillofac Implants. 1993;8:41-44.

141. Pomeroy BD, Keim LW, Taylor RJ. Preoperative hyperbaric oxygen therapy for radiation induced injuries. J Urol. 1998;159:1630-1632.

142. Sassler AM, Esclamado RM, Wolf GT. Surgery after organ preservation therapy: analysis of wound complications. Arch Otolaryngol Head and Neck Surg. 1995; 121(2):162-5.

143. Gray LH, Conger AD, Ebert M et al. The concentration of oxygen dissolved in tissues at the time of radiation as a factor in radiotherapy. Br J Radiol. 1953;26:638-48.

144. Churchill-Davidson I. The oxygen effect in radiotherapy: historical review. Front Radiat Ther Oncol. 1968.1:1-15.

145. Koshi K, Kinoshita Y, Imada H et al. Effects of radiotherapy after hyperbaric oxygenation on malignant gliomas. Br J Cancer. 1990;80:236-41n.

146. Beppu T, Kamada K Arai H et al. Change of oxygen pressure in glioblastoma tissue under various conditions. J Neurooncol. 2002;58:47-52.

147. Becker A, Kuhnt T, Liedtke H et al. Oxygenation measurements in head and neck cancers during hypervbaric oxygenation . Strahlenther Onkol. 2002;178:105-8.

148. Hartford AC, Davis TH, Buckey JC et al. Hyperbaric oxygen as radiation sensitizer for locally advanced squamous cell carcinoma of the oropharynz: a Phase 1 Dose-escalation study.

149. Personal communication with Mr. Richard E. Clarke, CHT. June 2018.

150. Allen BG, Bhatia SK, Anderson CM et al. Ketogenic diets as an adjuvant to cancer therapy: history and potential mechanism. Redox Biol. 2014;2:963-70.

151. Warburg O Wind F, Negelein E. The metabolism of tumors in the body. Journal of Physiol. 1926:519-30.

152. Poff AM, Ari C, Seyfried TN and D'Agostino DP. The ketogenic diet and hyperbaric oxygen therapy prolong survival in mice with systemic metastatic cancer. PLOS One. 2013.;8(6):1-9. |

153. Iyikesici MS, Slocum AK, Slocum A, et al. Efficacy of metabolically supported chemotherapy combined with ketogenic diet, hyperthermia and hyperbaric oxygen therapy for stageIV triple-negative breast cancer. Cureus. 2017;9(7):e1445.

154. Feldmeier J, Carl U,Hartmann K, Sminia P. Hyperbaric oxygen: Does it promote growth or recurrence of malignancy. UHM. 2003; 30(1):1-18.

155. Daruwalla J, Christophi C. Hyperbaroc oxygen therapy for malignancy. World J Surg. 2006;30:2112-31.

156. Moen I, Stuhr LE. Hyperbaric oxygen therapy and cancer-review. Targ Oncol. 2012;7:233-42.

157. Chong KT, Hampson NB, Bostwick DG, Vessella RL, Corman JM. Hyperbaric oxygen does not accelerate latent in vivo prostate cancer: implications for the treatment of radiation-induced haemorrhagic cystitis. BJU Int. 2004;94(9):1275-8.

158. Stuhr LE, Iverson VV, Straume O, Maehle BO, Reed RK. Hyperbaric oxygen alone or combined with 5-FU attenuates growth of DMBA induced rat mammary tumors. Cancer Lett. 2004;210(1):3540.

159. Sun TB, Chen RL, Hsu YH. The effect of hyperbaric oxygen on human oral cancer cells. Undersea Hyperb Med. 2004;31(2):251-60.

160. Shi Y, Lee CS, Wu J, Koch CJ, Thom SR, Maity A, Bernhard EJ. Effects of hyperbaric oxygen exposure on experimental head and neck tumor growth, oxygenation, and vasculature. Head Neck. 2005 May;27(5):362-9.

161. Granowitz EV, Tonomura N, Benson RM, Katz DM, Band V, Makari-Judson GP, Osborne BA. Hyperbaric oxygen inhibits benign and malignant human mammary epithelial cell proliferation. Anticancer Res. 2005;25:3833-42.

162. Daruwalla J, Christophi C. The effect of hyperbaric oxygen therapy on tumour growth in a mouse model of colorectal cancer liver metastases. Eur J Cancer. 2006 Dec;42(18):3304-11.

163. Haroon AT, Patel M, Al-Mehdi AB. Lung metastatic load limitation with hyperbaric oxygen. Undersea Hyperb Med. Int J Radiat Oncol Biol Bys. 2009;74(4):1077-82. 2007 Mar-Apr;34(2):83-90.

164. Eltorai I, Hart GB, Strauss MB. Et al. Does hyperbaric oxygen provoke an occult carcinoma in man? In Kindwall EP, ed. Proceedings of the eighth international congress on hyperbaric medicine. San Pedro, CA. 1987:18-29.

165. Bradfield JJ, Kinsella JB, Mader JT et al. Rapid progression of head and neck squamous carcinoma after hyperbaric oxygen. Otolaryngol Head and Neck Surg. 1996;114:793-7.

166. Lin HY, Ku CH, Liu DW et al. Hyperbaric oxygen therapy for late radiation-associated tissue necroses: Is it safe in patients with locoregionally recurrent and the successfully salvaged head-and-neck cancers? Int J Radiat Oncol Biol Phys. 2009;74:1077-82.

167. Elbers JBW, Veldhuis LI, Bhairosing PA et al. Salvage surgery for advanced stage head and neck squamous cell carcinoma following radiotherapy or chemoradiation. Eur Arch Otorhinolaryngol. 2019; Epub ahead of print.

CHAPTER 9

Sudden Sensorineural Hearing Loss

Tracy Leigh LeGros MD, PhD, and Heather Murphy-Lavoie MD

Introduction

Sudden sensorineural hearing loss (SSNHL) presents as the abrupt onset of hearing loss. Approximately 88% of SSNHL has no identifiable etiology and is termed idiopathic sudden sensorineural hearing loss (ISSHL).[1] Hearing specialists have investigated ISSHL since the 1970s. Over the past 30 years, more than 800 articles, or one every two weeks, have been published in the English medical literature.[2] ISSHL is the abrupt onset of hearing loss, usually unilaterally and upon wakening, that involves a hearing loss of at least 30 decibels (dB) occurring within three days over at least three contiguous frequencies.[3-4] As most patients do not present with premorbid audiograms, the degree of hearing loss is usually defined by the presentation thresholds of the unaffected ear.[4] Other associated symptoms include tinnitus, aural fullness, dizziness and vertigo.[4-5] The historical incidence of ISSHL ranges from 5–20 cases/100,000 population, with approximately 4,000 new cases per annum in the United States.[4,6] The true incidence is thought to be higher, as ISSHL is thought to be underreported. Interestingly, 4,000 cases annually calculate to 1.3 cases/ 100,000 in the United States; therefore, an incidence of 5–20/100,000 would translate to > 15,000 new ISSHL cases per annum in the United States. Recent literature has placed the annual ISSHL incidence in the United States as 27 cases/100,000, with a pediatric incidence of 11 cases/100,000.[7] Other studies report that the incidence is increasing (160/100,000), especially in the elderly (77/100,000), and conclude that ISSHL is no longer rare.[7-9] In 1984, Byl reviewed the literature and found the mean age of ISSHL presentation to be 46–49 years, with variation of incidence with age and an equal gender distribution.[6,10-13] The presentation of ISSHL does not appear to have seasonal variations, uneven distributions of presentation throughout the year, or an association with upper respiratory infections, either prior to or following symptom onset.[14] The spontaneous recovery is currently thought to be 30–60%.[15-17]

Etiopathogenesis of ISSHL

The first scientific reporting of ISSHL was published in 1944 in the Acta Oto-Laryngologica by De Kleyn.[18] To this day, otolaryngologists continue to investigate the etiologies and pathogenesis of ISSHL. Many mechanisms have been postulated, including: circulatory disturbances, ototoxicity, trauma, neoplasms, vascular occlusions, viral infections, labyrinthine membrane leaks, immune associated disease, abnormal cochlear stress response, abnormal tissue growth, and cochlear membrane damage.[1,19-21]

Early Experiments Investigating a Hypoxic Etiology for ISSHL

Early animal studies by Lamm and colleagues revealed that perilymph pO_2 of the scala tympani falls 50–80% during noise exposure.[22] Moreover, the compound action potential latency times are prolonged, and hair cell function declines by 60–70%. The authors opine that during noise exposure, the O_2 dependent sodium and potassium pumps of the organ of Corti (OOC) decompensate, resulting in intracellular sodium accumulations that cause microstructural damage. This damage is manifested in hair cell-cilia fusion, hair cell synaptic and dendritic swelling, hair cell contraction, and sustained depolarization.[23]

Circulatory Derangement Theories Regarding ISSHL

In 1980, Belal discussed the role of occlusive arterial disease (thrombotic, embolic or spastic) in the development of ISSHL and suggested a vascular etiology of ISSHL.[24] Vascular effects are the reasoning for the use of vasodilator drugs, stellate ganglion blocks, anticoagulants and rheological agents in the treatment of ISSHL. Animal studies show that labyrinthine artery occlusion results in severe degenerative changes, fibrosis, and new cochlear bone formation. This is similar to what occurs to the human cochlea deprived of its blood supply; there is progressive ossification of the cochlear spaces, loss of cochlear neurons, labyrinthine fibrosis, new bone formation, and endolymphatic hydrops.[25] In 2001, otolaryngologists at the University of Bologna investigated the blood pressures (BP) of a group of 23 young, untreated and otherwise healthy, ISSHL patients. They were compared with 20 age and sex matched, normotensive control subjects. Both groups underwent 24-hour BP monitoring. The authors found both systolic and diastolic BP measurements were significantly lower in the ISSHL group compared to the control group, leading them to conclude that systemic hypotension must be considered as a possible etiology of ISSHL in young healthy subjects.[26] The role of hypotension had been found in studies of ISSHL patient before, and these studies are important for several reasons.[27-30] First, they are in contradistinction to previous theories which suggested that sustained increases in BP are responsible for hemorrhagic and thrombotic events that may occur within the cochlea of ISSHL patients. Secondly, they provide plausible reasoning for how young, previously healthy patients, without known comorbidities, acquire ISSHL. Importantly, the implication that hypotension is a causative insult, would caution against the use of vasodilators in the treatment of those with lowered BP readings who acquire ISSHL. Moreover, the effects of hypotension may be prominently deleterious for the inner ear, which has significantly less circulatory autoregulation compared to cerebral blood flow.[31] The vascular hypothesis for ISSHL maintains that, as a result of vascular disruption and the resultant ischemia, the cochlear apparatus, cochlear nerve, or other components of the central auditory nervous system are damaged.

The Contribution of Comorbid Conditions to the Development of ISSHL

Interestingly, a recurrence of ISSHL has been observed in those with comorbid conditions, principally, diabetes (DM), hypertension (HTN), and dyslipidemia.[32] In 1996, Brant and others evaluated the relationship between age-associated hearing loss and several cardiovascular (CV) risk factors, including age, BP, alcohol use and cigarette smoking. They reviewed the records of 531 men participating in the Baltimore Longitudinal Study of Aging that began in 1965. They found that only systolic BP showed a significant relationship with hearing loss in the speech frequencies.[33] Others have theorized that atherosclerosis, and its associated risk factors, may play a role in the etiology of ISSHL.[34] In 2010, Aimoni and co-workers performed an observational case-control study of ISSHL patients (n = 141), matched for age and gender, with a control group (n = 271). They examined CV risk factors, including DM, HTN, smoking history, hypercholesterolemia, and hypertriglyceridemia. They found that DM and hypercholesterolemia were significantly more frequent in the ISSHL group compared to the control population and that the risk of ISSHL increased with the number of CV risk factors.[35] In 2012, Ciccone and colleagues studied 29 consecutive patients with ISSHL. The control subjects had no history of CV disease and normal hearing. Compared to the control group, the ISSHL patients had significantly higher total cholesterol, low density lipoprotein cholesterol (LDL-C) levels (early markers of atherosclerosis), and flow-mediated dilation (FMD) of the brachial artery, an early marker of endothelial dysfunction.[32] Moreover, ISSHL has been shown to be an early marker for an increased risk of stroke. Lin, et al., followed two cohorts of patients. One group consisted of all patients admitted for ISSHL (n = 1,423); the control group consisted of all patients admitted with appendicitis (n = 5,692). Both groups were followed for five years. The authors found a 12.7% stroke rate in the ISSHL group versus 8.7% of the appendicitis cohort. The stroke hazard was 1.64 times greater (p < 0.001) for the ISSHL patients, suggesting that ISSHL can be an early warning sign for stroke.[36] In 2014, Ozler investigated the neutrophil-lymphocyte ratio (NLR) levels in 40 ISSHL patients and compared them to 40 control subjects without evidence of auditory pathology. He found that all ISSHL patients, regardless of severity, had elevated NLR values compared to controls. The author suggests that high NLR values may be a predictor of other ischemic conditions, such as coronary or cerebral ischemia, and advocates that ISSHL patients be referred to cardiology and neurology specialists in follow up.[37]

Competing Multifactorial Theories for ISSHL

Gloddek and colleagues reviewed the differing theories regarding the pathogenesis of ISSHL, noting that a viral infection of the stria vascularis, OOC or spiral ganglion is alluded to in the American literature, while European scientists favor a vascular pathology with impaired inner ear perfusion.[38] A viral association with ISSHL has been suggested before, however, no specific serological profiles or response to antiviral treatment has been reported.[39] Gloddek's group melded the competing theories of immunologic, viral and vascular ISSHL etiologies. They hypothesize a virally stimulated, immunologically mediated perivasculitis, promoted by endothelial cell secretion of cytokines, results in circulating immunoglobulin deposition perivascularly, cochlear hypoperfusion and tissue hypoxia.[38] This is the basis of the immunopathological theory of ISSHL, which results in ischemia, stenosis, and atresia. There is additional evidence that ISSHL may be the result of abnormal activation of endocochlear nuclear factor κB, a molecular transcription factor that mediates the cellular responses to pathogenic stress, such as infections, mechanical stress, osmotic stress, and other insults.[40]

The Challenge in Treating ISSHL – Multi-Factorial Etiopathogenesis

More than 60 protocols have been put forth for the treatment of ISSHL, including the following: agents that decrease blood viscosity (osmotic diuretics, volume expanders, hydroxyethyl starch, rheologic agents, dextran, pentoxifylline, plasmapheresis, therapeutic phlebotomy, and normovolemic hemodilution); vasodilator drugs and procedures (histamine, papaverine, verapamil, procaine, cyclandelate, nifedipine, carbogen, dorsal sympathectomy, and stellate ganglion blocks); antiviral agents (acyclovir and valaciclovir); anticoagulants (sodium enoxaparin and heparin); free radical scavenging vitamins (B, C, and E); antibiotics; gingko biloba; magnesium; benzodiazepines; xanthinonictone, probanthine; lipoprostaglandin E1; IV lidocaine; repeated smallpox vaccinations; interferon alpha; ATP; betahistine; thrombolytics (tissue plasminogen activator, batroxibin); vinpocetine; bed rest; salt restriction; increased fluid intake; modification of cardiovascular risk factors; contrast dye (diatrizoate meglumine); corticosteroids; and HBO_2 therapy.[2,8] Of these many protocols, the one with the greatest efficacy is the combination of corticosteroids and HBO_2.

Rationale for the Use of Corticosteroids

The initial rationale for the use of corticosteroids in the treatment of ISSHL is their benefit in reducing both inflammation and edema. One theory assumes that the cochlear damage in ISSHL results from inflammatory triggers or an insult, and that corticosteroids counteract the inflammatory cascade, spare the cochlea further damage, and reverse some of the damage.[41] However, it is now known that corticosteroids have a primary role in protecting the cochlea from inflammatory mediators, specifically tumor necrosis factor alpha (TNF-α) and nuclear factor kappa-light-chain-enhancer (NF-κB).[38,41] TNF-α is a cell signaling protein (cytokine), and one of the initial components of the acute phase reaction of inflammation, which induces fever, apoptotic cell death, cachexia, the inflammatory response to tumorigenesis, viral replication, and the response to sepsis via interleukins. NF-κB is a protein complex that controls DNA transcription, cytokine production, and cell survival. It is produced in times of stress from cytokines, free radicals, and bacterial or viral antigens. Additionally, corticosteroids increase cochlear blood flow and ameliorate cochlear ischemia, favorably altering the inner ear milieu.[42-44] Corticosteroids also regulate protein synthesis within the inner ear. Inner ear glucocorticoid and mineralocorticoid receptors have been found within the inner ear, and steroid therapy may be affecting inner ear electrolyte and fluid balance.[42] It is within the inner ear, specifically at the vascular stria, where both sodium and potassium secretion are regulated to maintain the endocochlear membrane potential. This region is also the most frequent site of injury in those with ISSHL.[45] Systemic corticosteroids improve stria vascularis function and this may preserve its morphology in those that recover from ISSHL.[46]

Literature Review of Corticosteroids in the Treatment of ISSHL

In 2001, Alexiou and colleagues reported their retrospective review showing those with lower, middle or pancochlear hearing deficits had improved outcomes with corticosteroids and vasoactive agents.[47] In 2005, Slattery and colleagues conducted an unblinded, non-randomized, open-label clinical trial (n = 20) involving ISSHL patients who received four injections of intra-tympanic (IT) methylprednisolone within a two-week period, following failure of oral steroid therapy. The authors reported statistically significant improvement in four-frequency pure-tone average and speech discrimination score at one month follow up. Additionally, the improvements in tinnitus were statistically significant.[48] In 2008, Battaglia and colleagues performed a multicenter, double-blinded, placebo-controlled randomized study involving ISSHL patients who received either IT dexamethasone + placebo taper (Group A, n = 17), IT placebo injections + high dose prednisone taper (Group B, n = 18), or both steroid therapies (Group C, n = 16). They enrolled 51 patients with ISSHL with < six weeks of symptoms and followed them prospectively for three weeks. The combination group had an average improvement in speech discrimination of 44%, with a 40-dB improvement in pure tone average (PTA), significant improvement compared to prednisone taper only group (p < 0.05 and p < 0.02, respectively). Logistic regression analyses revealed the combination group demonstrated better odds of hearing recovery than patients in both of the other groups (p < 0.05) and recovered their hearing more quickly than the other groups (p < 0.05).[17] In 2011, Dispenza and others performed a prospective randomized trial comparing IT corticosteroids versus systemic corticosteroids in the treatment of ISSHL. They found both treatments resulted in hearing gains above that shown without treatment, however, there were no significant between group differences.[49] In the same year, Seggas and colleagues performed a comprehensive literature review on the use of IT corticosteroids for ISSHL. They identified the three main protocols for IT steroid administration, including the following: initial treatment, adjunctive treatment in combination with systemic corticosteroids, and as a salvage therapy after failure of systemic steroid (standard) treatment. The purpose of the review was to seek the best delivery technique and the optimal administration schedule. Randomized and non-randomized case control studies and case series studies were reviewed from 1996 to 2009. The authors concluded that topical corticosteroids can be a valuable treatment for ISSHL. However, the use of combination therapy yielded controversial results, and they were unable to determine whether this therapy could yield superior results to systemic corticosteroids. They also remarked upon the need for establishment of standard criteria for hearing recovery.[50] Another systematic review on the use of IT corticosteroids for ISSHL was also published in 2011 by Spears and Schwartz.[51] They identified 176 articles, of which, 32 were studies of initial or salvage IT corticosteroids for sudden hearing loss. These studies included six randomized trials and randomized control trials (RCTs). They found the vast majority of the studies of IT corticosteroids for salvage treatment at all levels demonstrated benefit. The higher quality studies imparted a 13.3 dB improvement, which is statistically significant. However, it was unclear to the authors if this difference was clinically significant. Moreover, initial IT steroid therapy was equivalent to standard therapy (systemic corticosteroids) in the existing literature of all qualities. The authors concluded that primary IT steroid therapy for ISSHL loss is equivalent to treatment with high-dose oral prednisone therapy. However, as a salvage therapy, IT corticosteroids offer the potential for some degree of additional hearing recovery.[51] In 2012, Ferri and coworkers investigated the use of IT corticosteroids in ISSHL patients who had failed 10 days of IV steroid therapy. They injected 0.5 mL of IT methylprednisolone up to seven times over 20 days. This salvage therapy resulted in improvement for 52.7% of patients. The authors surmised that the greatest positive influences on hearing recovery were early IT steroid therapy, hearing losses < 80 dB, and the involvement of low frequency deficits.[52]

Despite a reported ISSHL spontaneous recovery rate of 30–60%, the recovery in hearing in ISSHL patients is much poorer for those who have failed previous systemic steroid therapy.[16-17,48,53-56] The use of IT steroid therapy has several advantages over systemic therapy, including increasing intracochlear steroid concentrations and reducing the incidence of possible toxic side effects. IT steroid therapy also leads to much higher perilymphatic concentrations compared to system steroid therapy.[16,52,57] A substantial concentration gradient occurs in the scala tympani perilymph following round window application of IT corticosteroids.[57-58] Currently, the use of systemic corticosteroids is thought to impart a 50–80% recovery rate in the treatment of ISSHL.[52] However, there is concern regarding potential side effects, including the following: hyperglycemia (glucose intolerance), HTN, gastrointestinal bleeding, cataracts, adrenal suppression, psychosis, immunosuppression, and altered mental status. Currently, there is a paucity of data regarding the prevalence of these side effects with the relatively short courses of systemic steroid therapy used in the treatment of ISSHL.[59] In 2016, Gao and Liu reported their meta-analysis on the combined use of IT and systemic corticosteroids for ISSHL. They searched the literature databases for all available observational studies. They accepted eight studies for review, including seven prospective and one retrospective study. They reported that combination steroid therapy provides greater benefit than systemic steroid administration alone, and that those with severe-profound ISSHL would benefit more with combination therapy than mild-moderate patients for hearing outcomes but not recovery rate. They advocated that IT steroid therapy might serve as an alternative modality for seeking better outcomes.[60] In 2016, Qiang et al. published a meta-analysis, also comparing the use of systemic corticosteroids versus IT corticosteroids as initial therapy for ISSHL. They evaluated six RCTs and concluded that IT steroid groups exhibited better outcomes in PTA improvement and recovery rate than systemic steroid therapy, and that IT corticosteroids might be a potentially more beneficial modality for ISSHL patients regardless of the initial hearing loss severity.[61] IT corticosteroids have several advantages, including the following: assured compliance, therapy directed to the affected ear, high concentrations of corticosteroids in the perilymph, few side effects and complications, office-based procedure (no anesthesia), well tolerated, and more suitable for those in whom systemic corticosteroids are contraindicated or refused (DM, immunosuppressed states, and peptic ulcer disease).[2,16-17,48,50,53,62-68] Alternatively, there are disadvantages to IT steroid administration, including pain, tympanic membrane perforation, otitis media, vertigo (usually temporary), and hearing loss.[2]

Rationale for the Use of HBO$_2$ Therapy

The rationale for the use of HBO$_2$ therapy in the treatment of ISSHL is supported by an understanding of the rapid metabolism and vascular paucity of the cochlea and the structures within it. The stria vascularis and OOC, in particular, require an extremely high oxygen supply.[69] Moreover, a direct vascular supply to the OOC is minimal.[70] Tissue oxygenation to the cochlea occurs via oxygen diffusion from cochlear capillary networks into the perilymph and the cortilymph.[22] It is the perilymph that serves as the primary oxygen sources for structures within the cochlea. In 1983, Nagahara and colleagues studied the perilymph pO$_2$ in anesthetized human with hearing loss. The duration of hearing loss varied greatly (13 days to 15 years). However, they found that perilymph pO$_2$ tended to be lower in those with ISSHL than in those with otosclerosis, sudden cochleovestibular loss, or rapidly progressive sensorineural hearing loss. There was no correlation between the degree of hearing loss and the perilymph pO$_2$. However, these results led the authors to comment that some cases of ISSHL may be due to ischemia.[70] Later animal studies confirmed that while normobaric oxygen increases perilymph pO$_2$ 3.4-fold, HBO$_2$ increases perilymph pO$_2$ 9.4-fold.[22] Although normobaric hyperoxygenation increases intracochlear oxygen tensions, only HBO$_2$ therapy achieves the extremely high arterial perilymphatic oxygen concentrations differences required for efficacy.[22,71-72] Additional benefits of HBO$_2$ may be related to its obviation of ischemic reperfusion injury, edema reduction, and anti-inflammatory effects.

Literature Review: The Use of HBO₂ in the Treatment of ISSHL

Use of HBO₂ as a Primary Treatment for ISSHL

There is a scarcity of literature regarding the use of HBO₂ therapy as a primary treatment for ISSHL. HBO₂ is usually an adjunctive therapy with medical therapies or as salvage therapy following failure of medical therapy. In 1998, Schwab and colleagues reported the results of their RCT of 75 ISSHL patients treated within 14 days, with or without HBO₂ therapy (1.5 atmospheres absolute [ATA] 100% O₂ for 45 minutes daily for 10–20 sessions). There were 37 patients in the HBO₂ group and 38 in the control group. They found clinical and statistically significant improvement with the use of HBO₂ compared to the control group (15.6 dB versus 10.7 dB, respectively).[73] In 2001, Fatorri et al., published a RCT of 50 ISSHL patients who presented to their otolaryngology offices within 48 hours of symptom onset and were treated with either HBO₂ (2.2 ATA with 100% O₂ for 90 minutes daily for 10 sessions; n = 30) or medical therapy (IV buflomedil; n = 20). The HBO₂ group showed a statistically significant improvement in hearing compared to the medical therapy group (61.3 dB versus 24.0 dB, respectively) as well as a significantly greater response to therapy (73% vs 55%, respectively). They also found that those with pantonal hypoacusis responded significantly better than those with a milder presentation.[74] In 2003, Racic and colleagues compared HBO₂ (2.8 bar) with varying dosages of IV pentoxifylline infusion (n = 64). The HBO₂ group showed statistically significant improvement compared to IV pentoxifylline in overall hearing (46.35 dB versus 21.48 dB, respectively), attainment of physiological hearing values (47.1% versus 6.2%, respectively), and in moderate hearing gains (41.2% versus 12.5%), respectively.[75] In 2007, Dundar and colleagues prospectively compared ISSHL patients treated primarily with HBO₂ to those treated with medical therapy. The HBO₂ patients had statistically significant hearing gains across all frequencies, with tinnitus patients showing the greatest hearing improvement.[76]

The Use of HBO₂ as a Salvage Therapy for ISSHL

The literature supports that a significant number of patients, between 35–39%, do not respond to medical or placebo therapies. These patients may benefit from salvage therapy. One of the earliest studies was the 1995 RCT, presented by Hoffman and coworkers, evaluating 20 ISSHL patients treated with HBO₂ therapy 14 days after failing primary medical therapy. The primary medical therapy consisted of treatment with hydroxyethyl starch, pentoxifylline and cortisone. Half of these patients were then treated with HBO₂ therapy (10-20 sessions, once daily at 1.5 ATA for 45 minutes). The HBO₂ salvage therapy resulted in significant hearing gains compared to the control group (7.5 dB versus 0.7 dB, respectively).[77] In 1998, Lamm and colleagues analyzed more than 50 trials utilizing HBO₂ as an adjunctive therapy for ISSHL, acoustic trauma, noise-induced hearing loss and tinnitus. They also performed a subset analysis on the patients within these studies that failed to respond to any medical therapies (n = 4,109). In this group, they found that if HBO₂ was started between two to four weeks, 50% showed marked hearing gains (at least three frequencies of > 30 dB), 33% showed moderate improvement (10 dB – 20 dB), and 13% showed no improvement. If adjunctive HBO₂ was utilized between six weeks to three months, 13% showed definite improvement in hearing, 25% showed moderate improvement, and 62% had no improvement.[78] In 2000, Marchesi and others, retrospectively studied 95 patients, 80% of whom had previous ineffective medical treatment, and were then treated with HBO₂. Following HBO₂ therapy, 78.9% of patients had a mean improvement of 38.3 +/- 8.3 dB, and 41% gained > 20 dB. Complete recovery occurred in 11.6%. HBO₂ was most effective in those patients treated within 14 days.[79] That same year, Murakawa and colleagues reviewed 522 cases of ISSHL, occurring over a ten-year period, in patients unresponsive to medical therapies, who then received HBO₂ therapy. Following HBO₂ treatment, complete recovery occurred in 19.7%, with significant improvement in 34.9%, and slight improvement in 23.2%. Delay to treatment > 14 days, advanced age, and vertigo were associated with poorer outcomes.[80] In 2010, Muzzi et al. treated 19 ISSHL patients, who failed medical therapy, with HBO₂. The use of HBO₂ salvage therapy improved PTAs, particularly at the low frequencies. They also found better results with early HBO₂ therapy and in older patients.[81] In the same year, Ohno and colleagues compared ISSHL patients who had failed four weeks of medical treatment, and then treated with HBO$_2$, to a similar group treated with medical therapy alone. The mean hearing gains were not different between groups. However, those with profound hearing loss did show significantly higher hearing gains.[82] Importantly, in 2012, The American Academy of Otolaryngology – Head and Neck Surgery Foundation, published *their Clinical Practice Guidelines for Sudden Hearing Loss.* They recommended HBO$_2$ therapy for use within three months of symptom onset.[4]

In 2013, Cvorovic and colleagues published a randomized prospective trial utilizing IT corticosteroids and HBO$_2$ as salvage therapies for ISSHL. They enrolled 155 ISSHL patients at their tertiary referral center and treated them with the primary medical therapy of IV dexamethasone (40 mg daily for three days, followed by 10 mg for three days). They then enrolled the 50 patients who failed primary therapy (< 10 dB improvement in hearing gains), in a 1:1 fashion, to receive salvage therapy with either IT corticosteroids (four IT injections in 13 days) or HBO$_2$ therapy (2.0 ATA with 100% O$_2$ for 60 minutes daily for 20 days). They found that HBO$_2$ salvage therapy resulted in significant improvement in hearing thresholds at all tested frequencies. The IT steroid salvage therapy was found to be significantly beneficial at most frequencies (except 2 kHz). Their subgroup analyzes revealed that those patients with PTAs < 81 dB and those younger than 60 years had a better response to HBO$_2$ therapy, than did those who were profoundly deaf or the elderly.[83] During this same time, Yang and coworkers published their historical cohort study of ISSHL patients who received primary medical therapy. They then related in detail, a smaller subset of this group (n = 103) who, after failing primary systemic therapy, opted to participate in salvage therapy. All patients were initially admitted to the Kaohsiung Chang Gung Memorial Hospital in Taiwan and treated with IV dexamethasone in decreasing dosages. Over the next five days, they also received 30 mg oral prednisolone daily, radiopaque contrast (Hypaque 76, 10 ml IV daily), and a plasma expander (Dextran-40, 500 ml IV daily). Patients who were refractory to this regimen were then informed of 4 choices: IT corticosteroids (four injections of dexamethasone within two weeks); HBO$_2$ therapy (2.5 ATA for 120 minutes with 100% O$_2$ for 10 sessions within two weeks); combination of IT corticosteroids and HBO$_2$; and observation only without salvage therapy. The patients chose their treatment arms: IT corticosteroids (n=35); HBO$_2$ (n=22); IT Steroid + HBO$_2$ (n = 19); and control group (n = 27).

The authors reported no significant differences between groups regarding baseline characteristic, duration of symptoms, or initial hearing thresholds between the four groups. The hearing gains in PTA were significantly improved in those who received either IT corticosteroids, HBO$_2$, or both (IT corticosteroids + HBO$_2$) compared to the control group (p=0.02, 0.036, and 0.003, respectively). However, the hearing gain in dB between treatment groups was not statistically different. The combined therapy group (IT corticosteroids + HBO$_2$) also had statistically significant improvement in word recognition scoring (WRS) compared to the control group. The authors concluded that the combination of IT corticosteroids and HBO$_2$ as salvage therapy may be the most beneficial for the recovery of hearing.[84] In 2015, Pezzoli and colleagues reported their study of 135 ISSHL patients treated with primary therapy and their further investigations on the 23 patients who accepted salvage therapy with HBO$_2$. Over a roughly two-year period, they evaluated 168 ISSHL patients and excluded 33 patients. The remaining 135 patients were treated primarily with IV 4 mg betamethasone and osmotic diuretics (250 cc of IV mannitol 18%) for six consecutive days. Those failing primary therapy, were then treated with a seven-day course of oral dexamethasone (25 mg daily) and offered HBO$_2$ salvage therapy. Twenty-three patients were treated with oral dexamethasone and HBO$_2$ (2.5 ATA for 60 minutes for 15 treatments), and compared with the 21 patients who accepted oral steroid therapy but refused HBO$_2$ salvage therapy (non-randomized control group). There were no reported differences between these groups in baseline characteristics. The patients receiving HBO$_2$ had a significantly increased mean improvement of 15.6 dB versus the spontaneous mean improvement of the control group of 5.0 dB (p = 0.013). They also found that those with the worst hearing had the greatest degree of improvement, regardless of treatment onset (within 10 days or 11–30 days).[85] This study was unrandomized, had probable selection bias (inability to afford treatment at private facility) and an outcome measure based upon absolute values of hearing gains but not clinical improvement.

The Use of HBO₂ Therapy for Chronic Hearing Loss

The strength of evidence is weaker for the use of HBO_2 in the treatment of chronic hearing loss. In 1990, Schumann and colleagues treated 557 chronic hearing loss patients with 10 sessions of HBO_2. An improvement of > 10 dB was found in 27.8% of cases.[86] In 1995, Hoffman and colleagues presented their RCT of 44 ISSHL patients with symptoms lasting greater than six months. The HBO_2 group (n = 22) received 15 sessions (1.5 ATA with 100% oxygen for 45 minutes). The control group (n = 22) received 15 sessions of hyperbaric air (1.5 ATA air for 45 minutes). No significant differences were found between groups due to lack of inclusion of standard deviations (inestimable). The study was also limited by unclear randomization and allocation concealment and a lack of a sham true control group.[87] Importantly, this was, in fact, an RCT with two hyperbaric treatment groups and without a true control group. Hyperbaric oxygen therapy is a dual therapy treatment of both hyperoxygenation and pressure, and pressurized air is not physiologically inert.[88-89] In 1997, Kau and co-workers reported their use of HBO_2 salvage therapy in 359 ISSHL patients who failed primary medical therapy. In those with hearing loss between one and three months, noticeable improvement or complete recovery was seen in 13% (> 20 dB in at least three test frequencies), and moderate recovery occurred in 25.2% (10 dB–20 dB). Overall, 30% had an improvement of > 10 dB, but only 2% regained normal hearing.[90] The use of HBO_2 for those with chronic hearing loss does show some promise, but the best results occur with the use of early HBO_2 therapy combined with steroid administration.

The Use of HBO₂ With Medical Therapies in the Treatment of ISSHL

The use of HBO_2 in combination with various medical and procedural therapies has been extensively investigated. In this section, greater emphasis will be placed on larger and more recent studies that have not been discussed in detail elsewhere. In 1979, Giger published a prospective, randomized trial of 55 patients treated with either carbogen inhalation (95% O_2/5% CO_2) or IV infusion of papaverine and dextran. Although immediate differences were not found, audiogram testing at one year showed statistically better audiometric testing in those treated with carbogen, suggesting hyperoxygenation may improve ISSHL outcomes.[91] In the same year, Goto and co-workers compared medical therapy, stellate ganglion block (SGB) and HBO_2. They found that 100% of the patients treated with SGB and HBO_2 achieved > 10 dB PTA improvement, and 40% of these patients recovered to within 20 dB of their baseline hearing.[92] In 1985, Pilgramm and colleagues published a RCT (n=37) of ISSHL patients treated with medical therapy with or without HBO_2 therapy. All patients presented within 14 days of symptoms onset. The medical therapy group (n=19) received 500 ml of 10% dextran-40 and sorbitol 5%, 600 mg naftidrofuryl hydrogenaxalate and vitamin B orally for 14 days. The HBO_2 therapy included 10 sessions once daily (2.5 ATA for 60 minutes). The HBO_2 group (n = 18) had a significantly increased hearing gains when compared to the medical therapy group (29.2 dB versus 20.2 dB, respectively).[93] In 1993, French investigators conducted several studies evaluating the use of HBO_2 in combination with various medical therapies. They found HBO_2 to be a useful synergistic adjunct, with twice daily HBO_2 sessions reducing the length of therapy.[94,95] In 1996, Cavallazzi and coworkers published their RCT of 64 patients with ISSHL treated with either medical therapy or HBO_2. The authors did not relay the duration of patients' ISSHL symptomatology, so the acuity or chronicity of the ISSHL is unknown. The medical therapy group (n = 30) was treated with multiple drugs, including: heparin, betamethasone, nicotinic acid, flunarizine, cytidine, phosphocholine, dextran, vitamins, neurotropic and antiviral drugs. The doses for these medical therapies were also not provided. This medical group was considered the control group, and was compared to another group, who received the same medical therapies and HBO_2 group (n = 32). The HBO$_2$ therapy was provided for 15 sessions over three weeks (2.5 ATA with 100% O$_2$ for 60 minutes daily). The addition of HBO$_2$ conferred improvement in hearing gains compared to the control group (95% versus 71%, respectively). However, these differences were not statistically significant. This study is limited by the unknown duration of the subjects' hearing loss, unknown specifics regarding multiple medical therapies, possible selection bias (no mention of allocation concealment), and it was not blinded. Moreover, this study may not have been randomized, as randomization was not described.[96] Most importantly, due to the lack of specifics regarding the acuity or chronicity of the participants' ISSHL symptomatology, and the unknown dosages of the 10 drugs used in the medical therapy of both groups, this study cannot be replicated or validated, basic tenets required for ensuring the accuracy and meaningfulness of scientific inquiry. In 2002, Aslan et al. published their experience utilizing medical therapy combined with either SGB or HBO$_2$. A significant increase in hearing gains was found with the addition of HBO$_2$ therapy.[97]

In 2004, Topuz and others published an RCT of 51 ISSHL patients who presented within two weeks of symptomatology and treated with medical therapy with or without HBO$_2$. All patients were admitted and given primary medical therapy, which included: IV prednisone (1 mg/kg per day for 14 days), IV Rheomacrodex (a plasma expander dextran given as a 500-ml infusion over six hours daily for five days), diazepam (5 mg orally twice daily), IV pentoxifylline (200 mg twice daily), and salt restriction. The medical control group (n = 21) received no further therapy. Those patients randomized to the HBO$_2$ group (n = 30) received 25 sessions in total, applied at 2.5 ATA with 100% O$_2$ for 90 minutes twice daily for the first five days, then once daily for 15 days. For those with mild hearing loss, there was no difference between groups. However, for those with moderate hearing loss, the addition of HBO$_2$ significantly improved hearing gains compared to the medical control group (35.4 dB versus 16.2 dB, respectively). For those with severe hearing loss, the statistically superior results for the HBO$_2$ group were more impressive (50.7 dB versus 13 dB, respectively). The HBO$_2$ group displayed statistically significant improvement in hearing gains over all frequencies tested, except 2,000 Hz. Within the HBO$_2$ group, the mean hearing gains for those older than 50 years was greater than for those younger than 50 years.[98] In 2006, Narozny et al. reviewed two historical groups of ISSHL patients treated with combinations of medical therapy, corticosteroids, and HBO$_2$. The hearing gains were statistically significant for the HBO$_2$ group over all frequencies and in four ranges of frequencies for both relative and absolute values. Additionally, the combination of corticosteroids and HBO$_2$ resulted in statistically improved clinical outcomes. The authors found delay to treatment and flat hearing loss to be predictors of poor clinical outcomes. Linear regression analyses were also performed to identify prognostic factors related to hearing improvement. Favorable prognostic factors included treatment with high-dose corticosteroids + HBO$_2$ and early treatment (within 10 days). A poor prognosis was found with delayed treatment, labyrinth responsiveness disorders, and decreased TSH levels.[99] In 2008, Suzuki and coworkers reported on 196 consecutive ISSHL patients, comparing steroid or IV prostaglandin E1 (PGE1) combined with HBO$_2$. No differences were found between groups, indicating corticosteroids and PGE1 may be equally effective when combined with HBO$_2$ therapy. Additionally, PGE1 may be a potential alternative for steroid-intolerant patients.[100] In the same year, the same lead author published a similar trial, comparing ISSHL patients treated with IV PGE1 or SGB combined with HBO$_2$. In those with less severe hearing loss (< 80 dB), the outcomes were similar. However, for those with severe hearing loss (> 80 dB), the hearing rate was statistically superior in those treated with SGB and HBO$_2$.[101]

In 2009, Cekin, et al., conducted an RCT study evaluating 57 ISSHL patients treated with medical therapy with prednisolone (1 mg/kg tapering dose over three weeks) and famotidine (40 mg once daily) with or without HBO$_2$. There were 21 patients in the medical therapy group and 36 patients in the HBO$_2$ group. Hyperbaric therapy was applied with 2.5 ATA with 100% O$_2$ for 90 minutes for 10 sessions. Both groups had recovery rates above 70% (79.0% HBO$_2$ versus 71.3% medical therapy). However, there was no statistical differences between the groups.[102] The most interesting limitation of this study was that it lacked an intention to treat analysis. The lead author of this study was contacted regarding the size disparity between groups. The stated randomization was as follows: Subjects were allocated randomly, using a computer, into study and control groups. The author responded that some of the patients in the control group were not improving, and did not return. An intention to treat analysis would have been beneficial. In 2010, Liu and others reviewed their treatment of 120 ISSHL patients treated within two weeks with medical therapy, with or without HBO_2. The overall effectiveness was clinically and statistically superior for the HBO_2 patients. The most profound improvement occurred in those with moderate to severe deafness, and those with descending and flat types of audiograms.[103] In 2011, Korpinar and coworkers published their treatment of 80 ISSHL patients treated with medical therapy and HBO_2. They sought to identify factors that affect treatment outcomes. They found that hearing gains were significantly improved for those with early HBO_2, a higher number of HBO_2 treatments, the use of corticosteroids, low frequency-ascending and total audiogram configurations, and profound hearing loss.[104] In 2011, Holy and colleagues reviewed the outcomes of 61 ISSHL patients treated with IV vasodilation therapy and HBO_2. Hearing improvement occurred in 59.7% of patients. However, if HBO_2 was started within 10 days, significant or complete recovery was found in 65.9% of patients. In those treated with HBO_2 > 10 days from symptom onset, improvement was noted in only 38.9%.[105] In 2011, Liu and colleagues retrospectively reported their care of 465 ISSHL patients treated with either IV and oral corticosteroids, IV and oral corticosteroids plus dextran, or IV and oral corticosteroids, dextran and HBO_2. The addition of HBO_2 was found beneficial in those with initially profound hearing loss. The addition of dextran did not improve outcomes.[106]

Use of HBO_2 With Corticosteroids in the Treatment of ISSHL

The best outcomes in the literature are found when HBO_2 is combined with steroid therapy in the treatment of ISSHL. In 2007, Fujimura and colleagues published their work with 130 consecutive ISSHL patients treated with corticosteroids, with or without HBO_2. The HBO_2 group showed statistically improved rate of hearing recovery. A subset analysis of those with severe hearing loss (> 80 dB) showed that the HBO_2 groups had a statistically superior rate of hearing improvement.[107] In 2011, Suzuki and colleagues performed simple and multiple regression analysis on 174 consecutive ISSHL patients treated with hydrocortisone and HBO_2. They sought to develop a regression model for predicting hearing outcomes in ISSHL patients. They found significant inverse correlations between hearing improvement and days from onset to treatment, patient age, and the presence of vertigo.[108] In the same year, Alimoglu and others retrospectively reviewed their treatment of 217 ISSHL patients (219 ears) receiving various combinations of oral or IT corticosteroids and HBO_2. The most statistically superior hearing gains (highest mean gain among all groups and the greatest proportion of complete recovery) occurred with the use of both oral corticosteroids and HBO_2 therapy.[21] In 2012, Filipo and colleagues reported their prospective, randomized trial of 48 ISSHL patients with < 14 days of symptoms, who were recruited by the ENT emergency room staff of the Department of Sensory Organs of Sapienza University of Rome. The patients were grouped according to initial PTAs. Group I (n = 25) had severe hearing loss (70 dB – 90 dB), while Group II (n = 23) had profound hearing loss (> 90 dB). All patients received HBO_2 therapy (multiplace chamber, 2.4 ATA 100% O_2 for 75 minutes daily for 10 sessions). Intravenous corticosteroid (IV methylprednisolone, 1 mg/kg/day for seven days) was given to 13 patients in the severe group and 13 patients in the profound group. Intratympanic corticosteroids (IT prednisolone, 62.5 mg/ml day for three days, injected two hours prior to HBO_2 therapy) was given to 12 patients in the severe group and to 10 patients in the profound group. The authors reported positive additional benefit with the addition of HBO_2 therapy. They also found an increase in the success rate in the IT steroid + HBO_2 group. However, the results were not statistically significant.[109]

In 2015, Capuano and colleagues published a retrospective four-year cohort study of 300 patients, divided into three groups. Group A (IVS) received the IV steroid methylprednisolone, at decreasing doses of 40 mg for seven days, and 20 mg for another three days (n=100). Group B (HBO$_2$) received HBO$_2$ at 2.5 ATA for 90 minutes, week-days for 16 sessions (n=100). Group C (IVS + HBO$_2$) received both therapies (n=100). There were no statistically significant between group differences in baseline characteristics. The IVS + HBO$_2$ group had the highest response rate to therapy, compared to the HBO$_2$ group or the IVS group (84% versus 70% and 68%, respectively), as well as the highest rate of complete recovery (58% versus 24% and 20%, respectively) regardless of initial hearing levels. In all groups, those who began therapy within the first two weeks had significantly greater mean hearing gains, while those with hypercholesterolemia (> 240 mg/dL) had significantly worse responses.[110] Importantly, the title of this study asked if the routine application of HBO$_2$ was helpful in ISSHL. The authors concluded that the combination of HBO$_2$ and steroids was more effective than either alone.[110]

In 2016, Carneiro and coworkers published two case reports of ISSHL occurring following spinal anesthesia. These cases are illustrative in that they opine a mechanistic causation not usually discussed in ISSHL literature. They are considered to be the first cases of spinal anesthesia-related cases treated with HBO$_2$ to be published. The first case involved a healthy 27-year-old woman who received spinal anesthesia prior to a cesarean section. Six hours following surgery, the patient complained of left-sided hearing loss, which persisted for three days. She was diagnosed with profound left-sided ISSHL across the entire spectrum of frequencies and was treated with pentoxifylline and corticosteroids. The patient did not improve and began HBO$_2$ therapy 14 weeks after symptom onset. Following HBO$_2$ therapy, the patient had improvement in audiogram testing. The second case involved a 61-year-old man with HTN, dyslipidemia, hyperuricemia, left nephrectomy due to renal cell carcinoma, adrenal adenoma, and gonarthrosis, who underwent spinal anesthesia for a total knee replacement. Immediately following the surgery, the patient developed severe left-sided hearing loss and mild left-sided tinnitus. Audiogram results confirmed new left-sided moderate SSNHL in the lower frequencies. Speech discrimination was 60% on the left and 80% on the right. The patient was initially treated with conservative measures (bed rest and fluid intake) and corticosteroids. The patient began HBO$_2$ therapy on the 10th day from symptom onset. Following HBO$_2$ therapy, the PTA thresholds significantly improved, and speech discrimination was 100% on both sides. The authors discuss the possible etiologies of postoperative SSNHL following non-cardiac surgery and concluded that decreases in cerebrospinal fluid (CSF) pressure, more common after spinal anesthesia, were contributory in these cases. The anesthesia literature has been studying this phenomenon for some time and have evaluated the spinal needle design, type of spinal needle, size of the spinal needle, and the association of post-dural procedural headache (PDPH) and hearing loss. The current prevailing theory is that there is disruption of the endolymph/perilymph balance that is caused by the decrease in CSF pressure.[111] Cerebrospinal fluid dynamics are integral to auditory function of the inner ear. The puncture of the dura membrane results in a CSF leak, drop in CSF volume and pressure, and that reduced subarachnoid pressure is transmitted to the inner ear through a patent cochlear aqueduct, reducing perilymphatic pressure, resulting in an endolymphatic hydrops, which disrupts the hair cells on the basement membrane. Treatment relies on management of the PDPH and drugs or procedures to ensure adequate oxygenation.[111]

In 2017, Hosokawa and others retrospectively reviewed the clinical data of the 334 ISSHL patients presenting to Shizuoka Saiseikai General Hospital in Japan over a five-year period. All patients were treated with HBO$_2$ (2.0 ATA for 60 minutes once daily for 10 days) therapy and IV corticosteroids (hydrocortisone 400 mg, tapered over 10 days). They reported that improvement rates varied with the degree of initial hearing loss. Improvement rates for those with Grade 1 hearing loss (< 40 dB) were 44.7%; 60.5% for those with Grade 2 hearing loss (40 dB – 60 dB); 81.5% for those with Grade 3 hearing loss (60 dB – 90 dB); and 75.6% for those with Grade 4 hearing loss (> 90 dB.). The authors concluded that HBO$_2$ therapy has a significant additional effect when used in combination with IV corticosteroids for ISSHL. The study was limited by lack of a control group or blinding and no long-term outcomes.[112]

Literature Summary for the Treatment of ISSHL

The best evidence regarding improvement in hearing for those with ISSHL involves combination therapy with corticosteroids and HBO_2. Table 1 summarizes the retrospective and prospective case-controlled series for the treatment of ISSHL. These 15 studies represent 2,343 patients treated with a variety of medical therapies, HBO_2, or both.[21,75-76,82,84-85,92,97,99-101,103,106-107,110] All of these trials are level two evidence; however, most are adequately dosed and treated within 30 days of symptom onset. While acknowledging that level one evidence is preferred, it is important to remember the large amount of clinical treatments, in all realms of medicine and surgery, without any RCT support. Surgeons have argued for decades that sham surgeries are unethical, and large amounts of critical care and emergency medicine do not have RCTs for many common and lifesaving interventions. Specific to the application of HBO_2 and RCTs, it is not an overestimation to say that no one has devised an appropriate "sham control" for the use of HBO_2 therapy. Theories regarding the placebo effects of HBO_2 therapy abound. However, there have been no long-term studies to validate these presumptions. Lack of sham controls are a limitation of every comparative trial in the HBO_2 literature. One of the most beneficial advances that could be made in the field of hyperbaric medicine would be the development of a truly sham control protocol for future studies.

Table 1. Retrospective and Prospective Case-Controlled Studies of ISSHL and HBO_2

Study	Patient Groups	HBO_2	Hearing Gains
Capuano 2015 [110]	n = 300 IVS (n = 100) HBO_2 (n = 100) IVS + HBO_2 (n = 100)	2.5 ATA 90 minutes 16 sessions	Complete Recovery Regardless of Initial Levels 58% IVS + HBO_2* 24% HBO_2 20% IVS Response Rate to Therapy 84% IVS + HBO_2 70% HBO_2 68% IVS
Pezzoli 2014 [85]	n = 44 treatment applied after failing MT POS (n = 21) POS + HBO_2 (n = 23) POS group (controls)	2.5 ATA 60 minutes 15 sessions	Hearing Gains 15.6 dB POS + HBO_2* 5.0 dB POS those with worst hearing had greatest improvement with HBO_2, regardless of symptom onset
Yang 2013 [84]	n = 103 treatments applied after failing MT ITS (n = 35) HBO_2 (n = 22) ITS + HBO_2 (n = 19) observation only controls (n = 27)	2.5 ATA 120 minutes 10 sessions	Compared to Controls ITS (p = 0.02)* HBO_2 (p = 0.036)* ITS + HBO_2 (p =0.003)** no between group differences Word Recognition Scoring ITS + HBO_2 (p = 0.05)*
Alimoglu 2011 [21]	n = 219 HBO_2 (n = 57) POS (n = 58) ITS (n = 43) POS + HBO_2 (n = 61) POS & ITS (control groups)	2.5 ATA 120 minutes 20 sessions	Response to Therapy 86.9% POS / HBO_2* 63.8% POS 46.5% ITS 43.9% HBO_2 Complete Recovery 42.6% POS / HBO_2* 19.0% POS 17.5% HBO_2 11.6% ITS Highest Mean Hearing Gain POS + HBO_2*

Table 1. Retrospective and Prospective Case-Controlled Studies of ISSHL and HBO$_2$ (continued)

Study	Patient Groups	HBO$_2$	Hearing Gains
Liu 2011 [106]	n = 465 IVS & POS (n = 76) IVS & POS + Dex (n = 277) IVS & POS + Dex + HBO$_2$ (n = 112)	2.5 ATA 60 minutes 10 – 20 sessions	addition of HBO$_2$ improved good and fair recoveries significantly more than other groups* and is beneficial with profound initial hearing loss
Liu 2010 [103]	n = 120 treated < 14 d MT + HBO$_2$ (n = 60) MT only (n = 60) MT control (type unknown)	unknown	<u>Overall Effectiveness</u> 83.3% HBO$_2$* 60% MT
Ohno 2010 [82]	n = 92 HBO$_2$ (n = 48) MT only (n = 44) MT control (IVS, POS, vitamins, ATP) HBO$_2$ applied (mean 7.4 wks) following MT failure	2.0 ATA 60 minutes mean sessions 13.0	<u>HBO$_2$ Mean Hearing Gains</u> Initial Profound Loss 18.3 dB* Initial Severe Loss 4.4 dB Initial Moderate Loss 2.1 dB Initial Mild Loss 2.3 dB
Suzuki 2008 [100]	n = 196 POS + HBO$_2$ (n = 101) PEG1 & HBO$_2$ (n = 95) hearing loss ≥ 40 dB for ≤ 30 days unaffected ears (controls)	2.5 ATA 60 minutes 10 sessions	no between group differences PGE1 as an alternative for steroid intolerant
Suzuki 2008 [101]	n = 205 PGE1 + HBO$_2$ (n = 95) SBG + HBO$_2$ (n = 110) hearing loss ≥ 40 dB for ≤ 30 days unaffected ears (controls)	2.5 ATA 60 minutes 10 sessions	<u>Improvement Rate > 80 dB</u> SGB + HBO$_2$ 53.0%* PGE1 + HBO$_2$ 35.3%
Dundar 2007 [76]	n = 80 MT + HBO$_2$ (n = 55) MT only (n = 25) hearing loss ≥ 40 dB for < 30 days MT type unknown unaffected ears (controls)	unknown	HBO$_2$ gains across all frequencies* patients with tinnitus showed the highest hearing improvement but only with the addition of HBO$_2$
Fujimura 2007 [107]	n = 130 POS + HBO$_2$ (n = 67) POS only (n = 63) hearing loss ≥ 40 dB for ≤ 30 days unaffected ears (controls)	unknown	Severe Loss (≥ 80 dB) <u>Hearing Rate Improvement</u> 51.1% HBO$_2$* 27.1% controls <u>Rate of Recovery</u> 59.7% HBO$_2$* 39.7% controls
Narozny 2004 [134]	n = 133 MT + HBO$_2$ (n = 52) MT only (n = 81) HBO$_2$ + MT (VD, high dose steroid, vitamins & histamine analog) MT = VD, low dose steroid & vitamins	2.5 ATA 60 minutes 5 days a week unknown # sessions	Hearing Gain <u>In All Frequencies</u> MT + HBO$_2$* % Hearing Gain <u>In All Frequencies</u> MT + HBO$_2$*
Racic 2003 [75]	n = 115 HBO$_2$ (n = 51) MT (n = 64) MT control group (varying pentoxifylline infusion dosages)	2.8 ATA	<u>Improvement in Hearing</u> 46.4 dB HBO$_2$* 21.5 dB MT <u>Physiologic Hearing Values</u> 47.1% HBO$_2$* 6.2% MT <u>Moderate Hearing Gains</u> 41.2% HBO$_2$* 12.5% MT

Table 1. Retrospective and Prospective Case-Controlled Studies of ISSHL and HBO$_2$ (continued)

Study	Patient Groups	HBO$_2$	Hearing Gains
Aslan 2002 [97]	n = 50 MT + HBO$_2$ (n = 25) MT only (n = 25) MT (betahistine HCl, prednisone, SGB)	2.4 ATA 90 minutes 20 sessions BID x 7 days daily X 6 days	<u>Hearing Gains</u> 37.9 dB MT + HBO$_2$* 20.0 dB MT MT + HBO$_2$ <u>Mean Hearing Gains (Age)</u> 51.4 dB (< 50 years)* 23.3 dB (> 50 years) 48.9 dB (< 60 years)** 14.5 dB (> 60 years) HBO$_2$ effective within 14 days
Goto 1979 [92]	n = 91 MT + SGB + HBO$_2$ (n = 20) SGB + HBO$_2$ (n = 49) MT (n = 22) MT = VD, corticosteroids, and vitamins	2.4 ATA 90 minutes 20 sessions	<u>Treated < 7 d (PTA > 10 dB)</u> 100% MT + SGB + HBO$_2$ 83% SGB + HBO$_2$* 69% MT only <u>Treated < 14 d (PTA > 10 dB)</u> 100% MT + SGB + HBO$_2$** 69% SGB + HBO$_2$** 33% MT only Hearing Improvement <u>Initial Profound Hearing Loss</u> 100% MT + SGB + HBO$_2$** 83% SGB + HBO$_2$* 33% MT only

MT = Medical Therapy   POS = Oral Steroid   VD = Vasodilator
HBO$_2$ = Hyperbaric Oxygen   Dex = Dextran   ATP = Adenosine Tri Phosphate
IVS = Intravenous Steroid   PGE1 = Prostaglandin E1   *(p < 0.05)
ITS = Intratympanic Steroid   SGB = Stellate Ganglion Block   **(p < 0.01)

Table 2 highlights eight RCTs on the use of HBO$_2$ in the treatment of ISSHL.[83,73-74,77,93,98,102,109] This chapter has added several recently published RCTs and removed others. Specifically, the 1996 RCT by Cavallazzi and coworkers is excluded.[96] The study has possible selection bias for two reasons: a lack of information regarding allocation concealment and unclear randomization with possible random sequence generation.[113] It is also unblinded and lacks sham controls. Importantly, the study has fatal flaws involving the authors' exclusion of information. The authors did not report the study groups' duration of ISSHL symptomatology, making the acuity or chronicity of the ISSHL unknown. Additionally, medical therapy given to both groups involved pharmacological treatments with 10 drugs, including heparin, betamethasone, nicotinic acid, flunarizine, cytidine, phosphocholine, dextran, vitamins, neurotropic and antiviral drugs. However, the doses for these medical therapies were not provided. Both of these exclusions prohibit trial replication or validation, a basic tenet for ensuring the accuracy and meaningfulness of scientific inquiry. The 1995 RCT by Hoffman and coworkers is also excluded.[87] This study is limited by unclear randomization and allocation concealment, and it is unblinded.[113] Importantly, this RCT has fatal flaws. The first is the omission of standard deviations of their results. It makes interpretation of the data inestimable and puts into question their findings of no significant differences between groups. The second, and possibly most important flaw, is that this study is an RCT with two hyperbaric treatment groups and without a true control group. The control group was treated with hyperbaric air, which is not physiologically inert.[88,89] Finally, this RCT evaluated patients with chronic ISSHL. It has been shown in numerous studies that significant benefit is found with early HBO$_2$ therapy for those with ISSHL.[78-79,81,99,103-105,110,112-114] Other meta-analyses have included this RCT and it is an error. [113,115-117] This is the only RCT on the treatment of chronic ISSHL that is included in these meta-analyses; however, the patients are not similar. Simply continuing to include this RCT should cease.

2. Diagnose presumptive SSNHL if audiometry confirms a 30-dB hearing loss at three consecutive frequencies and an underlying condition cannot be identified by history and physical examination.

3. Evaluate patients with SSNHL for retrocochlear pathology by obtaining magnetic resonance imaging, auditory brainstem response, or audiometric follow up.

4. Offer intratympanic steroid therapy when patients have incomplete recovery from SSNHL after failure of initial management.

5. Obtain follow up audiometric evaluation within six months of diagnosis for those patients with SSNHL.

Patient Management

The most recent guidelines published by the American Academy of Otolaryngology strongly recommend the following:[4]

1. Complete physical examination and referral to an otolaryngologist to distinguish sensorineural hearing loss from conductive hearing loss.

2. Patient education regarding SSNHL, inclusive of the natural history of the condition, the benefits and risks of medical interventions, and the limitations of existing evidence regarding efficacy of treatment.

3. Counseling of patients with incomplete recovery of hearing about the possible benefits of amplifications and hearing assistive technologies and other supportive measures.

Treatment

Corticosteroid Therapy

Patients without contraindications to corticosteroid therapy should be treated with either IT corticosteroids or systemic oral corticosteroids. It is prudent to begin with oral steroid therapy along with urgent referral to an otolaryngologist for audiometric testing to confirm the diagnosis. It is reasonable to start oral steroid therapy with prednisone (1 mg/kg/day) with a slow taper over two to three weeks.[129] The decision to switch to either IT corticosteroids or to add IT corticosteroids should be made by the patient and the referring otolaryngologist.

For decades, the standard of care has been oral corticosteroids. However, many studies have shown the efficacy of IT steroid therapy, and the use of IT corticosteroids does result in higher steroid concentrations within the perilymph compared to oral steroid therapy.[16,52,56] Additionally, IT corticosteroids reduce the incidence of possible toxic side effects of systemic steroid regimens. Currently, there is a paucity of data regarding the prevalence of these side effects with the relatively short courses of systemic steroid therapy used in the treatment of SSNHL.[59] However, it may be that IT corticosteroids are a better option for those who are intolerant or refuse systemic steroid therapy.[16,17,48,50,53,62-68]

Hyperbaric Oxygen Therapy

Patients diagnosed with SSNHL who meet selection criteria and without contraindications to HBO_2 therapy may benefit from treatment. The recommended treatment profile is 100% O_2 at 2.0–2.5 ATA for 90 minutes daily for 10 to 20 sessions.[129]

Other Medical Therapies

The American Academy of Otolaryngology recommends *against* the routine use of anti-virals, thrombolytics, vasodilators, vasoactive substances or antioxidants for patients with SSNHL.[4] There are more than 60 protocols involving a multitude of medical therapies in the treatment of SSNHL. However, only two therapies have been shown to be efficacious: the use of corticosteroids and HBO_2 therapy. These two therapies have received the highest medical therapy recommendation in the Guidelines for the treatment of SSNHL, published by the American Academy of Otolaryngology. They are also the only two therapies endorsed by the UHMS Committee Report on the treatment of SSNHL.[129]

Follow-Up

Continued consultation and follow-up with an otolaryngologist are recommended. Additional testing and therapy may be recommended by the otolaryngologist, and the patient should continue to be followed by the otolaryngology specialist during and following HBO_2 therapy.[4,129]

Prognosis

Hearing loss imposes a significant burden for the patient. For those least affected (slight impairment range of 26 dB–40 dB), patients are able to hear and repeat words in a normal voice at 1 meter and may only require counseling. However, for those with hearing impairment in the moderate range (41 dB–60 dB) or the severe range (61 dB–80 dB), hearing aids are recommended, and lip reading and signing may be required.[131] The use of HBO_2 therapy imparts a 37.7 dB improvement in hearing gains for those with a severe hearing deficit and a 19.3 dB improvement with those with moderate hearing deficits.[116] These hearing improvements resolve the hearing loss toward the normal range and may significantly affect a patient's quality of life and obviate the need for lip reading, signing, or hearing adjuncts.

Cost Impact

The World Health Organization has detailed the cost impact of hearing loss worldwide. Hearing loss impairs the ability of a patient to obtain, perform or retain employment. These patients are often stigmatized and may become socially isolated. The cost of specialized education and lost employment imposes a heavy social and economic burden.[132] Adult onset hearing loss is the third leading cause of years lost to disability, and the 15th leading cause of burden of disease; it is projected to move up to seventh by the year 2030.[133] Remarkably, hearing loss is the most common cause of disability globally, just ahead of refractive errors, and well ahead of depression, cataracts, and accidental injuries, which round out the top five.[133] For those able to afford them, hearing aids cost between $1,500.00–$3,000.00 per pair. Many require replacement every three to five years and may not result in fully functional hearing.

Acknowledgment

Steven M. Piper DO contributed to the earlier editions of this review.

Figure 1. Flowchart for the Treatment of SSNHL
Details for management are described in the text.

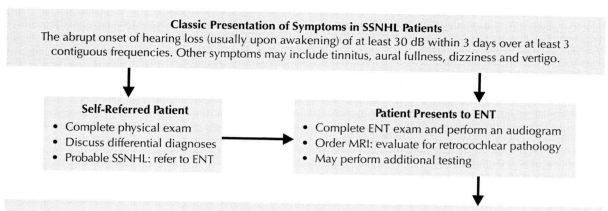

Classic Presentation of Symptoms in SSNHL Patients
The abrupt onset of hearing loss (usually upon awakening) of at least 30 dB within 3 days over at least 3 contiguous frequencies. Other symptoms may include tinnitus, aural fullness, dizziness and vertigo.

Self-Referred Patient
- Complete physical exam
- Discuss differential diagnoses
- Probable SSNHL: refer to ENT

Patient Presents to ENT
- Complete ENT exam and perform an audiogram
- Order MRI: evaluate for retrocochlear pathology
- May perform additional testing

Hyperbaric Medicine Consultation
- **Evaluate for SSNHL Selection Criteria:** a) Confirmed diagnosis of SSNHL; b) The SSNHL is moderate to profound ($\geq$40 dB); and c) The patient presents $\leq$14 days from symptom onset.*
- **Complete Exam and History:** Evaluate for any contraindications to HBO$_2$ therapy.
- **Call ENT:** Discuss dosing of oral prednisone (1 mg/kg/day) with a slow taper over 2-3 weeks; consider IT steroids; schedule repeat audiogram post-HBO$_2$ therapy.
- **Begin HBO$_2$ Therapy:** 100% O$_2$ at 2.0-2.5 ATA for 90 minutes daily for 10-20 sessions
- **When HBO$_2$ Therapy Is Completed:** Refer the patient back to ENT; timely follow-up with both

*The American Academy of Otolaryngology - Head and Neck Surgery Foundation recommends HBO$_2$ therapy up to three months from symptom onset.

References

1. Fetterman BL, Saunders JE, Luxford WM. Prognosis and treatment of sudden sensorineural hearing loss. Am J Otol. 1996 Jul; 17(4):529–536.
2. O'Malley MR, Haynes DS. Sudden hearing loss. Otolaryngol Clin N Am. 2008;41: 633–649.
3. Haberkamp TJ, Tanyeri HM. Management of idiopathic sudden sensorineural hearing loss. Am J Otol. 1999 Sept;20:587–592.
4. Stachler R, Chandrasekhar S, Archer S, Rosenfeld R, Schwartz S, Barrs D, Brown S, Fife T, Ford P, Ganiats T, Hollingsworth D, Lewandowski C, Montano J, Saunders J, Tucci D, Valente M, Warren B, Yaremchuk K, Robertson P. Clinical practice guidelines: sudden hearing loss. Otolayrgology – Head and Neck Surgery. 2012;146:S1-35.
5. Rauch SD. Idiopathic sudden sensorineural hearing loss. N Engl J Med. 2008 Aug 21;359(8):833–840.
6. Byl FM Jr. Sudden hearing loss: eight years' experience and suggested prognostic table. Laryngoscope. 1984 May; 94 (5 Pt 1): 647–661.
7. Alexander TH, Harris JP. Incidence of sudden sensorineural hearing loss." Otol Neurotol. 2013;34:1586–1589.
8. Teranishi M, Katayma N, Uchida Y, Tominaga M, Nakashima T. Thirty-year trends in sudden deafness from four nationwide epidemiological surveys in Japan. Acta Otolaryngol. 2007;127:1259–1265.
9. Klemm E, Deutscher A, Mosges R. A Present investigation of the epidemiology in idiopathic sudden sensorineural hearing loss." Larygorhinootologie. 2009;88:524 –527.
10. Hallberg OE. Sudden deafness of obscure origin. Laryngoscope.1956 Oct; 66(10):1237–1267.
11. Byl FM. Seventy-six cases of presumed sudden hearing loss occurring in 1973; prognosis and incidence. Laryngoscope. 1977 May;87(5 Pt 1):817–825.
12. Mattox DE, Simmons FB. Natural history of sudden sensorineural hearing loss. Ann Otol Rhinol Laryngol. 1977 Jul-Aug; 86(4 Pt 1):463–480.
13. Shaia FT, Sheehy JL. Sudden sensori-neural hearing impairment: a report of 1,220 cases. Layrngoscope. 1976 Mar; 86(3):389–398.
14. Jourdy DN, Donatelli LA, Victor JD, Selesnick SH. Assessment of variation throughout the year in the incidence of idiopathic sudden sensorineural hearing loss. Otol Neurotol. 2010 Jan;31(1):53–57.
15. Wilson WR, Byl FM, Laird N. The efficacy of steroids in the treatment of idiopathic sudden hearing loss. A double-blind clinical study." Arch Otolaryngol. 1980 Dec; 106(12):772–776.
16. Chandrasekhar SS. Intratympanic dexamethasone for sudden sensorineural hearing loss: clinical and laboratory evaluation. Otol Neurotol. 2001 Jan; 22(1):18 –23.
17. Battaglia A, Burchette R, Cueva R. Combination therapy (intratympanic dexamethasone + high-dose prednisone taper) for the treatment of idiopathic sudden sensorineural hearing loss." Otol Neurotol. 2008 Jun;29(4):453–460.
18. De Kleyn A. Sudden complete or partial loss of function of the octavus system in apparently normal persons. Acta Otolaryngologica. 1944(32):407–429.
19. Cole RR, Jahrsdoerfer RA. Sudden hearing loss: an update. Am J Otol. 1988 May; 9 (3):211–215.
20. Hughes GB, Freedman MA, Haberkamp TJ, Guay ME. Sudden sensorineural hearing loss. Otolaryngol Clin North Am. 1996 Jun; 29(3):393–405.
21. Alimoglu Y, Inci E, Edizer DT, Ozdilek A, Aslan M. Efficacy comparison of oral steroid, intratympanic steroid, hyperbaric oxygen and oral steroid and hyperbaric oygen treatments in idiopathic sudden sensorineural hearing loss cases. Eur Arch Otorhinolaryngol. 2011 Dec; 268(12):1735–1741.
22. Lamm C, Walliser U, Schumann K, Lamm K. Oxygen partial pressure measurements in the perilymph and the scala tympani in normo- and hyperbaric conditions. An animal experiment study. HNO. 1988 Sept;35(9):363–366.
23. Lamm K, Lamm C, Lamm H, Schumann K. Simultaneous determinations of oxygen partial pressure in the scala tympani, electrocochleography and blood pressure measurements in noise stress in guinea pigs. HNO. 1988 Sep; 36(9):367–372.
24. Belal A Jr. Pathology of vascular sensorineural hearing impairment. Laryngoscope. 1980 Nov;90(11 Pt 1):1831–1839.
25. Yoon TH, Paparella MM, Schachern PA, Alleva M. Histopathology of sudden hearing loss. Laryngoscope. 1990 Jul;100(7):707–715.
26. Pirodda A, Ferri GG, Modugno GC, Borghi C. Systemic hypotension and the development of acute sensorineural hearing loss in young healthy subjects." Arch Otolaryngol Head Neck Surg. 2001 Sep;127:1049–1052.
27. Lehnhardt E, Hesch RD. Causes of inner ear deafness: a critique of therapy. HNO. 1980;28:73–79.
28. Maass B. Autonomic nervous system and hearing. Adv Otorhinolaryngol. 1981;27:14–25.

29. Pirodda A, Saggese D, Giausa G, Ferri GG, Nascetti S, Gaddi A. Can hypotension episodes cause cochlear damage in young subjects? Med Hypotheses. 1997;48:195–186.

30. Pirodda A, Feri Gg, Modugno GC, Gaddi A. Hypotension and sensorineural hearing loss: a possible correlation. Acta Otolaryngol. 1999;119(7):758–762.

31. Kawakami M, Makimoto K, Fukuse S, Takahashi H. Autoregulation of cochlear blood flow. A comparison of cerebral blood flow with muscular blood flow. Eur Arch Otorhinolaryngol. 1991;248:471–474.

32. Ciccone MM, Cortese F, Pinto m, Di Teo C, Fornarelli F, Gesualdo M, Mezzina A, Sabatelli E, Scicchitano P, Quaranta N. Endothelial function and cardiovascular risk in patients with idiopathic sudden sensorineural hearing loss. Atherosclerosis. 2012;225:511–516.

33. Brant LJ, Gordon-Salant S, Pearson JD, Klein LL, Morrell CH, Metter EJ, Fozard JL. Risk factors related to age-associated hearing loss in the speech frequencies. J Am Acad Audiol. 1996;7:152–160.

34. Rudack C, Langer C, Stoll W, Rust S., Walter M. Vascular risk factors in sudden hearing loss. Thromb Haemost. 2006;95:454–561.

35. Aimoni C, Bianchini C, Borin M, Ciorba A, Fellin R, Martini A, Scanelli G, Volpato S. Diabetes, cardiovascular risk factors and idiopathic sudden sensorineural hearing loss: a case-control study. Audio Neurotol. 2010;15(2):111–115.

36. Lin HC, Chao PZ, Lee HC. Sudden sensorineural hearing loss increases the risk of stroke: a 5-year follow-up study. Stroke. 2008 Oct;39 (10):2744–2748.

37. Ozler GS. Increased neutrophil-lymphocyte ratio in patients with idiopathic sudden sensorineural hearing loss. J Craniofac Surg. 2014 May;25(3): e260–e263.

38. Gloddek B, Lamm K, Arnold W. Pharmacological influence on inner ear endothelial cells in relation to the pathogenesis of sensorineural hearing loss. Adv Otorhinolaryngol. 2002;59:75–83.

39. Merchant SN, Durand ML, Adams JC. Sudden deafness: is it viral? ORL J Otorhinolaryngol Relat Spec. 2008;70:52–62.

40. Merchant SN, Adams JC, Nadol JB Jr. Pathology and pathophysiology of idiopathic sudden sensorineural hearing loss. Otol Neurotol. 2005 Mar;26(2):151–160.

41. Stokroos RJ, Albers FW, Schirm J. The etiology of idiopathic sudden sensorineural hearing loss: experimental herpes simplex virus infection of the inner ear. Am J Otol. 1998 Jul;19(4):447–452.

42. Shirwany NA, Seidman MD, Tang W. Effect of transtympanic injection of steroids on cochlear blood flow, auditory sensitivity, and histology in the guinea pig. Am J Otol 1998; 19:230 –235.

43. Nagura M, Iwasaki S, Wu R, Mizuta K, Umemura K, Hoshino T. Effects of corticosteroid, contrast medium and ATP on focal microcirculatory disorders of the cochlea. Eur J Pharmacol. 1999 Jan 29;366(1):47–53.

44. Tabuchi K, Oikawa K, Uemaetomari I, Tsuji S, Wada T, Hara A. Glucocorticoids and dehydroepiandrosterone sulfate ameliorate ischemia-induced injury of the cochlea. Hear Res. 2003 Jun; 180(1-2):51–56.

45. Lin DW, Trune DR. Breakdown of stria vascularis blood-labyrinth barrier in C3H/lpr autoimmune disease mice. Otolaryngol Head Neck Surg. 1997 Nov;117(5):530– 534.

46. Trune DR, Wobig RJ, Kempton JB, Hefeneider SH. Steroid treatment improves cochlear function in the MRL. MpJ-Fas(lpr) autoimmune mouse. Hear Res. 1999 Nov;137(1-2):160–166.

47. Alexiou C, Arnold W, Fauser C, Schratzenstaller B, Gloddek B, Fuhrmann S, Lamm K. Sudden sensorineural hearing loss: does application of glucocorticoids make sense? Arch Otolaryngol Head Neck Surg. 2001, Mar; 127(3):253-258.

48. Slattery WH, Fisher LM, Iqbal Z, Friedman RA, Liu N. Intratympanic steroid injection for treatment of idiopathic sudden hearing loss. Otolaryngol Head Neck Surg. 2005 Aug; 133(2):251–259.

49. Dispenza F, Amodio E, De Stefano A, Gallina S, Marchese D, Mathur N, Riggio F. Treatment of sudden sensorineural hearing loss with transtympanic injection of steroids as single therapy: a randomized clinical study. Eur Arch Otorhinolaryngol. 2011 Sep;268(9):1273-1278.

50. Seggas I, Koltsidopoulos P, Bibas A, Tzonou A, Sismanis A. Intratympanic steroid therapy for sudden hearing loss: a review of the literature. Otol Neurotol. 2011 Jan; 32(1):29–35.

51. Spear SA, Schwartz SR. Intratympanic steroids for sudden sensorineural hearing loss. A systematic review. Otolaryngol Head Neck Surg. 2011 Oct;145(4):534–543.

52. Ferri E, Frisina A, Fasson AC, Armato E, Spinato G, and Amadori M. Intratympanic steroid treatment for idiopathic sudden sensorineural hearing loss after failure of intravenous therapy. ISRN Otolaryngology. 2012;1–6.

53. Haynes DS, O'Malley M, Cohen S, Watford K, Labadie RF. Intratympanic dexamethasone for sudden sensorineural hearing loss after failure of systemic therapy. Laryngoscope. 2007 Jan;117(1):3–15.

54. Cinamon U, Bendet E, Kronenberg J. Steroids, carbogen or placebo for sudden hearing loss: a prospective double-blind study. Eur Arch Otorhinolaryngol. 2001 Nov;258(9):477–480.

55. Zadeh MH, Storper IS, Spitzer JB. Diagnosis and treatment of sudden-onset sensorineural hearing loss: a study of 51 patients. Otolaryngol Head Neck Surg. 2003 Jan;128(1):92–98.

56. Parnes LS, Sun AH, Freeman DJ. Corticosteroid pharmacokinetics in the inner ear fluids: an animal study followed by clinical application. Laryngoscope. 1999 Jul; 109(7 Pt 2):1–17.

57. Bird PA, Begg EJ, Zhang M, Keast AT, Murray DP, Balkany TJ. Intratympanic versus intravenous delivery of methylprednisolone to cochlear perilymph. Otol Neurotol. 2007 Dec; 28(8):1124–1130.

58. Plontke SK, Biegner T, Kammerer B, Delabar U, Salt AN. Dexamethasone concentration gradients along scala tympani after application to the round window membrane. Otol Neurotol. 2008 Apr; 29(3):401–406.

59. Wei BPC, Stathopoulos D, O'Leary S. Steroids for idiopathic sudden sensorineural hearing loss. Cochrane Database of Systematic Reviews. 2013;Issue 7. Art. No.: CD003998.

60. Gao Y, Liu D. Combined intratympanic and systemic use of steroids for idiopathic sudden sensorineural hearing loss: a meta-analysis. Eur Arch Otorhinolaryngol. 2016; 273:3699–3711.

61. Qiang Q, Wu X, Yang T, Yang C, Sun H. A comparison between systemic and intratympanic steroid therapies as initial therapy for idiopathic sudden sensorineural hearing loss: a meta-analysis. Acta Oto-Laryngologica. 2016 Dec 6: 1–8 ISSN:0001-6489.

62. Ho HG, Lin HC, Shu MT, Yang CC, Tsai HT. Effectiveness of intratympanic dexamethasone injection in sudden-deafness patients as salvage treatment. Laryngoscope. 2004 Jul;114(7):1184–1189.

63. Xenellis J, Papadimitriou N, Nikolopoulos T, Maragoudakis P, Segas J, Tzagaroulakis A, Ferekidis E. Intratympanic steroid treatment in idiopathic sudden sensorineural hearing loss: a control study. Otolaryngol Head Neck Surg. 2006 Jun;134(6):940– 945.

64. Ahn JH, Han MW, Kim JH, Chung JW, Yoon TH. Therapeutic effectiveness over time of intratympanic dexamethasone as salvage treatment of sudden deafness. Acta Otolaryngol. 2008 Feb;128(2):128–131.

65. Kilic R, Safak MA, Oguz H, Kargin S, Demirci M, Samim E, Ozluoglu LN. Intratympanic methylprednisolone for sudden sensorineural hearing loss. Otol Neurotol. 2007 Apr;28(3):312–316.

66. Plaza G, Herraiz C. Intratympanic steroids for treatment of sudden hearing loss after failure of intravenous therapy. Otolaryngol Head Neck Surg. 2007 Jul;137(1): 74–78.

67. Hong SM, Park CH, Lee JH. Hearing outcomes of daily intratympanic dexamethasone alone as a primary treatment modality for ISSHL. Otolaryngol Head Neck Surg. 2009 Nov;141(5):579–583.

68. Tsai YJ, Liang JG, Wu WB, Ding YF, Chiang RP, Wu SM. Intratympanic injection with dexamethasone for sudden sensorineural hearing loss. J Laryngol Otol. 2011 Feb; 125(2):133–137.

69. Cavallazzi GM. Relations between O2 and hearing function. Eds: Marroni A, Oriani G, Wattel F. Proceedings of International Joint Meeting on Hyperbaric and Underwater Medicine. Milano, Italy. 1996a Sept 4–8; 633–645.

70. Nagahara K, Fisch U, Yagi N. Perilymph oxygenation in sudden and progressive sensorineural hearing loss. Acta Otolaryngol. 1983 Jul – Aug;96(1–2):57–68.

71. Lamm H. Der einfluss der hperbaren sauerstofftherapie auf den tinnitus und horverlust bei akuten und chronischen innenohrschaden. Otorhinolaryngol Nova. 1995; 5:161–169.

72. Tsunoo M, Perlman MB. Temporary arterial obstruction. Effects on perilymph oxygen and microphonics. Acta Otolaryngol. 1969;67:460–466.

73. Schwab B, Flunkert C, Heermann R, Lenarz T. HBO in the therapy of cochlear dysfunctions – first results of a randomized study. EUBS diving and hyperbaric medicine, collected manuscripts of XXIV Annual Scientific Meeting of the European Underwater and Baromedical Society. Stockholm: EUBS. 1998:40–42.

74. Fattori B, Berrettini S, Casani A, Nacci A, De Vito A, De Iaco G. Sudden hypoacusis treated with hyperbaric oxygen therapy: a controlled study. Ear Nose Throat J. 2001 Sept;80(9):655–660.

75. Racic G, Maslovara S, Roje Z, Dogas Z, Tafra R. Hyperbaric oxygen in the treatment of sudden hearing loss. ORL J Otorhinolaryngol Relat Spec. 2003 Nov–Dec;65(6): 317–320.

76. Dundar K, Gumus T, Ay H, Yetiser S, Ertugrul E. Effectiveness of hyperbaric oxygen on sudden sensorineural hearing loss: prospective clinical research. J Otolaryngol. 2007 Feb;36(1):32–37.

77. Hoffmann G, Bohmer D, Desloovere C. Hyperbaric oxygenation as a treatment for sudden deafness and acute tinnitus. Proceedings of the Eleventh International Congress on Hyperbaric Medicine. Flagstaff, AZ: Best Publishing Company; 1995. Pp:146–151.

78. Lamm K, Lamm H, Arnold W. Effect of hyperbaric oxygen therapy in comparison to conventional or placebo therapy or no treatment in idiopathic sudden hearing loss, acoustic trauma, noise-induced hearing loss and tinnitus. A Literature Survey. Adv Otorhinolaryngol. 1998;54:86–89.

79. Marchesi G, Valetti TM, Amer M, Ross M, Tiberti R, Ferani R, Mauro G Di. The HBO effective in sudden hearing loss treatment. UHMS Meeting Abstracts, 2000. http://archive.rubicon-foundation.org/6781.

80. Murakawa T, Kosaka M, Mori Y, Fukazawa M, Misaki K. Treatment of 533 patients with sudden deafness performed oxygenation at high pressure. Nihon Jibiinkoka Gakkai Kaiho. 2000 May;103(5):506–515.

81. Muzzi E, Zennaro B, Visentin R, Soldano F, Sacilotto C. Hyperbaric oxygen therapy as salvage treatment for sudden sensorineural hearing loss: review of rationale and preliminary report. J Laryngol Otol. 2010;124(2):e2.

82. Ohno K, Noguchi Y, Kawashima Y, Yagishita K, Kitamura K. Secondary hyperbaric oxygen therapy for idiopathic sudden sensorineural hearing loss in the subacute and chronic phases. J Med Dent Sci. 2010;57(2):127–132.

83. Cvorovic L, Jovanovic MG, Milutinovic Z, Arsovic N, Djeric D. Randomized prospective trial of hyperbaric oxygen therapy and intratympanic steroid injection as salvage treatment of sudden sensorineural hearing loss. Otol and Neurotology. 2013;34(6):1021–1026.

84. Yang CH, Wu RW, Hwang CF. Comparison of intratympanic steroid injection, hyperbaric oxygen and combination therapy in refractory sudden sensorineural hearing loss. Otol and Neurotology. 2013;34:1411–1416.

85. Pezzoli M, Magnano M, Maffi L, Pezzoli L, Marcato P, Orione M, Cupi D, Bongioannini G. Hyperbaric oxygen therapy as salvage treatment for sudden sensorineural hearing loss: a prospective controlled study. Eur Arch Otorhinolaryngol. 2015 Jul; 272(7):1659–1666.

86. Schumann K, Lamm K, Hettich M. Effect and effectiveness of hyperbaric oxygen therapy in chronic hearing disorders. Report of 557 cases 1989. HNO. 1990 Nov; 38(11):408–411.

87. Hoffman G, Bohmer D, Desloovere C. Hyperbaric oxygenation as a treatment of chronic forms of inner ear hearing loss and tinnitus. Proceedings of the Eleventh International Congress on Hyperbaric Medicine. Flagstaff, AZ: Best Publishing Company; 1995. Pp.141–145.

88. Kramer MR, Springer C, Berkman N, Glazer M, Bubil M, Bar-Yishay E, Godfrey S. Rehabilitation of hypoxemic patients with COPD at low altitude at the dead sea, the lowest place on earth. Chest. 1998 Mar;113(3):571–575.

89. Dean JB, Mulkey DK. Continuous Intracellular recordings from mammalian neurons exposed to hyperbaric helium, oxygen, or air. J Appl Physiol. 2000 Aug 89 (2):807–822.

90. Kau RJ, Sendtner-Gress K, Ganzer U, Arnold W. Effectiveness of hyperbaric oxygen therapy in patients with acute and chronic cochlear disorders. ORL J Otorhinolarygnol Relat Spec. 1997 Mar–Apr; 59(2):78-83.

91. Giger HL. Therapy of sudden deafness with O2 / CO2 inhalation. HNO. 1979 Mar; 27(3):107–109.

92. Goto F, Fujiita T, Kitani Y, Kanno M, Kamei T, Ishii H. Hyperbaric oxygen and stellate ganglion blocks for idiopathic sudden hearing loss. Acta Otolaryngol. 1979;88(5– 6):335–342.

93. Pilgramm M, Lamm H. Schumann K. Hyperbaric oxygen therapy in sudden deafness. Laryngol, Rhinol, Otol. 1985 Jul;64(7):351–354.

94. Dauman R, Poisot D, Cros AM, Zennaro O, Bertrand B, Duclos JY, Esteban D, Milacic M, Boudey C, Bebear JP. Sudden deafness: a randomized comparative study of 2 administration modalities of hyperbaric oxygenotherapy combined with naftidrofuryl. Rev Laryngol Otol Rhinol (Bord). 1993;114(1):53–58.

95. Zennaro O, Dauman R, Poisot A, Esteben D, Duclose JY, Bertrand B, Cros AM, Milacic M, Bebear JP. Value of the association of normovolemic dilution and hyperbaric oxygenation in the treatment of sudden deafness. A retrospective study. Ann Otolaryngol Cir Cervicofac. 1993;110(3):162–169.

96. Cavallazzi G, Pignataro L, Capaccio P. Italian experience in hyperbaric oxygen therapy for idiopathic sudden sensorineural hearing loss. Proceedings of the International Joint Meeting on Hyperbaric and Underwater Medicine. Bologna: Grafica Victoria; 1996. Pp: 647–649.

97. Aslan I, Oysu C, Veyseller B, Baserer N. Does the addition of hyperbaric oxygen therapy to the conventional treatment modalities influence the outcome of sudden deafness? Otolaryngol Head Neck Surg. 2002 Feb;126(2):121–126.

98. Topuz E, Yigit O, Cinar U, Seven H. Should hyperbaric oxygen be added to treatment in idiopathic sudden sensorineural hearing loss? Eur Arch Otorhinolaryngol. 2004 Aug;261(7)393–396.

99. Narozny W, Kuczkowski J, Kot J, Stankiewicz C, Sicko Z, Mikaszeweski B. Prognostic factors in sudden sensorineural hearing loss: our experience and a review of the literature. Ann Otol Rhinol Laryngol. 2006 Jul;115(7):553–558.

100. Suzuki H, Fujimura T, Shiomori T, Ohbuchi T, Kitamura T, Hashida K, Udaka T. Prostaglandin E1 versus steroid in combination with hyperbaric oxygen therapy for idiopathic sudden sensorineural hearing loss. Auris Nasus Larynx. 2008 Jun;35 (2):192–197.

101. Suzuki H, Fujimura T, Ikeda K, Shiomori T, Udaka T, Ohbuchi T, Nagatani G. Prostaglandin E1 in combination with hyperbaric oxygen therapy for idiopathic sudden sensorineural hearing loss. Acta Otolaryngol. 2008 Jan;128(1):61–65.

102. Cekin E, Cincik H, Ulubil SA, Gungor A. Effectiveness of hyperbaric oxygen therapy in management of sudden hearing loss. J Laryngol Otol. 2009;123:609–612.

103. Liu Y, Sun D, Shao S, Jiang W, Sun Z, Li Z. The effect of hyperbaric oxygen therapy to different degree of hearing loss and types of threshold curve in sudden deafness patients. Lin Chung Er Bi Yan Hou Tou Jing Wai Ke Za Zhi. 2010 Oct; 24(19):890– 894.

104. Korpinar S, Alkan Z, Yigit O, Gor AP, Toklu AS, Cakir B, Soyuyuce OG, Ozkul H. Factors influencing the outcome of idiopathic sudden sensorineural hearing loss treated with hyperbaric oxygen therapy. Eur Arch Otorhinolaryngol. 2011 Jan; 268 (1):41–47.

105. Holy R, Navara M, Dosel P, Fundova P, Prazenica P, Hahn A. Hyperbaric oxygen therapy in idiopathic sudden sensorineural hearing loss (ISSHL) in association with combined treatment. Undersea Hyperb Med. 2011 Mar – Apr;38(2):137–142.

106. Liu SC, Kang BH, Lee JC, Lin YS, Huang KL, Liu DW, Su WF, Kao CH, Chu YH, Chen HC, Wang CH. Comparison of therapeutic results in sudden sensorineural hearing loss with/without additional hyperbaric oxygen therapy: a retrospective review of 465 audiologically controlled cases. Clin Otolaryngol. 2011 Apr;36(2):121–128.

107. Fujimura T, Suzuki H, Shiomori T, Udaka T, Mori T. Hyperbaric oxygen and steroid therapy for idiopathic sudden sensorineural hearing loss. Eur Arch Otorhinolaryngol. 2007 Aug;264(8):861–866.

108. Suzuki H, Mori T, Hashida K, Shibata M, Nguyen KH, Wakasugi T, Hohchi N. Prediction model for hearing outcome in patients with idiopathic sudden sensorineural hearing loss. Eur Arch Otorhinolaryngol. 2011;268(4):497–500.

109. Filipo R, Attanasio G, Viccaro M, Russo FY, Mancini P, Rocco M, Pietropaoli P, Covelli E. Hyperbaric oxygen therapy with short duration intratympanic steroid therapy for sudden hearing loss. Acta Otolaryngol. 2012 May;132(5):475–481.

110. Capuano L, Cavaliere M, Parente G, Damiano A, Pezzuti G, Lopardo D, Lemma M. Hyperbaric oxygen for idiopathic sudden hearing loss: is the routine application helpful? Acta Oto-Laryngologica. 2015 Jul;135(7):692–697.

111. Carneiro SN, Guerreiro DV, Cunha AM, Camacho OF, Aguiar IC. Hyperbaric oxygen therapy in sudden sensorineural hearing loss following spinal anesthesia: case reports. Undersea Hyperb Med. 2016;43(2):153 –159.

112. Hosokawa S, Sugiyama K, Takashashi G, Takebayashi S, Mineta H. Prognostic factors for idiopathic sudden sensorineural hearing loss treated with hyperbaric oxygen therapy and intravenous steroids. J Laryngol and Otol. 2017;131:77–82.

113. Bennett MH, Kertesz T, Perleth M, Yeung P, Lehm JP. Hyperbaric oxygen for idiopathic sudden sensorineural hearing loss and tinnitus. Cochrane Database Syst Rev. 2012; Issue 10. Art. No.:CD004739.

114. Yildirim E, Murat Ozcan K, Palah M, Ali Cetin M, Ensari S, Dere H. Prognostic effect of hyperbaric oxygen therapy starting time for sudden sensorineural hearing loss. Eur Arch Otorhinolaryngol. 2015;272:23–28.

115. Bennett MH, Kertesz T, Yeung P. Hyperbaric oxygen for idiopathic sudden sensorineural hearing loss and tinnitus. Cochrane Database Syst Rev. 2005 Jan 25 (1):CD004739.

116. Bennett MH, Kertesz T, Yeung P. Hyperbaric oxygen for idiopathic sudden sensorineural hearing loss and tinnitus. Cochrane Database Syst Rev. 2007 Jan 24 (1):CD004739.

117. Bennett MH, Kertesz T, Matthias P, Yeung P. Hyperbaric oxygen for idiopathic sudden sensorineural hearing loss and tinnitus. Cochrane Database Syst Rev. 2010 Jan 20(1):CD004739.

118. Conlin AE, Parnes LS. Treatment of sudden sensorineural hearing loss. A systematic review. Arch Otolaryngol Head Neck Surg. 2008 Jun;133:573–581.

119. Agarwal L, Pothier Dd. Vasodilators and vasoactive substances for idiopathic sudden sensorineural hearing loss. Cochrane Database Syst Rev. 2009 Oct 7;(4): CD003422.

120. Tucci DL, Farmer JC, Kitch RD, Witsell DL. Treatment of sudden sensorineural hearing loss with systemic steroids and valaciclovir. Otol Neurotol. 2002;23:301– 308.

121. Stokroos RJ, Albers FWJ, Tenvergert EM. Antiviral treatment of idiopathic sudden sensorineural hearing loss: a prospective, randomized, double-blinded clinical trial. Acta Otolaryngol. 1998b;118: 488–485.

122. Westerlaken BO, Stokroos RJ, Dhooge IJ, Wit HP, Albers FW. Treatment of idiopathic sudden sensorineural hearing loss with antiviral therapy: a prospective, randomized, double-blind clinical trial. Ann Otol Rhinol Laryngol. 2003;112:993– 100.

123. Uri N, Doweck I, Cohen-Kerem R, Greenberg E. Acyclovir in the treatment of idiopathic sudden sensorineural hearing loss. Otolaryngol Head Neck Surg. 2003; 128:544–549.

124. Awad Z, Huins C, Pothier DD. Antivirals for idiopathic sudden sensorineural hearing loss. Cochrane Database Syst Rev. 2012 Aug 15;(8):1–22.

125. Wei BP, Mubiru S, O'Leary S. Steroids for idiopathic sudden sensorineural hearing loss. Cochrane Database Syst Rev. 2006 Jan 25;(1):CD003998.

126. Nosrati-Zarenoe R, Hultcrantz E. Corticosteroid Treatment of Idiopathic Sudden sensorineural hearing loss: randomized triple-blind placebo-controlled trial. Otol Neurotol. 2012 Jun; 22(4):523–531.

References

1. Brouwer MC, Tunkel AR, McKhann GM, 2nd, van de Beek D. Brain abscess. N Engl J Med. 2014;371(5):447-56.
2. Brouwer MC, Coutinho JM, van de Beek D. Clinical characteristics and outcome of brain abscess: systematic review and meta-analysis. Neurology. 2014;82(9):806-13.
3. Tunkel AR. Brain abscess. In: Bennett JE, Dolin R, Blaser MJ, editors. Mandell, Douglas, and Bennett's Principles and Practice of Infectious Diseases, Updated Edition. 8 ed. Philadelphia, PA: Elsevier Saunders; 2015. p. 1164-76.
4. Tekkok IH, Erbengi A. Management of brain abscess in children: review of 130 cases over a period of 21 years. Childs Nerv Syst. 1992;8(7):411-6.
5. Udayakumaran S, Onyia CU, Kumar RK. Forgotten? Not Yet. Cardiogenic Brain Abscess in Children: A Case Series-Based Review. World Neurosurg. 2017;107:124-9.
6. Gelfand MS, Stephens DS, Howell EI, Alford RH, Kaiser AB. Brain abscess: association with pulmonary arteriovenous fistula and hereditary hemorrhagic telangiectasia: report of three cases. Am J Med. 1988;85(5):718-20.
7. Press OW, Ramsey PG. Central nervous system infections associated with hereditary hemorrhagic telangiectasia. Am J Med. 1984;77(1):86-92.
8. Chang YT, Lu CH, Chuang MJ, Huang CR, Chuang YC, Tsai NW, et al. Supratentorial deep-seated bacterial brain abscess in adults: clinical characteristics and therapeutic outcomes. Acta Neurol Taiwan. 2010;19(3):178-83.
9. Sukoff MH, Ragatz RE. Hyperbaric oxygenation for the treatment of acute cerebral edema. Neurosurgery. 1982;10:29-38.
10. Mader JT, Brown GL, Guckian JC, Wells CH, Reinarz JA. A mechanism for the amelioration by hyperbaric oxygen of experimental staphylococcal osteomyelitis in rabbits. J Infect Dis. 1980;142:915-22.
11. Siddiqui A, Davidson JD, Mustoe TA. Ischemic tissue oxygen capacitance after hyperbaric oxygen therapy: a new physiologic concept. Plast Reconstr Surg. 1997;99(1):148-55.
12. Price JC, Stevens DL. Hyperbaric oxygen in the treatment of rhinocerebral mucormycosis. Laryngoscope. 1980;90:737-47.
13. Ferguson BJ, Mitchell TG, Moon R, Camporesi EM, Farmer J. Adjunctive hyperbaric oxygen for treatment of rhinocerebral mucormycosis. Rev Infect Dis. 1988;10(3):551-9.
14. Roden MM, Zaoutis TE, Buchanan WL, Knudsen TA, Sarkisova TA, Schaufele RL, et al. Epidemiology and outcome of zygomycosis: a review of 929 reported cases. Clin Infect Dis. 2005;41(5):634-53.
15. Verklin RM, Jr., Mandell GL. Alteration of effectiveness of antibiotics by anaerobiosis. J Lab Clin Med. 1977;89(1):65-71.
16. Madsen ST. Sepsis, endocarditis, and brain abscess. Scand J Gastroenterol Suppl. 1983;85:48-54.
17. Kaide CG, Khandelwal S. Hyperbaric oxygen: applications in infectious disease. Emerg Med Clin North Am. 2008;26(2):571-95, xi.
18. Larsson A, Engstrom M, Uusijarvi J, Kihlstrom L, Lind F, Mathiesen T. Hyperbaric oxygen treatment of postoperative neurosurgical infections. Neurosurgery. 2008;62 Suppl 2:652-71.
19. Bartek J, Jr., Jakola AS, Skyrman S, Forander P, Alpkvist P, Schechtmann G, et al. Hyperbaric oxygen therapy in spontaneous brain abscess patients: a population-based comparative cohort study. Acta Neurochir (Wien). 2016;158(7):1259-67.
20. Kutlay M, Colak A, Yildiz S, Demircan N, Akin ON. Stereotactic aspiration and antibiotic treatment combined with hyperbaric oxygen therapy in the management of bacterial brain abscesses. Neurosurgery. 2008;62 Suppl 2:540-6.
21. Lampl LA. Hyperbaric oxygen in intracranial abscess. In: Whelan HT, Kindwall EP, editors. Hyperbaric Medicine Practice. 4th ed. North Palm Beach, FL: Best Publishing Company; 2017. p. 467-83.
22. Baechli H, Schmutz J, Mayr JM. Hyperbaric oxygen therapy (HBO) for the treatment of an epidural abscess in the posterior fossa in an 8-month-old infant. Pediatr Neurosurg. 2008;44(3):239-42.
23. Kohshi K, Abe H, Mizoguchi Y, Shimokobe M. Successful treatment of cervical spinal epidural abscess by combined hyperbaric oxygenation. Mt Sinai J Med. 2005;72(6):381-4.
24. Kurschel S, Mohia A, Weigl V, Eder HG. Hyperbaric oxygen therapy for the treatment of brain abscess in children. Childs Nerv Syst. 2006;22(1):38-42.
25. Nakahara K, Yamashita S, Ideo K, Shindo S, Suga T, Ueda A, et al. Drastic therapy for listerial brain abscess involving combined hyperbaric oxygen therapy and antimicrobial agents. J Clin Neurol. 2014;10(4):358-62.

CHAPTER 11

Necrotizing Soft Tissue Infections

Caesar A. Anderson MD, MPH, Irving Jacoby MD, FACP, FACEP, FAAEM, FUHM

Rationale

Necrotizing soft tissue infections (NSTIs) remain among the highest sources of morbidity and mortality. Confirmed cases within the United States approximate the overall mortality rate at 20%.[1] They are often considered one of the most difficult disease entities facing treating physicians and surgeons. Their ability to produce considerable tissue damage in a rapidly progressive manner underscores the importance of timely recognition and initiation of aggressive therapeutic interventions. Hyperbaric oxygen therapy is a recognized accepted adjunct to early judicious surgical debridement(s), appropriate broad-spectrum parenteral antibiotic therapy and a multidisciplinary approach to the management of necrotizing soft tissue infections.[2-6] Moreover, reducing post survival morbidity while optimising survivor quality of life and societal reintegration are facets often neglected in the overall long-term trajectory of care of individuals affected by this devastating disease entity.[7]

It is relevant to approach any therapeutic discussion of a disease state of such high mortality by exploring its underlying pathophysiology, biomechanics, and risk to benefit stratification. Though surgical debridement remains the mainstay of current therapy despite adequate randomized controlled studies or specifics regarding extent or frequency of debridements required, it remains a prudent option.[8] Review of the literature also reflects the wide variability in antibiotic selection and duration.[9] Despite these apparent discrepancies, therapeutic efforts to debulk necrotic tissue and combat systemic infection remain critical principles of care. Of equal consideration must be orchestrated efforts which further target the pathophysiologic contributions of underlined widespread tissue hypoxia and inflammation characterized by necrotizing soft tissue infections with the use of adjunctive hyperbaric oxygen therapy.

A number of clinical scenarios, specific lesions and syndromes have been described over the years, based on the affected tissues and location of infection, the etiologic organism or combination of organisms involved in the infection, and particular host immunologic and vascular risk factors. In all of these clinical situations, there appears to be the common denominator of the development of hypoxia resulting in tissue necrosis.

Hypoxia is known to impair phagocytosis by polymorphonuclear leukocytes.[10] After an infective process is initiated, metabolic products of aerobic and anaerobic metabolism tend to lower the oxidation-reduction potential (E_h), leading to a drop in pH, which creates a milieu for growth of strict and facultative anaerobic organisms. When the blood supply to the skin is affected by involvement within a phlegmon, with edema and necrosis in the deep fascial layers in which they reside, the decreased perfusion pressure and ischemia predispose to rapid progression and advancement of the infectious process within the skin and subcutaneous tissues, exacerbated by the dysfunctional polymorphonuclear leukocytes. Local hypoxia occurs, with up-regulation of endothelial adherence molecules, resulting in leukocyte adhesion and endothelial cytotoxicity. Leukocytes may become sequestered in vessels, impairing local immunity, and incomplete substrate oxidation results in hydrogen and methane accumulation in the tissues. Tissue necrosis occurs, with purulent discharge and gas production. Quantities of gas within tissues are frequently seen in gas gangrene, crepitant anaerobic necrotizing cellulitis, and necrotizing fasciitis.

Hyperbaric oxygen therapy can reduce the amount of hypoxic leukocyte dysfunction occurring within an area of hypoxia and infection, and provide oxygenation to otherwise ischemic areas, thus limiting the spread and progression of infection.[11-12] The diffusion of oxygen dissolved in plasma in the circulation, where it is initially carried in large vessels, proceeds to areas of poorly perfused tissue, from regions of very high O_2 saturation down a gradient to lower oxygen levels in tissue. Integrin inhibition decreases leukocyte adherence, reducing systemic toxicity.[13]

In cases where the antibiotic being used requires oxygen for transport across bacterial cell walls, hyperbaric oxygen therapy can act to enhance antibiotic penetration into target bacteria. Enhancement of the post-antibiotic effect by hyperbaric oxygen has been demonstrated for aminoglycosides and Pseudomonas.[14]

Clinical classification of the necrotizing infections of soft tissues is easiest early in the course of infection, when anatomic levels of involvement of skin, superficial or deep fascia, and muscle involvement can be assessed either during exploration, on punch biopsy, or by radiologic investigation. However, as infection progresses, distinction between some of the clinical entities may become blurred as full thickness necrosis extends into muscle late, after having extended through skin, fat, fascia, and into muscle via direct extension of infection. At presentation, it may be difficult to differentiate these necrotizing soft tissue infections one from another, or from clostridial myositis and myonecrosis, until either Gram stain or cultures are available. Considering their historical differences and evolution, it remains useful to examine each category of infection separately in order to anticipate pathways of extension, anticipate complications, and identify when adjunctive hyperbaric oxygen therapy should be considered.

Introduction

Dr. Joseph Jones, surgeon of the Confederate Army in 1871, coined the initial terminology used to describe 2,642 cases of necrotizing infections as "hospital gangrene."[15] Later in 1883, Dr. Jean-Alfred Fournier characterised necrotizing infections to the perineum. Necrotizing fasciitis was initially described and named "hemolytic *streptococcal* gangrene" by Meleney in 1924.[16] He described an illness characterized by gangrene of subcutaneous tissues, followed by rapid necrosis of the overlying skin from involvement of the blood vessels supplying the skin, which are found in the affected fascial layers. All his patients grew hemolytic streptococci on cultures, and the patients were all seriously ill. Surgical extirpation appeared to be the therapeutic approach. The actual term "necrotizing fasciitis" was credited to Dr. Wilson much later in 1952.[17]

Necrotizing fasciitis is an acute, potentially fatal infection of the superficial and deep fascia of the skin and soft tissues, which progresses to ischemic dermal necrosis after involvement of the dermal blood vessels which traverse the fascial layers. The popular media often refer to this entity as infection with "flesh-eating bacteria." The incidence of NSTI is estimated at approximately 1,000 cases per year in the United States. Though extremely rare, this clinical entity has had an increase in incidence for reasons which remain unclear. Some experts suggest higher case reporting coupled with raised disease awareness, increased numbers of immune-suppressed patients on newer immune-supressing drugs, rising antimicrobial resistance, along with more virulent strains of bacteria.[18]

Etiology of Disease

Necrotizing fasciitis and necrotizing myositis present some diagnostic complexity considering the possibility of both skeletal muscle and fascia involvement with both conditions. Necrotizing fasciitis chiefly involves the fascia whereas necrotizing myositis involves skeletal muscle. The rapidly progressive destruction of muscle fascia seen in necrotizing fasciitis is a direct result of deep soft tissue hypoxia as a direct result of a hypoxic infectious insult. The characteristically poor blood supply of the muscle fascia stands in stark contrast to the more abundant arterial supply to the muscle. This phenomenon has been well described in the earlier Archives of Surgery by Gozal et al.[19] The characteristic level of infection is at the deep fascia. Because infection with necrosis is noted to spread along fascial planes deep to the skin, it is not an uncommon event for there to be minimal skin signs early on. Pain out of proportion to findings could be an early tip off to the presence of deep fascial infection. Since blood vessels supplying overlying skin travel thru fascia, it is the involvement of these vessels by infection that leads to rapid progression to dermal necrosis. Microbiologically, groups A, C, or G beta-hemolytic *streptococci* can be isolated from tissue specimens in 50 to 90% of case series, with one or two more organisms often also accompanying the *streptococci* in up to half the cases. The occurrence of *Staphylococcus aureus* plus anaerobic *streptococci* is also known as Meleney's synergistic gangrene. Commonly isolated organisms include *Enterobacteriaceae, Enterococci, Bacteroides* species, and *Peptococcus* species. *Candida* species have also been reported.[20] Necrotizing fasciitis is also reported to be caused by community-acquired strains of methicillin-resistant *Staphylococcus aureus* (CA-MRSA) alone.[21] In many cases, infection is polymicrobial, with *Enterobacteriaceae* and anaerobes frequently isolated.

Necrotizing soft tissue infections can be subdivided into three bacteriologic classes based on microbial etiology, susceptible host populations and presentation.[22] However, disease course along with associated morbidity and mortality do not appear to differ among classes.

Type I NSTIs are typically polymicrobial with at least one anaerobic species isolated along with an aerobe. Anaerobes such as *Clostridium, Bacteroides,* or *Peptostreptococcus* are most commonly cultured with *Enterobacteriaceae* and one or more facultative anaerobic *streptococci* species other than group A streptococcus (GAS).[23] Perineum and trunk dominate anatomical infectious loci with host characterised by greater medical comorbidities, older age, without frank trauma history. Antecedent perforation, abscess or bacterial translocation are thought responsible for the initial disruption in tissue integrity.

Though rare secondary to hygiene and sanitation improvements, involvement of clostridial species warrants strong consideration when subcutaneous injection of "black tar" heroin is seen within the IV drug abusing population.[24] The lethality of clostridia rests primarily with its alpha and theta toxins. Alpha toxin is thought to be prothrombotic in the early stages of disease by serving as a potent platelet agonist.[25] Local tissue hypoxia ensues at the sites of infection with subsequent reduction in tissue pH further favouring bacterial proliferation. Locally absorbed alpha toxin also contributes to neutrophil dysfunction by impeding diapedesis directly and their adherence to platelets.[25] This underscores the low or negligible levels of neutrophils from Gram stains obtained from clostridial infections. Both alpha and theta toxin act synergistically to disrupt effective phagocytosis while also promoting intravascular hemolysis, decreased vascular tone and endothelial cell integrity.[25]

Fournier's gangrene and necrotizing infection of the head and neck are also included with Type I NSTI classification. Mouth anaerobes (*Bacteroides, Fusobacteria,* and spirochetes) are causative agents for head and neck NSTIs, whereas facultative organisms (*Klebsiella, enterococci, E.coli*) combined with anaerobes (*Bacteroides, Clostridium,* anaerobic or microaerophilic *streptococci*) are responsible for Fournier's gangrene infections.[26] In patients with cervical necrotizing fasciitis, where the chief complication typically involves descending infections with mediastinal involvement, diabetes has been the systemic illness most often associated.[27] Case series review of patients with cervical necrotizing fasciitis treated with HBO$_2$ found statistically significant decrease in hospital stay.[28]

Type II NSTIs are considered monomicrobial with isolation of group A *streptococcus* (GAS) or other beta-hemolytic *streptococci* or *Staphylococcus aureus*. Infected hosts are characteristically healthier, younger, with a clear history of trauma or surgery. Hematogenous translocation from the throat to the area of direct trauma is thought responsible for Type II NSTIs without clear portal of bacterial entry.[29] The lethality of GAS rests primarily with its M proteins though several other microbiologic mechanisms augment its toxicity. M proteins allow for more effective bacterial adherence and avoidance of phagocytosis. Moreover, M proteins elicit a robust inflammatory response by presenting superantigens to T cell receptors thus activating 20% rather than the usual 0.1% of T cells. This leads to catastrophic shock and eventual death secondary to massive stimulation of IL-6, TNF alpha, and IL-1 release.[30] M protein types 1 and 3 are associated with *streptococcal* toxic shock syndrome in over 50% of cases.[31]

Type III NSTIs have isolates of gram-negative marine bacteria such as *Vibrio vulnificus*. Like Type II NSTIs, this category of disease results in earlier signs of systemic toxicity with shock occurring more rapidly despite wide area of disease involvement. Though infection is usually through an open wound, host infection has also been described from ingestion of colonized oysters by cirrhotics.[32-33]

Risk Factors

The most common risk factors associated with necrotizing fasciitis are traumatic breaks in the skin, most commonly lacerations, insect bites, burns, deep abrasions, puncture wounds, or following surgery, particularly those involving bowel perforations. Diabetes appears to be a strong risk factor, as are obesity, alcoholism, smoking, liver disease, and intravenous drug abuse. Reports of necrotizing fasciitis as a result of infection of otherwise typical lesions of chickenpox have been published.[34] Both the use of sodium-glucose cotransporter 2 inhibitors used in management of type 2 diabetes and NSAIDS have been implicated as potential risk factors in the development of NSTIs.[35-37] It's important to note that although a direct causal relationship by NSAIDS, which remain ubiquitous in use, seems unlikely, there does exist a relationship between NSAID use and NSTI. NSAIDs are cyclooxygenase inhibitors and may have an adverse effect on neutrophil killing and cell-mediated immunity. NSAIDs are reported to inhibit monocyte superoxide production.[38] Their mode of action, in the clinical setting of NSTI, may relate to a dampened immunomodulatory effect on leukocyte adhesion, chemotaxis, granulocyte functions, and bactericidal control.[39] Most recently, Nizet et al. reported that patients with rheumatoid arthritis taking a medication, anakinra, a drug that dampens autoimmunity by inhibiting interleukin-1ß, are >300 times more likely to experience invasive Group A *streptococcal* infections than patients not on the drug.[40]

Most common sites of occurrence of necrotizing fasciitis are the lower extremities, while an increased incidence in the upper extremities is seen in the parenteral drug abuse population. However, any location of the body can be affected, including the abdominal wall of neonates, in association with omphalitis.[41] Involvement of the scrotum and perineum in the male is known as Fournier's gangrene, which is essentially necrotizing fasciitis of the superficial perineal fascia, also known as Colles' fascia; which can spread infection to the penis and scrotum via Buck's fascia or Dartos' fascia; or Scarpa's fascia, which connects to, and can spread infection to, the abdominal wall. Perianal or perirectal infection may also spread into these areas, and undrained or inadequately drained perirectal abscesses are often cited as a source of Fournier's gangrene. Perineal necrotizing fasciitis can also occur in the female. Diabetes mellitus remains a strong risk factor in this particular form of necrotizing fasciitis as well. Fournier's gangrene is more likely to have multiple mixed organisms cultured, particularly *Enterobacteriaceae*, Group D *streptococci*, and anaerobic organisms, such as *Bacteroides fragilis*.

Differential Diagnosis

Clearly a goal when making the diagnosis of necrotizing fasciitis is to make it as early as possible so as to be able to start appropriate treatments and avoid rapid spreading and the onset of sepsis. Time is tissue. The main differential diagnosis includes standard cellulitis, which may be a precursor of necrotizing fasciitis in some cases; and erysipelas, with its erythematous well-delineated border. Additional entities which should be considered include clostridial myositis and myonecrosis; non-clostridial myositis and myonecrosis; toxic shock syndrome, which may accompany necrotizing fasciitis; Zygomycotic gangrenous cellulitis; mixed aerobic/anaerobic necrotizing cellulitis; toxic epidermal necrolysis (TEN), also known as Lyell's disease, usually due to exposure to particular medications; and *staphylococcal* scalded skin syndrome, also known as Ritter's disease, due to exfoliative toxins produced by *staphylococci*, with the latter two entities being most common in neonates and children under 5 years of age. In the neonate with omphalitis, violaceous discoloration of the skin appears to be a strong marker for the emergence of necrotizing fasciitis. *Vibrio vulnificans* infections cause blistering infection quite commonly, and are seen in patients who have either been swimming in waters, along the Gulf of Mexico, or have been eating shellfish from that area. Aeromonas infections also occur following open wounds acquired in sea water. Cutaneous anthrax may present with a blackened central area and surrounding edema.

Clinical Presentation

The patient with necrotizing fasciitis will typically present with an acute combination of pain and swelling, which may or may not be accompanied by fever and chills. There may already be a focus of cellulitis apparent, but in some instances early on, there may be very few skin changes. In some patients, there may be pain out of proportion to the skin findings, which may not be unexpected considering that the initial level of infection is the fascia, not necessarily the skin. In others, manifestations of a large phlegmon may be quite obvious, although at times the area of infection may have been assumed to be cellulitis and not a more serious form of infection. Pain may proceed to numbness, as a result of compression of nerves which also pass through the fascia. With time however, the infection will rapidly proceed to cause areas of blistering and bullae formation. Hints of darkening of the skin may appear as perfusion decreases, until obvious areas of dermal ischemia appear, making the skin appear dusky, grayish or frankly black. Upon exploration of the process, a clinical diagnosis can be confirmed at the time of biopsy or debridement, when the fascia is grossly observed by the surgeon to be necrotic, and will give way easily to a probing finger or surgical clamp, giving the sensation of "thunking" of the skin against the underlying muscle layers, instead of remaining tight and crisply defined. It has been suggested that limbs of patients with necrotizing fasciitis, as opposed to those with cellulitis only, may be observed to have markedly reduced tissue oxygen saturations as measured by near-infra-red spectroscopy throughout the involved site, with oxygen saturations in the 52% ±18% range, compared to control measurements of 86% ±11% in uninvolved sites.[42]

In the neonate, necrotizing fasciitis of the abdominal wall can be seen as a complication of omphalitis in 10 to 16% of cases,[43] and appears to carry over a 50% mortality rate even when treated with aggressive debridement of involved skin, subcutaneous tissue and fascia.[44]

Diagnostic Considerations

Raised clinical suspicion remains essential. However, a number of diagnostic observations have been made to enable confirmation of the diagnosis of necrotizing fasciitis. Immunocompromised patients add to the diagnostic complexity in that they have atypical clinical presentations when compared to immune-competent patients. Such variability often leads to further delays in initializing prompt treatment and supportive care. Hence, a two-fold increase in mortality is often seen with Immunocompromised NSTI patients.[45]

Frozen section soft-tissue biopsy early in the evolution of a suspect lesion may provide definitive diagnosis.[46] Cultures of deep tissue at the time of debridement for aerobes, anaerobes and fungi, are imperative as up to 75% of patients in some series' have demonstrated polymicrobial etiologies. Fungal cultures are particularly important in the immunocompromised, diabetic and cancer populations and in patients who have not responded to standard antibacterial antibiotics.

Imaging studies should not delay surgical intervention, especially with clinical signs of crepitus or a worsening physical examination. CT scan is considered the best initial diagnostic modality to obtain with NSTIs due to its high specificity and relative expediency and availability. It also offers greater detection of soft tissue gas when compared to MRI.[47] Moreover, MRI has been shown to overestimate deep tissue involvement blurring the distinction between necrotizing cellulitis and deeper tissue infection.

Asymmetrical fascial thickening that was at least twice the contralateral side and associated with fat stranding was seen in 80% of 20 patients with necrotizing fasciitis. Gas tracking along fascial planes was seen in 55%, characteristically did not involve muscle and was not associated with abscess formation.[48] The authors note that the areas of black, gangrenous skin were far smaller than the widespread infection in the underlying fascial planes. Also of note was that 7 of the 20 patients had associated deep space abscesses requiring immediate surgical drainage, which demonstrates the need for CT studies to assess extent of disease, particularly in patients who do not appear to be responding to therapy.

Magnetic resonance imaging (MRI) also demonstrates the extent of affected tissue well, is able to differentiate fluid and gas through differential signal intensities, and is useful in differentiating cellulitis from necrotizing fasciitis after injection of gadolinium contrast. But in a study of 15 patients, MRI overestimated the extent of deep fascial involvement in one patient who only had cellulitis, following IM injections which showed up on MRI as thickening of both superficial and deep fascia of the deltoid muscle.[49]

The Laboratory Risk Indicator for Necrotizing Fasciitis (LRINEC) score has gained wider use in helping to detect the presence of NSTIs early though it has not yet been validated. It utilizes six laboratory indicators to predict the likelihood of disease. Admission serum glucose (< or >180), C-reactive protein (< or >150), creatinine (< or >1.6), white cell count (< 15 or >25), hemoglobin (>13.5 or <11.5), and sodium (< or >135) values scored individually. Positive predictive value is reported at 92% with a 96% Negative predictive value on a LRINEC score > or = to 6.[50] Its use alone as a diagnostic tool is not advocated. LRINEC fails to consider age, clinical presentation, comorbidities and other parameters often included in APACHE II or GLASGOW type scoring systems.[51] Borschitz et al. have suggested a modified LRINEC with inclusion of additional clinical and laboratory parameters which address some of the apparent flaws of the LRINEC.[52] Preliminary work on Pentraxin-3, an early inflammatory biomarker, may also assist in early diagnosis of NSTI.[53] More recent studies appear to suggest LRINEC use more akin to predicting associated NSTI mortality and amputation risk rather than diagnosing NSTIs.[54-55] Nevertheless, it remains a useful tool when coupled with raised clinical suspicion and diagnostic uncertainty.

Clinical Management with Adjunctive Hyperbaric Oxygen Therapy

Prompt surgical debridement and empiric antibiotic coverage remains essential to early management of NSTIs. Figure 1 illustrates the need for risk stratification of patients in order to triage their care. However, evidence based best practice guidelines following the use of antibiotics and surgical debridement for the management of NSTIs do not exist.

Initial use of broad-spectrum antibiotics is advocated for all patients after blood cultures but *prior* to obtaining direct tissue cultures once operatively debrided. Empiric adult regimens should target anaerobes, gram-positive, and gram-negative organisms: beta-lactamase inhibitor (piperacillin-tazobactam, ampicillin-sulbactam) or carbapenem (imipenem, meropenem) along with MRSA coverage and clindamycin (600–900 mg iv q8h) for coverage against toxin-releasing species of *streptococci* or *staphylococci*.[56] Review of literature suggests continuing the antibiotic regimen until no further debridements are required or patient reaches hemodynamic stability. Premature cessation of antibiotics should be avoided given NSTI proclivity for rapid deterioration and/or relapse. Faraklas et al. noted within their multi-center review of 341 patients that an extended duration of antibiotic therapy did not equate to better therapeutic outcomes.[57] This further echoes the complexity and lack of current evidence-based guidelines on antibiotic use.

The use of post exposure prophylaxis (10 days of penicillin 250 mg orally q4h) for immunosuppressed close contacts remains uncertain though reasonable for those exposed to NSTI patients with (GAS) group A *streptococcus*[58] It is with this category of GAS infected patients that IVIG has shown any promise though its routine use remains to be validated.[59]

Adjunctive hyperbaric oxygen therapy is most often indicated in the treatment of conditions with underlying tissue hypoxia. Its ability to augment oxygen delivery is best explained with an understanding of ideal gas laws which describe the direct relationship of dissolved gas in solution and partial pressure. The dissolved oxygen content of 6 ml/dl, which is adequate enough to provide resting tissue oxygen demands *irrespective* of hemoglobin-bound oxygen, can be achieved with delivery of hyperbaric oxygen at 3 atm.

Table 1. Literature Summary: Therapeutic Survival Outcomes for Hyperbaric Oxygen Therapy and NSTIs

Author	Study Type	Study Group	Sample Size	Control	Treatment Regimen	HBO₂ Therapy vs. No-HBO₂ In-Hospital Survival Rates
Stevens et al. (2017)	Systematic review	Type I, II	n=57	n/a	Not described.	Not described. Notes significant survival in recent US and Australian study.
Levett et al. (2015)	Meta-analysis	Type I, II, and III	n=673	n/a	Not described.	Not described.
Wang et al. (2003)	Systematic review	Type I, II, and III	n=17 clostridial studies; n=9 non-clostridial	n/a	n=17, 2-3 atm, 4 to 44 HBO₂ therapy, n=9, 2-3 atm, 90 mins O₂/tx, 5-7 HBO₂ therapy	Summary estimates unobtainable. Poor study quality.
Shaw et al. (2014)	Retrospective, 14 multi-centers	Type I (non-clostridial, clostridial)	1583	n=1466	n=117, not specified	95% vs 88%, In-hospital survival: p=0.028
Li et al. (2014)	Retrospective	Type I (non-clostridial)	28	n=12	n=16, 2.5 atm, 90-120 mins O₂/tx, bid HBO₂ therapy	87.5% vs 66%, In-hospital survival: p<0.05

Table 1. Literature Summary: Therapeutic Survival Outcomes for Hyperbaric Oxygen Therapy and NSTIs (continued)

Author	Study Type	Study Group	Sample Size	Control	Treatment Regimen	HBO$_2$ Therapy vs. No-HBO$_2$ In-Hospital Survival Rates
Massey et al. (2014)	Retrospective	Type I (non-clostridial)	80	n=48	n=32, 2-2.8 atm, 45 mins O$_2$/tx, 1-8 HBO$_2$ therapy	84.4% vs 81.2%, In-hospital survival: p<0.77
Mehl et al. (2010)	Retrospective	Type I (non-clostridial, clostridial)	40	n=14	n=26, 2-2.5 atm, 120 mins O$_2$/tx, 6-20 HBO$_2$ therapy	88.5% vs 64.3%, In-hospital survival: p=0.07
George et al. (2009)	Retrospective, multicenter	Type I and II (non-clostridial, GAS), 5 patients clostridial	78	n=30	n=48,3 atm, 90 mins O$_2$/tx, tid then bid HBO$_2$ therapy	91.7% vs 86.7%, In-hospital survival: p=0.48; aOR 0.98 (0.18-5.42)
Ayan et al. (2005)	Retrospective	Type I (non-clostridial)	41	n=23	n=18,2.5 atm, 90 mins O$_2$/tx, 3-10 HBO$_2$ therapy	100% vs 61%, In-hospital survival: p=0.013
Escobar et al. (2005)	Retrospective	Type I (Non-Clostridia)	42	n/a	n=42,2-2.5 atm, 90-120 mins O$_2$/tx, bid then qd HBO$_2$ therapy	88.1% vs 66%, In-hospital survival: p=0.013
Wilkinson et al. (2004)	Retrospective	Type I (Non-Clostridia)	44	n=11	n=33,2.8 atm, 60 mins O$_2$/tx, tid then bid HBO$_2$ therapy	94% vs 64%, In-hospital survival: p=0.03
Hollabaugh et al. (1998)	Retrospective	Type I (non-clostridial, clostridial)	26	n=12	n=12,2.4 atm, 90 mins O$_2$/tx, bid x 7 days HBO$_2$ therapy the qd	93% vs 58%, In-hospital survival:

Numerous studies have continued to demonstrate the beneficial effect of adjunctive hyperbaric oxygen therapy in the management of NSTIs (Refer to Table 1). In 2012, Soh et al. launched a large retrospective review of 45,913 NSTI cases from a nationwide database (Nationwide Inpatient Sample) within the United States. They found a statistically significant reduction in mortality among patients treated with HBO$_2$ (4.5% vs 9.4 %). Further analysis controlling for confounders and other predictors of mortality did not alter results, demonstrating a survival advantage in the HBO$_2$ treated group (odds ratio [OR] 0.49;95% CI 0.29-0.83).[60]

Wilkinson and Doolette[61] reported a five-year retrospective cohort Australian study of 44 patients with necrotizing soft tissue infection, between 1994 and 1999, looking at the primary outcome of survival to hospital discharge, and secondary outcomes of limb salvage and long-term survival after hospital discharge. Logistic regression analysis determined the strongest association with survival was the intervention of hyperbaric therapy (p=.02). Hyperbaric oxygen therapy increased survival with an odds ratio of 8.9 (95% confidence interval, 1.3-58.0) and a number of three needed to treat to benefit. Hyperbaric oxygen therapy also reduced the incidence of amputation (p=.05) and improved long-term outcome (p=.002).

In the series by Escobar et al., there were no further amputations beyond those already done prior to transfer, once hyperbaric oxygen therapy was initiated in their series of 42 patients.[62] The negative study by Brown at al. which purports to be a multi-center retrospective review of treatment at three facilities over 12 years, of 54 patients, had numerous discrepancies in the demographics of their two groups.[63] Half of the hyperbaric-oxygen-treated group of 30 patients, all from one institution, were noted to have clostridial infections, while the non-hyperbaric treated group had only four of 24 patients (17%) with clostridial infection. Six of the 30 in the hyperbaric group are noted to have the diagnosis of clostridial myositis and myonecrosis, whereas only one of the non-hyperbaric oxygen treated patients were so diagnosed. Hence this clearly shows the same diseases were not being compared in this study. Additionally, as is pointed out in a subsequent letter to the editor, 80% of the patients received four or fewer treatments, the remaining 20% received between five and seven treatments, and the timing of these treatments is not specified.[64] If the guideline of treating three times in the first 24 hours were followed, and then twice per day until the patient is stable and shows no relapse of toxicity between treatments, the gas gangrene patients in this study were treated for less than a day and a half, which is a shorter period of time than most other studies, and the others were treated for around two days.

In the Wilkinson study, patients received a median of 8 treatments, which is more than that received by the patient with the greatest number of treatments in Brown et al. The authors state that the mortality difference between the two groups (9/30, or 30% of the hyperbaric group, versus 10/24, or 42% in the non-hyperbaric group) was not statistically significant. Thus the Brown et al study should not be used as an argument that the use of hyperbaric oxygen for truncal necrotizing fasciitis is "controversial," because these mortality statistics are not comparable, with a different mix of diagnoses in the two, compounded by the fact that the numbers themselves are small, resulting in a study that had insufficient power to demonstrate a statistically significant result. Furthermore, the study does not add to the literature of necrotizing fasciitis involving the limbs and other non-truncal sites.

Amputation rates of 26% up to 50% are reported in cases of necrotizing fasciitis of the extremities, without hyperbaric therapy.[65-66] Mortality in reported series range from 16.9% up to 66% without the use of hyperbaric oxygen. Mortality is often associated with delayed diagnosis, underlying immunocompromise, and underlying heart disease, degree of leukocytosis, septic shock and severe underlying metabolic abnormalities.

In the neonate, necrotizing fasciitis is reported as a complication of omphalitis, balanitis, mastitis, postoperative infection, and fetal monitoring.[67] Four of six cases found in a literature review who received hyperbaric oxygen therapy survived, while the overall mortality rate was 39/66 (59%). In a group of neonatal omphalitis patients with abdominal wall necrotizing fasciitis reported from Children's Hospital in Los Angeles, seven out of eight cases died, for a mortality rate of 87% without hyperbaric oxygen therapy.[68] In a series of 32 cases of omphalitis from Seattle over a 10-year period, seven developed necrotizing fasciitis, and five of the seven died. The two patients who did survive, out of the four who had hyperbaric oxygen treatments, were noted to have resolved their systemic sepsis more rapidly, and had healthier granulation tissue on the perimeter of the debridement. Neither survivor treated with hyperbaric oxygen required any further debridements before their wounds were closed.[69]

Gozal et al. treated necrotizing fasciitis patients with combined antibiotics, radical surgery and hyperbaric oxygen, and reduced the historic mortality rate from 38% to 12.5%. Of 29 patients reported retrospectively by Riseman et al., 12 were treated by surgical debridement and antibiotics only, and 17 received hyperbaric oxygen treatments in addition.[70-71] Both groups had similar parameters of age, race, sex, wound bacteriology and antimicrobial therapy. Body surface area was also similar. However, perineal involvement (53% vs. 12 %) and septic shock (29% vs. 8%) were more common in the hyperbaric group, yet the overall mortality was significantly lower at 23%, versus 66% in the non-hyperbaric oxygen treated group. Additionally, only 1.2 debridements per patient in the hyperbaric treatment group were performed, vs. 3.3 debridements per patient in the surgery plus antibiotics-only group.

Fortunately, Fournier's gangrene cases in the literature are usually studied and reported as a distinct group. Due to the difficulty in making direct comparisons of clinical series, a Fournier's gangrene Severity Index Score was developed in order to assess a number of variables rather than the presence of the disease itself.[72] The score uses degrees of deviation from normal of physiologic variables to generate a score that correlates with patient mortality. It is clear that the amount of disease, related by some to body surface area of involvement, may be a significant variable. The Duke University analysis of 50 consecutive patients seen at their institution over a 15-year period had a 20% overall mortality.[73] Three statistically significant predictors of outcome were identified when examined using univariate analysis: extent of infection, depth of the necrotizing infection, and treatment with hyperbaric oxygen. However, the same data using multivariate regression analysis identified only the extent of the infection as the only statistically significant independent predictor of outcome in the presence of other co-variables. Patients with disease involving a body surface area of 3.0% or less all survived. The numbers of patients with disease extent greater than 3%, where hyperbaric oxygen would thus be expected to play a role, became smaller, and with small numbers of patients, the power of the study to demonstrate a significant response was not present. Using multivariate analysis, the p value for statistical significance for hyperbaric oxygen treatments was equal to .06.

Aside from early surgical debridement and empiric antibiotic coverage in the management of Fournier's gangrene, adjunctive hyperbaric oxygen therapy has been advocated by several authors. HBO_2 therapy has been shown to halt tissue laden anaerobic bacterial growth, limit tissue necrosis, and minimise systemic toxicity.[74] Hollabaugh et al. reported a retrospective series of 26 cases from the University of Tennessee's five hospitals.[75] Of the 15 patients with identifiable sources for their infections, eight had urethral disease or trauma, five had colorectal disease, and two had penile prosthesis. All patients were managed with prompt surgical debridement and broad-spectrum antibiotics. Procedures performed included urinary diversion, fecal diversion, and multiple debridements. Fourteen of the 26 were additionally treated with hyperbaric oxygen. The group treated with hyperbaric oxygen had a mortality rate of 7%, versus 42% in the group not receiving hyperbaric oxygen (p=.04), with a combined overall mortality rate of 23%. The one patient who died while receiving hyperbaric oxygen therapy had been progressing well without evidence of ongoing infection, but suffered an acute MI not thought to be related to the underlying disease process. In the non-hyperbaric group, deaths were usually attributed to ongoing or fulminant sepsis. Relative risk for survival was 11 times greater in the group receiving hyperbaric oxygen therapy. This study did not show a decrease in the number of debridements by HBO_2 therapy, but was confounded due to the larger number of patients who died and thus were not able to get further debridements. Delay to treatment was not a factor in the different groups.

Additional series include that of the Genoa, Italy group who treated 11 patients without any deaths, and all delayed corrective procedures healed without infectious complications.[76] Another 33 patients were reported in a series from Turku, Finland.[77] These patients were treated at 2.5 atmospheres absolute (ATA), in conjunction with antibiotics and surgery. Three patients died, for a mortality rate of 9%. Hyperbaric oxygenation was observed to reduce systemic toxicity, prevent extension of the necrotizing process, and increased demarcation, improving overall outcomes. Two of the three patients who died were moribund upon arrival to their facility. Management included diverting colostomies for those patients with a perirectal or perineal source, and orchiectomy, although sometimes reported in all series, is not routinely done since the blood supply to the testes is from the spermatic vessels which do not perfuse the scrotum and penis. Suprapubic cystostomy was indicated and performed when the source of the infection was genitourinary.

of the infection, initial symptoms would be similar to routine sinusitis with sinus pain, congestion, and drainage. The infection then accelerates, extending into adjacent structures and tissues with development of erythema, progressing to violaceous or dusky to frankly black tissue in the nares, turbinates, palate, or orbit. The organisms appear to have a predilection for invasion of arteries, lymphatics, and nerves. Invasion of vascular structures leads to a fibrin reaction and development of a *Mucor* thrombus within vessels, which leads to infarction. The infarcted tissue becomes acidotic and permissive for even further fungal ingrowth and proliferation. Lack of perfusion prevents antibiotic penetration into affected tissues. Extension into adjacent periorbital and orbital structures is often found even early on.

Clinical manifestations can include periorbital edema, tearing, and proptosis. Involvement of the optic nerve will be marked by blurring followed by loss of vision. Abnormalities of eye movement may occur as markers of cranial nerve involvement. Extension can also move inferiorly into the hard palate via the maxillary sinuses. Black, necrotic ulcers may be found on the palate, and the nasal turbinates may appear black and necrotic. Infection may extend into the cranial vault, either via the ethmoid sinus and through the cribriform plate, or through the orbital apex into the area of the cavernous sinus, producing the orbital apex syndrome. This consists of ophthalmoplegia and fifth cranial nerve involvement, progressing to cavernous sinus thrombosis, and thrombosis of the internal carotid artery and results in major hemispheric stroke and altered consciousness. Due to the propensity for angioinvasion, fungemia can occur, disseminating the infection systemically. Rhinocerebral mucormycosis has a very high mortality rate. Standard treatment consists of the antifungal antibiotic amphotericin B lipid complex or liposomal amphotericin B in a dose of 5 mg/kg daily and surgical debridement when indicated. Survivors have usually had earlier diagnosis and surgical debridements.

Pulmonary involvement is the second most common type of zygomycosis overall, seen particularly in patients with leukemia and lymphoma.[95] Isolated solitary nodular lesions, lobar involvement, cavitary lesions, and disseminated lesions have all been reported.[96] Erosion of the fungus into mediastinal structures, particularly the pulmonary artery, with massive hemoptysis, is a fatal occurrence. Wedged infarctions of the lung may be seen as a manifestation of thrombosed pulmonary vessels from angioinvasion.[97]

One of the manifestations of cutaneous infection includes a rapidly progressive, ascending, necrotizing infection consistent with necrotizing fasciitis, which can involve an extremity or the torso. Aerial hyphae can sometimes be grossly visualized in wounds infected with zygomycosis organisms as a loose, whitish cottony exudate covering the surface of open wounds. Risk factors for the development of cutaneous and subcutaneous involvement include various types of breakdown of the skin barrier including puncture wounds, other trauma, and burn wounds. Mortality rates of 30 to 70% are reported in necrotizing fasciitis with these organisms, depending on the underlying condition associated with the infection. Since diabetic ketoacidosis is a treatable condition, reversal of the acidosis affords an opportunity for the host response to reconstitute, and thus may have a decreased mortality compared to the patients with non-reversible conditions.

The GI syndrome is characterized by abdominal pain and distention associated with nausea and vomiting. Fever and hematochezia may occur. Stomach, ileum, and colon are most commonly affected. Most such diagnoses are made postmortem, but if suspected, may require laparotomy to manage the bowel infarctions that may occur.[98]

Differential Diagnosis

Upon initial presentation, rhinocerebral mucormycosis may be misidentified as the more common routine bacterial sinusitis due to usual Gram-positive or anaerobic organisms, although there should not be any necrotic lesions in those cases. However, once evidence of necrosis is apparent, or in the proper clinical settings, there should be no hesitation in ordering a biopsy looking for the various characteristic fungal forms (e.g. wide, non-septate hyphae branching off at right angles), and signs of angioinvasive processes should be sought. Affected tissue usually has neutrophilic infiltrates, and inflammatory vasculitis is seen involving both arteries and veins. Cultures for routine aerobic, anaerobic, and fungal organisms should always be sent. Cavernous sinus thrombosis can occur as an extension of suppurative, usually staphylococcal, facial cellulitis or abscess, but there would not be the typical lesions in the nose or sinuses. Radiological studies such as plain films or CT scans may show more extensive bone necrosis than was anticipated. Orbital cellulitis and bacterial osteo- myelitis of the frontal bone or orbit are other entities, which may clinically resemble this form of zygomycosis.

Lung involvement may be non-specific and can look like other cases of atelectasis, pneumonia, and granulomatous disease or, particularly in patients with cancer, infection due to *Aspergillus* species. Use of radiologic studies may hasten the diagnosis. In a retrospective analysis of CT findings in 16 cases of pulmonary zygomycosis vs. 29 cases of invasive pulmonary aspergillosis at the University of Texas M.D. Anderson Cancer Center, logistic regression analysis of clinical characteristics demonstrated that concomitant sinusitis and voriconazole prophylaxis were significantly associated with pulmonary zygomycosis.[99] CT scan findings of multiple (≥10) nodules and pleural effusion were both independent predictors of pulmonary zygomycosis, suggesting potential clues in differentiating the two types of infections. Pulmonary mucormycosis can also be confused with standard pulmonary embolism. Gastrointestinal disease must be differentiated from other bowel infections, perforation, and staphylococcal necrotizing enterocolitis seen in infants.

Rationale for Use of HBO$_2$

From a physiological viewpoint, mechanistic steps are only now being discovered to explain the virulence and invasiveness of the filamentous fungi in causing disease. Each of these mechanisms, as discovered, would well be worth testing in the presence of hyperbaric oxygen to assess potential roles for hyperbaric oxygen therapy. Filamentous fungi are aerobic, and thus it is not expected that there would be a direct effect on fungi under clinical hyperbaric conditions.

Hyperbaric oxygen therapy in the setting of zygomycosis could be beneficial in a number of ways. The angioinvasive character of these infections creates areas of hypoxia, ischemia, and subsequent necrosis, which will directly affect neutrophilic killing of organisms as phagocytosis becomes inefficient. Areas of tissue that are ischemic due to partial loss of perfusion can be made normoxic during hyperbaric therapy and restore immune mechanisms that have become dysfunctional due to hypoxia.

The neutrophil has a significant role in defending against filamentous fungi despite the larger size of the hyphae. Engulfment by neutrophils and damage to hyphae is correlated with response to infection. Both mononuclear and polymorphonuclear white cells of normal hosts kill *Rhizopus* by generation of oxidative metabolites and cationic peptide defensins.[100-102] Comparison of antifungal function of human polymorphonuclear leukocytes against hyphae of *Rhizopus oryzae* and *Rhizopus microsporus*, the most frequently isolated zygomycetes, with that of *Absidia corymbifera* have shown that oxidative burst responses by PMNs and PML-induced hyphal damage were significantly lower in response to the *Rhizopus* species than to the *Absidia* species, and that hyphal damage increased when PMLs were incubated with interferon-gamma and granulocyte-macrophage colony stimulating factor (GM-CSF).[63] Mouse bronchoalveolar macrophages prevent germination of spores in vitro and in vivo in a murine model, and this ability is blocked by corticosteroid therapy. Correction of hypoxia for such critical cells should enhance oxidative killing of fungi.

The significant hallmark of zygomycoses is their ability to invade blood vessels causing blood vessel inflammation, thrombosis, and tissue necrosis in many different tissues and subsequent hematogenous dissemination to other organs. Penetration of endothelial cells lining blood vessels must be a key step in the pathophysiology of zygomycosis. Studies examining these steps are crucial in defining additional steps to treat infection by blocking fungal dissemination. It has been demonstrated that *Rhizopus oryzae* spores adhere to subendothelial matrix proteins better than hyphae, but spores and hyphae adhere equivalently to human umbilical vein endothelial cells.[103] Phagocytosis of *Rhizopus oryzae* by endothelial cells was also shown to damage the endothelial cells, raising the question of whether such steps could be related to subsequent thromboses. Hyperbaric oxygen research has not begun to delve into these neutrophil and fungal/endothelial interactions, but studies are sorely needed.

Much of the surgery required to manage the necrotizing aspects of infection involving sinuses, orbit, and skull is quite deforming, and the addition of hyperbaric oxygen to wound management would facilitate generation of granulation tissue, epithelialization, and bone healing. Additionally, there are other non-specific mechanisms that are still being worked out for several forms of sepsis which appear to be positively affected by hyperbaric oxygen.[104-105] Standard therapy involves the use of antifungal antibiotics and definitive debridement of necrotic tissue. Hyperbaric oxygen clinical studies to date have generally been either isolated case reports or retrospective case series and literature reviews. John et al.[67] reported such a literature review of 28 published cases that had received hyperbaric oxygen treatments. Among the Mucorales isolates, there were 11 cases of *Rhizopus* species, followed by three cases of *Apophysomyces* species, and two cases each of *Mucor* and *Absidia*. Three isolates from entomophthoramycoses were *Conidiobolus* species. Risk factors in these patients were a spectrum of the typically seen range, with 17/28 (61%) being diabetics, 10 of whom had keto-acidosis; five patients (18%) developed their infections after trauma; one patient was on systemic steroids; three (11%) had hematological malignancies or bone marrow transplants; and three (11%) had no known risk factors for zygomycosis. The overall survival rate was 86%, which encompassed a 94% survival rate in diabetic patients, but only a 33% survival rate in patients with hematological malignancies or bone marrow transplants. All patients except for two had also received amphotericin B. Despite the range of cases, all groups were small, and there were no case controls to which to compare the case responses.

In a large series of all cases of zygomycosis found in the literature since 1885, 929 cases of zygomycosis were reported and analyzed by Roden et al.[106] Survival rates were reported by type of treatment received. Forty-four patients were identified as having received hyperbaric oxygen therapy, and in that group 64% of patients survived. Other treatments identified and their survival rates were amphotericin B deoxycholate recipients, 324 of 532 patients (61%); amphotericin B lipid formulation, 80 of 116 patients (69%); itraconazole, ketoconazole, or posaconazole, 10 of 15 patients (67%); no antifungal therapy at all, 59 of 333 patients (18%); surgery alone, 51 of 90 patients (57%); surgery plus antifungal therapy, 328 of 470 cases (70%); granulocyte colony stimulating factor, 15 of 18 patients (83%); and granulocyte transfusion, two of seven cases (29%). In patients who received no therapy at all, there were eight survivors out of 241 cases (3%).

Major difficulties arise with the data, particularly since it usually does not differentiate between intent to treat studies vs. salvage therapy when standard treatments, which range from use of antibiotics, surgery, or hyperbaric oxygen therapy, appear to be failing. This is an observed difficulty in interpreting large numbers of individual case reports and series.[107] An example is the case reported by Bentur et al. of mucormycosis of the fourth finger of the hand in a diabetic with ketoacidosis.[108] In this case, hyperbaric oxygen therapy is begun only after other modalities have been tried, including amphotericin B, amputation of the affected finger followed by wide debridement of the hand, and fasciotomy of the forearm, and the disease continued to progress. After receiving 29 hyperbaric treatments, the infection appeared improved and the patient went on to heal her wounds.

Similarly, the case of an Entomophthorales infection in the medial orbit of an 18-month-old is another example of hyperbaric oxygen therapy used as salvage therapy in conjunction with radical surgery when the organism was found to be resistant to all available antifungal antibiotics.[109] Thus, any future database of cases of zygomycoses treated with hyperbaric oxygen therapy should document classification of cases by whether hyperbaric oxygen was used as an early adjunct at the time of initial institution of therapy, or as "rescue" or "salvage" therapy. In addition, hyperbaric oxygen would normally be considered an adjunct to use of antibiotics and indicated surgery, and such subgroup analysis was not done in the Roden et al. report. It is unfair to compare the results if hyperbaric oxygen therapy were started late in the treatment course as salvage therapy, when an initial course of antibiotics and surgical debridement have been determined to have failed and infection is progressing and considered to be refractory, as opposed to surgery and antibiotics started early on without hyperbaric oxygen. Appropriate comparisons can be made when hyperbaric therapy is added as an adjunct to the initial management of surgery and antibiotics.

A strong argument for controlling for such variables in different studies is well-advised and comparable to the discussions in the medical literature related to other salvage interventions, such as with a new antibiotic, where the answers to the questions of how much of the treatment effect is attributable to the commencement of therapy and how much is attributable to the natural history of partially-treated disease, can rarely be separated out.[110] In the setting of a rare, relatively unusual infection, it is a given that randomized studies would be unrealistic, and those authors recommend that carefully selected, matched, contemporaneous control subjects are likely to be the most useful alternative. Although these comments were made in reference to use of newer antifungal antibiotics, the same observations would apply to the analysis of hyperbaric oxygen therapy.

Treatment

Antibiotic treatment should be commenced with an amphotericin B preparation. The fungus is relatively refractory to standard medical therapy, thus maximally tolerated doses of amphotericin B deoxycholate should be used, usually 1–1.5 mg/kg/day. Lipid complex forms of amphotericin B doses are better tolerated and doses are higher. The dose of amphotericin B lipid complex (Abelcet) and liposomal amphotericin B (AmBisome) is 5 mg/kg/day. It has been observed that the use of voriconazole as fungal prophylaxis in the hematopoietic stem cell transplant population is a risk factor for developing zygomycosis and should be avoided.[111] Other currently available azoles such as ketoconazole, itraconazole, fluconazole, or miconazole are not efficacious either. Posaconazole, a newer extended-spectrum oral azole, has demonstrated in vitro and in vivo activity against zygomycetes and has been used as salvage therapy for 24 patients with zygomycetes infections who were intolerant of, or whose infections were resistant to, standard antifungal therapy.[112] Surgical debridement should be considered based on area of involvement and sequential debridements may be necessary to control spread. Frozen-section guided debridement has been advocated to assure adequate margins.[113] Reconstructive surgery may also be necessary once the infection has been cleared. Intense management of the underlying predisposing cause of infection is also a marker for successful therapy. In diabetics with reversible acidosis, recovery rates are higher than in those patients with underlying malignancy and immunosuppression. Immunosuppressive drugs should be reduced in dosage or discontinued if possible during attempts to control the infection.

Hyperbaric oxygen therapy should be considered as adjunctive therapy and does not replace adequate antifungal therapy or surgical debridements. There are no clinical data that might suggest a specific treatment pressure to use in the setting of zygomycosis infection. It would be appropriate to commence hyperbaric oxygen treatments early in the course rather than as salvage therapy, in the 2.4 to 3 ATA (243.18–303.98 kPa) range of pressures, twice a day during the acute phase of the illness to enhance the immune response to the fungal hyphae and protect borderline ischemic areas from progression of ischemia to necrosis. Many of the successful cases have been treated with up to 30 total treatments, although there are no controlled studies that would suggest a specific treatment duration or pressure. Due to the rarity of the infection, it is unlikely that a prospective controlled trial could ever be done at a single institution, and thus adequate data would likely require multicenter studies controlling for intent-to-treat vs. salvage therapy, timing of hyperbaric therapy, depth and duration of treatments, as well as extent of infection at time of diagnosis, number and degree of debridements necessary, and category of predisposing factor, along with other standard parameters.

Evidence-Based Review

From a physiological viewpoint, all necrotizing soft tissue infections should benefit from hyperbaric oxygen treatments, considering all the physiologic steps that enhance host response to infection.

Although some authors and organizational committees claim that hyperbaric oxygen therapy remains controversial for use to treat necrotizing fasciitis due to lack of prospective, randomized, blinded, or double-blinded controlled studies comparing hyperbaric oxygen treatments vs. no hyperbaric treatments, other authors have concluded that the improvements in morbidity and mortality as compared to the historical data would make it unethical to perform such randomized clinical trials on patients, as it would deny a well-substantiated adjunctive treatment for a disease with a high rate of morbidity and mortality with generally few risks of complications from the treatments. There are in fact no prospective, randomized, controlled trials either using just surgery or surgery and antibiotics for necrotizing fasciitis, yet these interventions are widely used without question based on retrospective studies and clinical series as well. Thus, the argument against using hyperbaric oxygen therapy because of a lack of randomized controlled trials cannot be seriously entertained.[114] There are numerous clinical series that do show reduced morbidity and mortality when hyperbaric oxygen has been used for numerous forms of necrotizing fasciitis, including Fournier's gangrene. This would make it a highly recommended adjunct to antibiotics and surgical debridements.

For necrotizing fasciitis related to the zygomycoses, the very high incidence of morbidity, disfigurement, and mortality in a population that is overall usually quite compromised leads to the conclusion that early institution of hyperbaric oxygen therapy is indicated when the diagnosis is made rather than waiting until signs of failure to respond to what is seemingly standard therapy, and then attempting to use hyperbaric oxygen treatments in a salvage mode when the chances of success would seem less likely. Numerous case reports of success, even when hyperbaric oxygen treatments have been used in a salvage mode, support this recommendation. The disease process, which involves angio-invasive infection leading to ischemia, infarction, and extension of infection, appears to be one to which hyperbaric oxygen treatments should be beneficial.

Utilization Review

Twice-a-day hyperbaric oxygen treatments during the acute phase of necrotizing soft tissue infections are advised until extension of necrosis has been halted. This is often seen within seven to 10 treatments. Due to the natural history of often relentless progression and undetected foci of necrosis, these treatments would then be followed by once-daily treatments over an extended period until the infection is well controlled, which may take up to 30 treatments. Utilization review should be requested after 30 treatments.

Cost Impact

Under a diagnosis-related group system, where reimbursement is based on an admitting diagnosis and confounding existing conditions, the cost of the treatments may be borne by the hospital while the patient is an inpatient. Due to the tissue-, limb-, and life-threatening aspects of these infections, the cost impact of hyperbaric treatments can well be justified. Adjunctive use of hyperbaric oxygen therapy may reduce the length of hospital stay and the number of procedures needed to attain infection control. However, limb salvage could generate additional costs and procedures in the rehabilitation phase of recovery. In the Soh et al. Nationwide Inpatient Sample Study discussed above, surviving patients who had been treated with hyperbaric oxygen therapy for necrotizing infections had longer hospital stays (14.1 days, 95% CI 12.9–15.4 days) compared to that of surviving patients who did not receive hyperbaric oxygen (10.7 days, 95% CI 10.6–10.9 days).

Higher hospital cost of hospitalization was reported to go along with the higher survival rates for the HBO_2 treated patients. In this retrospective analysis, it was difficult to attribute the longer hospital stay solely to the hyperbaric oxygen treatments since the patients treated with hyperbaric oxygen therapy were more likely to be at urban non-teaching centers rather than in rural or urban teaching facilities; it is also unclear whether the length of stay and cost data were controlled for performance of amputations vs. reconstructive procedures, as patients undergoing amputation may be discharged earlier than patients who are undergoing limb salvage with flaps after infection has been controlled. More studies that analyze such indirect costs are needed.

References

1. Kao LS, Lew DF, et al. Local variations in the epidemiology, microbiology, and outcome of necrotizing soft tissue infections: a multicenter study. Am J Surg 2011;202:139.
2. Wilkinson D, Doolette D. Hyperbaric Oxygen treatment and survival from necrotizing soft tissue infection. Arch Surg. 2004;139:1339 -1345.
3. Escobar SJ, Slade JB. Adjuvant hyperbaric oxygen therapy for treatments of necrotizing fasciitis reduces mortality and amputation rates. Undersea and Hyperb Med. 2006;32(6):437-443.
4. Anaya DA, Predictors of mortality and limb loss in necrotizing soft tissue infections. Arch Surg. 2005.
5. Shupak A, Shoshani O, Goldberg I, et al. Necrotizing fasciitis: An indication for hyperbaric oxygen therapy? Surgery. 1995;118:873-878.
6. Shaw JJ, Psoinos C, Emhoff TA, et al. Not just full of hot air: Hyperbaric oxygen therapy increases survival in cases of necrotizing soft tissue infections. Surg Infect (Larchmt). 2014;15:328-335.
7. Hakkarainen TW, Kopari NM, Pham TN, Evans HL. Necrotizing soft tissue infections: Review and current concepts in treatment, systems of care, and outcomes. Curr Probl Surg. 2014 August;51(8):344-362.
8. Sudarsky LA, Laschinger JC, et al. Improved results from a standardized approach in treating patients with necrotizing fasciitis. Ann Surg. 1987;206:661-665.
9. Faraklas I, Yang D, et al. A Multicenter Review of Care Patterns and Outcomes in Necrotizing Soft Tissue Infections. Surgical Infections. 2016;Volume 17(6).
10. Mandell G. Bacteriacidal activity of aerobic and anaerobic polymorphonuclear neutrophils. Infect Immun. 1974;9:337-341.
11. Mader JT, Adams KR, Sulton TE. Infectious diseases: pathophysiology and mechanisms of hyperbaric oxygen. J Hyperbaric Med. 1987;2:133-140.
12. Hunt TK, Linsey M, Grislis G, et al. The effect of differing ambient oxygen tension on wound infection. Ann Surg. 1975 Jan;181(1):35-39.
13. Thom SR, Mendiguren I, Hardy K, Bolotin T, Fisher D, Nebolon M, et al. Inhibition of human neutrophil beta2-- integrin-dependent adherence by hyperbaric O_2. Am J Physiol. 1997 Mar;272(3 Pt 1):C770-777.
14. Park MK, Muhvich KH, Myers RA, Marsella L. Hyperoxia prolongs the aminoglycoside-induced postantibiotic effect in Pseudomonas aeruginosa. Antimicrob Agents Chemother. 1991;35(4):691-695.
15. Jones J. Surgical Memoirs of the War of the Rebellion. Investigation Upon the Nature, Causes, and Treatment of Hospital Gangrene as Prevailed in the Confederate Armies 1861-1865. United States Sanitary Commision;New York, NY. p.1871.
16. Meleney FL. Hemolytic streptococcus gangrene. Arch Surg. 1924;9:317-364.
17. Wilson B. Necrotizing fasciitis. Am Surg.1952;18:416-431.
18. Simonsen E, Orman E, et al.Cellulitis incidence in a defined population. Epidemiol Infect. 2006;134(2):293-299.
19. Gozal D, Ziser A, et al. Necrotizing fasciitis. Arch Surg. 1986;121:233.
20. Anaya DA, Patchen Dellinger E. Necrotizing soft-tissue infection: diagnosis and management. Clin Infect Dis. 2007;44:705-710.
21. Miller LG, Perdreau-Remington F, Rieg G, Mehdi S, Perlroth J, Bayer AS, Tang AW, Phung TO, Spellberg B. Necrotizing fasciitis caused by community-associated methicillin-resistant Staphylococcus aureus in Los Angeles. N Engl J Med. 2005;352:1445-1453.
22. Giuliano A, Lewis F, et al. Bacteriology of necrotizing fasciitis. Am J Surg.1977;1134(1):52-57.
23. Miller L, Carrick M, et al. Necrotizing fasciitis caused by community associated methicillin-resistant Staphylococcal aureus in Los Angeles. N Engl J Med. 2005;352(14):1445-1453.
24. Bryant AE, Stevens DL, et al. clostridial myonecrosis: new insights in pathogenesis and management. Curr Infect Dis Rep. 2010;12(5):383-391.
25. Stevens DL, Aldape MJ, et al. Life threatening clostridial infections. Anaerobe. 2011;18(2):254-259.
26. Eke N. Fournier's gangrene: a review of 1726 cases. Br J Surg. 2000;87:718.
27. Toro C, Castillo A, et al. Cervical necrotizing fasciitis: Report of 6 cases and review of literature. European Annals Otorhinolaryngology, Head and Neck Diseases. 2014;131:357-359.
28. Flanagan C, Daramola O, et al. Surgical debridement and adjunctive hyperbaric oxygen in cervical necrotizing fasciitis. Otorhinolaryngology, Head and Neck Diseases. 2009;140 (5):730-4.h
29. Stevens DL, Bryant AE. Necrotizing soft tissue infections. N Engl J Med. 2017;377:2253.
30. Shiroff A, Herlitz G, Gracias V. Necrotizing soft tissue infections. J Intensive Care Med. 2014;29(3):138-144.
31. Darenberg J, Luca-Harari B, et al. Molecular and clinical characteristics of invasive GAS infection in Sweden. Clin Infect Dis. 2007;45:450.

32. Goodell J, Jordan M, et al. Rapidly advancing necrotizing fasciitis caused by Phytobacterium (Vibrio) damsel: a hyperaggressive variant. Crit Care Med. 2004;32(1):278-281.

33. Hau V, Ho CO. Necrotizing fasciitis caused by Vibrio vulnificans in the lower limb following exposure to seafood on the hand. Hong Kong Med J. 2011;17:335.

34. Brogan TV, Nizet V, Waldhausen JHT, Rubens CE, Clarke W. Group A streptococcal necrotizing fasciitis complicating primary varicella: a series of fourteen patients. Pediatr Infect Dis J. 1995;14:588-594.

35. https://www.fda.gov/downloads/drugs/drugsafety/ucm618466.pdf

36. Stevens DL, Bryant AE, et al. Necrotizing soft tissue infections. N Engl J Med. 2017;377:2253.

37. Hamilton SM, Bayer CR, Stevens DL, and Bryant AE. Effects of selective and nonselective nonsteroidal anti-inflammatory drugs on antibiotic efficacy of experimental Group A Streptococcal myonecrosis. Jour Infect Dis. 2014; 209:1429-1435.

38. Bell AL, Adamson H, Kirk F, McCaigue MD, Rotman H. Diclofenac inhibits monocyte superoxide production ex vivo in rheumatoid arthritis. Rheumatol Int. 1991;11:27-30.

39. Stevens DL. Could nonsteroidal anti-inflammatory drugs (NSAIDS) enhance the progression of bacterial infections to toxic shock syndrome? Shock. 2013;21(4):977-980.

40. LaRock CN, Todd J, LaRock DL et al. IL-1ß is an innate immune sensor of microbial proteolysis. Sci. Immunol. 2016;1,eaah3539.

41. Sawin RS, Schaller RT, Tapper D, Morgan A, Cahill J. Early recognition of neonatal abdominal wall necrotizing fasciitis. Am J Surg. 1994;167:481-484.

42. Wang TL, Hung CR. Role of tissue oxygen saturation monitoring in diagnosing necrotizing fasciitis of the lower limbs. Ann Emerg Med. 2004;44:222-228.

43. Lally KP, Atkinson JB, Wooley MM, Mahour GH. Necrotizing fasciitis: a serious sequela of omphalitis in the newborn. Ann Surg. 1984;199:101-103.

44. Sawin RS, Schaller RT, Tapper D, Morgan A, Cahill J. Early recognition of neonatal abdominal wall necrotizing fasciitis. Am J Surg. 1994;167:481-484.

45. Keung E, Liu X, et al. Immunocompromised status in patients with necrotizing soft tissue infections. JAMA Surg. 2013;148(5):419-426.

46. Stamenkovic I, Lew PD. Early recognition of potentially fatal necrotizing fasciitis: the use of frozen-section biopsy. N Engl J Med. 1984;310:1689-1693.

47. Carbonetti F, Cremona A, et al. The role of contrast enhanced computed tomography in the diagnosing of necrotizing fasciitis and comparison with the Laboratory risk indicator for Necrotizing fasciitis (LRINEC). Radiol Med. 2016 Feb;121(2):106-121.

48. Wysoki MG, Santora TA, Shah RM, Friedman AC. Necrotizing fasciitis: CT characteristics. Radiology. 1997;203:859-863.

49. Schmid MR, Kossman T, Duewell S. Differentiation of necrotizing fasciitis and cellulitis using MR imaging. Am J Roentgenol. 1998;170:615-620.

50. Wong C, Khin L, et al. The LRINEC (laboratory risk indicator for necrotizing fasciitis) score: a tool for distinguishing necrotizing fasciitis from other soft tissue infections. Crit Care Med. 2004;32(7):1535-1541.

51. Bechar J, Sepehripour S, et al. Laboratory risk indicator for necrotizing fasciitis (LRINEC) score for the assessment of early necrotizing fasciitis: a systematic review of the literature. Ann R Coll Surg Engl. 2017;99:341-346.

52. Borschitz T, Schlicht S, et al. Improvement of a clinical score for necrotizing fasciitis: 'pain out of proportion' and high CRP levels aid the diagnosis. PLoS One 2015;10(7):e0132775.

53. Hansen M, Rasmussen L, et al. Pentraxin-3 as a marker of disease severity and risk of death in patients with necrotizing soft tissue infections: a nationwide, prospective, observational study. Critical Care. 2016;(20)40.

54. Su YC, Chen HW, et al. Laboratory risk indicator for necrotizing fasciitis score and outcomes. ANZ J Surg. 2008;78:968-972.

55. Hansen MB, Rasmussen LS, et al. Association between cytokine response, the LRINEC score and outcome in patients with necrotizing soft tissue infection: a multicenter, prospective study. Sci Rep. 2017; 7:42179.

56. Stevens DL, Bisno AL, et al. Practice guidelines for the diagnosis and management of skin and soft tissue infections:2014 update by the infectious diseases society of America. Clin Infect Dis. 2014;59:147.

57. Faraklas I, Yang D, et al. A Multicenter Review of Care Patterns and Outcomes in Necrotizing Soft Tissue Infections. Surgical Infections. 2016; Volume 17(6).

58. Sablier F, Slaouti T, et al. Nosocomial transmission of necrotizing fasciitis. Lancet. 2010;375:1052.

59. Bilbault P, Castelain V, et al. Life threatening cervical necrotizing fasciitis after a common dental extraction. Am J Emerg Med. 2008;26:5-7

60. Soh CR, Pietroban R, Freiberger JJ, et al. Hyperbaric Oxygen therapy in necrotizing soft tissue infections:a study of patients in the US Nationwide Inpatient sample. Intensive Care Med. 2012;38:1143.

61. Wilkinson D, Doolette D. Hyperbaric oxygen treatment and survival from necrotizing soft tissue infection. Arch Surg. 2004;139:1339-1345.

62. Escobar SJ, Slade JB, Hunt TK, Cianci P. Adjuvant hyperbaric oxygen therapy (HBO$_2$) for treatment of necrotizing fasciitis reduces mortality and amputation rate. Undersea Hyperb Med. 2006;32(6):437-443.

63. Brown DR, Davis NL, Lepawsky M, Cunningham J, Kortbeek J. A multicenter review of the treatment of major truncal necrotizing infections with and without hyperbaric oxygen therapy. Am J Surg. 1994;167:485-489.

64. Monestersky JH, Myers RAM. Letter to the editor: hyperbaric oxygen treatment of necrotizing fasciitis. Am J Surg. 1995;169:187-188.

65. Anaya DA, McMahon K, Nathens AB, Sullivan SR, Foy H, Bulger E. Predictors of mortality and limb loss in necrotizing soft tissue infections. Arch Surg. 2005;140:151-157.

66. McHenry CR, Piotrowski JJ, Petrinic D, Malangoni MA. Determinants of mortality for necrotizing soft-tissue infections. Ann Surg. 1995;221:558-563.

67. Hsieh WH, Yang, PH, Chao HC, Lai JY. Neonatal necrotizing fasciitis: report of 3 cases and review of the literature. Pediatrics. 1999;103(4):e53. Available at: http://pediatrics.aappublications.org/cgi/content/full/103/4/e53

68. Lally KP, Atkinson JB, Wooley MM, Mahour GH. Necrotizing fasciitis: a serious sequela of omphalitis in the newborn. Ann Surg. 1984;199:101-103.

69. Sawin RS, Schaller RT, Tapper D, Morgan A, Cahill J. Early recognition of neonatal abdominal wall necrotizing fasciitis. Am J Surg. 1994;167:481-484.

70. Gozal D, Ziser A, Shupak A, Ariel A, Melamed Y. Necrotizing fasciitis. Arch Surg. 1986;121:233-235.

71. Riseman JA, Zamboni WA, Curtis A, Graham DR, Konrad HR, and Ross DS. Hyperbaric oxygen therapy for necrotizing fasciitis reduces mortality and the need for debridements. Surgery. 1990;108:847-850.

72. Laor E, Palmer LS, Tolia BM. Outcome prediction in patients with Fournier's gangrene. J Urol. 1995;154:89-92.

73. Dahm P, Roland FH, Vaslef SN, Moon RE, Price DT, Georgiade GS, Viewig J. Outcome analysis in patients with primary necrotizing fasciitis of the male genitalia. Urol. 2000;56:31-36.

74. Mallikarjuna M, Vijayakumar A, et al. Fournier's gangrene: current practices. ISRN Surgery 2012(ID 942437):1-8.

75. Hollabaugh RS, Dmochowski RR, Hickerson WL. Fournier's gangrene: therapeutic impact of hyperbaric oxygen. Plast Reconstr Surg. 1998;101:94-100.

76. Pizzorno R, Bonini F, Donelli A, Stubinski R, Medica M, Carmignani G. Hyperbaric oxygen therapy in the treatment of Fournier's disease in 11 male patients. J Urol. 1997;158:837-840.

77. Korhonen K, Him M, Niinikoski J. Hyperbaric oxygen in the treatment of Fournier's gangrene. Eur J Surg. 1998;164:251-255.

78. Willy C, Rieger H, et al. Hyperbaric oxygen therapy for NSTI. Chirug 2012;83:960.

79. Eggerstedt M, Gamelli RL, et al. The care of necrotizing soft tissue infections. Patterns of definitive intervention at a large referral center. J Burn Care Res. 2015;36:105-110.

80. Holena DN, Mills AM, et al. Transfer status: A risk factor for mortality in patients with necrotizing fasciitis. Surgery. 2011;150:363-370.

81. Davaney B, Frawley G, et al. Necrotising soft tissue infections: the effect of hyperbaric oxygen on mortality. Anaesth Intensive Care. 2015;43:6.

82. Gore M. Odontogenic necrotizing fasciitis: a systematic review of the literature. BMC Ear, Nose and Throat Disorders. 2018;18:14.

83. Shaw JJ, Psoinos C, Emhoff TA, et al. Not just full of hot air: Hyperbaric oxygen therapy increases survival in cases of necrotizing soft tissue infections. Surg Infect (Larchmt). 2014;15:328-335.

84. Torp KD, Carraway MS. Safe administration of hyperbaric oxygen after bleomycin:a case series of 15 patients. Undersea Hyperb Med. 2012;39:873.

85. Karagoz B, Suleymanoglu S, et al. Hyperbaric Oxygen therapy does not potentiate doxorubicin-induced cardiotoxicity in rats. Basic Clin Pharmacol Toxicol. 2008;102:287.

86. Stone HH, Martin JD. Synergistic necrotizing cellulitis. Ann Surg. 1972;175:702-711.

87. Bessman AN, Wagner W. Nonclostridial gas gangrene. JAMA. 1975;233:958.

88. Cullen TS. A progressively enlarging ulcer of abdominal wall involving the skin and fat, following drainage of an abdominal abscess, apparently of appendiceal origin. Surg Gynecol Obstetr. 1924;38:579-582.

89. Ledingham IM, Tehrani MA. Diagnosis, clinical course and treatment of acute dermal gangrene. Br J Surg. 1975;62:364-372.

90. Chayakulkeeree M, Ghannoum MA, Perfect JR. Zygomycosis: the re-emerging fungal infection. Eur J Clin Microbiol Infect Dis. 2006;25:215-229.

91. McNulty JS. Rhinocerebral mucormycosis: predisposing factors. Laryngoscope. 1982;92:1140-1143.
92. Windus DW, Stokes TJ, Julian BA, Fenves AZ. Fatal Rhizopus infections in hemodialysis patients receiving deferoxamine. Ann Int Med. 1987;107:678-680.
93. Boelaert JR, Van Roost GF, Vergauwe PL, Verbanck C, De Vroey C, Segaert MF. The role of deferoxamine in dialysis-associate mucormycosis: report of three cases and review of the literature. Clin Nephrol. 1988; 29:261-266.
94. Cocanour CS, Miller-Crouchett P, Reed RL, Johnson PC, Fischer RP. Mucormycosis in trauma patients. J Trauma. 1992;32:12-15.
95. Tedder MJ, Spratt JA, Anstadt MP, Hegde SS, Tedder SD, Lowe JE. Pulmonary mucormycosis: results of medical and surgical therapy. Ann Thorac Surg. 1994;57:1044-1050.
96. Ribes JA, Vanover-Sams CL, Baker DJ. Zygomycetes in human disease. Clin Microbiol Revs. 2000;13:236-301.
97. Murray HW. Pulmonary mucormycosis with massive fatal hemoptysis. Chest. 1975;68:65-68.
98. Michalak DM, Cooney DR, Rhodes KH, Telander RL, Kleinberg F. Gastrointestinal mucormycosis in infants and children: a cause of gangrenous intestinal cellulitis and perforation. J Pediatr Surg. 1980;15:320-324.
99. Chamilos G, Marom EM, Lewis RE, Lionakis MS, Kontoyiannis DP. Predictors of pulmonary zygomycosis versus invasive pulmonary aspergillosis in patients with cancer. Clin Infect Dis. 2005;41:60-66.
100. Diamond RD, Haudenschild CC, Erickson III NF. Monocyte-mediated damage to Rhizopus oryzae hyphae in vitro. Infect Immun. 1982;38:292-297.
101. Waldorf AR. Pulmonary defense mechanisms against opportunistic fungal pathogens. Immunol Ser. 1989;47: 243-271.
102. Waldorf AR, Ruderman N, Diamond RD. Specific susceptibility to mucormycosis in murine diabetes and bron-choalveolar macrophage defense against Rhizopus. J Clin Invest. 1984;74:150-160.
103. Ibrahim AS, Spellberg B, Avanessian V, Fu Y, Edwards, Jr. E. Rhizopus oryzae adheres to, is phagocytosed by, and damages endothelial cells in vitro. Infect Immun. 2005;73:778-783.
104. Imperatore F, Cuzzocrea S, De Lucia D, Sessa M, Rinaldi B, Capuano A, Liguori G, Filippelli A, Rossi F. Hyperbaric oxygen therapy prevents coagulation disorders in an experimental model of multiple organ failure syndrome. Intensive Care Med. 2006;32:1881-1888.
105. Buras JA, Holt D, Orlow D, Belikoff B, Pavlides S, Reenstra WR. Hyperbaric oxygen protects from sepsis mortality via an interleukin-10-dependent mechanism. Crit Care Med. 2006;34(10):2624-2629.
106. Roden MM, Zaoutis TE, Buchanan WL, Knudsen TA, Sarkisova TA, Schaufele RL, Sein M, Sein T, Chiou CC, Chu JH, Kontoyiannis DP. Epidemiology and outcome of zygomycosis: a review of 929 reported cases. Clin Inf Dis. 2005;41:634-653.
107. Almyroudis NG, Konoyiannis DP, Sepkowitz KA, De Pauw BE, Walsh TJ, Segal BH. Issues related to the design and interpretation of clinical trials of salvage therapy for invasive mold infection. Clin Inf Dis. 2006;43:1449-1455.
108. Bentur Y, Shupak A, Ramon Y, Abramovich A, Wolfin G, Stein H, Krivoi N. Hyperbaric oxygen therapy for cutaneous/soft-tissue zygomycosis complicating diabetes mellitus. Plastic and Reconstr Surg. 1998;102:822-824.
109. Temple ME, Brady MT, Koranyi KI, Nahata MC. Periorbital cellulitis secondary to Conidiobolus incongruous. Pharmacotherapy. 2001;21(3):351-354.
110. Powers JH. Salvage therapy trials in fungal disease: challenges and opportunities. Clin Inf Dis. 2006;43:1456-1459.
111. Trifilio SM, Bennett CL, Yarnold PR, McKoy JM, Parada J, Mehta J, Chamilos G, Palella F, Kennedy L, Mullane K, Tallman MS, Evens A. Scheetz MH, Blum W, Kontoyiannis DP. Breakthrough zygomycosis after voriconazole administration among patients with hematologic malignancies who receive hematopoietic stem-cell transplants or intensive chemotherapy. Bone Marrow Transplant. 2007;39:425-429.
112. Greenberg RN, Mullane K, van Burick J-AH, Raad I, Abzug MJ, Herbrecht R, Langston A, Marr KA, Schiller G, Schuster M, Wingard JR, Gonzalez CE, Revankar SG, Corcoran G, Kryscio RJ, Hare R. Posaconazole as salvage therapy for zygomycosis. Antimicrob Agents and Chemother. 2006;50(1):126-133.
113. Langford JD, McCartney DL, Wang RC. Frozen section-guided surgical debridement for management of rhino--orbital mucormycosis. Am J Ophthalmol. 1997;124:265-267.
114. Jallali N, Withey S, Butler PE. Hyperbaric oxygen as adjuvant therapy in the management of necrotizing fasciitis. Am J Surg. 2005;189(4):462-466.

CHAPTER 12

Refractory Osteomyelitis

Brett B. Hart MD

Abstract

Refractory osteomyelitis is defined as a chronic osteomyelitis that persists or recurs after appropriate interventions have been performed or where acute osteomyelitis has not responded to accepted management techniques.[1] To date, no randomized clinical trials examining the effects of hyperbaric oxygen (HBO$_2$) therapy on refractory osteomyelitis exist, and the number of new osteomyelitis clinical trials conducted over the past decade has been limited. However, based on a comprehensive review of the scientific literature, the addition of HBO$_2$ therapy to routine surgical and antibiotic treatment of *previously refractory* osteomyelitis appears to be both safe and ultimately improves infection resolution rates. In most cases, the best clinical results are obtained when HBO$_2$ treatment is administered in conjunction with culture-directed antibiotics and initiated soon after clinically indicated surgical debridement. Where extensive surgical debridement or removal of fixation hardware is relatively contraindicated (e.g. cranial, spinal, sternal, or pediatric osteomyelitis), a trial of culture-directed antibiotics and HBO$_2$ therapy prior to undertaking more than limited surgical interventions provides a reasonable prospect for osteomyelitis cure. HBO$_2$ therapy is ordinarily delivered on a once daily basis, five-seven days per week, for 90–120 minutes using 2.0–3.0 atmospheres absolute (ATA) pressure. Where prompt clinical improvement is seen, the existing regimen of antibiotics and HBO$_2$ therapy should be continued for approximately four to six weeks. Typically, 20–40 HBO$_2$ sessions are required to achieve sustained therapeutic benefit. In contrast, if prompt clinical response is not noted or osteomyelitis recurs after this initial treatment period, then continuation of the current antibiotic and HBO$_2$ treatment regimen is unlikely to be effective. Instead, clinical management strategies should be reassessed and additional surgical debridement and/or modification of antibiotic therapy considered. Subsequent reinstitution of HBO$_2$ therapy will again help maximize the overall chances for treatment success in these persistently refractory patients.

Mechanistic Rationale for Use

Initial evidence for a beneficial therapeutic effect of HBO$_2$ in managing osteomyelitis stemmed from reports collected during the 1960s[2-5]. In vitro and in vivo studies have subsequently uncovered several contributory mechanisms of action. Common to each of these mechanisms is the restoration of normal to elevated oxygen tensions in the infected bone. Mader and Niinikoski demonstrated that the decreased oxygen tensions typically associated with bony infections can be returned to normal or above normal levels while breathing 100% oxygen in a hyperbaric chamber.[6-7] Achieving such elevations has important consequences for the hypoxic milieu of osteomyelitic tissues.[8]

Neutrophils require tissue oxygen tensions of 30–40 mmHg to destroy bacteria by oxidative killing mechanisms.[9-10] Leukocyte-mediated killing of aerobic gram-negative and gram-positive organisms, including *Staphylococcus aureus*, is restored when the low oxygen tensions intrinsic to osteomyelitic bone are increased to physiologic or supraphysiologic levels. Mader et al. confirmed this finding in an animal model of *S. aureus* osteomyelitis, demonstrating that phagocytic killing markedly decreased at a pO$_2$ of 23 mmHg, improved at 45 and 109 mmHg, but was most effective at 150 mmHg.[7] In this study, animals exposed to air achieved a mean pO$_2$ of 21 mmHg and 45 mmHg in infected and uninfected bone, respectively. When the same animals were exposed to 100%

263

oxygen at 2 ATA, mean pO_2 levels of 104 and 321 mmHg in infected and noninfected bone were respectively achieved.

Subsequent animal studies by Esterhai reconfirmed these infection and pO_2-dependent results, measuring mean oxygen tensions in infected bone of 16±3.8 mmHg in sea level air, 17.5±2.7 mmHg in sea level oxygen, 198.4±19.7 mmHg in 2 ATA oxygen and 234.1±116.3 mmHg at 3 ATA oxygen, respectively.[11] Corresponding values for noninfected bone were 31±4.6 mmHg in sea level air, 98.8±22.0 mmHg in sealevel oxygen, 191.5±47.9 mmHg in 2 ATA of oxygen and 309.3±29.6 mmHg at 3 ATA oxygen.

In addition to enhanced leukocyte activity, HBO_2 helps augment the transport of certain antibiotics across bacterial cell walls. Aminoglycoside transport across the bacterial cell wall is both oxygen-dependent and impaired in a hypoxic environment. More specifically, active transport of antibiotics (e.g. gentamicin, tobramycin, amikacin) across bacterial cell walls does not occur if tissue oxygen tensions are below 20 to 30 mmHg.[12] Therefore, HBO_2 exposures can enhance this transport and augment the efficacy of antibiotic action.[12-14] This synergistic effect has also been shown for the cephalosporin class of antibiotics, where the combination of cefazolin and HBO_2 therapy produced a 100-fold greater reduction in bacterial counts than either antibiotics or HBO_2 therapy alone.[15-16]

Comparable effects are also seen with HBO_2 in mitigating localized soft tissue infections. Sugihara et al. demonstrated a 46% reduction in infection resolution time from a mean of 13 to only six days when HBO_2 therapy was added to antibiotics in the management of soft tissue infections.[17] As infected soft tissues often act as conduits for initiating and sustaining cortical bone infections, HBO_2 therapy's parallel benefit in ameliorating soft tissue infections may be critical to its overall efficacy in refractory osteomyelitis.[18]

Separately, HBO_2 therapy has been noted to exert a direct suppressive effect on anaerobic infections.[3,8] This effect can be clinically important, as anaerobes make up approximately 15% of the isolates in chronic, non-hematogenous osteomyelitis.

There is also evidence that HBO_2 enhances osteogenesis.[19-23] Animal data suggest that bone mineralization and healing can be accelerated by intermittent exposure to HBO_2.[24-25] Remodeling of bone by osteoclasts is an oxygen-dependent function. Consequently, inadequate oxygen tensions inhibit microscopic debridement of dead, infected bone by osteoclasts. As previously noted, HBO_2 can restore physiologic or induce supraphysiologic oxygen tension in hypoxic bone environments, enhancing osteoclast function in infected bone. This stimulatory effect of HBO_2 on osteoclasts has been confirmed in animal models.[26-27] Furthermore, as demarcation between healthy and necrotic bone is not always clear at the time of surgery, osteoclast enhancement may improve the overall quality of bony debridement and reduce the chances that local infections will recur.[28]

Finally, the pathophysiology of chronic osteomyelitis is characterized by both acute and chronic sources of ischemia. HBO_2 therapy has been shown to be effective in acutely reducing tissue edema, lowering intra-compartmental pressures, and ameliorating the detrimental effects of inflammatory reactions.[29-32] Over the longer term, HBO_2 can be used to promote new collagen formation and capillary angiogenesis in both hypoxic bone and surrounding tissues.[33-36] This neovascularization works to counter the less easily reversible consequences of osteomyelitis, such as surgical trauma, tissue scarring, and nutrient blood vessel occlusion. By creating a sustained increase in arterial perfusion of previously hypoxic bone and soft tissues, HBO_2 can reduce future susceptibility of these tissues to recurrent infection and necrosis.

Patient Selection Criteria

Failure of Standard Therapy

Depending upon the timing of osteomyelitis presentation, source of infection, identified organism, degree of bony involvement, and overall status of the host, osteomyelitis can be considered either a primarily medical or surgical disease.[37-39] Initial management efforts typically center on starting culture-directed antimicrobial therapy. Where present, infected sinus tracts, sclerotic bone, and sequestra should be debrided.[16,40] Various authors also suggest removal of internal fixation hardware and other foreign materials that do not directly contribute to the osseous stability of the site.[41-47] Others, particularly in complex spinal cases, have suggested that hardware removal is not necessarily required.[46,48-52] Advances in surgical technique, such as microvascular free muscle grafts and Ilizarov procedures, have decreased the incidence of postoperative infection in long bone fractures. However, these procedures often entail long durations of surgical therapy and significant expense.[28,53-55]

Overall, resolution rates for primary osteomyelitis treated with surgery and antibiotics range between 35–100%.[38,56-72] Despite the wide range of reported results, it can be estimated that a 70-80% cure rate can be achieved using routine surgical and antibiotic management techniques.[40,59,73-76] This finding is in agreement with corresponding estimates for long-term osteomyelitis recurrence, which range between 20 and 30%.[77-78]

It is when appropriate surgical and antibiotic interventions fail and osteomyelitis progresses, recurs, or presents a high probability for morbidity or mortality that HBO$_2$ therapy should be considered for inclusion in the patient's treatment regimen.

Defining Refractory Osteomyelitis

Clinical opinion differs as to what constitutes "appropriate interventions" and "accepted management techniques." Therefore, defining specific time frames for the terms "chronic" or "refractory" osteomyelitis is not straightforward. Classically, chronic osteomyelitis differs from acute or subacute osteomyelitis by exceeding an arbitrary time limit of four to six weeks clinical duration.[39,79-80] Accordingly, osteomyelitis is considered refractory when it fails to respond to definitive surgical debridement and a period of four to six weeks of appropriate antibiotic therapy.[81] From the mechanistic standpoint, this treatment period was selected to ensure antibiotic coverage is continued throughout the time necessary for surgically debrided bone to undergo revascularization.[82] While some authors have advocated longer courses of antibiotic treatment, others argue that failure to achieve infection resolution after six weeks of culture-directed therapy is primarily due to inadequate surgical debridement, rather than an incomplete course of antibiotics.[40,75,81-82]

Further, the traditional mandate that parenteral antibiotics need be administered throughout this four- to six-week period has been questioned. A number of authors report equivalent success with conversion from intravenous to oral antibiotic agents after one to two weeks.[56,83-87] Comparable results have also been reported in children, although these studies focused principally on acute, rather than chronic, osteomyelitis treatment.[88-90] Regardless, it appears that as long as adequate antibiotic serum and bone concentrations are maintained throughout this four- to six-week coverage period, antibiotic specificity and compliance with the prescribed treatment regimen are more important than the route of administration.[42,81]

Additional factors that need be considered when deeming a case of osteomyelitis refractory include the site of involvement and medical status of the host.[40] Indeed, osteomyelitis has been considered refractory *before* completion of the traditional antibiotic period when the infection is not responding promptly or the sternum, vertebrae, base of the skull or other sites critical to function and survival are involved.[71,91-93] This caveat is particularly germane when the overall health of the patient is compromised by coexisting disease.[18,37]

Patient Classification

The Cierny-Mader classification of osteomyelitis can be used as a guide to determine which patients will most likely benefit from adjunctive HBO₂ therapy.[16] Although alternative classification strategies have been proposed, Cierny-Mader staging functionally incorporates the related elements of infectious etiology, anatomic location, and host physiology into a single system that is valuable in guiding clinical treatment.[82, 94-100]

Under the Cierny-Mader staging paradigm, osteomyelitis is anatomically segregated into four distinct groups based on the following: whether the infection involves the bone's intramedullary surfaces: superficial cortical aspects and adjacent soft tissues; full-thickness, but localized, segments of the cortex; or diffuse, through-and-through

Figure 1. Cierny-Mader's Anatomic Staging.

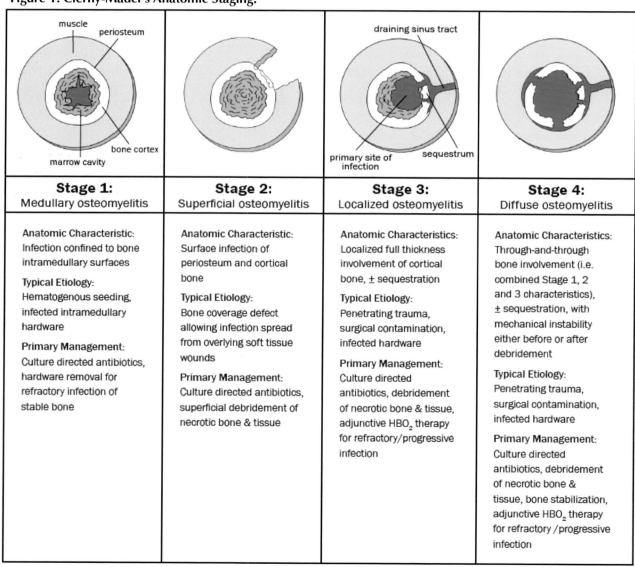

Stage 1: Medullary osteomyelitis	Stage 2: Superficial osteomyelitis	Stage 3: Localized osteomyelitis	Stage 4: Diffuse osteomyelitis
Anatomic Characteristic: Infection confined to bone intramedullary surfaces	Anatomic Characteristic: Surface infection of periosteum and cortical bone	Anatomic Characteristics: Localized full thickness involvement of cortical bone, ± sequestration	Anatomic Characteristics: Through-and-through bone involvement (i.e. combined Stage 1, 2 and 3 characteristics), ± sequestration, with mechanical instability either before or after debridement
Typical Etiology: Hematogenous seeding, infected intramedullary hardware	Typical Etiology: Bone coverage defect allowing infection spread from overlying soft tissue wounds	Typical Etiology: Penetrating trauma, surgical contamination, infected hardware	Typical Etiology: Penetrating trauma, surgical contamination, infected hardware
Primary Management: Culture directed antibiotics, hardware removal for refractory infection of stable bone	Primary Management: Culture directed antibiotics, superficial debridement of necrotic bone & tissue	Primary Management: Culture directed antibiotics, debridement of necrotic bone & tissue, adjunctive HBO₂ therapy for refractory/progressive infection	Primary Management: Culture directed antibiotics, debridement of necrotic bone & tissue, bone stabilization, adjunctive HBO₂ therapy for refractory /progressive infection

portions of the bone.[101-102] These anatomic distinctions are respectively termed medullary, superficial, localized, and diffuse osteomyelitis and are correspondingly designated as Stages 1, 2, 3, and 4. Cierny-Mader's anatomic staging is summarized in Figure 1. In Table 1, patients are further classified by their host status as an A host (normal), B host (compromised) or C host (those for whom the treatment of the disease is worse than the disease). B hosts are subdivided according to whether they are compromised systemically (B_S), locally at the site of osteomyelitis (B_L) or both (B_{LS}). Examples of systemic and local factors that can compromise the host are listed in Table 2.

Using the Cierny-Mader classification, Stage 1 disease is managed primarily with antibiotics. Similarly, Stage 2 disease generally responds well to appropriate antibiotics and superficial debridement of the affected cortical bone and soft tissues. It is those patients with Stage 3 or 4 osteomyelitis, particularly when complicated by adverse local or systemic risk factors, who are most likely to benefit from HBO_2 therapy as an adjunct to continued antibiotics and repeat surgical debridement.[16] Ultimately, Cierny-Mader staging serves as a predictor of treatment success and, regardless of classification, adjunctive HBO_2 therapy should be considered for inclusion in the patient's overall treatment regimen whenever the associated osteomyelitis proves either refractory or progressive despite the application of standard of care interventions.

Special Indications

As previously alluded, due to their central neuraxial location and propensity for generating life-threatening infections, certain cases of refractory osteomyelitis deserve special consideration. Specific areas of concern include the sternum, vertebrae, cranium, and other central bony structures.

Table 1. Host Physiologic Class

A Host	B Host	C Host
Normal Physiology	Systemic Compromise (B_S)	Osteomyelitis treatment or physiologic outcome is worse for host than ongoing disease
	Local Compromise (B_L)	
	Concurrent Local and Systemic Compromise (B_{LS})	

Table 2. Class B Host Compromising Factors

Systemic Factors (B_S)	Local Factors (B_L)
Malnutrition	Chronic lymphedema
Renal failure	Venous stasis
Diabetes mellitus	Major vessel compromise
Chronic hypoxia	Arteritis
Malignancy	Extensive scarring
Immune deficiency	Radiation fibrosis
Immunosuppression	Small vessel disease
Extremes of age	Complete loss of local sensation
Tobacco abuse	

Sternal osteomyelitis after median sternotomy is an uncommon (0.4%-8.4%) but often fatal condition. Despite extensive surgical debridement and complex grafting procedures, recurrence ranges between 3–8%. [103-104] More aggressive methods, though capable of eradicating sternal infection, are associated with high rates of mortality (20–35%).[105-106] Complications associated with vertebral osteomyelitis are equally concerning. Fully 25% of individuals treated nonsurgically for vertebral infections experience medical failure.[107] For the majority of these cases, extensive surgical debridement and removal of retained fixation hardware have been described as necessary to eradicate the disease.[92] Postoperative morbidity and mortality from vertebral osteomyelitis has been reported to be 29% and 12%, respectively.[52] Cranial osteomyelitis, comprising about 1.5% of all osteomyelitis cases, occurs in approximately 2-9% of patients following craniotomy.[92,108-111] While the corresponding direct surgical morbidity and mortality approximate 13% and 7%, respectively,[112] secondary mortality from complications associated with cranial bone infections has been reported to be as high as 20–40%.[108]

Malignant external otitis represents a special subcategory of otitis-associated skull base infections that are often lethal.[113] As with other central bone infections, the standard methods of treatment have involved the use of antibiotics, local treatments, and, where necessary, surgical excision of necrotic tissue.[114] Despite advances in antibiotic therapy, these approaches do not always provide a complete cure and overall mortality remains in the 10–20% range.[115]

What is clear in these cases of central-structure osteomyelitis is that aggressive clinical management is vital to limiting associated morbidity and mortality.[116] Consequently, each of these special indications have earned independent consideration in the subsection of this chapter entitled Human Study Data.

Clinical Management

As noted in the previous section on Patient Selection Criteria, the initial treatment of osteomyelitis depends on the classification of the patient's clinical disease. Generally, patients with Cierny-Mader Stage 1 and 2 disease may be primarily managed with antibiotics and limited surgical debridement. In contrast, patients with refractory, Stage 3B and 4B osteomyelitis should be considered candidates for adjunctive HBO_2 therapy. In situations where alternative clinical classification systems more effectively apply (e.g. Wagner classification of diabetic foot ulcers or Tisch classification of malignant external otitis), these systems may similarly be used to guide decisions to include HBO_2 therapy. Regardless, the principal determinant for adding HBO_2 treatment to the overall management of the patient's osteomyelitis remains their clinical response to standard of care interventions.

If not already initiated, culture-directed antibiotic therapy should be restarted. For most cases of extremity or miscellaneous site osteomyelitis, initiation of HBO_2 therapy should coincide as closely as possible with plans for pre-HBO_2 surgical debridement. In certain clinical settings, such as osteomyelitis affecting children or bony structures adjacent to the central nervous system or other vital organs, a trial of combined HBO_2 and antibiotic therapy should be considered prior to patients undergoing extensive surgical debridement or procedures associated with a high risk for morbidity or mortality. A summary of AHA Class recommendations for HBO_2 treatment of osteomyelitis relative to specific anatomic site and clinical setting is provided in Table 3.

In determining an ideal hyperbaric treatment pressure, the primary goal is to restore oxygen tensions to normal or above-normal levels in the infected bone. Based on Mader's previously reviewed work, a target oxygen tension of ≥150 mmHg is recommended.[7] Animal models suggest that a minimum of 2 ATA is necessary to achieve this goal.[7,11] Given that mean bone oxygen tensions in Mader's model reached only 104 mmHg while exposed to oxygen at 2.0 ATA, treatment pressures greater than 2.0 ATA may be required to achieve the desired clinical effects. When considering the practical range of osteomyelitis treatment pressures, all clinical studies included

Table 3. Summary of AHA Class Recommendations for HBO$_2$ Treatment of Osteomyelitis

	Patient descriptors	Treatment method combination	AHA class recommendation
Long bone / non-specified	Adult	HBO$_2$, antibiotics and debridement	Class IIa
	Adult	HBO$_2$ and antibiotics	Class IIb
	Adult	HBO$_2$ alone	Class III
	Before debilitating surgery / amputation	HBO$_2$, antibiotics and limited debridement	Class IIa
Mandibular	Adult	HBO$_2$, antibiotics and debridement	Class IIa
	Adult	HBO$_2$ and antibiotics	Class IIb
	Adult	HBO$_2$ alone	Class III
	Child	HBO$_2$, antibiotics and limited debridement	Class IIa
	Child	HBO$_2$ and antibiotics	Class IIa
Spinal	Before debridement surgery / hardware removal	HBO$_2$ and antibiotics	Class IIa
	All patients	HBO$_2$, antibiotics and limited debridement	Class IIa
Cranial	Before debridement surgery / hardware removal	HBO$_2$ and antibiotics	Class IIa
	All patients	HBO$_2$, antibiotics and limited debridement	Class IIa
Malignant otitis external	Tisch Stage III or IV	HBO$_2$, antibiotics and debridement	Class IIa
	Tisch Stage I or II	HBO$_2$, antibiotics and debridement	Class IIb
Sternal	All patients	HBO$_2$, antibiotics and limited debridement	Class IIa
Diabetic ulcers	Wagner Grade 3 or 4	HBO$_2$, antibiotics and limited debridement	Class I

in this review reported HBO$_2$ treatment at pressures between 2.0–3.0 ATA. However, the majority of successful treatment responses were associated with studies employing chamber pressures between 2.4–2.5 ATA. Thus, in the absence of noninvasive clinical methods that effectively guide bone pO$_2$ titration, initial HBO$_2$ treatment of refractory osteomyelitis at 2.4–2.5 ATA may provide physicians with the best physiological balance between clinical efficacy and oxygen toxicity risk.

Variability in HBO$_2$ treatment session duration and frequency also exists. Each HBO$_2$ treatment is generally delivered over a period of 90–120 minutes. Most clinicians provide HBO$_2$ therapy on a once-daily basis, five to seven times per week. However, some advocate twice-daily treatment during the first two to three postoperative days, the goal being to aggressively prevent bacterial recolonization and maximize other associated benefits of postoperative HBO$_2$ therapy (i.e., mitigation of ischemia, edema, inflammation, and reperfusion injury). This more aggressive initial treatment has also been suggested in cases of osteomyelitis involving the central nervous system and other structures, where significant morbidity or mortality would be incurred if the infection were to progress.

Similarly, the total number of required treatments varies with the severity and location of the patient's infection, the presence or absence of coexisting diseases and the patient's individual responsiveness to treatment. In the studies available for review, treatments ranged from 14 to over 100 total sessions, with the majority of studies reporting between 20 and 50 total sessions. As would be expected from the preceding discussions, variability in clinical presentations and concurrent management strategies render specific treatment number recommendations impractical. Instead, it is recommended that clinicians carefully consider each patient's disease severity, clinical responsiveness, and risk for osteomyelitis recurrence in guiding such determinations.

Where initial treatment with indicated surgical debridement, appropriate antibiotics, and concurrent HBO$_2$ is met with prompt clinical improvement, the regimen of antibiotic and HBO$_2$ therapy should be continued until the surgically debrided bone becomes adequately revascularized. [81-82] As noted previously, this regenerative period usually corresponds to approximately four to six weeks. Depending upon the prescribed frequency of HBO$_2$ treatment, a total of 20–40 postoperative HBO$_2$ sessions will typically be delivered during this interval. After this point, as long as no occult nidus for reinfection exists (i.e., retained sequestra or unsterile fixation hardware), the bony milieu should be sufficiently recovered to prevent infection recurrence. In cases where removal of fixation hardware or extensive surgical debridement may be relatively contraindicated (e.g., cranial, spinal, sternal or pediatric osteomyelitis), a trial of culture-directed antibiotics, HBO$_2$ therapy, and limited surgical debridement, prior to implementing more radical surgical interventions, provides a reasonable prospect for osteomyelitis cure. Again, a course of four to six weeks of combined therapy should be sufficient to achieve the desired clinical results. Although co-existing local and systemic processes, such as Cierny-Mader B factors, may slow the expected rate of infection resolution, extension of HBO$_2$ and antibiotic treatment beyond one to two more weeks is unlikely to provide definitive benefit. Indeed, if osteomyelitis fails to resolve or recurs after a total of six to eight weeks of continuous culture-directed antibiotics and HBO$_2$ treatment (i.e., 30–40 sessions), then additional surgical debridement will likely be required to eradicate residual infection.

Figure 2 illustrates the general flow and decision tree for adjunctive HBO$_2$ treatment of refractory osteomyelitis.

Figure 2. Flowchart for HBO₂ Management of Refractory Osteomyelitis

Details of management are described in the text.

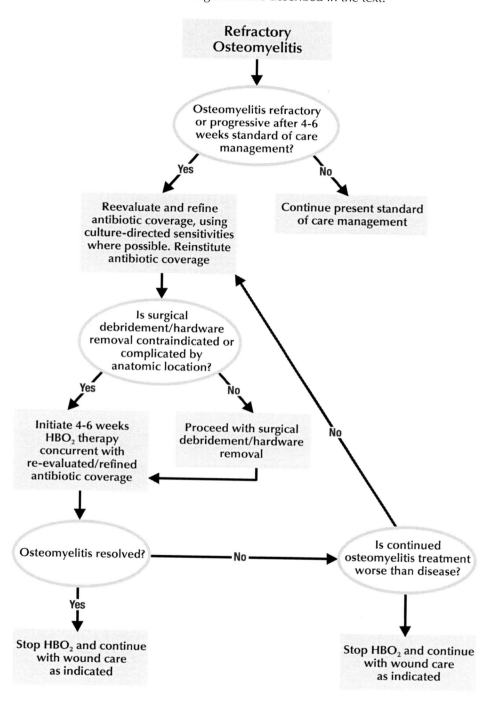

Evidence-Based Review

Review Methodology

This evidence-based review has been updated to include new studies not previously incorporated into the *UHMS Hyperbaric Oxygen Therapy Indications 13th edition*.[166] Congruous with that review's methodology, all studies identified through online searches using the terms "hyperbaric oxygen" and "osteomyelitis" were abstracted. This search methodology subsequently returned an updated total of 293 articles, spanning the period from 1965 through the present. Of the accumulated English language studies, 106 studies contained original data on HBO_2 treatment of osteomyelitis in human (96) or animal (10) subjects; the balance consisted of literature reviews, foreign language articles, previously reported data or papers not directly addressing the effects of systemic HBO_2 therapy on the disease. Similarly, studies that co-mingled osteomyelitis and nonosteomyelitis patient treatment data or lacked distinction between HBO_2- and non-HBO_2-treated patients were also excluded. For the purposes of this review, studies having fewer than three patients were considered case reports and excluded from further analysis. This left a total of 44 studies (9 animal and 35 human) that could be evaluated in accordance with American Heart Association guidelines for this evidence-based review.

Animal Studies

Quality

Nine prospective animal studies examining the effects of HBO_2 on experimentally induced bone infection were reviewed. The overall quality of the studies was considered good, with three studies found to be excellent in terms of their methodological design and control. However, none of the studies included concurrent bony debridement as part of their overall management. This is unfortunate, as bony debridement is frequently considered an essential part of refractory osteomyelitis management; consequently, an important parallel with clinical management was missed. Nevertheless, the results and import of these studies are presented in the following section.

Data

From the mechanistic standpoint, the ability of HBO_2 to increase intramedullary oxygen tensions was demonstrated by Esterhai.[11] Specifically, he showed that oxygen tensions could be elevated to levels at or above that required for normal phagocytic function. As previously discussed in the section entitled Rationale, Esterhai's study provided early objective evidence validating a primary physiologic effect of HBO_2 therapy in osteomyelitis.[7]

Two early studies evaluating osteomyelitis in animal models reported increases in bone healing after exposure to HBO_2.[4,117] Specifically, Hamblin showed 70% primary healing in the HBO_2-treated group vs. 26% in controls. Similarly, Triplet demonstrated improved fracture stability in 75% of HBO_2-treated animals vs. 12.5% of controls. In 2012, Shandley et al. reported results from a prospective murine trial evaluating HBO_2 as a stand-alone treatment for implant-associated long bone osteomyelitis.[160] However, as none of these authors included antibiotic therapy or surgical debridement in their treatment models, these studies demonstrated a neutral effect of HBO_2 on bacterial colony counts.

In contrast, the complimentary effect of combined HBO_2 and antibiotic therapy on bacterial growth was prospectively evaluated in five separate studies.[13,15,118-120] Relative to nontreated controls, each study reported a statistically significant benefit in terms of improved wound healing and/or decreased bacterial colony counts after treatment with either HBO_2 or antibiotics therapy. Further, the two most recent studies demonstrated significant synergy between HBO_2 and antibiotics relative to either agent being used alone.[15,118] Specifically, combination therapy reduced colony counts relative to controls by a factor of 10^2-10^4 after two weeks and 10^3-10^6 after four weeks of continuous therapy, respectively. Perhaps most importantly, Mendel showed that, when HBO_2 therapy was combined with antibiotics and debridement of overlying infected soft tissues, complete eradication of osteomyelitis could be achieved.[118]

Conclusions

It can be concluded from these controlled animal trials that, while neither antibiotics nor HBO_2 alone reliably impede bacterial growth in infected bone, the synergy between these two agents produces significant reductions in bacterial colony counts. However, it is when HBO_2 and antibiotics are combined with surgical debridement that the most efficacious results are achieved. Thus, the sum of animal data suggests that a management triad of culture-directed antibiotics, thorough surgical debridement, and concurrent HBO_2 therapy is the strategy most likely to achieve clinical cure in refractory osteomyelitis.

Human Studies

Quality

The significant majority of the available human study data included in this review was derived from clinical case series. Consequently, 29 of 35 reports were classified as AHA Level 5 evidence. Six studies made use of either a nonrandomized cohort (three) or control group (three), therefore achieving AHA Level 4 and Level 3 classifications, respectively. The overall quality of the studies was judged to be intermediate between the AHA descriptors of fair and good. Whereas six studies were considered excellent and 14 studies good in their design and result documentation, the remaining 15 studies were judged as being less well designed. If only the 27 studies specifically reporting refractory osteomyelitis were considered, the median quality of the studies was assessed to be good. Unfortunately, variations in the extent and location of involved bone, identified infective organisms, coexisting diseases, and strategies for antibiotic and surgical intervention made the direct comparison of clinical management strategies difficult. Further, conceptual differences existed in the application of terminology such as "cure," "arrest," "improvement," and "failure," clouding interpretation of eventual clinical outcomes. [14]

The above caveats are not limited to HBO_2 studies. Indeed, they are common to all osteomyelitis treatment modalities.[71] By way of example, Lazzarini et al. attempted to determine the most appropriate approach to antibiotic therapy in osteomyelitis.[42] After completing a retrospective analysis of 93 clinical trials, Lazzarini's group concluded that the available literature on treatment of osteomyelitis is inadequate to determine the best agent(s), route or duration of antibiotic therapy.

When one considers that the majority of clinical series evaluating the effects of HBO_2 therapy on osteomyelitis are conducted in patients who have previously failed attempts to control infection with one or more courses of antibiotics and/or surgical debridement, the relative benefit of combining HBO_2 therapy with these standard of care therapies is more readily perceived.

Cohort and Controlled Trials

In a large nonrandomized series of 689 osteomyelitis patients, Kawashima reported differential outcomes for patients treated with antibiotics, debridement and closed irrigation vs. treatment with adjunctive HBO_2 therapy.[171] For the cohort of 256 patients receiving no HBO_2 therapy, the results of treatment were 88.3% "good," 2.7% "fair" and 9% "poor" responders. In contrast, the cohort of 433 patients treated with HBO_2 was reported as having 91.9% "good," 2.3% "fair" and 5.8% "poor" responders. The difference between these two groups was noted to be statistically significant ($p<0.01$). Unfortunately, it is not possible to determine from the data presented whether or not the term "good" represented complete healing. Additionally, there is no information provided regarding statistical uniformity of the two cohorts. Thus, although significant differences in outcome were reported between the two groups, the power of this study to determine a differential treatment effect is limited.

In a second large retrospective analysis, Roje et al. reported their combat-related experience in a series of 388 patients sustaining Gustilo type III A, B and C war wounds to the upper and lower extremities (i.e., fractures involving extensive damage to the soft tissues, including muscle, skin, and neurovascular structures).[162] In this 2008 retrospective analysis, osteomyelitis developed in 74% of patients who received only standard of care treatment in accordance with North Atlantic Treaty Organization (NATO) surgical strategies vs. 63% of patients who additionally received HBO_2 treatment ($p= 0.030$). Although the study more accurately reflects the use of HBO_2 therapy to prevent osteomyelitis rather than treat it, the results of this study in complex long bone infections remain noteworthy.

Reporting results from a recent retrospective analysis, Yu et al. compared treatment outcomes in 12 patients: six HBO_2-treated and six case-matched controls, all of whom developed sternal osteomyelitis after undergoing median sternotomy for cardiothoracic procedures.[165] While all of these patients received primary treatment with antibiotics and indicated surgical debridement, six patients additionally received HBO_2 treatment. Although the total number of debridements required and hospital length of stay did not differ between groups, the six patients who additionally received HBO_2 therapy experienced significant decreases in length of ICU stay (8.7 ± 2.7 vs. 48.8 ± 10.5 days, $p<0.05$); shortened duration of mechanical ventilation (4 ± 1.5 vs. 34.8 ± 8.3 days, $p<0.05$) or positive pressure support (4 ± 1.9 vs. 22.3 ± 6.2 days, $p<0.05$); and overall reduced mortality (0 vs. 3 cases, $p<0.05$).

In a nonrandomized, prospective analysis of 28 patients, Esterhai et al. reported no benefit from the use of adjunctive HBO_2 therapy.[121] In this study, a total of four patients from both the control and experimental groups, all with tibial infections, failed to clear their disease. These failures occurred, in the author's opinion, because of the inability to remove sufficient necrotic, infected bone. Given this procedural complication and the fact that Esterhai experienced only four total treatment failures (three in the HBO_2-treated group and one in the non-treated group), the power of the study to statistically distinguish outcomes between the two groups was limited. Further, with an osteomyelitis arrest rate of more than 90% in the nontreated control group, questions are raised as to whether patients in this study met criteria for refractory osteomyelitis. Indeed, as an author and co-author on two subsequent manuscripts, Esterhai reported control group infection arrest rates of only 62%.[122-123] Thus, while Esterhai's attempt at a prospective cohort trial was welcomed, it fell short of being clinically reliable.

Barili et al. conducted a prospective trial in 32 patients designed to evaluate the effect of HBO_2 therapy on post-operative sternal infections after median sternotomy.[124] Group 1 ($n=14$) included patients who accepted and were able to undergo HBO_2 therapy; Group 2 ($n=18$) included 16 patients who refused HBO_2 therapy secondary to claustrophobia and two patients originally assigned to the HBO_2 treatment group who were excluded by persistent medical contraindications (i.e., postoperative pneumothorax). From anatomic descriptions provided by the primary author, all patients were considered to have the equivalent of Cierny-Mader Class 4 infection. Though not strictly randomized, the two groups were well matched in terms of preoperative clinical characteristics, operative factors, duration, and quality of their chronic sternal infection. Upon completion of the treatment period, Barili found that infection relapse rates were significantly lower in the HBO_2-treated group relative to nontreated controls (0% vs. 33.3%, p=0.024). Moreover, the duration of intravenous antibiotic use (47.8+/-7.4 vs. 67.6+/-25.1 days, p=0.036) and total hospital stay (52.6+/- 9.1 vs. 73.6+/-24.5 days, p=0.026) were both significantly shorter in the HBO$_2$-treated group. As this prospective study's design was uncomplicated by variability in infection site, disease severity, and surgical approach, the power of the trial to delineate an HBO$_2$ treatment effect is superior to all other studies considered in this review. Thus, Barili's investigation provides the most rigorous evidence available to date documenting improvements in clinical outcome when HBO$_2$ is added to standard of care treatment of refractory osteomyelitis.

Two recent prospective, nonrandomized trials also reported results in location-specific osteomyelitis cohorts. Onen et al. evaluated HBO$_2$ treatment of 19 patients found to have iatrogenic spinal infections refractory to a minimum of three weeks of antibiotic therapy.[167] The majority of these spinal infections involved the lumbar region, occurring after spinal instrumentation in 12 cases and microdiscectomy in seven cases. An average of 20 hyperbaric sessions was administered (range 10–40). By the completion of HBO$_2$ treatment, all 19 spinal infections had resolved. Of particular note, no surgical revisions or removal of hardware were required to achieve infection resolution in any of the 12 patients who had undergone spinal instrumentation. Separately, in a paper primarily focused on assessing long-term delivery of antibiotics via femoral central lines, Coulson and colleagues reported cure rates in a series of eight patients presenting with diabetic foot ulcers and underlying osteomyelitis that were refractory to healing after at least four weeks of antibiotic therapy and routine wound care.[168] Combining IV vancomycin with a course of 40 HBO$_2$ sessions, osteomyelitis resolution and ulcer healing was achieved in 75% of these previously refractory patients. The two patients who did not achieve treatment success were noted to be noncompliant with their prescribed treatment regimen.

Long Bone and Miscellaneous Sites

The earliest reports of HBO$_2$ therapy being applied to patients with chronic, long bone osteomyelitis were presented by Slack et al.[3] In this series of five patients treated with antibiotics and HBO$_2$, 80% responded with clearance of infection. However, these cases were a mix of patients with both chronic and refractory disease and varied in terms of types of concurrent treatment.

Similarly, Welsh et al. reported the outcomes of five patients treated with HBO$_2$ for osteomyelitis. After an average of 34 treatments, the application of HBO$_2$ in concert with antibiotics resulted in four of five (80%) assorted site infections being healed.[125] However, as osteomyelitis was not the prime focus of Welsh's retrospective study, specifics regarding whether the infections were refractory in nature and the extent of concurrent clinical management were not defined.

In contrast, a number of authors reported their experience with treating refractory cases of osteomyelitis. Specifically, Perrins et al. first described using HBO$_2$ to treat patients who had previously failed to heal with conservative antibiotic and/or surgical management.[2] Combining an average 20 days of HBO$_2$ treatment with antibiotics and occasional sequestrectomy, Perrins was able to achieve complete healing in 19/24 (79%) and improvement in two (8.3%), limiting treatment failure to only three (12.5%) patients. On follow-up, four cases relapsed, yielding an overall cure rate of 62%. In this series, concurrent debridement was not uniformly provided during this study and the osteomyelitis cases involved a variety of bony sites.

Further demonstrating the variety of osteomyelitis sites amenable to HBO$_2$ treatment, Eltorai et al. described results in managing 44 spinal cord-injured patients.[126] Of these, osteomyelitis developed secondary to pressure ulcers in 88%, while the remainder were secondary to trauma and/or surgical sources. After a follow-up period ranging between six months and nine years, HBO$_2$ was found to be a useful adjunct in resolving bone infections and encouraging wound healing in two-thirds of the affected patients. Of note, none of these patients underwent surgical debridement in conjunction with their course of HBO$_2$ therapy. Eltorai subseqeuntly attributed the majority of treatment failures to concomitant vascular disease, presumably due to generating suboptimal elevations in bone oxygen tensions during HBO$_2$ therapy. Nevertheless, all five cases of spinal osteomyelitis cleared despite this lack of surgical debridement, a seminal finding that has been additionally corroborated by others. (See Human Studies - Spinal osteomyelitis section.)

Bingham and Hart addressed potential differences in HBO$_2$ treatment response depending upon the specifically involved osteomyelitis site.[69] In their series of 70 patients with a mix of refractory cranial, torsal, upper and lower extremity bone infections, an overall osteomyelitis clearance rate of 61% was achieved. Whereas infections in all patients were noted to have been arrested or improved, significant differences in relative response by infection location were found. For tibial infections, the respective arrest and improvement rates were 73% and 27%. In the femur, arrest and improvement rates were reversed (40% and 60%), as they were for the hip (38% and 62%). Consistent with the series by both Perrins and Eltorai, all patients received concurrent antibiotic therapy. However, it is again unclear whether Bingham and Hart's patients underwent concurrent surgical debridement.

Reporting more definitive data on concurrent surgical management, Morrey et al. detailed the effects of HBO$_2$ in 40 patients with surgery and antibiotic-refractory long bone osteomyelitis.[72] Prior to HBO$_2$ initiation, all patients were treated with three or more surgical debridements and concomitant antibiotics over an average period of 30 months. Coincident with the initiation of HBO$_2$ treatment, all patients received a new course of parenteral antibiotics and surgical debridement. An average of 42 HBO$_2$ sessions were provided and, after 23 months' average follow-up, 34 of 40 (85%) patients remained disease-free. Re-evaluation at the seven- to 10-year point demonstrated continued symptom resolution in 75%.[71]

In a subsequent series of 38 patients, Davis et al. reported HBO$_2$ treatment outcomes in patients presenting with refractory, nonhematogenous osteomyelitis of the long bones.[71] All patients had failed at least one or more previous attempts at sterilization with combined surgery and antibiotics. An average of 45 HBO$_2$ treatments were provided in conjunction with debridement and antibiotics. After nearly three years of mean follow-up, 34 of 38 (89%) remained infection-free.

Chen and colleagues, in their 2008 retrospective analysis, described use of adjunctive HBO$_2$ in an attempt to eradicate diffuse tibial/humeral bone infections in a series of 10 hemodialysis-dependent patients.[161] Importantly, each patient met criteria for refractory osteomyelitis, in that the infection had persisted for at least one month, failed a minimum of one surgical debridement, and endured despite concomitant treatment with a course of parenteral antibiotics. Employing a combination of surgical debridement, antibiotics, and 20 HBO$_2$ treatment sessions, the multimodal therapy promoted osteomyelitis resolution in 80% of these systemically compromised patients, with only two of 10 ultimately requiring limb amputation to control their disease.

More recently, as part of a larger retrospective report of their experience with using HBO$_2$, Skeik et al. reported their success with adding HBO$_2$ treatment to the management of refractory osteomyelitis.[169] During the four-year assessment period encompassed by Skeik's review, 23 of 181 patients who received HBO$_2$ were treated for refractory, nondiabetic ulcer-related infections of various bony sites. By the authors' assessment, 82.6% of these patients achieved either infection eradication or improvement in clinical outcome. Unfortunately, detail relative to the nature of improvement attained was not available.

For completeness, Esterhai's nonrandomized, prospective analysis of 28 patients with long bone osteomyelitis is reiterated in this section.[121] Although Esterhai reported no benefit from the adjunctive use of HBO_2 therapy, the power of his study was severely limited by patient refusals to undergo indicated surgical debridement. Thus, in truth, the effectiveness of HBO_2 could not be equitably evaluated in the context of Esterhai's study.

Combining HBO_2 treatment with autogenous microsurgical muscle transplantation, Maynor et al. reported long-term success in patients with refractory osteomyelitis of the tibia.[127] The median delay from osteomyelitis diagnosis to initiation of HBO_2 therapy was 12.5 months. Additionally, all subjects had previously received treatment with parenteral antibiotics and an average of 8.3 failed surgical procedures. Prior to commencing HBO_2 therapy, all patients were restarted on culture-directed antibiotics and underwent one additional open debridement. Twenty patients (59%) were given vascularized muscle flaps as part of their overall treatment. An average of 35 HBO_2 sessions were provided. After three months of follow-up, 28 of 34 (82%) patients were drainage-free. At 24 and 60 months respectively, 21 of 24 (81%) and 12 of 15 (80%) of the patients available for follow-up were still without drainage. At 84 months the previously stable rate of resolution dropped to 63%. It is unclear, however, whether this fall in sustained resolution represents delayed osteomyelitis recurrence or statistical bias introduced by follow up of only a limited proportion of the original study group (i.e., ≤ 22%).

Using a well-defined set of inclusion criteria, orthopedic surgeons from the Chang Gung Memorial Hospital, Taiwan, reported HBO_2 treatment effects in three separate prospective trials involving refractory long bone osteomyelitis.[128-130] Specifically, each study required eligible patients to meet the following criteria: demonstrated persistent infection for at least six months; failed at least three previous surgical procedures designed to eliminate the infection; and received concurrent treatment with parenteral antibiotics on each sequential attempt. Additionally, all patients were expressly categorized as having Cierny-Mader Stage 3 or 4 infections. In the first study by Chao-Yu Chen et al., 13 of 15 (86%) patients with refractory tibial osteomyelitis were successfully treated with surgical debridement, parenteral antibiotics, and an average of 26 HBO_2 treatments.[128] No recurrences among treatment responders were noted after a mean follow-up of 17 months. In a follow-on study using the same methodology, Chin-En Chen et al. demonstrated resolution of tibial infection in 11 of 14 (79%) previously refractory osteomyelitis patients.[129] Finally, Chin-En Chen's group used this same treatment paradigm to manage 13 patients with refractory osteomyelitis of the femur.[130] After an average of 50 HBO_2 treatments and a mean follow-up period of 22 months, 12 of 13 (92%) of the patients remained infection-free. Although these three prospective trials were not controlled, the specificity of the inclusion criteria, as well as these same surgeons' failure to achieve osteomyelitis resolution after three or more previous attempts at infection control strongly support a beneficial effect of adjunctive HBO_2 in refractory osteomyelitis management.

In summary, for refractory osteomyelitis involving the long bones and nonspecified sites, nonsurgical management with combined HBO_2 therapy and antibiotics appears to provide cures in approximately 60–70% of cases. Unfortunately, in the absence of concurrent surgical debridement, HBO_2 does not confer a selective advantage over the 70–80% primary cure rates anticipated using standard of care management. Consequently, for the majority of osteomyelitis cases involving the long bones and miscellaneous sites, HBO_2 therapy alone or in combination with antibiotics garners only an AHA Class IIb recommendation and is not a preferred alternative to repeat surgical debridement and appropriate antibiotic therapy. In contrast, when HBO_2 is combined with appropriate antibiotics and concurrent surgical debridement, overall cure rates in refractory osteomyelitis of the long bones and miscellaneous sites range between 80-90%. This meets or exceeds outcomes expected for standard of care therapy. Thus, HBO_2 should be considered an AHA Class IIa intervention when combined with proximate surgical debridement and appropriate antibiotic treatment. Similarly, in refractory osteomyelitis patients facing potential extremity amputation or debilitating surgery, prior to implementing these radical surgical resections, a trial of adjunctive HBO$_2$ may be considered an AHA Class IIa supplement to limited surgical debridement and continued, culture-directed antibiotic therapy.

Mandibular Osteomyelitis

A review of the available literature concerning the treatment of mandibular osteomyelitis yields as much variation in applied protocols as it does in the clinical response to the prescribed interventions. Overall cure rates of 30% to 100% have been reported.[131]

In terms of HBO$_2$ therapy for mandibular osteomyelitis, Jamil reported results in 16 patients with treatment-resistant infections. HBO$_2$ therapy alone induced lasting resolution in only six of 16 (37%) patients.[132] This low response rate is in concurrence with the HBO$_2$-only interventions previously discussed for refractory long-bone osteomyelitis. Similarly, Handschel attempted to manage a mix of primary and refractory osteomyelitis cases using HBO$_2$ alone.[133] In patients with no history of antibiotic pretreatment, seven of 13 (54%) patients were relapse-free after receiving 40 HBO$_2$ treatments. In patients previously refractory to antibiotics and surgical debridement, only four of nine (44%) patients were rendered relapse-free after completing a course of HBO$_2$ treatment. It is interesting to note, however, that superior results were achieved in younger patients. In this subset of osteomyelitis patients relapsing after receiving antibiotics alone, three of four (75%) experienced sustained resolution of their infection. Lentrodt's recent experience with refractory mandibular osteomyelitis in three other children tends to confirm this differential response in younger patients.[134] Despite the recurrent nature of each child's disease, the combination of HBO$_2$ and antibiotic therapy was effective in clearing three of three (100%) of these refractory infections.

Control of mandibular osteomyelitis by combined debridement, antibiotics, and HBO$_2$ was reported by Mainous et al.[135] Although distinctions between primary and refractory osteomyelitis were not reported, osteomyelitis resolution was achieved in 23 of 24 (96%) patients. The use of this trimodality approach to mandibular osteomyelitis management was further supported by Van Merkesteyn.[136] In his series of 16 patients, only one of nine (11%) patients improved after bimodality therapy with HBO$_2$ and antibiotics. In contrast, seven of seven (100%) patients treated concurrently with decortication, antibiotics and HBO$_2$ therapy were cured. The authors concluded that in patients with refractory osteomyelitis, the coordinated use of HBO$_2$, antibiotics, and surgery tended to provide the best overall chance for cure.

In an interesting departure from the majority of osteomyelitis studies utilizing mainly postoperative HBO$_2$ treatment, Aitasalo used a series of 10 preoperative and five to seven post-operative HBO$_2$ treatments along with antibiotics to induce osteomyelitis resolution in 26 of 33 (79%).[137] Despite the fact that these patients were previously refractory to "conservative therapy with antibiotics alone, the author concluded that coordinated HBO$_2$ therapy allowed for a reduction in overall treatment duration. One might hypothesize that Aitasalo's 79% treatment success may have been further improved if the total number of postoperative treatments were increased to more closely align with typical HBO$_2$ protocols. Nonetheless, Aitasalo's study provided additional support for a trimodality approach to osteomyelitis treatment. Further, his work highlights the potential benefit of scheduling surgical debridement proximate to antibiotic and HBO$_2$ therapy.

Based on the results of these published series, HBO$_2$ cannot be recommended as a monotherapy for the management of mandibular osteomyelitis (i.e., AHA Class III). When combined with antibiotics in the treatment of adult primary or refractory mandibular osteomyelitis, HBO$_2$ therapy can be elevated to an AHA Class IIb intervention. In child and adolescent subpopulations, where the potential risk for disfigurement and impaired bone growth is high, a trial of HBO$_2$ and antibiotics prior to major debridement surgery may be considered an

AHA Class IIa intervention. In adults, treatment of mandibular osteomyelitis with the combination of antibiotics, surgical debridement, and HBO₂ appears to maximize the potential for infection clearance, particularly in recurrent or refractory cases.

While the wide variability in reported cure rates inhibits statistical comparison, the lack of viable clinical alternatives to this trimodality treatment approach earns HBO₂ therapy an AHA Class IIa designation in the management of refractory mandibular osteomyelitis.

Spinal Osteomyelitis

In a study of 44 patients evaluating the efficacy of antibiotics alone in vertebral osteomyelitis, 27% of patients failed to respond to this conservative approach.[138] Extending antibiotic coverage to an average of 142 days, Priest was able to achieve a higher rate of infection cure, clearing hematogenous vertebral infections in 24 of 29 (83%). However, a full 50% of Priest's treated population still suffered infection-related sequelae.[75] Kovalenko was able to further increase the resolution rate of hematogenous osteomyelitis, however his 91% primary cure success required radical reconstructive surgery and was still associated with 6% recurrence and 2% perioperative mortality.[139] In a series of technically more complex cases involving spinal fusion, Talmi was able to achieve infection resolution in only four of six (66%) patients when using combined surgical debridement and antibiotic therapy. These results persisted despite treatment with one or more drainage procedures and the removal of hardware in two of six (33%).[51] Chen also reported refractory deep space infections in a series of 36 patients after undergoing thoracic and lumbar instrumentation.[46] Despite extensive debridement, antibiotics, and a course of continuous irrigation treatment, recurrence was noted in 11% of patients.

In contrast to the above non-HBO₂ treated cases, Eltorai et al. reported success using HBO₂ and antibiotics to eradicate osteomyelitis in five of five (100%) cases of adult lumbar osteomyelitis.[126] Similarly, Ahmed et al. used adjunctive HBO₂ therapy to treat six patients with complicated spinal osteomyelitis.[163] In four patients, the osteomyelitis developed subsequent to antecedent spinal surgery, whereas two cases derived from hematogenous seeding. In each case, the infections were noted to be either refractory or progressive despite appropriate antibiotic treatment. Combining HBO₂ therapy with continued antibiotics and, in two cases, removal/revision of previously placed spinal instrumentation, osteomyelitis resolution was achieved in five of six cases. Ahmed noted no recurrence of infection during an average follow-up period of 1.6 years (range five months to three years).

Larsson similarly reported benefit from combined HBO₂ and antibiotic therapy in patients suffering from osteomyelitis subsequent to spinal surgery and implantation of fixation material.[92] After an average of 30 HBO₂ treatments, seven of seven (100%) of his patients' infections resolved. Of note, spinal fixation material was maintained in situ for five of seven (71%) patients. The success of this primarily nonoperative approach compares favorably with others who achieved osteomyelitis eradication in patients with retained spinal instrumentation. However, with no infection recurrence after treatment with adjunctive HBO₂ therapy (vs. 11% for antibiotics alone), Larsson's nonsurgical success exceeds the outcomes experienced by Chen.

Extending this nonoperative HBO₂ treatment success were the recent findings of Onen et al. in eradicating iatrogenic spinal infections in 19 adult patients who proved refractory to a minimum of three weeks of antibiotic therapy alone.[167] As previously noted, the majority of the spinal infections involved the lumbar region, occurring after spinal instrumentation in 12 cases and microdiscectomy in seven cases. By the completion of HBO₂ treatment (mean 20, range 10–40 sessions), all 19 spinal infections had resolved. Of greatest import to patient clinical management, no surgical debridement, revision, or hardware removal was required achieve infection resolution.

When combined with antibiotics, the ability of HBO$_2$ to eliminate spinal osteomyelitis and obviate hardware removal in the majority of patients suggests that a trial of HBO$_2$ therapy prior to scheduling patients for extensive surgical debridement is warranted. This is particularly true for patients where removal of surgical hardware is relatively contraindicated or associated with significant postsurgical morbidity or mortality. Thus, the addition of HBO$_2$ therapy to antibiotics and, if clearly indicated, limited surgical debridement should be considered an AHA Class IIa recommendation in patients with spinal osteomyelitis.

Cranial Osteomyelitis

Following craniotomy, the bone flap generated is devascularized and devitalized, increasing its susceptibility to infection.[92] This increase in infection risk also applies to procedures involving the implantation of cranial prosthetics. Overall, a 5-9% postoperative infection rate can be anticipated.[109-111] Cures can subsequently be affected, but antibiotics, surgical debridement, and, frequently, removal of the infected bone flaps or prostheses are required.[140-143]

Sandner et al. examined the effects of adjunctive HBO$_2$ in managing 10 patients with refractory, skull base osteomyelitis.[164] By combining antibiotics and surgical debridement with HBO$_2$ therapy, Sandner was able to achieve infection clearance in 80% of these previously refractory patients. In what appears to be a recurring theme in HBO$_2$ treatment failures, the two patients who failed to clear their refractory skull base infections were remarkable for having refused further therapy (after receiving only two and five HBO$_2$ treatments, respectively) and ultimately succumbed to their disease. Thus, Sandner's effective infection control rate in patients completing prescribed antibiotic, surgical and HBO$_2$ therapy was 100%.

Of potentially greater import, Larsson reported primary success with HBO$_2$ in a series of patients previously failing to resolve cranial osteomyelitis with antibiotic therapy.[92] Prior to the initiation of HBO$_2$, none of his patients had undergone attempts at surgical debridement. Based on the presence or absence of confounding risk factors, Larsson divided the patients into two groups. Group 1 patients manifest uncomplicated free cranial bone flap osteomyelitis, with no known risk factors for delayed healing. Group 2 patients presented with additional risk factors, such as repeated surgical procedures, retained foreign material, malignant disease, or previous radiotherapy. Of the patients in Group 1, 12 of 15 (80%) resolved their bone flap infection without a need for surgical intervention; 20% recurred. In Group 2, after excluding analysis of two patients with early death secondary tumor progression, 10 of 16 (62%) refractory infections were resolved nonsurgically. Furthermore, three of four (75%) and three of six (50%) of bone and acrylic flaps were retained in each group, respectively. If cures achieved subsequent to removal of the bone and acrylic sequestra are included, 15 of16 (94%) of Group 2 patients resolved their infections. When overall success criteria are defined as clearance of infection vs. avoidance of surgery, Larsson was able to achieve a cure in 97% of his patients with refractory osteomyelitis. Interestingly, data regarding HBO$_2$-associated treatment costs were also provided, with primary cures using HBO$_2$ therapy conferring a 48-66% savings over repeat craniotomy.

Consequently, a combination of HBO$_2$ therapy, antibiotic and, where indicated, limited surgical debridement appears to be very effective in eradicating refractory cranial osteomyelitis. Given the potential for HBO$_2$-induced, nonsurgical cure rates approaching 70 to 100%, as well as the concurrent ability to minimize both the risks and costs associated with repeat craniotomy, a trial of HBO$_2$ therapy prior to undergoing major cranial debridement should be considered. Accordingly, in the setting of antibiotic refractory cranial osteomyelitis, HBO$_2$ can be recommended as AHA Class IIa therapeutic adjunct to standard of care interventions.

Malignant External Otitis

Malignant external otitis is an invasive form of osteomyelitis with a tendency to extend beyond the external auditory canal, potentially producing lethal results.[113] In an early series, Lucente reported mortality rates in antibiotic-treated patients of over 30%.[113] Fortunately, advances in antibiotic therapy have increased projected survival rates to approximately 80-90%.[115,144-146] However, in these series, the extent of bony versus merely soft tissue involvement and the number of cases requiring surgical debridement were not clear. Thus, it is hypothesized that many of these treatment successes occurred in patients with less severe disease.

Addressing this potential variation in infection severity, Tisch employed a classification system similar to Cierny-Mader's to stratify his patients into four categories:[114] Specifically, patients with superficial cortical disease only; local invasion without cranial nerve involvement; local invasion with zygomatic bone or cranial nerve involvement; and diffuse involvement of the cranium with meningitis or sepsis were classified as being Stage I, II, III, and IV patients, respectively. Using this classification system, reported mortality after treatment with antibiotics and surgery was 14%, 50%, and 70%, respectively, for Stage I-II, Stage III, and Stage IV disease.

Comparing these malignant external otitis cure rates to those attainable with the addition of HBO_2 therapy is instructive. In a series of 22 nonsurgically managed cases, Martel achieved resolution in 95% of cases after combining HBO_2 therapy with antibiotic treatment.[147] These cases were, however, not specifically reported as being previously refractory to antibiotics.

Focusing wholly on the management of antibiotic refractory patients, Narozny demonstrated resolution of infection in seven of eight (87.5%) patients using HBO_2.[148] Only one patient required concurrent surgical debridement, and his single treatment failure was associated with a fungal etiology. Extending these findings, Davis treated 16 cases, including six advanced cases, that were previously refractory to multiple courses of antibiotics.[149] After completing a 30-day course of HBO_2 combined with antibiotic therapy, all patients experienced resolution of their infection. This curative success persisted without recurrence throughout his one- to four-year follow-up period. In a retrospective case series of 23 patients with malignant external otitis refractory to primary treatment with antibiotics and surgical debridement, Yeheskeli et al. evaluated adding HBO_2 treatment as a rescue intervention in 23 patients.[170] Although four patients eventually died from the disease, one was lost to follow-up, and three subsequently required re-hospitalization and a secondary course of HBO_2 treatment for infection control, Yeheskeli was able to achieve infection resolution in 78% of these previously treatment refractory patients. Similarly, after adding HBO_2 to his overall management strategy, Tisch achieved cures in 21 of 22 (95%) patients with antibiotic refractory malignant external otitis. Although this resolution rate is comparable to that reported for quinolone antibiotic therapy in nonstratified cases, Tisch's success is remarkable given that 59% of his patients had either Stage III or IV involvement.

It is concluded that, while malignant external otitis generally responds well to primary management with antibiotics and minimal surgical debridement, HBO_2 appears to be effective in cases refractory to standard therapy. This appears particularly true for more extensive Stage III and IV disease, where extensive debridement and historically high mortality rates can potentially be avoided. Thus, for Stage I and Stage II cases of malignant external otitis, HBO_2 should be considered AHA Class IIb therapy. In refractory cases, as well as those with higher stage malignant external otitis, HBO_2 can be recommended as an AHA Class IIa intervention.

Sternal Osteomyelitis

In a large series of patients undergoing coronary artery bypass grafting, the incidence of sternal osteomyelitis was reported to be 2.1%.[150] Of these cases, 89% required surgical intervention to obtain control of the infection.

Even so, 30% still failed this primary surgical debridement and required secondary, more extensive procedures to eradicate the residual infection.

Adjunctive HBO$_2$ therapy seems to improve upon these historical results. In a small series of patients undergoing lung transplantation, four patients with sternal osteomyelitis were adjunctively treated with HBO$_2$ therapy.[91] Despite the immunosuppressed status of these patients, two of four patients healed completely without the need for any surgical intervention. One additional patient's infection was cleared but required skin grafting to close a residual soft tissue defect. The fourth patient, who refused further HBO$_2$ therapy after three uncomplicated sessions, subsequently died from complications of sepsis. Thus, of three patients completing a course of HBO$_2$ therapy, all were able to clear their infections without the need for surgical debridement.

As previously discussed, Yu et al. compared treatment outcomes in 12 patients with sternal osteomyelitis after undergoing median sternotomy for cardiothoracic procedures.[165] Although total debridements and hospital stay length did not differ between groups, the six patients who additionally received HBO$_2$ therapy logged significant decreases in length of ICU stay (8.7 ± 2.7 *vs.* 48.8 ± 10.5 days, $p<0.05$); shortened duration of mechanical ventilation (4 ± 1.5 vs. 34.8 ± 8.3 days, $p<0.05$) and/or positive pressure support (4 ± 1.9 vs. 22.3 ± 6.2 days, $p<0.05$); and overall reduced mortality (0 vs. 3 cases, $p<0.05$).

Also previously discussed was the prospective study by Barili, which provides even stronger support for the use of HBO$_2$ in controlling sternal infections.[124] In Barili's trial, the addition of HBO$_2$ therapy to the overall treatment regimen resulted in significantly lower infection relapse rates (0% vs. 33.3%, $p=0.024$), shortened antibiotic therapy durations (47.8 +/- 7.4 vs. 67.6 +/- 25.1 days, $p=0.036$) and reduced hospital stay lengths (52.6 +/- 9.1 vs. 73.6 +/- 24.5 days, $p=0.026$) relative to matched controls managed only with antibiotics and surgical debridement. Though few in number, these series demonstrate that HBO$_2$ is effective in reducing the need for sternal debridement and/or extensive surgical interventions. Consequently, HBO$_2$ therapy should be considered an AHA Class IIa adjunct in the management of sternal osteomyelitis.

Diabetic Patients

Although covered extensively in another chapter of this publication, the majority of patients presenting for treatment of refractory osteomyelitis are those with comorbid diabetic foot wounds.[28] Indeed, several authors contend that concurrent osteomyelitis can be assumed to be present in virtually all diabetic patients presenting with plantar foot ulcers, particularly when the wound exposes the underlying bone.[18,151-152]

It is from the body of literature evaluating management strategies for Wagner Grade 3 and 4 diabetic ulcers that HBO$_2$ therapy derives some of its highest level of evidence support for use in refractory osteomyelitis. Citing five randomized controlled trials involving patients with diabetic ulcers (118 patients), Roeckl-Wiedmann concluded from pooled data that adjunctive HBO$_2$ treatment confers a significant reduction in the risk of major amputation (RR: 0.31; CI 0.13 to 0.71).[153] Further, others have noted in randomized prospective trials that HBO$_2$ can improve the mean rate of healing in diabetic foot ulcers.[154-156] Consequently, HBO$_2$ is both recommended and accepted as an AHA Class I therapy for refractory osteomyelitis associated with diabetic foot ulcers.[157]

Safety Considerations

While HBO$_2$ therapy is generally safe and well tolerated, exposures have been associated with known adverse side effects. A description of these side effects, expected incidence rates, and associated risk factors are discussed in detail elsewhere in this publication. However, in the setting of refractory osteomyelitis, reports of adverse,

HBO$_2$-related sequelae have been rare. As with most clinical HBO$_2$ treatments, the most common events reported were middle ear and sinus barotrauma. Typically, these pressure-related events were both mild and self-limiting. Although a few authors did report the need for tympanostomy tube placement to help facilitate continuation of HBO$_2$ therapy, no patient being treated for osteomyelitis discontinued HBO$_2$ therapy secondary to barotraumas.

In considering potential side effects associated with repeated exposure to elevated oxygen partial pressures, only transient myopia was reported to occur. As is characteristic for this clinical phenomenon, all cases of myopia spontaneously resolved after completion of HBO$_2$ therapy. More permanent visual changes, such as cataract formation, were not reported in this patient population. Similarly, no reports of CNS or pulmonary oxygen toxicity could be found.

Evidence-Based Conclusions

The bulk of available human data on refractory osteomyelitis was abstracted from retrospective clinical case series, thus representing primarily AHA Level 5 quality evidence. Five studies did make use of either a control or comparative cohort group, providing the literature's only AHA Level 3 and Level 4 reports addressing HBO$_2$ treatment of osteomyelitis. That said, the overwhelming majority of available studies supported the use of HBO$_2$ as a beneficial adjunct in the management of refractory osteomyelitis. Specifically, the highest-reported osteomyelitis cure rates were obtained when HBO$_2$ therapy was combined with culture-directed antibiotics and concurrent surgical debridement.

As these treatment success rates generally exceeded that found in the literature for standard of care therapy using antibiotics and surgical debridement alone, HBO$_2$ therapy can be generally recommended as an AHA Class II intervention in refractory osteomyelitis. In certain clinical settings, such as osteomyelitis involving children or bony structures adjacent to the central nervous system or other vital organs, a favorable risk-benefit balance appears to support a trial of HBO$_2$ and antibiotictherapy prior to attempting extensive surgical debridement (AHA Class IIa).

For patients with refractory diabetic ulcers, adjunctive HBO$_2$ therapy can be definitively regarded as an AHA Class I intervention. In contrast, the combination of HBO$_2$ and antibiotics in most other forms of uncomplicated primary, extremity or miscellaneous site osteomyelitis typically garners only AHA Class IIb support. This variability in HBO$_2$ treatment recommendations is to be expected, however, given similar location-dependent irregularity in osteomyelitis treatment success with standard of care therapies.

Finally, while one prospective study did report a neutral benefit from the use of adjunctive HBO$_2$ treatment, no study reported significant negative treatment effects from adding HBO$_2$ to standard of care therapies. As the addition of HBO$_2$ to osteomyelitis treatment regimens was not associated with reports of significant adverse side effects, adjunctive HBO$_2$ should be considered a safe, well-tolerated intervention in the management of refractory osteomyelitis.

Utilization Review

As discussed in the preceding sections, no specific recommendations can be made for the total number of HBO$_2$ treatments required. Consequently, the duration of HBO$_2$ therapy must be judged on the basis of each patient's clinical response. If a patient responds to initial management with appropriate antibiotics, indicated surgical debridement, and HBO$_2$, then continuation of antibiotics and HBO$_2$ therapy for a period of approximately four to six weeks should be considered a Class II intervention. Although mitigating clinical circumstances exist that would suggest treatment continuation beyond this point, utilization review is generally indicated after completion of 30–40 HBO$_2$ treatment sessions.

In contrast, if a patient does not respond with prompt clinical improvement or progressive healing progress stalls, then the existing antibiotic and HBO$_2$ regimen is unlikely to be clinically effective and continuation without modification should be considered an AHA Class III intervention. Instead, clinical management strategies should be reassessed and additional surgical debridement and/or adjustment of antibiotic therapy implemented without delay. Subsequent to these treatment modifications, the clinical evidence accumulated to date suggests that reinstitution of adjunctive HBO$_2$ therapy will still help maximize the overall chances of achieving resolution of refractory bone infections.

Cost Impact

When used within the above guidelines, adjunctive HBO$_2$ can decrease overall health care costs in patients with refractory osteomyelitis. Analyzing a series of complicated osteomyelitis cases, Strauss reported an average expenditure of $204,000 on hospitalization and treatment prior to the initiation of HBO$_2$ therapy (n.b.: All U.S. dollar values in these examples have been normalized to present-day equivalents).[1] Once HBO$_2$ was combined with surgery and antibiotic therapy for control of the infection, expenditures on these previously refractory cases were limited to an additional $35,500 per patient. While this did represent a one-time, 17% increase in total cost, it was projected that these patients would have experienced equal or greater costs in association with continued standard of care interventions. Consequently, cost-effectiveness was calculated as being five-fold in favor of adjunctive HBO$_2$ therapy in refractory osteomyelitis.[158]

Strauss' results were seconded in a series of patients with infected cranial bone flaps, where Larsson demonstrated that treatment with HBO$_2$ therapy was effective in resolving cranial infection and preventing the need for revision cranioplasty.[92] Citing per-case surgical costs of 130,000-210,000 SEK versus an average 71,000 SEK for HBO$_2$ therapy, the adjunctive use of HBO$_2$ resulted in a two- to threefold savings over standard of care surgical treatment. (Monetary figures are reported in Swedish *kroner*, as the exchange rate at the time of the study is unknown.)

In a separate cost analysis, Riddick et al. evaluated patients undergoing HBO$_2$ treatment for sternal wound infections realized a relative reduction in hospital length of stay and pharmacy costs.[159] Calculated savings of $11,154 per case or approximately 12% were reported.

Finally, in a Canadian technology assessment, Sheps noted that while overall management costs for chronic osteomyelitis are high (ranging from $144,000- 360,000), the subset of costs associated with HBO$_2$ account for only 5% of the total cost per case.[40,73]

Although not specifically reporting cost figures, per se, two sternal osteomyelitis studies provide insight into potential cost savings. Specifically, Yu et al. demonstrated that despite no change in required number of debridements or hospital length of stay, patients who additionally received HBO$_2$ therapy logged significant decreases in length of ICU stay (8.7 ± 2.7 vs. 48.8 ± 10.5 days, $p<0.05$); shortened duration of mechanical ventilation (4 ± 1.5 vs. 34.8 ± 8.3 days, $p<0.05$) or positive pressure support (4 ± 1.9 *vs.* 22.3 ± 6.2 days, $p<0.05$); and overall reduced mortality (0 vs. 3 cases, $p<0.05$) [165]. Barili's prospective, controlled trial extended these results, noting that patients who received HBO$_2$ therapy as part of their overall management required shorter courses antibiotic therapy (47.8 +/- 7.4 vs. 67.6 +/- 25.1 days, $p=0.036$) and reduced hospital stay lengths (52.6 +/- 9.1 vs. 73.6 +/- 24.5 days, $p=0.026$) relative to non- HBO$_2$-treated controls.[124]

In sum, while HBO$_2$ therapy can be costly, its addition to the management of patients with refractory osteomyelitis appears to be associated with a reduction in total need for surgical procedures, required courses of antibiotic therapy, duration of intensive care/inpatient management, and, hence, overall health care expenditures.

Review Conclusions

Animal studies have demonstrated basic mechanisms by which HBO$_2$ enhances the body's ability to inhibit bacterial growth. Specifically, HBO$_2$ therapy elevates oxygen tensions in infected bone to normal or supranormal levels. Elimination of hypoxia restores bacterial phagocytosis and oxidative killing by neutrophils. Further, active transport of aminioglycoside and cephalosporin antibiotics across bacterial cell walls is improved. When combined, antibiotic, and HBO$_2$ therapy can produce a 100-fold reduction in bacterial cell counts relative to the use of either agent alone.

In clinical practice, this antibacterial synergy has resulted in numerous case reports and clinical series describing effective control of osteomyelitis in previously refractory patients. Over the last decade, these results have also been confirmed by prospective trials. While variations in host status, bony involvement, pathogenic organisms, antibiotic regimens, and surgical techniques still complicate the analysis of HBO$_2$ therapy's effectiveness, the infection arrest rates achieved when adjunctive HBO$_2$ therapy is added remain superior to standard of care interventions alone. Thus, the weight of accumulated clinical evidence supports HBO$_2$ therapy as an AHA Class II adjunct to routine surgical and antibiotic management of refractory osteomyelitis. In particular, for patients with Cierny-Mader Class 3B or 4B disease, adjunctive HBO$_2$ therapy should be considered an AHA Class IIa intervention. For the subset of patients with Wagner Grade 3 or 4 diabetic ulcers, adjunctive HBO$_2$ should be regarded as an AHA Class I intervention. When refractory osteomyelitis involves children or bony structures adjacent to the CNS or other vital organs, a favorable risk-benefit balance earns AHA Class IIa support for combined HBO$_2$ and antibiotic therapy prior to extensive surgical debridement. In contrast, in the absence of adequate surgical debridement, such combined therapy for the management of uncomplicated primary, extremity or miscellaneous site osteomyelitis typically garners only an AHA Class IIb recommendation.

In terms of dosing, HBO$_2$ therapy is usually applied on a once-daily basis, five to seven times per week, and timed to begin just after the most recent surgical debridement. However, some clinicians advocate twice-daily treatment during the first two to three postoperative days to more aggressively prophylax against bacterial recolonization and maximize the secondary benefits of postoperative HBO$_2$ therapy. Further, individual HBO$_2$ treatment sessions are most frequently delivered over a period of 90–120 minutes. Although treatment pressures ranging from 2.0–3.0 ATA are clinically appropriate, initial treatment at 2.4–2.5 ATA may provide the best theoretical balance between clinical efficacy and oxygen toxicity risk.

Where prompt clinical improvement is seen, the present antibiotic and HBO$_2$ treatment regimen should be continued for approximately four to six weeks. In those cases where removal of fixation hardware or extensive surgical debridement is relatively contraindicated (e.g., cranial, spinal, sternal or pediatric osteomyelitis), a trial of limited debridement, culture-directed antibiotics, and HBO$_2$ prior to radical surgical intervention will provide a reasonable chance for osteomyelitis cure. Again, a course of four to six weeks of combined therapy is indicated. Depending upon the frequency of prescribed HBO$_2$ treatment, a total of 20–40 postoperative HBO$_2$ sessions will be required to attain the desired clinical results. After this point, the bony milieu should be sufficiently revascularized to prevent infection recurrence. Although co-existing diseases may slow the rate of infection resolution, extension of this treatment regimen beyond one to two additional weeks does not appear to provide definitive benefit. Indeed, if osteomyelitis fails to resolve or recurs after a total of six to eight weeks of continuous culture-directed antibiotics and HBO$_2$ treatment (i.e., 30–40 sessions), then a nidus of reinfection, such as an occult sequestra or fixation hardware refractory to sterilization, should be suspected. Therefore, further surgical debridement or removal of fixation hardware will likely be required to eradicate any residual infection.

Similarly, if initial antibiotic and HBO_2 treatment do not result in prompt clinical improvement or healing progress is noted to stall, then continuation of the current regimen should be considered an AHA Class III intervention. Instead, patient management strategies should be reassessed and additional surgical debridement and/or adjustment of antibiotic therapy implemented without delay. Subsequent to these interventions, the reinstitution of HBO_2 will help maximize overall chances for treatment success. Regardless of the clinical presentation, utilization review is generally recommended after a total of 30–40 treatments.

In conclusion, while no randomized clinical trials exist, the overwhelming majority of published animal data, human case series, and prospective trials support HBO_2 therapy as a safe and effective adjunct to the management of refractory osteomyelitis. Further, when used appropriately, HBO_2 therapy appears to reduce the total need for surgical procedures, required antibiotic therapy, and, consequently, overall health care expenditures.

References

1. Strauss MB. Refractory osteomyelitis. J Hyperbaric Med. 1987;2:147-159.
2. Perrins DJD, et al. OHP in the management of chronic osteomyelitis. In third international conference on hyperbaric medicine. Washington D.C.: National Academy of Sciences-National Research Council;1966.
3. Slack WK, Thomas DA, Perrins D. Hyperbaric oxygenation chronic osteomyelitis. Lancet. 1965;14:1093-4.
4. Hamblen DL. Hyperbaric oxygenation. Its effect on experimental staphylococcal osteomyelitis in rats. J Bone Joint Surg Am. 1968;50(6):1129-41.
5. Sippel HW, Nyberg CD, Alvis HJ. Hyperbaric oxygen as an adjunct to the treatment of chronic osteomyelitis of the mandible: report of case. J Oral Surg. 1969;27(9):739-41.
6. Niinikoski J, Hunt TK. Oxygen tensions in healing bone. Surg Gynecol Obstet. 1972;134(5):746-50.
7. Mader JT, et al. A mechanism for the amelioration by hyperbaric oxygen of experimental staphylococcal osteomyelitis in rabbits. J Infect Dis. 1980;142(6):915-22.
8. Park MK, Myers RA, Marzella L. Oxygen tensions and infections: modulation of microbial growth, activity of antimicrobial agents, and immunologic responses. Clin Infect Dis. 1992;14(3):720-40.
9. Hohn DC. Oxygen and leukocyte microbial killing, in hyperbaric oxygen therapy. Davis JC, Hunt TK eds. Bethesda, Maryland: Undersea Medical Society; 1977. Pp.101-10.
10. Kindwall EP. Uses of hyperbaric oxygen therapy in the 1990s. Cleve Clin J Med. 1992;59(5):517-28.
11. Esterhai Jr, JL, et al. Effect of hyperbaric oxygen exposure on oxygen tension within the medullary canal in the rabbit tibial osteomyelitis model. J Orthop Res.1986;4(3):330-6.
12. Verklin Jr, RM, Mandell GL. Alteration of effectiveness of antibiotics by anaerobiosis. J Lab Clin Med. 1977;89(1):65-71.
13. Mader JT, Adams KR, Couch LA. Potentiation of tobramycin by hyperbaric oxygen in experimental Pseudomonas aeruginosa osteomyelitis. In 27th interscience conference on antimicrobial agents and chemotherapy. New York;1997.
14. Mader JT, et al. Hyperbaric oxygen as adjunctive therapy for osteomyelitis. Infect Dis Clin North Am.1990;4(3):433-40.
15. Mendel V, et al. Therapy with hyperbaric oxygen and cefazolin for experimental osteomyelitis due to Staphylococcus aureus in rats. Undersea Hyperb Med. 1999;26(3):169-74.
16. Mader J, Shirtliff M, Calhoun JH. The use of hyperbaric oxygen in the treatment of osteomyelitis. In hyperbaric medicine practice. Kindwall EP, Whelan HT, eds. Flagstaff, AZ: Best Publishing Company, 1999. Pp.603-616.
17. Sugihara A, et al. The effect of hyperbaric oxygen therapy on the bout of treatment for soft tissue infections. J Infect. 2004;48(4):330-3.
18. Mader JT, Ortiz M, Calhoun JH. Update on the diagnosis and management of osteomyelitis. Clin Podiatr Med Surg. 1996;13(4):701-24.
19. Coulson DB, Ferguson Jr, AB, Diehl Jr, RC. Effect of hyperbaric oxygen on the healing femur of the rat. Surg Forum. 1966;17:449-50.
20. Niinikoski J, Penttinen R, Kulonen K. Effect of hyperbaric oxygenation on fracture healing in the rat: a biochemical study. Calcif Tissue Res. 1970:p.Suppl:115-6.
21. Penttinen R. Biochemical studies on fracture healing in the rat, with special reference to the oxygen supply. Acta Chir Scand Suppl. 1972;432:1-32.
22. Yablon IG, Cruess RL. The effect of hyperbaric oxygen on fracture healing in rats. J Trauma. 1968;8(2):186-202.
23. Steed DL. Enhancement of osteogenesis with hyperbaric oxygen therapy. A clinical study. J Dent Res.1982;61A: 288.
24. Ueng SW, et al. Bone healing of tibial lengthening is enhanced by hyperbaric oxygen therapy: a study of bone mineral density and torsional strength on rabbits. J Trauma.1998;44(4):676-81.
25. Sawai T, et al. Histologic study of the effect of hyperbaric oxygen therapy on autogenous free bone grafts. J Oral Maxillofac Surg.1996;54(8):975-81.
26. Jones Jr, JP. The effect of hyperbaric oxygen on osteonecrosis. Anaheim, CA: Orthopaedic Research Society;1991.
27. Strauss MB. Effect of hyperbaric oxygen on bone resorption in rabbits. In seventh annual conference on the clinical applications of hyperbaric oxygen. Anaheim, CA; 1982.
28. Strauss MB, Bryant B. Hyperbaric oxygen. Orthopedics. 2002;25(3):303-10.
29. Skyhar MJ, et al. Hyperbaric oxygen reduces edema and necrosis of skeletal muscle in compartment syndromes associated with hemorrhagic hypotension. J Bone Joint Surg Am. 1986;68(8):1218-24.
30. Strauss MB, et al. Reduction of skeletal muscle necrosis using intermittent hyperbaric oxygen in a model compartment syndrome. J Bone Joint Surg Am. 1983;65(5):656-62.

31. Zamboni WA, et al. Morphologic analysis of the microcirculation during reperfusion of ischemic skeletal muscle and the effect of hyperbaric oxygen. Plast Reconstr Surg. 1993;91(6):1110-23.
32. Nylander G, et al. Reduction of postischemic edema with hyperbaric oxygen. Plast Reconstr Surg. 1985;76(4):596-603.
33. Hunt TK, Halliday B, Knighton DR.. Impairment of microbicidal function in wounds: correction with oxygenation, in soft and hard tissue repair. Hunt TK, Heppenstall RB, Pines E, eds. Praeger: New York; 1984;455-68.
34. Hohn DC, et al. Effect of O2 tension on microbicidal function of leukocytes in wounds and in vitro. Surg Forum. 1976;27(62):18-20.
35. Hunt TK, Pai MP. The effect of varying ambient oxygen tensions on wound metabolism and collagen synthesis. Surg Gynecol Obstet.1972;135(4):561-7.
36. Connolly WB, et al. Influence of distant trauma on local wound infection. Surg Gynecol Obstet. 1969;128:713-8.
37. Wald ER. Risk factors for osteomyelitis. Am J Med. 1985;78(6B):206-12.
38. Le Saux N, et al. Shorter courses of parenteral antibiotic therapy do not appear to influence response rates for children with acute hematogenous osteomyelitis: a systematic review. BMC Infect Dis. 2002;2:16.
39. Lew DP, Waldvogel FA. Osteomyelitis. Lancet. 2004;364(9431):369-79.
40. Davis JC, Heckman JD. Refractory osteomyelitis, in problem wounds: the role of oxygen. Davis JC, Hunt TK, eds. New York: Elsevier Science Publishing Co., Inc.; 1988. Pp.125-142.
41. Attinger C, Cooper P. Soft tissue reconstruction for calcaneal fractures or osteomyelitis. Orthop Clin North Am. 2001;32(1):135-70.
42. Lazzarini L, Lipsky BA, Mader JT. Antibiotic treatment of osteomyelitis: what have we learned from 30 years of clinical trials? Int J Infect Dis. 2005;9(3):127-38.
43. Zalavras CG, Singh A, Patzakis MJ. Novel technique for medullary canal debridement in tibia and femur osteomyelitis. Clin Orthop Relat Res. 2007;461:31-4.
44. Thonse R, Conway J. Antibiotic cement-coated interlocking nail for the treatment of infected nonunions and segmental bone defects. J Orthop Trauma. 2007;21(4):258-68.
45. Kocaoglu M, et al. Reconstruction of segmental bone defects due to chronic osteomyelitis with use of an external fixator and an intramedullary nail. J Bone Joint Surg Am.2006;88(10):2137-45.
46. Chen F, et al. [The treatment of deep wound infection after posterior thoracic and lumbar instrumentation]. Zhonghua Wai Ke Za Zhi. 2005;43(20):1325-7.
47. Varzos PN, et al. Chronic osteomyelitis associated with monofilament wire fixation. J Foot Surg.1983;22(3):212-7.
48. Chang WC, et al. Successful treatment of extended epidural abscess and long segment osteomyelitis: a case report and review of the literature. Surg Neurol. 2008 Feb;69(2):117-20. Note original 2007 citation was for an Epub.
49. Barbarossa V, et al. Treatment of osteomyelitis and infected non-union of the femur by a modified Ilizarov technique: follow-up study. Croat Med J.2001;42(6):634-41.
50. Pappou IP, et al. Postoperative infections in interbody fusion for degenerative spinal disease. Clin Orthop Relat Res. 2006;444:120-8.
51. Talmi YP, et al. Postsurgical prevertebral abscess of the cervical spine. Laryngoscope. 2000;110(7):1137-41.
52. Przybylski GJ, Sharan AD. Single-stage autogenous bone grafting and internal fixation in the surgical management of pyogenic discitis and vertebral osteomyelitis. J Neurosurg. 2001;94(1 Suppl):1-7.
53. May Jr. JW, Gallico III, GG, Lukash FN. Microvascular transfer of free tissue for closure of bone wounds of the distal lower extremity. N Engl J Med. 1982;306(5):253-7.
54. Steinlechner CW, Mkandawire NC. Nonvascularised fibular transfer in the management of defects of long bones after sequestrectomy in children. J Bone Joint Surg Br. 2005;87(9):1259-63.
55. Simard S, Marchant M, Mencio G. The Ilizarov procedure: limb lengthening and its implications. Phys Ther. 1992;72(1):25-34.
56. Daver NG, et al. Oral step-down therapy is comparable to intravenous therapy for Staphylococcus aureus osteomyelitis. J Infect. 2007;54(6):539-44.
57. Aneziokoro CO, et al. The effectiveness and safety of oral linezolid for the primary and secondary treatment of osteomyelitis. J Chemother. 2005;17(6):643-50.
58. Cole WG, Dalziel RE, Leitl S. Treatment of acute osteomyelitis in childhood. J Bone Joint Surg Br. 1982;64(2):218-23.
59. Gentry LO. Overview of osteomyelitis. Orthop Rev.1987;16(4):255-8.
60. Ketterl R, et al. Use of ofloxacin in open fractures and in the treatment of post-traumatic osteomyelitis. J Antimicrob Chemother. 1988;22 (Supp.C):159-66.
61. Lamp KC, et al. Clinical experience with daptomycin for the treatment of patients with osteomyelitis. Am J Med. 2007;120(10 Sup p.1):S13-20.
62. Miller,DJ, Mejicano GC, Vertebral osteomyelitis due to Candida species: case report and literature review. Clin Infect Dis. 2001;33(4):523-30.

63. Petersen S, et al. Acute haematogenous osteomyelitis and septic arthritis in childhood. A 10-year review and follow-up. Acta Orthop Scand.1980;51(3):451-7.

64. Powers T, Bingham DH. Clinical and economic effect of ciprofloxacin as an alternative to injectable antimicrobial therapy. Am J Hosp Pharm. 1990;47(8):1781-4.

65. Rayner CR et al. Linezolid in the treatment of osteomyelitis: results of compassionate use experience. Infection. 2004;32(1):8-14.

66. Schurman DJ, Dillingham M. Clinical evaluation of cefoxitin in treatment of infections in 47 orthopedic patients. Rev Infect Dis.1979;1(1):206-9.

67. Stefanovski N, Van Voris LP. Pyogenic vertebral osteomyelitis: report of a series of 23 patients. Contemp Ortho. 1995;31(3):159-64.

68. Stratov I, Korman TM, Johnson PD. Management of Aspergillus osteomyelitis: report of failure of liposomal amphotericin B and response to voriconazole in an immunocompetent host and literature review. Eur J Clin Microbiol Infect Dis. 2003;22(5):277-83.

69. Bingham EL, Hart GB. Hyperbaric oxygen treatment of refractory osteomyelitis. Postgrad Med. 1977;61(6):70-6.

70. Depenbusch FL, hompson RE, Hart GB. Use of hyperbaric oxygen in the treatment of refractory osteomyelitis: a preliminary report. J Trauma. 1972;12(9):807-12.

71. Davis JC, et al. Chronic non-hematogenous osteomyelitis treated with adjuvant hyperbaric oxygen. J Bone Joint Surg Am. 1986;68(8):1210-7.

72. Morrey BF, et al. Hyperbaric oxygen and chronic osteomyelitis. Clin Orthop Relat Res.1979(144):121-7.

73. Sheps SB. Hyperbaric oxygen for osteomyelitis and osteoradionecrosis. Vancouver: University of British Columbia;1992. Pp.1-21.

74. Senneville E, et al. Effectiveness and tolerability of prolonged linezolid treatment for chronic osteomyelitis: a retrospective study. Clin Ther. 2006;28(8):1155-63.

75. Priest DH, Peacock, Jr JE. Hematogenous vertebral osteomyelitis due to Staphylococcus aureus in the adult: clinical features and therapeutic outcomes. South Med J. 2005;98(9):854-62.

76. Gomez J, et al. [Orthopedic implant infection: prognostic factors and influence of long-term antibiotic treatment on evolution. Prospective study, 1992-1999]. Enferm Infecc Microbiol Clin. 2003;21(5):232-6.

77. Eckardt JJ, Wirganowicz PZ, Mar T. An aggressive surgical approach to the management of chronic osteomyelitis. Clin Orthop Relat Res.1994(298):229-39.

78. Hall BB, Fitzgerald, Jr.,RH, Rosenblatt JE. Anaerobic osteomyelitis. J Bone Joint Surg Am. 1983;65(1):30-5.

79. Marx RE. Chronic osteomyelitis of the jaws. Oral Maxillofac Surg Clin North Am.1991;3:367-81.

80. Mercuri LG. Acute osteomyelitis of the jaws. Oral Maxillofac Surg Clin North Am.1991;3:355-65.

81. Mader JT, et al. Antimicrobial treatment of chronic osteomyelitis. Clin Orthop Relat Res.1999(360):47-65.

82. Waldvogel FA, Medoff G, Swartz MN. Osteomyelitis: a review of clinical features, therapeutic considerations and unusual aspects (second of three parts). N Engl J Med. 1970;282(5):260-6.

83. Gomis M, et al. Oral ofloxacin versus parenteral imipenem-cilastatin in the treatment of osteomyelitis. Rev Esp Quimioter.1999;12(3):244-9.

84. Mader JT, Cantrell JS, Calhoun J. Oral ciprofloxacin compared with standard parenteral antibiotic therapy for chronic osteomyelitis in adults. J Bone Joint Surg Am. 1990;72(1):104-10.

85. Gentry LO, Rodriguez-Gomez G. Ofloxacin versus parenteral therapy for chronic osteomyelitis. Antimicrob Agents Chemother. 1991;35(3):538-41.

86. Jauregui LE, Hageage G, Martin M. Oral enoxacin versus conventional intravenous antimicrobial therapy for chronic osteomyelitis. J Chemother.1989;1(4 Suppl):735-6.

87. Swiontkowski MF, et al. A comparison of short- and long-term intravenous antibiotic therapy in the postoperative management of adult osteomyelitis. J Bone Joint Surg Br. 1999;81(6):1046-50.

88. Spencer,CH. Bone and joint infections in children. Curr Opin Rheumatol. 1998;10(5):494-7.

89. Tetzlaff TR, McCracken Jr. GH, Nelson JD. Oral antibiotic therapy for skeletal infections of children. II. Therapy of osteomyelitis and suppurative arthritis. J Pediatr. 1978;92(3):485-90.

90. Wall EJ. Childhood osteomyelitis and septic arthritis. Curr Opin Pediatr. 1998;10(1):73-6.

91. Higuchi T, et al. Preliminary report of the safety and efficacy of hyperbaric oxygen therapy for specific complications of lung transplantation. J Heart Lung Transplant.2006;25(11):1302-9.

92. Larsson A,et al. Hyperbaric oxygen treatment of postoperative neurosurgical infections. Neurosurgery. 2002;50(2): 287-95; discussion 295-6.

93. Lucente FE, Parisier SC, Som PM. Complications of the treatment of malignant external otitis. Laryngoscope.1983; 93(3):279-81.

94. Waldvogel FA, Medoff G, Swartz MN. Osteomyelitis: a review of clinical features, therapeutic considerations and unusual aspects. N Engl J Med.1970;282(4):198-206.
95. Waldvogel FA, Medoff G, Swartz MN. Osteomyelitis: a review of clinical features, therapeutic considerations and unusual aspects. Osteomyelitis associated with vascular insufficiency. N Engl J Med. 1970;282(6):316-22.
96. Ger R. Muscle transposition for treatment and prevention of chronic post-traumatic osteomyelitis of the tibia. J Bone Joint Surg Am. 1977;59(6):784-91.
97. Gordon L, Chiu EJ. Treatment of infected nonunions and segmental defects of the tibia with staged microvascular muscle transplantation and bone-grafting. J Bone Joint Surg Am. 1988;70(3):377-86.
98. Kelly PJ. Infected nonunion of the femur and tibia. Orthop Clin North Am. 1984;15(3):481-90.
99. May Jr. JW, et al. Clinical classification of posttraumatic tibial osteomyelitis. J Bone Joint Surg Am. 1989;71(9):1422-8.
100. Weiland AJ, Moore JR, Daniel RK. The efficacy of free tissue transfer in the treatment of osteomyelitis. J Bone Joint Surg Am. 1984;66(2):181-93.
101. Mader JT, Shirtliff M, Calhoun JH. Staging and staging application in osteomyelitis. Clin Infect Dis. 1997;25(6): 1303-9.
102. Cierny III G, Mader JT, Penninck JJ. A clinical staging system for adult osteomyelitis. Clin Orthop Relat Res. 2003(414):7-24.
103. Fanning WJ, Vasko JS, Kilman JW. Delayed sternal closure after cardiac surgery. Ann Thorac Surg. 1987;44(2): 169-72.
104. Clarkson JH, et al. Our experience using the vertical rectus abdominis muscle flap for reconstruction in 12 patients with dehiscence of a median sternotomy wound and mediastinitis. Scand J Plast Reconstr Surg Hand Surg. 2003;37(5):266-71.
105. Farinas MC, et al. Suppurative mediastinitis after openheart surgery: a case-control study covering a seven-year period in Santander, Spain. Clin Infect Dis. 1995;20(2):272-9.
106. Athanassiadi K, et al. Omental transposition: the final solution for major sternal wound infection. Asian Cardiovasc Thorac Ann. 2007;15(3):200-3.
107. Rezai AR, et al. Contemporary management of spinal osteomyelitis. Neurosurgery. 1999;44(5):1018-25; discussion 1025-6.
108. Osei-Yeboah C, et al. Osteomyelitis of the frontal bone. Ghana Med J. 2007;41(2):88-90.
109. Blomstedt GC. Craniotomy infections. Neurosurg Clin N Am. 1992;3(2):375-85.
110. Malone DG, et al. Osteomyelitis of the skull base. Neurosurgery. 1992;30(3):426-31.
111. Stieg PE, Mulliken JB. Neurosurgical complications in craniofacial surgery. Neurosurg Clin N Am. 1991;2(3): 703-8.
112. Gallagher RM, Gross CW, Phillips CD. Suppurative intracranial complications of sinusitis. Laryngoscope. 1998;108(11 Pt 1):1635-42.
113. Lucente FE et al. Malignant external otitis: a dangerous misnomer? Otolaryngol Head Neck Surg.1982;90(2):266-9.
114. Tisch M, Maier H. [Malignant external otitis]. Laryngorhinootologie. 2006;85(10):763-9; quiz 770-3.
115. Bhandary, S, Karki P, Sinha BK. Malignant otitis externa: a review. Pac Health Dialog. 2002;9(1):64-7.
116. Slattery III, WH. Brackmann DE. Skull base osteomyelitis. Malignant external otitis. Otolaryngol Clin North Am. 1996;29(5):795-806.
117. Triplett RG, et al. Experimental mandibular osteomyelitis: therapeutic trials with hyperbaric oxygen. J Oral Maxillofac Surg.1982;40(10):640-6.
118. Mendel V, Simanowski HJ, Scholz H. Synergy of HBO2 and a local antibiotic carrier for experimental osteomyelitis due to Staphylococcus aureus in rats. Undersea Hyperb Med.2004;31(4):407-16.
119. Mader JT, et al. Therapy with hyperbaric oxygen for experimental osteomyelitis due to Staphylococcus aureus in rabbits. J Infect Dis. 1978;138(3):312-8.
120. Triplett RG, Branham GB. Treatment of experimental mandibular osteomyelitis with hyperbaric oxygen and antibiotics. Int J Oral Surg. 1981;10(Sup p.1):178-82.
121. Esterhai Jr. JL, et al. Adjunctive hyperbaric oxygen therapy in the treatment of chronic refractory osteomyelitis. J Trauma. 1987;27(7):763-8.
122. Esterhai Jr. JL, et al. Treatment of chronic osteomyelitis complicating nonunion and segmental defects of the tibia with open cancellous bone graft, posterolateral bone graft, and soft-tissue transfer. J Trauma. 1990;30(1):49-54.
123. MacGregor RR, Graziani AL, Esterhai JL. Oral ciprofloxacin for osteomyelitis. Orthopedics. 1990;13(1):55-60.
124. Barili F, et al. Role of hyperbaric oxygen therapy in the treatment of postoperative organ/space sternal surgical site infections. World J Surg. 2007;31(8):1702-6.

Evidence-Based Review

In medical resuscitative intervention, the AHA evidence-based criteria is widely accepted to guide clinical therapeutic intervention.[17] NBO_2 is considered a class I indication while HBO_2 may be a class IIb indication. Controlled animal studies support this assumption, as referenced in Table 1.

Table 1. Evidence-Based Evaluation (29 studies found for review)

AHA		NCI-PDQ *	BMJ **
Level	**Class**		
6a[18–39] (decisive control groups)	IIb (acceptable and useful)[18–29,31,32,36–39]	NA	NA
6b[40–45] (not decisive control group)	IIb (acceptable and useful)[40–42]		
	Indeterminate[43–46]		

* National Cancer Institute Patient Data Query evidence-based criteria (NCI-PDQ)47

** *British Medical Journal* evidence-based criteria (BMJ)48

Rather consistently, this body of literature confirms over and over again better survival in animal models of both hemorrhage to a predetermined mean arterial pressure (Wiggers model)[49] or fixed-volume hemorrhage.[50] Both increased short-term and long-term survival for HBO_2 groups over normobaric air (NBA) or NBO_2 groups.

Published human case reports and case series allow similar evidence-based acceptance. Published case reports or case series are referenced in Table 2.

Table 2. Evidence-Based Evaluation of Human Case Reports/Series

AHA		NCI-PDQ	BMJ
Level	**Class**		
5 (case series and case reports)	IIb (acceptable and useful) [54] Indeterminate [13,16,51–54,57]	3iii (case series or presentation neither consecutive or population based) [13,16,51–55,57]	Most likely beneficial [13,16,51–55,57]
6	IIb[56]	NA	NA

A more detailed report of the above tabulated findings has been published in a focused journal review article on the use of HBO_2 in acute blood loss anemia.[58]

In a recent controlled prospective human trial, the use of postoperative hyperbaric oxygen therapy with restriction of transfusions in patients undergoing a partial hepatectomy for cancer of the liver resulted in improved outcome in the hyperbaric group compared to the non-hyperbaric group (control group *n*=21, HBO_2 group *n*=20). The results suggested that acute HBO_2 therapy after hepatectomy, aimed at reducing perioperative erythrocyte transfusions, may successfully be employed for overcoming deficiencies in systemic and hepatic oxygen supply, thereby diminishing postoperative complications.[59]

In summary, both by the support of animal work and human clinical experience, evidence-based analysis firmly supports the use of HBO_2 as a treatment option in severe anemia using AHA, NCI-PDQ, and *British Medical Journal* evidence-based criteria.

Utilization Review

In review, HBO_2 should be considered in severe anemia when patients cannot receive blood products for medical, religious, or strong personal preferential reasons or situational blood inavailability. Its use should be guided by the patient's calculated accumulating oxygen debt rather than by waiting for signs or symptoms of systemic or individual end-organ failure. HBO_2 should be considered as a bridge therapy until severe life-threatening acute anemia can be resolved.

HBO_2 therapy can be administered rapidly at pressures up to 200–300 kPa for periods of three or four hours three times a day to four times a day if intra-treatment patient air breaks are used. Hematinics should be co-administered along with nutritional support to correct protein energy malnutrition. HBO_2 therapy should be continued with taper of both individual treatment to the time and frequency of treatment tables until RBCs have been replaced adequately by patient regeneration or patient acceptance of transfusion if possible.

Cost Impact

A single HBO_2 treatment table cost is comparable to the cost of one unit of packed RBCs.[13] Side effects of HBO_2 are few and infrequent,[60-63] and safety of hospital-based HBO therapy in the United States has been very good to date.

Summary

In summary, hyperbaric-administered oxygen allows oxygen to be dissolved in increased concentration in red blood cell-poor plasma or crystalloid/colloid-diluted intravascular fluids in a volume-resuscitated patient. Additionally, in both subacutely and chronically anemic patients, pulsed, intermittently provided normobaric, or hyperbaric oxygen induces an increase in red blood cell/hemoglobic mass. Transfusions of separate donor red blood cells are transplantations of tissue not uncomplicated by immunomodulatory reactions. In the long term, autologous blood products may be less problematic than transfused, homologous packed red blood cells to reduce patient oxygen debt in illness or injury. Hyperbaric oxygen can reduce oxygen debt decisively in the polar clinical extremes of exsanguinations with cardiopulmonary arrest all the way to resuscitation of the severely anemic patient who cannot be transfused with red blood cells for religious reasons, immunologic reasons, or blood availability problems.[64] A hyperbaric oxygen treatment is equivalent in wholesale cost to a unit of packed red blood cells in the Western world.

Hyperbaric oxygen provides a low-technology, cost-competitive means of pharmacologically reducing accumulated oxygen debt in the anemic, injured, or critically ill patient with little side effect. To address severe anemia in trauma or illness, the future may well afford the use of hyperbaric oxygen therapy in the military far-forward, in pre-hospital EMS settings, in trauma center emergency departments, in operative and recovery units, and in intensive care units of hospitals.[65,70-72]

Hyperbaric oxygen provides availability in the form of bridge therapy to avoid the dangers from hastily given multiple units of blood for severely inflicted anemia by medical, surgical or traumatic bleeds. After stabilization of the patient, a more measured administration of blood products in lesser quantity becomes an option.

Figure 1. Flowchart of Severe Anemia
Details of management are described in the text.

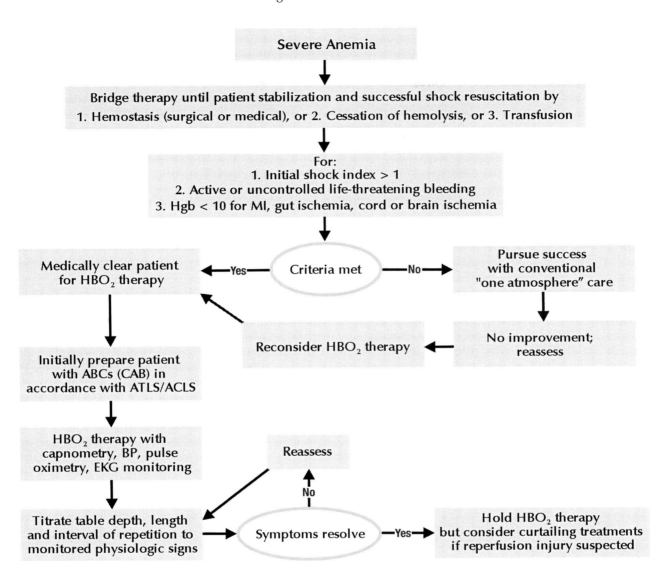

References

1. Van Slyke DD, Neill JM. The determination of gases in blood and other solutions by vacuum extraction and manomet- ric measurement. J Biol Chem. 1924;61:523-573.

2. Chance EM, Chance B. Oxygen delivery to tissue: calculation of oxygen gradient in the cardiac cell. Adv Exp Med Biol. 1988;222:69-75.

3. Fick A. Uber die messung des blut quantums in der herzventrikeln. SB Phys-Med Ges Wurzburg. 1870:16.

4. Shoemaker WC, Appel PL, Kram HB. Tissue oxygen debt as a determinant of lethal and nonlethal post-operative organ failure. Crit Care Med. 1988;16:1117-1120.

5. Goodnough LT, Schander A, Brecher ME. Transfusion medicine: looking into the future. Lancet. 2003;361:161-169.

6. Johnson JL, Moore EE, Gonzalez RJ, et al. Alteration of the post-injury hyperinflammatory response by means of resuscitation with a red cell substitute. J Trauma. 2003;54:133-140.

7. Vamvakas EC. Transfusion associated cancer recurrence and post-operative infection: meta-analysis of randomized controlled clinical trials. Transfusion. 1996;36:175-186.

8. Winslow RM. Blood substitutes. Curr Opin Hematol. 2002;9:146-151.

9. Cohn C, Cushing M. Oxygen therapeutics: perfluorocarbons and blood substitute safety. Crit Care Med. 2009;25:399-414.

10. Kindwall EP, editor. Hyperbaric oxygen therapy: a committee report. Bethesda, MD: Undersea and Hyperbaric Medical Society; 1977.

11. Hampson NB, editor. Hyperbaric oxygen therapy: a committee report. Bethesda, MD: Undersea and Hyperbaric Medical Society; 1999. Pp. 35-36.

12. Hart GB. Hyperbaric oxygen and exceptional blood loss anemia. In: Kindwall EP, Whelan HT, editors. Hyperbaric medicine practice. 2nd ed. revised. Flagstaff, AZ: Best Publishing Co.; 2002. Pp. 741-751.

13. DeBets D, Theunissen S, Devriendt J, et al. The normobaric oxygen paradox: does it increase hemoglobin. Diving and Hyperbar Med. 2012;42(2):67-71.

14. Brozak J, Grande F. Body composition and basal metabolism in man correlation analysis versus physiologic approach. Human Biol. 1955;27:22-31.

15. Boerema I, Meyne NG, Brummelkamp WH, et al. Life without blood. Arch Chir Neerl. 1959;11:70-84.

16. McLoughlin PL, Cope TM, Harrison JC. Hyperbaric oxygen therapy in management of severe acute anemia in a Jehovah's witness. Anesthesia. 1999;54:879-898.

17. Cummins RO, Hazinski MF, Kerber RE, et al. Low-energy biphasic waveform defibrillation: evidence-based review applied to emergency cardiovascular care guidelines. Circulation. 1998;97:1654-1667.

18. Burnet W, Clark RG, Duthie HL, et al. The treatment of shock by oxygen under pressure. Scot Med J. 1959;4:535-538.

19. Cowley RA, Attar S, Esmond WG, et al. Electrocardiographic and biochemical study in hemorrhagic shock in dogs treated with hyperbaric oxygen. Circulation. 1963;27:670-675.

20. Blair E, Henning G, Esmond WG, et al. The effect of hyperbaric oxygenation (OHP) on three forms of shock – traumatic, hemorrhagic, and septic. J Trauma. 1964;4:652-663.

21. Clark RG, Young DG. Effects of hyperoxygenation and sodium bicarbonate in hemorrhagic hypotension. Brit J Surg. 1965;52:705-708.

22. Cowley RA, Attar S, Blair E, et al. Prevention and treatment of shock by hyperbaric oxygenation. Ann NY Acad Sci. 1965;117:673-683.

23. Elliot DP, Paton BC. Effect of 100% oxygen at 1 and 3 atmospheres on dogs subjected to hemorrhagic hypotension. Surg. 1965;57:401-408.

24. Attar S, Scanlan E, Cowley RA. Further evaluation of hyperbaric oxygen in hemorrhagic shock. In: Brown IW, Cox B, editors. Proceedings of the third international congress on hyperbaric medicine. Washington DC: NAS/NRC; 1965. Pp. 417-424.

25. Jacobson YG, Keller ML, Mundth ED, et al. Hyperbaric oxygen therapy in experimental hemorrhagic shock. In: Brown IW, Cox B, editors. Proceedings of the third international congress on hyperbaric medicine. Washington DC: NAS/NRC; 1966. Pp. 425-431.

26. Jacobson YG, Keller ML, Mundth ED, et al. Hemorrhagic shock: influence of hyperbaric oxygen on metabolic parameters. Calif Med. 1966;105:93-96.

27. Navarro RU, Ferguson CC. Treatment of experimental hemorrhagic shock by the combined use of hyperbaric oxygen and low-molecular weight dextran. Surg. 1968;63:775-781.

28. Doi Y, Onji Y. Oxygen deficit in hemorrhagic shock under hyperbaric oxygen. In: Wada J, Iwa JT, editors. Proceedings of the fourth international congress on hyperbaric medicine. Baltimore, MD: Williams and Wilkins; 1970. P. 181-184.

29. Necas E, Neuwirt J. Lack of erythropoietin in plasma of anemic rats exposed to hyperbaric oxygen. Life Sci. 1969;8:1221-1228.

30. Oda T, Takeori M. Effect of viscosity of the blood on increase in cardiac output following acute hemodilation. In: Wada J, Iwa JT, editors. Proceedings of the fourth international congress on hyperbaric medicine. Baltimore, MD: Williams and Wilkins; 1970. Pp. 191-196.

31. Norman JN. Hemodynamic studies in total blood replacement. Biblio Haema. 1975;41:203-208.

32. Luenov AN, Yakovlev VN. Role played by cerebral nitrogen metabolism in the mechanism of the therapeutic oxygen effects under high pressure in the hemorrhagic shock. Biull Eksp Biol Med. 1977;83:418-420.

33. Gross DR, Moreau PM, Jabor M, Welch DW, Fife WP. Hemodynamic effects of dextran-40 on hemorrhagic shock during hyperbaria and hyperbaric hyperoxia. Aviat Space Environ Med. 1983;54:413-419.

34. Gross DR, Moreau PM, Chaikin BN, et al. Hemodynamic effects of lactated Ringers' solution on hemorrhagic shock during exposure to hyperbaric air and hyperbaric hyperoxia. Aviat Space Environ Med. 1983;54:701-708.

35. Gross DR, Dodd KT, Welch DW, Fife WP. Hemodynamic effects of 10% dextrose and of dextran-70 on hemorrhagic shock during exposure to hyperbaric air and hyperbaric hyperoxia. Aviat Space Environ Med. 1984;55:1118-1128.

36. Bitterman H, Reissman P, Bitterman N, et al. Oxygen therapy in hemorrhagic shock. Circ Shock. 1991;33:183-191.

37. Wen-Ren L. Resection of aortic aneurysms under 3 ATA of hyperbaric oxygenation. In: Bakker DJ, Cramer JS, editors. Proceedings of the tenth international congress of hyperbaric medicine. Flagstaff, AZ: Best Publishing Co.; 1992. Pp. 94-95.

38. Adir Y, Bitterman N, Katz E, et al. Salulary consequences of oxygen therapy or long-term outcome of hemorrhagic shock in awake, unrestrained rats. Undersea Hyperb Med. 1995;22:23-30.

39. Yamashita M, Yamashita M. Hyperbaric oxygen treatment attenuates cytokine induction after massive hemorrhage. Am J Physiol Endocrin Metab. 2000;28:E811-E816.

40. Boerema I, Meyne NG, Brummelkamp WH, et al. Life without blood: a study of the influence of high atmosphere pressure and hypothermia on dilution of the blood. J Cardiovasc Surg. 1960;1:133-146.

41. Attar S, Esmond WG, Cowley RA. Hyperbaric oxygenation in vascular collapse. J Thoracic Cardiovasc Surg. 1962;42:759-770.

42. Trytyshnikov IM. Effect of acute massive blood loss during hyperbaric oxygen therapy on nucleic and metabolism in the albino rat liver. Biull Eksp Biol Med. 1974;77:23-25.

43. Frank HA, Fine J. Traumatic shock V: a study of the effect of oxygen on hemorrhagic shock. J Clin Invest. 1943;22:305-314.

44. Whalen RE, Moor GF, Mauney FM, et al. Hemodynamic responses to "Life Without Blood." In: Brown IW, Cox B, editors. Proceedings of the third international congress on hyperbaric medicine. Washington DC: NAS/NRC; 1965. Pp. 402-408.

45. Barkova EN, Petrov AV. The effect of oxygen barotherapy on erythropoeisis in the recuperative period following hemorrhagic collapse. Buill Eksp Biol Med. 1976;81:156-158.

46. Marzella L, Yin A, Darlington D, et al. Hemodynamic responses to hyperbaric oxygen administration in a rat model of hemorrhagic shock. Circ Shock. 1992;37:12.

47. Cancer.Net. Levels of evidence: explanation in therapeutic studies (PDQ). Internet Service of the National Cancer Institute, 1999.

48. Barton S, editor. Clinical evidence. London: BMJ Publishing Group; 2001.

49. Wiggers CJ, Werle JM. Exploration of method for standardizing hemorrhagic shock. Proc Soc Exper Biol Med. 1942;49:604.

50. Bellamy RF, Maningas PA, Wenger BA, et al. Current shock models and clinical correlations. Ann Emerg Med. 1986;15:1392-1395.

51. Ledingham IM. Hyperbaric oxygen in shock. Anes Clin. 1969;7:819-839.

52. Amonic RS, Cockett ATK, Lonhan PH, et al. Hyperbaric oxygen therapy in chronic hemorrhagic shock. JAMA. 1969;208:2051-2054.

53. Hart GB. Exceptional blood loss anemia. JAMA. 1974;228:1028-1029.

54. Myking O, Schreinen A. Hyperbaric oxygen in hemolytic crisis. JAMA. 1974;227:1161-1162.

55. Hart GB, Lennon PA, Strauss MB. Hyperbaric oxygen in exceptional acute blood loss anemia. J Hyperbar Med. 1987;2:205-210.

56. Meyerstein N, Mazor D, Tsach T, et al. Resistance of human red blood cells to hyperbaric oxygen under therapeutic conditions. J Hyperbar Med. 1989;4:1-5.

57. Young BA, Burns JR. Management of the severely anemic Jehovah's Witness. Ann Int Med. 1992;119:170.

58. Van Meter KW. A systematic review of the literature reporting the application of hyperbaric oxygen in the treatment of exceptional blood loss anemia: an evidence-based approach. Undersea Hyperb Med. 2005;32(1):61-83.

59. Hillard JR. Severe claustrophobia in a patient requiring hyperbaric oxygen treatment. Psychosomatics. 1990;31:107-108.

60. Ross ME, Yolton DP, Yolton RL, et al. Myopia associated with hyperbaric oxygen therapy. Optometry and Vision Sci. 1996;73:487-494.

61. Ueno S, Sakoda M, Kurahara H, et al. Safety and efficacy of early post-operative hyperbaric oxygen therapy with restriction of transfusionsin patient with HCC who have undergone partial hepatectomy. Arch Surg. 2011;396:99-106.

62. Blanchard J, Toma A, Bryson P, et al. Middle ear barotrauma in patients undergoing hyperbaric oxygen therapy. Clin Otolaryn. 1996;21:400-403.

63. Youngberg JT, Myers AM. Complications from hyperbaric oxygen therapy. Ann Emerg Med. 1990;19:1356-1357.

64. Van Meter KW, Harch PG. HBO in emergency medicine. In: Jain KK, editor. Textbook of hyperbaric medicine. Cambridge, MA: Hogrefe & Huber Publishers; 1996. Pp. 453-481.

65. Van Meter KW. Hyperbaric oxygen therapy as an adjunct to pre-hospital advanced life support. Surg Technol Int. 2011 Dec 1;XXI:61-73.

66. Donat A, Damani E, Zuccan S, et al. Effects of short-term hyperoxia on erythropoietin levels and microcirculation in critically ill patients: a prospective, observational pilot study. MMC Anesthesiology 2017;17:49-59

67. Van Meter K. Van Meter KW. The effect of hyperbaric oxygen on severe anemia. Undersea Hyperb Med. 2012;39(5):937-42.

68. Saa P, Proctor M, Foster-Getal. Investigational testing for Zika virus among US blood donors. NEJM 2018;378:1778-1788.

69. Harrington T, Kuehnent MJ, Kamel H, et al. West Nile virus infection transmitted by blood transfusion. Transfusion 2004;3:1018-1022.

70. Graffeo C, Dishong W. Severe blood loss anemia in a Jehovah's Witness treated with adjunctive hyperbaric oxygen therapy. American Journal of Emergency Medicine. 2013;31:756.e3-756.e4.

71. Gutierrez G, Brotherton J. Management of severe anemia secondary to menorrhagia in a Jehovah's Witness: a case report and treatment algorithm. American Journal of Obstetrics & Gynecology. 2011;205(2):e5-8.

72. Wright JK, Ehler W, McGlasson DL, Thompson W. Facilitation of recovery from acute blood loss with hyperbaric oxygen. Archives of Surgery. 2002;137:850-853.

CHAPTER 14

Adjunctive Hyperbaric Oxygen Therapy in the Treatment of Thermal Burns

Paul Cianci MD, FAC, FUHM (Corresponding Author), Ronald M. Sato MD, Julia Faulkner

Abstract / Rationale

A significant and consistently positive body of evidence from animal and human studies of thermal injury supports the use of hyperbaric oxygen as a means of preventing dermal ischemia, reducing edema, modulating the zone of stasis, preventing partial- to full-thickness conversion, preserving cellular metabolism and promoting healing. The vast majority of clinical reports have shown reduction in mortality, length of hospital stay, number of surgeries and cost of care. Hyperbaric oxygen has been demonstrated to be safe in the hands of those thoroughly trained in rendering this therapy in the critical care setting and with appropriate monitoring precautions. Careful patient selection is mandatory.

Background

The National Burn Repository reviewed the combined data of acute burn admissions for the time period between 2006 through 2015. The key findings included data from 96 hospitals, 36 states, and the District of Columbia, totaling 205,033 records. Male patients outnumber female patients considerably. The bimodal distribution with the greatest prevalence in the pediatric age range from 1-15 compromised 30% of total burns, while the adult age group from 20-59 comprised 54% of burns. Patients age 60 or older represented 14% of burn cases. More than 75% of reported total burn cases involved less than 10% total body surface area and resulted in a mortality of 0.6%. The mortality rates were 3.3% for all cases and 5.8% for fire/flame injuries.

Seventy-three percent of burn injuries have occurred in the home. Nearly 95% of all reviewed burn injuries were identified as accidents, with 14% reported as work-related cases. Just over 2% were suspected of abuse, and 1% were self-inflicted. During the 10-year period from 2006-2015, the average length of stay for females declined from 9.3 days to 7.9 days while that for males declined less significantly, from 9.1 to 8.8 days. The mortality rate for females declined from 4.1% to 2.9%, while in males, the decline was 3.9% to 3%.

Deaths from burn injury increased with advancing age and burn size as well as presence of inhalation injury. A 20-39% burn in patients below 60 confers a morality rate of 2.5%. In the presence of inhalation injury, mortality rate increases to 14%. The same injury in a 60-year-old shows a mortality of 32%, which increases to 55.8% in the presence of inhalation injury. Thus, age and inhalation injury, as well as burn size, are important factors in burn injury survival. Pneumonia was the most frequent, clinically-related complication, occurring in 5.4% of fire/flame or flame-injured patients. The frequency of pneumonia and respiratory failure was greater in patients with four days or greater of mechanical ventilation. The rate of complications also increased with age.

For survivors, the length of stay was slightly greater than one day per percent total body surface area burn. For patients who died, the total hospital days were two times that of survivors on the average. However, this trend was reversed in patients with less than 20% total body surface burns. Eighty-seven percent of patients were discharged to home, while 3% were transferred to rehab facilities. Overall, charges for patients who died were three times greater than those who survived. However, this result was greatly affected by the large number of patients with less than 10% total body surface area burns. For this group, total charges averaged $257,582 for survivors, while nonsurvivors' charges averaged $340,474.

Burn care is extraordinarily expensive. Charges for a 50-59% total body surface area averaged $1,066,254 in 2015. A 60–70% burn averaged $1,168,006 during the same time frame. Workers compensation or automobile insurance were involved in approximately 10% of reviewed cases, while "no information provided" or self-insured is indicated in 29% of cases.

Significant morbidity attaches to burn injury: pneumonia, cellulitis, respiratory failure, urinary tract infection, wound infection, and sepsis are still the most frequently reported complications adding to mortality.[1] Therapy of burns, therefore, is directed to minimizing edema, preserving marginally viable tissue in the zone of stasis, protecting the microvasculature, enhancing host defenses, and providing the essential substrates necessary to maintain viability. The ultimate goals of burn therapy include survival of the patient, rapid wound healing, minimization of scarring or abnormal pigmentation, prevention of long-term problems such as chronic pain, and cost effectiveness. Optimal outcome, obviously, is restoration, as nearly as possible, to the pre-burn quality of life.[2,4]

A recent report by Wolf et al., summarized problems and research priorities in burns for the coming decade.[3] A major and continuing clinical problem is the innate inflammatory response induced by genetic factors such as those common in neutrophils and macrophages which are massively increased while the T-cell adaptive responses are downregulated. The latter are, perhaps, responsible for late effects of severe burns such as viral and fungal infections. Hyperbaric oxygen therapy has been shown to modulate white cell adherence and be helpful in the initial stages of inflammation. This could be an area of fruitful investigation. In fact, the burn injury may be "the universal trauma model." Wolf and colleagues point out control of the hypermetabolic response and the massive inflammation will be important to improvement in burn care.

Despite the advances of early excision in accelerating healing, we seem to have plateaued in this regard. The authors suggest it may be time to visit the notion of whether healing times can be accelerated. This is another area of potential benefit of hyperbaric oxygen. A continuing problem in burn therapy and one for future investigation, again suggested by Wolf et al., is the elimination of pain, both acute and chronic. Neuropathic pain is typically difficult to treat and thought to occur in a large percentage of those suffering severe burns.

Pathophysiology

Physiologic responses to a major burn include a fall in arterial pressure, tachycardia, and a progressive decrease in cardiac output and stroke volume. Metabolic responses are complex and include metabolic acidosis and hyperventilation. Cellular adenosine triphosphate levels fall, resting cell membrane potential decreases, and an intracellular accumulation of sodium, calcium and water is paralleled by a loss of cellular potassium.

Immunologic responses include alteration of macrophage function and perturbation of cellular and humoral immunity.[5] The burn wound is a complex and dynamic injury characterized by a zone of coagulation, surrounded by an area of stasis, and bordered by an area of erythema.[6] The zone of coagulation or complete capillary occlusion may progress by a factor of 10 during the first 48 hours after injury. This phenomenon is three-dimensional; thus, the wound can increase in size and depth during this critical period.

Local microcirculation is compromised to the greatest extent during the 12 to 24 hours post-burn. Burns are in this dynamic state of flux for up to 72 hours after injury.[5] Ischemic necrosis quickly follows. Hematologic changes include platelet microthrombi and hemoconcentration in the post-capillary venules. Edema formation is rapid in the area of injury secondary to increased capillary permeability, decreased oncotic pressure, increased interstitial oncotic pressure, changes in the interstitial space compliance and lymphatic damage.[7] Edema is most prominent in directly involved burned tissues but also develops in distant uninjured tissue, including muscle, intestine and lung. Changes occur in the distant microvasculature, including red cell aggregation, white cell adhesion to venular walls and platelet thromboemboli.[8]

Inflammatory mediators are elaborated locally, in part from activated platelets, macrophages and leukocytes. This contributes to the local and systemic hyper-permeability of the microcirculation, appearing histologically as gaps in the venular and capillary endothelium.[9] This progressive process may extend dramatically during the first early days after injury.[10-11]

The ongoing tissue damage in thermal injury is due to multiple factors, including the failure of surrounding tissue to supply borderline cells with oxygen and nutrients necessary to sustain viability.[6] Impediment of the circulation below the injury results in dessication of the wound, as fluid cannot be supplied via the thrombosed or obstructed capillaries. Topical agents and dressings may reduce, but cannot prevent, the dessication of the burn wound and the inexorable progression to deeper layers. Altered permeability is not caused by heat injury alone; oxidants and other mediators (prostaglandins, kinins and histamine) all contribute to vascular permeability.[12]

Neutrophils are a major source of oxidants and injury in the ischemia/reperfusion mechanism. This complex may be favorably affected by several interventions. Therapy is focused on the reduction of dermal ischemia, reduction of edema and prevention of infection. During the period of early hemodynamic instability, edema reduction has a markedly beneficial effect as well as modulating later wound conversion from partial- to full-thickness injury.[13]

Infection

Infection remains the leading overall cause of death from burns. Susceptibility to infection is greatly increased due to the loss of the integumentary barrier to bacterial invasion, the ideal substrate present in the burn wound, and the compromised or obstructed microvasculature, which prevents humoral and cellular elements from reaching the injured tissue.

Additionally, the immune system is seriously affected, demonstrating decreased levels of immunoglobulins, serious perturbations of polymorphonuclear leukocyte function,[14-15] including disorders of chemotaxis, phagocytosis and diminished killing ability. These functions greatly increase morbidity and mortality. Certain patients with specific polymorphisms in the tumor necrosis factor and bacterial recognition genes may have a higher incidence of sepsis than the burn injury alone would predict.[16] More recently, fungal infections have become a therapeutic challenge.[17]

Regeneration cannot take place until equilibrium is reached; hence, healing is retarded. Prolongation of the healing process may lead to excessive scarring. Hypertrophic scars are seen in about 4% of cases taking 10 days to heal, 14% of cases taking 14 days or less, 28% of cases taking 21 days to heal, and up to 40% of cases taking longer than 21 days to heal.[18]

Figure 1. Tissue Oxygen Tension

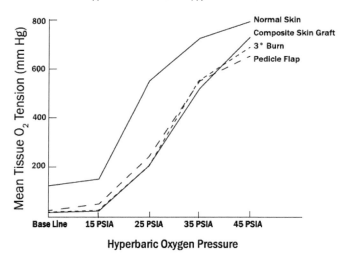

Mean oxygen tension of normal skin and various hypoxic tissues as a function of hyperbaric oxygen pressure. Note: Oxygen tension rises in burned skin only with increasing pressure. (With permission.)

Figure 2. Capillary State: Control vs. HBO$_2$

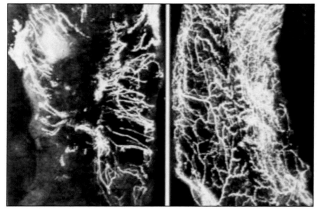

Left panel: Capillary disorganization, inflammation and leakage of contrast agent in control.

Right panel: Restoration organized capillary arcades and intact circulation in HBO$_2$-treated animal.

(With permission.)

Experimental Data

The efficacy of hyperbaric oxygen (HBO$_2$) in the treatment of thermal injury is supported by animal studies and human clinical data. Edema reduction with HBO$_2$ therapy has been demonstrated in burned rabbits,[19] rats,[20] mice[21] and guinea pigs.[22-23] Improvement in healing time has been reported in burned rabbits[24] and rats.[25-26] Decreased infection rates were an additional observation noted in these models.[24-25]

In a seminal study in 1970 Gruber (Figure 1) demonstrated that the area subjacent to a third-degree burn was hypoxic when compared to normal skin and that the tissue oxygen tension could be raised only by oxygen administered at pressure.[27] Ketchum, in 1967, reported an improvement in healing time and reduced infection in an animal model.[24] He later demonstrated dramatic improvement in the microvasculature of burned rats treated with hyperbaric oxygen therapy.[25] (Figure 2)

In 1974, Hartwig[20] confirmed these findings and additionally noted less inflammatory response and suggested hyperbaric oxygen might be a useful adjunct to the technique of early debridement. Wells and Hilton (Figure 3), in a carefully designed and controlled experiment, reported a marked decrease (35%) in extravasation of fluid in 40% of flame-burned dogs.[28] The effect was clearly related to oxygen, and not simply to increased pressure. A reduction in hemoconcentration and improved cardiac output were also noted.

Nylander (Figure 4)[21] in a well-accepted animal model showed that hyperbaric oxygen therapy reduced the generalized edema associated with burn injury.

Kaiser (Figure 5) reported that hyperbaric oxygen treatment resulted in shrinkage of third-degree (full-thickness) injury in a rabbit model. Untreated animals demonstrated the expected increase in wound size during the first 48 hours. At all times treated animal wounds remained smaller than those of the controls. A reduction in subcutaneous edema was also observed.[22-23] Stewart and colleagues subjected rats to controlled burn wounds resulting in deep partial-thickness injury. Both experimental groups were treated with topical agents. The hyperbaric

Figure 3. Plasma Volume Losses

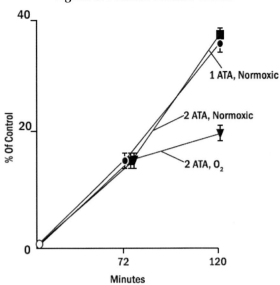

Plasma volume losses after burn in untreated animals (1 atmosphere absolute [ATA], normoxic), animals exposed to hyperbaric oxygen (2 ATA, O$_2$) and to pressure alone (2 ATA, normoxic). (With permission.)

Figure 4. Water Content of the Contralateral Unburned Ear

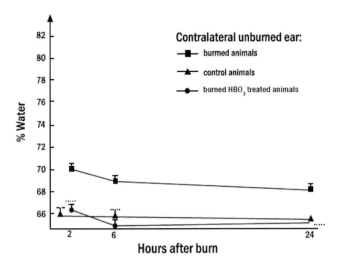

Water content (+) of the contralateral unburned ear in burned animals with and without HBO$_2$ treatment. (With permission.)

oxygen-treated animals showed preservation of dermal elements, no conversion of partial- to full-thickness injury, and preservation of adenosine triphosphate (ATP) levels. The untreated animals demonstrated marked diminution in ATP levels and conversion of partial- to full-thickness injury (Figures 6,7).[29-30]

These studies may relate directly to the preservation of energy sources for the sodium pump in cellulary physiology. Failure of the sodium pump is felt to be a major factor in the ballooning of the endothelial cells, which occurs after burn injury and subsequent massive fluid losses.[10] Germonpré reported decreased extension of burn injury with HBO$_2$.[31] HBO$_2$ has also been shown to dramatically improve the microvasculature of burned rats (Hartwig, Ketchum[20,25]). In guinea pigs, earlier return of capillary patency ($p<0.05$) was demonstrated using an India ink technique.[32]

Miller and Korn reported faster re-epithelialization ($p<0.001$) from these regenerative sites in guinea pigs treated with HBO$_2$ vs. controls. The observed decrease in wound desiccation in the HBO$_2$-treated group was due to preservation of capillary integrity in the zone of stasis.[12] Saunders similarly reported improved dermal circulation, preservation of dermal elements, and less collagen denaturation with HBO$_2$ treatments.[33]

Figure 5. Tissue Oxygen Tension

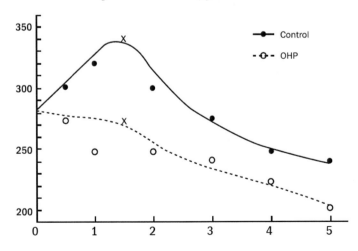

Kaiser and colleagues have recently demonstrated a significant reduction of subcutaneous edema in burned animals treated with HBO$_2$. He reported progression of the burn wound in controls, while in the hyperbaric-treated animal wound size decreased.[21] (With permission.)

Figure 6. Rat Burns Treated with Sulfadiazine Dressing

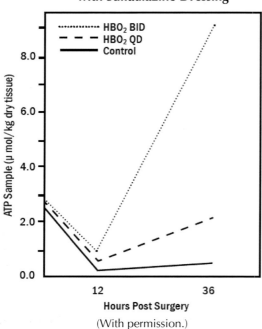

(With permission.)

Figure 7. Partial-Thickness Burns

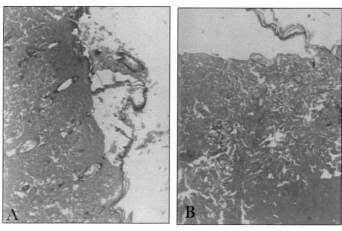

Biopsy of experimental partial thickness burns at 5 days.

A. Left: HBO₂-treated animals show preservation of the dermal elements.

B. Right: Nontreated animals show coagulations necrosis.

(With permission.)

On the other hand, Perrins, in a porcine scald model, failed to demonstrate modification of progressive tissue destruction. However, oxygen was administered at 2 atmospheres absolute (ATA) for only one hour, and treatment occurred over only a one-day period. No vascular studies were undertaken. It was also noted that the porcine model may not be appropriate given the following features about pigs: natural resistance to skin infection; skin that does not form a blister following scald wound injury; and lack of many shared dermal elements with humans, including cutaneous sweat glands.[34]

Also highlighting a further study, Niccole reported that HBO₂ provided no advantage in the treatment of full-thickness and partial-thickness burns alone or in combination with topical antibiotic therapy in controlling bacterial counts in a rat model. However, despite a treatment delay of 12 hours, hyperbaric oxygen significantly reduced the time to complete epithelialization in a partial-thickness burn injury.[26]

The pathophysiologic changes within the burn wound show a striking similarity to those noted in the ischemia reperfusion injury, i.e., depletion of ATP, production of xanthine oxidase, lipid peroxidation, activation of polymorphonuclear cells with subsequent endothelial adherence and generation of reactive oxygen species (ROS).[35-38]

Recent data regarding HBO₂ cardiac preconditioning (inducing cellular tolerance and protection from ischemia) and adaptive responses resulting in cardioprotection and attenuation of ischemia-reperfusion injury are mediated by HBO₂-induced ROS (e.g., superoxide and hydrogen peroxide) that stimulate the production of nitric oxide. HBO₂-induced reactive oxygen species (ROS) are known to initiate gene expression and reduce neutrophil adhesion (via a decrease in CDl1a/18 function, *P*-selectin and down-regulation of intracellular adhesion molecule-1). HBO₂ also decreases lipid peroxidation, stimulates neovascularization and increases antioxidants, thus resulting in cardioprotection.[39] Elucidation of these mechanisms for cardioprotection may provide further understanding of the mechanisms whereby hyperbaric oxygen is of benefit in acute thermal injury.

In a model of reperfusion injury, Zamboni demonstrated that hyperbaric oxygen is a potent blocker of white cell adherence to endothelial cell walls in skeletal muscle, interrupting the cascade that causes vascular damage.[40] The mechanism is felt to be an inhibitory effect on the CD18 locus.[41] As discussed by Wasiak et al.,[42] inhibition of beta 2-integrin activation of intracellular adhesion molecule one (ICAM-1)[43] enables tissues to maintain microvascular flow in areas otherwise subject to the well-described "secondary injury" following a thermal burn.[8] This effect persists for some hours, as demonstrated by both Ueno[44] and Milijkovic-Lolic;[45] Germonpré's data support this observation and may explain the beneficial effect of hyperbaric oxygen therapy on the microcirculation previously observed.[20,29-31,33]

Shoshani reported no benefit of HBO_2 in a rat burn model where all animals received standard sulfadiazine treatment.[46] There was no difference in burn wound size, re-epithelialization rate, Doppler blood flow or healing. In this report, the author erroneously stated that this was the first study utilizing standard burn care (topical agents). Compared to the earlier study by Stewart's group, which utilized silver sulfadiazine dressings and confirmed preservation of dermal elements[29-31] these contradictory findings might be explained by methodological differences.

Bleser and Benichoux, in a very large controlled study in a rat model of 30% body surface area (BSA) burns, reported reduced burn shock and a fourfold increased survival in HBO_2-treated animals vs. controls.[47] Tenenhaus and colleagues showed reduction in mesenteric bacterial colonization ($p<0.005$) in an HBO_2-treated burned mouse model.[48] Bacterial translocation is felt to be a major source of burn wound infection.

In 2005 Magnotti et al. proposed an evolution from bacterial translocation to gut ischemia-reperfusion injury after burn injury as the pathogenesis of multiple organ dysfunction syndrome. Systemic inflammation, acute lung injury and multiple organ failure after a major thermal injury are relatively common causes of morbidity and mortality. In the normal host, the intestinal mucosa functions as a major local defense barrier, a component of multiple defense mechanisms that helps prevent gut bacteria, as well as their products, from crossing the mucosal barrier. After a major thermal injury, and in other clinical and experimental situations, this intestinal barrier function becomes overwhelmed or impaired, resulting in the movement of bacteria and/or endotoxin to the mesenteric lymph nodes and systemic tissues, defined as bacterial translocation. The importance of this intestinal barrier function becomes clear when considering that the distal small bowel and colon contain 10^{10} concentrations of anaerobes and 10^5 to 10^8 each of Gram-positive and Gram-negative aerobic and facultative microorganisms per gram of tissue, and enough endotoxin to kill the host thousands of times over.[49]

Loss of gut barrier function and a resultant gut inflammatory response lead to the production of proinflammatory factors; this can cause a septic state, leading to distant organ failure. Splanchnic hypoperfusion leading to gut ischemia-reperfusion injury appears to be the dominant hemodynamic event, triggering the release of biologically active factors into the mesenteric lymphatics. The benefits of the early use of hyperbaric oxygen in burn victims may in part be mediated through amelioration of gut reperfusion injury.

The beneficial effects of HBO_2 in ischemic-reperfused tissues have been demonstrated in intestine,[50] skeletal muscle,[40,51] brain[52-54] and testicular tissue,[55] and myocardium.[39,56-58] In a study of severely burned humans (>30% TBSA), HBO_2-treated patients compared to controls had increased levels of serum-soluble interleukin-2 receptor ($p<0.05$) and decreased plasma fibronectin ($p<0.01$), resulting clinically in a lower incidence of sepsis ($p<0.05$).[59]

Total enteral nutrition, starting as early as possible after thermal injury, is recommended for burn patients. It results in decreased morbidity and mortality, and supports intestinal structure and function. Studies of intestinal barrier function biology, pathophysiology and consequences of gut barrier failure demonstrate that the ischemic and/or stressed gut can become a proinflammatory organ,[60] and gut-derived factors liberated after periods of splanchnic hypoperfusion can lead to acute distant organ, cellular dysfunction and activation of neutrophils and other proinflammatory cells.[61]

Reduction of PMNL-killing ability in hypoxic tissue has been well documented.[62-63] The ability of hyperbaric oxygen to elevate tissue oxygen tension and the enhancement of PMNL killing in an oxygen-enriched animal model as demonstrated by Mader[63] suggest that this may be an additional benefit of HBO$_2$. Hussman and colleagues have shown no evidence of HBO$_2$-induced immunosuppression in a carefully controlled animal model.[65]

In a 2005 randomized controlled study, Bilic evaluated the effects of HBO$_2$ on burn wound healing. Standard deep second-degree burns were produced in male Wistar rats treated with silver sulfadiazine and then randomly assigned to either a normoxic, placebo gas or to 2.5 atmospheres absolute (ATA) HBO$_2$ for 60 minutes for a total of 21 sessions. HBO$_2$ had a beneficial effect on post-burn edema ($p=0.022$), neoangiogenesis ($p=0.009$), numbers of regenerative active follicles ($p=0.009$), and time to epithelial regeneration ($p=0.048$). There were no significant differences in necrosis staging or margination of leukocytes. The authors conclude that the data support earlier conclusions that HBO$_2$ is of benefit in the healing of burn wounds.[66]

Turkaslan et al.[67] reported that hyperbaric oxygen treatment reduced progression of the zone of stasis in the first 24 hours after injury and accelerated the healing process by supporting neoangiogenesis. Prevention of progression in the zone of stasis is a major goal in burn therapy. This report lends further credence to the previously cited work of Miller, Korn, Hartwig and Ketchum.

HBO$_2$ has been shown to mobilize stem/progenitor cells in both humans and mice by stimulating bone marrow stromal cell type 3 (endothelial) nitric oxide synthase.[68-72] Findings indicate that some of the mobilized cells will home to peripheral sites where they function as de novo endothelial progenitor cells (EPCs), contributing to wound vasculogenesis, a complement to local angiogenesis. Additionally, at peripheral sites HBO$_2$ stimulates stem cell growth and differentiation by engaging a physiological autocrine loop responsive to oxidative stress, much the same as lactate.[73-75]

HBO$_2$ stimulates peripheral site EPCs recruitment and differentiation via a pathway involving thioredoxin-1, hypoxia-inducible factors-1 (HIF-1) and HIF-2. These findings provide new insight into possible mechanisms for the known clinical benefits of hyperbaric oxygen.

The overwhelming body of evidence in a large number of controlled animal studies demonstrates that hyperbaric oxygen reduces dermal ischemia, reduces edema, prevents conversion of partial- to full-thickness injury, preserves the microcirculation, and preserves ATP and cellular integrity. Additional benefits may be enhancement of PMNL killing and modulation of ischemia reperfusion injury, resulting in improved survival.

Clinical Experience

In 1965, Wada observed improved healing of burns in coal miners being treated for carbon monoxide poisoning with HBO$_2$. Later clinical series by Ikeda, Wada, Lamy, Tabor and Grossman[19,75-80] showed improved healing,[75] decreased length of hospital stay,[80] decreased mortality,[80-81] decreased overall cost of care,[80-82] improved morbidity,[80] decreased fluid requirements (30-35%),[81] and decreased number of surgeries ($p<0.041$).[82] Niu reported a very large clinical outcome series showing a statistically significant reduction in mortality ($p=0.028$) in 266 seriously burned patients who received HBO$_2$ when compared to 609 control patients.[81] The author also observed a lower incidence of infection and stated that HBO$_2$ allowed the burn surgeon more time to more accurately define the extent of injury.

Figure 8. Maximum Weight Gain/3 Days

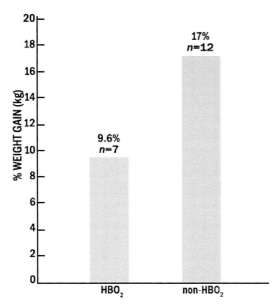

Maximum weight gain at three days expressed as percentage of admission weight. HBO_2 treated patients showed a 45 percent reduction in weight gain ($p<0.03$).[87] (With permission.)

Figure 9. Maximum Length as Function of Time

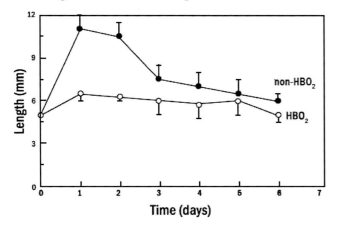

Maximum length (including edema adjacent to the wound) (mean ± s.d.) of u.v.-irradiated (●) and HBO_2-treated U.V.-irradiated (○) blister wounds as a function of time. The value on a) is approximately the diameter of the suction cup used to create the blister ($p<0.05$). (With permission.)

Cianci has shown a significant reduction in length of hospital stay in burns up to 39% TBSA.[83] Additionally noted was a reduction in the need for surgery, including grafting, in a series of patients with 40-80% burns when compared to non-HBO_2-treated controls. HBO_2-treated patients showed an average savings of 36% ($120,000) per case.[82] Adjusted for inflation, this would represent a saving of $227,000 per case in 2016 U.S. dollars.

Hart reported a sham controlled randomized series showing reduced fluid requirements, mean healing time ($p<0.005$), mortality and morbidity in 10-50% TBSA burn patients treated with HBO_2 when compared to controls and to United States National Burn Information Exchange Standards.[85]

Frequently cited as a negative study, a retrospective paired controlled series of burn patients treated with HBO_2, Waisbren reported increased sepsis, reduced renal function and decreased circulating white blood cells in HBO_2-treated patients. The author stated he could demonstrate neither a salutory nor deleterious effect on mortality.[86] Despite these negative conclusions, it should be noted that there was an important 75% reduction in the need for grafting ($p<0.001$) in the hyperbaric group.

In a randomized controlled study of 37 partial-thickness burn patients treated with HBO_2 vs. 37 controls, Merola reported increased granulation, faster healing and decreased scarring.[87]

Cianci observed similar results in a series of patients averaging 28% TBSA burns.[88] In a small blinded review, Cianci's group reported a 25% reduction in resuscitative fluid requirements ($p<0.07$) and maximum (and percent) weight gain ($p<0.012$) in seriously burned (40-80% TBSA) patients treated with adjunctive HBO_2 vs. controls at a regional burn center[82,84] (Figure 8).[89]

In a controlled pilot series, Maxwell reported reduced surgery, resuscitative weight gain, intensive care days, total hospitalization time, wound sepsis and cost of hospitalization in the HBO_2 group.[90] Cianci reported reduced surgeries ($p<0.03$), length of hospital stay (53%) and cost of care (49%) in 40-80% TBSA burns.[91] Hammarlund and colleagues showed reduced edema and wound exudation in a controlled series of human volunteers with UV-irradiated blister wounds[92] (Figure 9).

In a subsequent similar study, Niezgoda (Figure 10) demonstrated reduced wound size ($p<0.03$), laser Doppler-measured hyperemia ($p<0.05$) and wound exudate ($p<0.04$) in the HBO$_2$-treated group. This study was the first prospective randomized, controlled, double-blinded trial comparing HBO$_2$ with sham controls in a human burn model.[93]

In a study purporting to conclude limited positive impact of hyperbaric oxygen therapy for burn patients, Brannen et al. in 1997[94] reported a randomized prospective trial of hyperbaric oxygen in the treatment of burn injury. Sixty-three patients received hyperbaric oxygen and 62 served as controls. One-third of the hyperbaric-treated patients

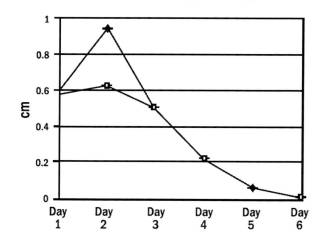

Figure 10. Hyperbaric Oxygen Therapy for Burns

Wound size measurements (cm) of ultraviolet-irradiated suction blister wounds in control group (□) and hyperbaric oxygen group (♦). Graph courtesy of Dr. Jeffrey A. Niezgoda.

received their first treatment within eight hours of injury. However, the average time to treatment was 11.5 hours after the burn injury. The authors noted no difference in the outcome measures of mortality, number of operations, or length of stay, stating they were unable to demonstrate any significant benefit to burn patients from the use of hyperbaric oxygen.

There were serious limitations in this study. Two-thirds of patients did not receive their first treatment until more than eight hours after burn injury, with a mean of 11.5 hours. Results in the subset of patients receiving earlier treatment were not examined separately. Important outcome measures not studied were functional and cosmetic aspects of facial, hand and perineal burns. Length of stay, number of surgeries, and extent of grafting are subject to a variety of confounding influences, including economic (e.g., hospital and insurance, utilization management, physician reimbursement) and social considerations (e.g., lack of adequate housing, caregivers and rehabilitation efforts).

Despite randomization for age, burn size and inhalation injury, the populations were still heterogeneous. Comorbidity was not examined. Further, all patients underwent exceedingly early and aggressive excisional therapy with rapid discharge to a lesser level of care. While the authors failed to conclude there were significant benefits of HBO$_2$ for burn patients in this study, the authors did observe less fluid loss, drier wounds, which necessitated fewer dressing changes, and earlier healing. Further analysis also showed a significant reduction in hospital costs in the hyperbaric group.

Recent Perspectives

Pain Management

There is a substantial body of evidence reporting the use of hyperbaric oxygen therapy in pain attenuation. Sutherland and colleagues[95] have done an excellent review of the literature and conclude that hyperbaric oxygen therapy has been proven to demonstrate a significant antinociceptive effect. They state early clinical research indicates that hyperbaric oxygen therapy may be useful in modulating human pain; however, further studies are required to determine whether HBO_2 is a safe and efficacious treatment modality.

A particularly difficult problem for some burn patients is that opioid overuse contributes to adaptive immune suppression, and this may be associated with poorer outcomes. Neuropathic pain is typically difficult to treat and thought to occur in a large percentage of those suffering severe burns. Rasmussen and colleagues[96] have reported a series of 17 patients who underwent a controlled first-degree burn. One group was treated at atmospheric pressure $FiO_2 = 0.21$ during hyperbaric treatment. Another group was treated at 2.4 ATM breathing 100% O_2. Patients who underwent chamber treatment demonstrated attenuation of secondary hyperalgesia, i.e., an antinociceptive effect. The authors state that post-burn hyperbaric oxygen therapy has a potent antinociceptive effect that works at a central desensitization level. The authors suggest this thermal injury model may give impetus to future neurophysiologic studies exploring the central effects of hyperbaric oxygen treatment.

Chong et al.[97] reported a group of 17 burn patients who were treated with hyperbaric oxygen or routine burn care. They noted no difference in inflammatory cytokines or depth of burns, though patients in both groups either increased or reduced estimated depth of injury. There were fewer positive biopsies for bacterial colonization in the hyperbaric group. They also related this was a preliminary study and of insufficient power to determine any real statistical significance, as 40 patients would have been required to achieve this goal. It was unclear as to the average time from injury to the provision of hyperbaric oxygen therapy. However, it was stated that patients were treated during "routine hyperbaric treatment sessions" and that the HBO_2 patients received two treatments within the first 22 hours. It would be more appropriate to treat as soon as the patient is stable as reported by others.

Jones et al.[98] have reported a series of diabetic patients suffering foot burns. Transcutaneous O_2 studies were performed, and those patients who had low TcO_2s and responded to an oxygen challenge underwent hyperbaric oxygen therapy in addition to standard care. There were 18 patients in the hyperbaric study group. All healed, with one amputation. The authors compared this to a group of 68 patients treated with traditional care. Eleven patients in this cohort suffered 31 amputations. The authors reported the observations of their burn surgeons that, with a larger sample size, a definite benefit could be demonstrated. Of note, three of the patients who were scheduled for grafting healed spontaneously with HBO_2 alone.

Immunity and Infection

A major and continuing clinical problem is the innate inflammatory response induced by genetic factors such as those common in neutrophils and macrophages, which are massively increased while the T-cell adaptive responses are downregulated. Zhang and colleagues[99] have shown that hyperbaric oxygen attenuates apoptosis and decreases inflammation in an ischemic wound model. The effect of hyperbaric oxygen on modulation of white cell adherence to endothelium has been described. Thom et al. have studied the effect of hyperbaric oxygen and demonstrated that HBO_2 additionally does not alter platelet function but inhibits Beta 2 integrin adhesion to endothelium at pressures of 2.8 or more. This would have a beneficial effect on the early stages of burn injury.[100]

Stem Cell Effects

Thom et al. have reported that hyperbaric oxygen increases marrow stem cell populations, and these cells migrate to areas of wounding.[101-102] The previously reported preservation of dermal elements, specifically, hair follicles, may represent an additional area for recruitment of native stem cells in the healing of burns. This has been described by Stewart et al.[103-104] These should be areas of fruitful research in burn patients where prolonged healing is a major problem.

Antioxidant Effects

Concern about oxygen toxicity is valid. However, Sureda and colleagues[105] have studied the effect of hyperbaric oxygen therapy in chronic wounds and reported that this modality actually enhanced plasma antioxidant defenses and contributed to the activation of healing resolution, angiogenesis, and vascular tone regulation by increasing the VEGF and IL-6 release and the endothelin-1 decrease. These may be significant factors in simulating wound healing. In clinical practice, acute oxygen toxicity is very rare and usually associated with prolonged treatments utilized in decompression sickness.

Inhalation Injury

Considerable attention has been given to the use of HBO_2 in inhalation injury due in part to fear that HBO_2 may cause worsening of pulmonary damage, particularly in those patients maintained on high levels of inspired oxygen. The more extensive the burn injury, the higher the incidence of an inhalation injury.[106] Pulmonary injury caused by smoke inhalation is a major cause of fire-related deaths.[107] The airway injury can be worsened by a variety of chemical pyrolysis products, depending on the material burned.[108]

Grim studied products of lipid peroxidation in the exhaled gases in HBO_2-treated burn patients and found no indication of oxidative stress.[109] In comparison with a comparable size burn alone, the combination of a body burn and smoke inhalation injury results in a marked increase in mortality and morbidity, in hemodynamic instability, in burn wound edema, a 30-50% increase in initial fluid requirements and an accentuation of lung dysfunction.

Ray analyzed a series of severely burned patients being treated for concurrent inhalation injury, thermal injury and adult respiratory distress syndrome.[110] The author noted no deleterious effect of HBO_2, even in those on continuous high levels of inspired oxygen. More rapid weaning from mechanical ventilation was possible in the HBO_2-treated group (5.3 days vs. 26 days, $p<0.05$). There was a significant reduction in cost of care per case of $67,000 in the HBO_2-treated patients ($p<0.05$). Adjusted to 2016 U.S. dollars, this figure would be $121,000. There is no current evidence to controvert these studies.

2009 Cochrane Review

In a 2009 Cochrane Data Base systemic review of the efficacy of HBO_2 for thermal burns, Villanueva et al. identified four randomized controlled studies, of which two satisfied their inclusion criteria.[111]

In the first trial in 1974,[85] Hart reported reduced fluid requirements and mean healing time ($p<0.005$), and reduced mortality and morbidity when compared to controls. There was also a reduction in mortality and morbidity when compared to the National Burn Information Exchange standards.

Because of heterogeneity, the studies could not be pooled, although Hart reported mean healing time as significantly shorter (19.7 vs. 43.8 days ($p<0.001$)). The authors suggested that the Hart study was particularly constrained by lack of power to detect useful clinical differences. The Brannen study,[94] reporting no difference in mortality, length of stay or surgeries, was constrained by the previously mentioned limitations. The authors state that while there are promising results from non-random clinical reports, there is insufficient evidence to recommend or refute the routine use of hyperbaric oxygen for the treatment of thermal burns. The authors further suggest that large multicenter randomized study of sufficient power would be needed to address these shortcomings. The Cochrane report did not consider several outcome studies with matched controls showing reduced length of stay, reduction in fluid requirements and edema, reduction of surgery and cost effectiveness.

While these reports certainly had limitations, they represent valid analysis of the benefits of early treatment in thermal injury and underscore that the observations of skilled and experienced physicians remain an important component of determining therapeutic efficacy. A well-designed, randomized, blinded control study with sham treatment and sufficient power is certainly desirable yet remains to be performed. Most centers see very few large burns; only 4% of burn admissions are for burns >40% TBSA, certainly necessitating a multicenter format. Attempts at organizing such a study have so far been unsuccessful.

Clinical Management

Surgical Perspectives

Over the past 40 years, the pendulum has swung to an aggressive surgical management of the burn wound, i.e., early tangential or sequential excision and grafting of the deep second-degree and probable third-degree burns, especially to functionally important parts of the body.[112-116] Hyperbaric oxygen, as an adjunctive therapy, has allowed the surgeon yet another modality of treatment for these deep second-degree burns, especially including those to the hands and fingers, face and ears, and other areas where the surgical technique of excision is often imprecise and coverage is sometimes difficult.

These wounds, not obvious third-degree, are then best treated with topical antimicrobial agents, bedside and enzymatic debridement, wound care, including biological dressings, and adjunctive hyperbaric oxygen therapy, allowing the surgeon more time for healing to take place and for definition of the extent and depth of injury (Figures 11-13).

Figure 11. Burn Victim's Recovery

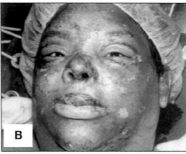
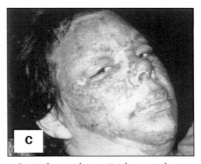

A. 23-year-old white female with facial burns from flaming gasoline and tar 12 hours after injury.

B. 24 hours later (36 hours after injury) after two HBO$_2$ treatments. Note resolution of edema.

C. 72 hours later (84 hours after injury) after six HBO$_2$ treatments.

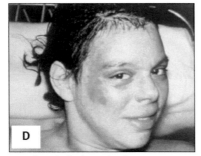
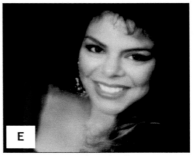

D. Shortly before discharge.

E. Four years after discharge.

Note: Consent to use these photos was obtained prior to publication.

Figure 12. Burn Victim's Recovery

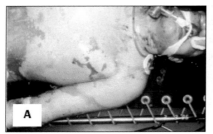

A. 19-year-old white male with deep partial-to full-thickness burns from flame burn. TBSA 70%. Photo taken pre-HBO₂.

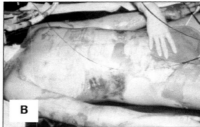

B. Patient six days later after HBO₂ twice daily.

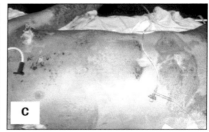

C. 30 days later with HBO₂. No skin grafts required on chest and torso.

Note: Consent to use these photos was obtained prior to publication.

Figure 13. Burn Victim's Recovery

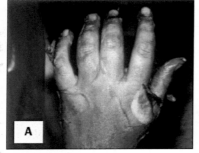

A. A deep partial-thickness burn to hand of 30-year-old male with 60 TBSA burn and inhalation injury. Taken on admission.

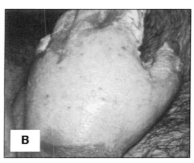

B. Patient six days later.

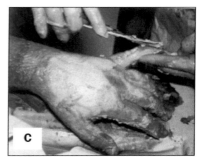

C. At surgery, light debridement.

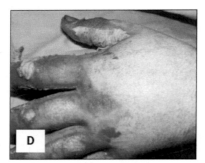

D. Immediately after surgery. Note preservation of dermal appendages.

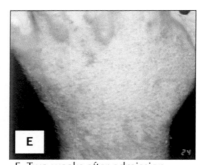

E. Two weeks after admission. Note re-epithelialization.

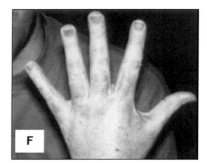

F. Appearance on discharge 25 days post-injury. Healed without grafting.

Note: Consent to use these photos was obtained prior to publication.

Adjunctive hyperbaric oxygen therapy has drastically reduced the healing time in the major burn injury, especially if the wounds are deep second-degree.[81-83,88] There is theoretical benefit of HBO$_2$ therapy for obviously less well-defined third-degree burns.[23] Fourth-degree burns, most commonly seen in high-voltage electrical injuries,[117] are benefited by reduction in fascial compartment pressures, as injured muscle swelling is lessened by preservation of aerobic glycolysis and, later, by a reduction of anaerobic infection.

Finally, reconstruction utilizing flaps, full-thickness skin and composite grafts, i.e., ear-to-nose grafts, has been greatly facilitated using adjunctive HBO$_2$.[121] Often the decision to use HBO$_2$ therapy has been made intraoperatively when a surgeon is concerned about a compromised cutaneous or myocutaneous flap. Patients are, in many instances, prepared preoperatively about the possibility of receiving adjunctive HBO$_2$ therapy immediately postoperatively.

Units planning treatment of burn patients should be experienced in management of critical-care patients in the hyperbaric setting and specific problems of burn patients prior to initiation of a therapy program. Preferably, personnel should be certified in burn care and hyperbaric oxygen therapy. The hyperbaric department should function as an extension of the burn unit and participate in the team approach to burn management.

Hyperbaric Oxygen

Hyperbaric oxygen therapy is begun as soon as possible after injury, often during initial resuscitation. Treatments are attempted three times within the first 24 hours and twice daily thereafter on a regimen of 90 minutes of 100% oxygen delivery at 2.0–2.4 ATA. Early experience in treating children recommended 45 minutes twice daily,[78] but more recent extensive clinical use of HBO$_2$ in children demonstrates that adult protocols are safe.

Patients are monitored during initial treatment and as necessary thereafter. Blood pressure can be monitored via transducers or non-invasively using blood pressure cuffs designed for use in monoplace chambers. Patients can be maintained on ventilator support during treatment, which is frequently the case in larger burns with concurrent inhalation injury.

Careful attention to fluid management is mandatory. Initial requirements may be several liters per hour, and pumps capable of this delivery at pressure must be utilized in order to maintain appropriate fluid replacement in the hyperbaric chamber. In larger burn injuries, adequate fluid and electrolyte resuscitation during the first 24 hours can be problematic. Certain patients can develop hypotension shortly after exiting the chamber. Careful volume replacement and assessment of fluid status is mandatory prior to, during, and immediately after HBO$_2$ treatment. Increasing fluids during ascent may help compensate for any hypovolemia unmasked after hyperbaric oxygen exposure.

Maintenance of a comfortable, ambient temperature must be accomplished. Thermal instability may be a problem within one to two hours of burn wound cleansing and dressing change (depending on the methods used), especially in large TBSA burns. These patients should be carefully assessed prior to an HBO$_2$ exposure. Febrile patients must be closely monitored and fever controlled, as oxygen toxicity is reported to be more common in this group.

In large burns of 40% TBSA or greater, treatment is rendered for 10–14 days in close consultation with the burn surgeon. Many partial-thickness burns will heal without surgery during this time frame and obviate the need for grafting. Treatment beyond 20-30 sessions is usually utilized to optimize graft take. While there is no absolute limit to the total number of hyperbaric treatments, it is rare to exceed 40–50 sessions, and utilization review is recommended.

Concern has been expressed about the use of the carbonic anhydrase inhibitor mafenide acetate (Sulfamylon) and its removal recommended prior to HBO_2 treatment based on the potential for CO_2 buildup, which can lead to vasodilatation.[122] Sulfamylon is less frequently utilized in burn centers, and rarely used at the authors' facility except in select cases (small TBSA, severe infection and/or contraindication to silver sulfadiazine). Its limited use in this setting has not resulted in any observed untoward effects.[123] Silver sulfadiazine is the most widely used topical therapy because of its relatively low toxicity and ease of use.[9]

In larger TBSA burns, especially of the head and neck, otic barotrauma may be a problem, and careful attention should be given to this potential complication. The HBO_2 team should make use of early ENT consultation when indicated.

Patients may be treated in a multiplace or monoplace configuration. Movement over long distances is not recommended; therefore patients should not be transported to a hyperbaric chamber that is not within the same facility as the burn center.[124]

Patient Selection Criteria

Hyperbaric oxygen therapy is recommended to treat serious burns, i.e., greater than 20% total body surface area and/or with involvement of the hands, face, feet or perineum that are deep partial- or full-thickness injury. Patients with superficial burns or those not expected to survive are not accepted for therapy. Transfer of patients for HBO_2 treatment should be considered carefully and should be sent only to a facility that has both a hyperbaric chamber and a burn unit.

Utilization Review

Utilization review is recommended after 30 hyperbaric oxygen sessions.

Cost Impact

Burn care is expensive. During 1997-98, in a Northern California regional burn center (Doctors Medical Center Burn Center), hospital costs for 20 burn patients averaged $253,000 ($393,000 in 2016 U.S. dollars).[125] This includes the cost of hyperbaric oxygen that averaged $6360 ($10,000 in 2016 U.S. dollars) per patient.

American Burn Association National Burn Repository 2017 Update indicated that charges for patients who died were over three times greater than those who survived, although this was greatly affected by the large number of patients with burns <10% TBSA. For burns >10% TBSA, total charges for surviving patients averaged $269,523 and for non-survivors, $361,342.1[1]

Although not calculated, cost savings as a result of the use of HBO_2 in acute thermal injury are implied in all of the 22 clinical studies in this report by demonstrating reductions in healing time, hospital length of stay, and numbers of surgeries including grafting. In six of the studies, the authors specifically analyzed costs of care in thermal injury with and without adjunctive HBO_2, estimating a range of average savings in patients treated with HBO_2 from $76,000 to $120,000 per case.

Discussion

Despite the many advances in burn therapy, including early excision, nutritional support, improved ventilation and infection control, since the mid-1980s there appears to have been little change in mortality except for patients over 65 with larger burns. Early excision seems to have decreased mortality and overall length of stay in smaller burns and for patients not suffering concurrent inhalation injury.[126] Engrav, in a review of 35 years' experience at the Harborview Burn Center in Seattle, Washington, reported that early excision did not decrease length of stay for larger burns, with little change since 1990.[127] It has also been suggested that burn care may have already achieved "a floor of survival."[128] Thus, further improvement in burn care, length of stay, mortality and cost containment must be addressed by additional therapeutic developments. Adjunctive hyperbaric oxygen therapy has been shown to reduce length of stay and cost of care in conjunction with early excision and comprehensive burn management. The reader is directed to a comprehensive and recent review on priorities of burn research.[129]

Summary

Hyperbaric oxygen in the treatment of burns has been demonstrated in numerous animal studies and human reports over the last 40 years. Observations utilizing hyperbaric oxygen therapy after burns have shown reversal of the zone of stasis, reduction of ischemia and ischemic necrosis, prevention of progression of partial- to full-thickness injury, moderation of inflammation, lessening of the capillary leak, preservation of dermal elements, a reduced need for grafting, shortened hospital stay, and a reduction in cost of care.

The burn community has pointed out the need for improvement in our control of pain, speed of healing, and scarring. Wolf and Engrav have both reported the limited progress in burn therapy that has been made in the last 20 years, especially in the control of the inflammatory state, the hypermetabolic syndrome, infection, and scarring. Perhaps the time has come for the burn community to routinely consider hyperbaric oxygen therapy in the treatment of clinical burns.

"It is clear from review of collected research and clinical data that hyperbaric oxygen therapy provides a unique environment for wound recovery and tissue regeneration for thermal injury that cannot be comparably achieved by our current surgical and medical therapies. Evidence of the reduction in patient morbidity and length of hospital stay are observed in the majority of clinical observations of the use of HBO_2 therapy in burn management and should be expected to be gained from carefully structured programs utilizing these methods. The scientific evidence of the efficacy of HBO_2 therapy as an effective tool for wound healing has made exceptional gains over the past three decades and provides us with a firm biological and physiologic basis for the use of this therapy in patients with complex wounds and burns. The scientific gains made from the observations of HBO_2 therapy-related mechanisms for stem progenitor cell signaling and wound healing have also been significant. Finally, research documenting the vulnerary effects of HBO_2 therapy at the cellular and molecular level also suggest that this therapy has the potential to provide a much-needed elevation of the "floor of survival" for burn victims and should provide for substantial enhancements in their wound healing and quality of life."[130]

Additional clinical evidence for the efficacy of hyperbaric oxygen therapy in burns would ideally result from a well-designed, multicenter, randomized study of sufficient power. While we await more data,[129] we should remember that the observations of seasoned clinicians also remain a valid test of efficacy.

Current data show that hyperbaric oxygen therapy, when used as an adjunct in a comprehensive program of burn care, is a cost-effective modality that can significantly improve morbidity and mortality, reduce length of hospital stay, and lessen the need for surgery. It has been demonstrated to be safe in the hands of those thoroughly trained in rendering hyperbaric oxygen therapy in the critical-care setting and with appropriate monitoring precautions. Careful patient selection and screening are mandatory.

Given our current understanding of the uniquely beneficial effects of hyperbaric oxygenation on the cellular and molecular mechanisms of wound healing, it is suggested that the formal integration of hyperbaric oxygen therapy in early burn wound management be thoughtfully considered, as well as further investigated in well-designed multicenter studies that may provide data for burn wound healing and burn patient outcomes supportive of this role.

Acknowledgments

The authors wish to thank Ms. Helen Doughty, medical librarian at John Muir Medical Center, Walnut Creek, California, for her invaluable contributions to this manuscript.

John B. Slade Jr. contributed to the earlier editions of this review.

Conflict of Interest Statement

The authors have no conflict of interest to declare.

Summary of Treatment Guidelines

- Patient referred by burn surgeon.

- 20% or greater TBSA and/or hands, face, feet, or perineum.

- Determine fitness to tolerate treatment and that there are no contraindications.

- Patient should be stable and accepting of hyperbaric treatment.

- Ensure critical care staff available.

- Treat at 2.0 or 2.4 ATA for 90 minutes at depth + descent and ascent time (travel time as patient tolerates).

- Monitor closely throughout treatment.

- Attempt three treatments in first 24 hours if possible, then twice daily thereafter.

- Daily dialog with surgeon and wound inspection, if possible.

- Continue treatment as burn surgeon requests.

- When grafting, provide one to two treatments at 2.0 or 2.4 ATA prior to surgery; twice daily thereafter until graft take (usually three to five days).

- Careful attention to fluid status, monitor carefully, hypovolemia may be masked by HBO_2. Additional fluids may be needed during and after decompression.

- Treatment may be discontinued after consultation with burn surgeon. Rare to exceed 40 treatments but not contraindicated to go beyond that point on a case by case basis.

Caveats

- Be prepared for side effects, i.e., barotrauma (16%) in head and neck burns.

- Be prepared to provide fluids ordered by surgeon during treatment.

- Maintain critical care standards at all times.

References

1. American Burn Association Report of Data from 2008-2017 National Burn Repository 2017 Update. Available from http://ameriburn.org/wp-content/uploads/2018/04/2017_aba_nbr_annual_report_summary.pdf.
2. American Burn Association, National Burn Repository Version 12.0. 2016.
3. Wolf SE, Tompkins RG, Herndon DN. On the Horizon – Research Priorities in Burns for the Next Decade. Surg Clin N Am. 2014;94:917-930.
4. Burd F, Chiu T. Allogenic skin in the treatment of burns. Clin Dermatol. 2005;23:376-387.
5. Atiyeh BS, Gunn SW, Hayek SN. State of the art in burn treatment. World J Surg. 2005;29(2):131-148.
6. Arturson G. Pathophysiology of the burn wound. Ann Chir Gynaecol. 1980;69:178-190.
7. Demling RH. The burn edema process: current concepts. J Burn Care Rehabil. May/June 2005;26:207-227.
8. Boykin JV, Eriksson E, Pittman RN. In vivo microcirculation of a scald burn and the progression of postburn dermal ischemia. Plast Reconstr Surg. 1980;66:191-198.
9. Monafo WW. Initial management of burns. NEJM. 1996;335(21):1581-1586.
10. Arturson G. The pathophysiology of severe thermal injury. J Burn Care Rehabil. 1985;6(2):129-146.
11. Heggers JP, Robson MC, Zachary LS. Thromboxane inhibitor for the prevention of progressive dermal ischemia due to the thermal injury. J Burn Care Rehabil. 1985;6:466-468.
12. Miller TA, Korn HN. Epithelial burn injury and repair, In: Davis JC, Hunt TK, editors. Hyperbaric oxygen therapy. Bethesda, MD: Undersea Medical Society, Inc.; 1977. P. 251.
13. Demling RH. Burns and other thermal injuries. In: Way LW, Doherty GM, editors. Current surgical diagnosis and treatment. 11th ed. New York, NY: McGraw-Hill Medical; 2003. P. 267.
14. Alexander JW, Meakins JL. A physiological basis for the development of opportunistic infections in man. Annals of Surgery. 1972;176:273.
15. Alexander JW, Wixson D. Neutrophil dysfunction and sepsis in burn injury. Surg Gynec Obstet. 1970;130:431.
16. Barber RC, Aragaki CC, Rivera-Chavez FA. TLR4 and TNF-alpha polymorphisms are associated with an increased risk for severe sepsis following burn injury. J Med Genet. 2004;41:808-813.
17. Church D, Elsayed S, Reid O, Winston B, Lindsay R. Burn wound infections. Clin Microbiol Rev. 2006;19(2): 403-434.
18. Deitch EA, Wheelahan TM, Rose MP, Clothier J, Cotter J. Hypertrophic burn scars: Analysis of variables. J Trauma. 1983;23:895-898.
19. Ikeda K, Ajiki H, Nagao H, Karino K, Sugii S, Iwa T, Wada J. Experimental and clinical use of hyperbaric oxygen in burns. In: Wada J, Iwa JT, editors. Proceedings of the fourth international congress on hyperbaric medicine. Baltimore, MD: Williams and Wilkins; 1970. P. 370.
20. Hartwig J, Kirste G. Experimentele untersuchungen uber die revaskularisierung von verbrennungswunden unter hyperbarer sauerstofftherapie. Zbl Chir. 1974;99:1112-1117.
21. Nylander G, Nordstrom H, Eriksson E. Effects of hyperbaric oxygen on oedema formation after a scald burn. Burns Incl Therm Inj. 1984 Feb;10(3):193-196.
22. Kaiser W, Schnaidt U, von der Leith H. Auswirkungen hyperbaren sauerstoffes auf die fresche brandwunde. Handchir Mikrochir Plast Chir. 1989;21:158-163.
23. Kaiser W, Voss K. Influence of hyperbaric oxygen on the edema formation in experimental burn injuries. Iugoslaw Physiol Pharmacol Acta. 1992;28(9):87-98.
24. Ketchum SA, Zubrin JR, Thomas AN, Hall AD. Effect of hyperbaric oxygen on small first, second and third degree burns. Surg Forum. 1967;18:65-67.
25. Ketchum SA, Thomas AN, Hall AD. Angiographic studies of the effect of hyperbaric oxygen on burn wound revascu-larization. In: Wada J, Iwa JT, editors. Proceedings of the fourth international congress on hyperbaric medicine. Tokyo: Igaku Shoin Ltd.; 1970. P. 388.
26. Niccole MW, Thornton JW, Danet RT, Bartlett RH, Tavis MJ. Hyperbaric oxygen in burn management: a controlled study. Surgery. 1977;82:727-733.
27. Gruber RP, Brinkley B, Amato JJ, Mendelson JA. Hyperbaric oxygen and pedicle flaps, skin grafts, and burns. Plast and Recon Surg. 1970;45:24-30.
28. Wells CH, Hilton JG. Effects of hyperbaric oxygen on post-burn plasma extravasation. In: Hunt TK, Davis JC, editors. Hyperbaric oxygen therapy. Bethesda, MD: Undersea and Hyperbaric Medical Society; 1977. P. 259.
29. Stewart RJ, Yamaguchi KT, Cianci PE, Knost PM, Samadani S, Mason SW, Roshdieh B. Effects of hyperbaric oxygen on adenosine triphosphate in thermally injured skin. Surg Forum. 1988;39:87.

30. Stewart RJ, Yamaguchi KT, Cianci PE, Mason WW, Roshdieh BB, Dabbassi N. Burn wound levels of ATP after exposure to elevated levels of oxygen. In: Proceedings of the American Burn Association, New Orleans, LA; 1989. P. 67.

31. Germonpré P, Reper P, Vanderkelen A. Hyperbaric oxygen therapy and piracetam decrease the early extension of deep partial thickness burns. Burns. 1996;22(6):468-473.

32. Korn HN, Wheeler ES, Miller TA. Effect of hyperbaric oxygen on second-degree burn wound healing. Arch Surg. 1977;112:732-737.

33. Saunders J, Fritz E, Ko F, Bi C, Gottlieb L, Krizek T. The effects of hyperbaric oxygen on dermal ischemia following thermal injury. In: Proceedings of the American Burn Association. New Orleans, LA; 1989. P. 58.

34. Perrins DJD. Failed attempt to limit tissue destruction in scalds of pig's skin with hyperbaric oxygen. In: Wada J, Iwa T, editors. Proceedings of the fourth international congress on hyperbaric medicine. Tokyo, Japan: Igaku Shoin Ltd.; 1970. P. 381.

35. Traystman RJ, Kirsch JR, Koehler RC. Oxygen radical mechanisms of brain injury following ischemia and reperfusion. J Appl Physiol. 1991;71:1185-1195.

36. Ward PA, Mulligan MS. New insights into mechanisms of oxyradical and neutrophil mediated lung injury. Klin Wochenschr. 1991;69:1009-1011.

37. Ward PA, Till GO. The autodestructive consequences of thermal injury. J Burn Care Rehabil. 1985;6:251-255.

38. McCord JM. Oxygen-derived free radicals in postischemic tissue injury. N Engl J Med. 1985;312:159-163.

39. Yogaratnam JZ, Laden G, Madden LA, Griffin S, et al. Hyperbaric oxygen: a new drug in myocardial revascularization and protection? Cardiovasc Revasc Med. 2006 Jul-Sep;7(3):146-154.

40. Zamboni WA, Roth AC, Russell RC, Graham B, Suchy H, Kucan JO. Morphological analysis of the microcirculation during reperfusion of ischemic skeletal muscle and the effect of hyperbaric oxygen. Plast Reconstr Surg. 1993;91: 1110-1123.

41. Zamboni WA, Stephenson LL, Roth AC, Suchy H, Russell RC. Ischemia-reperfusion injury in skeletal muscle: CD18 dependent neutrophil-endothelial adhesion. Undersea Hyperb Med. 1994;21(Suppl):53.

42. Wasiak J, Bennett M, Cleland H. Hyperbaric oxygen as adjuvant therapy in the management of burns: can evidence guide clinical practice? Burns. 2006;32:650-652.

43. Buras JA, Stahl GL, Svoboda KK, Weenstra WR. Hyperbaric oxygen down regulates ICAM-1 expression induced by hypoxia and hypoglycemia: the role of NOS. Am J Physiol Cell Physiol. 2000;278:C292-302.

44. Ueno S, Tanabe G, Kihara K et al. Early post-operativehyperbaric oxygen therapy modifies neutrophile activation. Hepatogastroenterology. 1999;46:1798-1799.

45. Miljkovic-Lolic M, Silbergleit R, Fiskum G, Rosenthal RE. Neuroprotective effects of hyperbaric oxygen treatment in experimental focal cerebral ischemia are associated with reduced brain leukocyte myeloperoxidase activity. Brain Res. 2003 May 2;971(1):90-94.

46. Shoshani O, Shupak A, Barak Y, Ullman Y, Ramon Y, Lindenbaum E, Peled Y. Hyperbaric oxygen therapy for deep second degree burns: an experimental study in the guinea pig. Brit J Plast Surg. 1998;51:67-73.

47. Bleser F, Benichoux R. Experimental surgery: The treatment of severe burns with hyperbaric oxygen. J Chir (Paris). 1973;106:281-290.

48. Tenenhaus M, Hansbrough JF, Zapata-Sirvent R, Neumann T. Treatment of burned mice with hyperbaric oxygen reduces mesenteric bacteria but not pulmonary neutrophil deposition. Arch Surg. 1994;129:1338-1342.

49. Magnotti LJ, Deitch EA. Burns, bacterial translocation, gut barrier function, and failure. J of Burn Care Rehab. 2005;26(5):383-391.

50. Yamada T, Taguchi T, Hirata Y, Suita S, Yugi H. The protective effect of hyperbaric oxygenation on the small intestine in ischemia-reperfusion injury. J Pediatr Surg. 1995;30:786-790.

51. Nylander G, Nordstrom H, Lewis D, Larsson J. Metabolic effects of hyperbaric oxygen in postischemic muscle. Plast Reconstr Surg. 1987;79:91-97.

52. Takahashi M, Iwatsuki N, Ono K, Koga Y. Hyperbaric oxygen therapy accelerates neurologic recovery after 15-minute complete global cerebral ischemia in dogs. Crit Care Med. 1992;20(11):1588-1594.

53. Thom SR. Functional inhibition of leukocyte B2 integrins by hyperbaric oxygen in carbon monoxide-mediated brain injury in rats. Toxicol Appl Pharmacol. 1993;123:248-256.

54. Veltkamp R, Siebing DA, Schwab S, Schwaninger M. Hyperbaric oxygen reduces blood-brain barrier damage and edema after transient focal cerebral ischemia. Stroke. 2005;36:1679-1683.

55. Kolski JM, Mazolewski PJ, Stephenson LL, Zamboni WA. Effect of hyperbaric oxygen therapy on testicular ischema- reperfusion injury. J of Urology. Aug 1998;160:601-604.

56. Shandling AH, Ellestad MH, Hart GB, et al. Hyperbaric oxygen and thrombolysis in myocardial infarction: The hot MI pilot study. Am Heart J. 1997;134:544-550.

57. Sharifi M, Fares W, Abdel-Karim I, Koch JM, Sopko J, Adler D; Hyperbaric Oxygen Therapy in Percutaneous Coronary Interventions Investigators. Usefulness of hyperbaric oxygen therapy to inhibit restenosis after percutaneous coronary intervention for acute myocardial infarction or unstable angina pectoris. Am J Cardiol. 2004 Jun 15;93(12):1533-1535.

58. Thomas MP, Brown LA, Sponseller DR, et al. Myocardial infarct size reduction by synergistic effect of hyperbaric oxygen and recombinant tissue plasminogen activator. Am Heart J. 1990 Oct;120(4):791-800.

59. Xu N, Li Z, Luo X. Effects of hyperbaric oxygen therapy on the changes in serum sIL-2R and Fn in severe burn patients. Zhonghua Zheng Xing Shao Shang Wai Ke Za Zhi. 1999;15(3):220-223.

60. Deitch EA, Xu DZ, Franko L, et al. Evidence favoring the role of the gut as a cytokine generating organ in rats subjected to hemorrhagic shock. Shock. 1994:1:141-146.

61. Deitch EA. Role of the gut lymphatic system in multiple organ failure. Current Opin Crit Care. 2001;7:92-98.

62. Hohn DC, McKay RD, Halliday B, Hunt TK. Effect of oxygen tension on the microbicidal function of leukocytes in wounds and in vitro. Surg Forum. 1976;27:18-20.

63. Allen DB, Maguire JJ, Mahdavian M, et al. Wound hypoxia and acidosis limit neutrophil bacterial killing mechanisms. Arch Surg. 1997;132:991-996.

64. Mader JT, Brown GL, Guckian JC, et al. A mechanism for the amelioration by hyperbaric oxygen of experimental staphylococcal osteomyelitis in rabbits. J Infect Dis. 1980;142:915-922.

65. Hussman J, Hebebrand D, Erdmann D, Moticka J. Lymphocyte subpopulations in spleen and blood after early wound debridement and acute/chronic treatment with hyperbaric oxygen. Hanchir Mikrochir Plast Chir. 1996;28(2):103-107.

66. Bilic I, Petri NM, Bota B. Effects of hyperbaric oxygen therapy on experimental burn wound healing in rats: A randomized controlled study. Undersea Hyperb Med. 2005;32(1):1-9.

67. Turkaslan T, Yogum N, Cimsit M, Solakoglu S, Ozdemir C, Ozsoy Z. Is HBOT treatment effective in recovering zone of stasis? An experimental immunohistochemical study. Burns. 2010;36(4):539-544.

68. Gallagher KA, Goldstein LJ, Thom SR, Velazquez OC. Hyperbaric oxygen and bone marrow-derived endothelial progenitor cells in diabetic wound healing. Vascular. 2006;14(6):328-337.

69. Gallagher KA, Liu ZJ, Xiao M, Chen H, Goldstein LJ, Buerk DG, Nedeau A, Thom SR, Velazquez OC. Diabetic impairments in NO-mediated endothelial progenitor cell mobilization and homing are reversed by hyperoxia and SDF-1 alpha. J Clin Invest. 2007;117:1249-1259.

70. Thom SR, Bhopale VM, Velazquez OC, Goldstein LJ, Thom LH, Buerk DG. Stem cell mobilization by hyperbaric oxygen. Am J Physiol Heart Circ Physiol. 2006;290:H1378-1386.

71. Goldstein LJ, Gallagher KA, Bauer SM et al. Endothelial progenitor cell release into circulation is triggered by hyperoxia-induced increases in bone marrow nitric oxide. Stem Cells. 2006;24:2309-2318.

72. Thom SR, Milovanova TN, Yang M, Bhopale VM, Sorokina EM, Uzun G, Malay DS, Troiano MA, Hardy KR, Lambert DS, Logue CJ, Margolis DJ. Vasculogenic stem cell mobilization and wound recruitment in diabetic patients: increased cell number and intracellular regulatory protein content associated with hyperbaric oxygen therapy. Wound Repair Regen. 2011;19(2):149-161.

73. Milovanova TN, Bhopale VM, Sorokina EM, Moore JS, Hunt TK, Hauer-Jensen M, Velazquez OC, Thom SR. Hyperbaric oxygen stimulates vasculogenic stem cell growth and differentiation in vivo. J Appl Physiol. 2009;106:711-728.

74. Milovanova TN, Bhopale VM, Sorokina EM, Moore JS, Hunt TK, Hauer-Jensen M, Velazquez OC, Thom SR. Lactate stimulates vasculogenic stem cells via the thioredoxin system and engages an autocrine activation loop involving hypoxia-inducible factor 1. Mol Cell Biol. 2008;28:6248-6261.

75. Wada J, Ikeda T, Kamata K, Ebuoka M. Oxygen hyperbaric treatment for carbon monoxide poisoning and severe burn in coal mine (hokutanyubari) gas explosion. Igakunoaymi (Japan). 1965;5:53.

76. Ikeda K, Ajiki H, Kamiyama T, Wada J. Clinical application of oxygen hyperbaric treatment. Geka (Japan). 1967;29:1279.

77. Wada J, Ikeda K, Kagaya H, Ajiki H. Oxygen hyperbaric treatment and severe burn. Jap Med J. 1966;13:2203.

78. Lamy ML, Hanquet MM. Application opportunity for OHP in a general hospital - a two year experience with a monoplace hyperbaric oxygen chamber. In: Wada J, Iwa JT, editors. Proceedings of the fourth international congress on hyperbaric medicine. Tokyo: Igaku Shoin Ltd.; 1970. P. 517.

79. Tabor CG. Hyperbaric oxygenation in the treatment of burns of less than forty percent. Korean J Intern Med. 1967;10(4):267-275.

80. Grossman AR, Grossman AJ. Update on hyperbaric oxygen and treatment of burns. Hyperbaric Oxygen Review. 1982;3:51.

81. Niu AKC, Yang C, Lee HC, Chen SH, Chang LP. Burns treated with adjunctive hyperbaric oxygen therapy: A comparative study in humans. J Hyperbar Med. 1987;2:75.

82. Cianci P, Lueders H, Lee H, Shapiro R, Sexton J, Williams C, Green B. Adjunctive hyperbaric oxygen reduces the need for surgery in 40-80% burns. J Hyperbar Med. 1988;3:97.

83. Cianci P, Lueders HW, Lee H, Shapiro RL, Sexton J, Williams C, Sato R. Adjunctive hyperbaric oxygen therapy reduces length of hospitalization in thermal burns. J Burn Care Rehabil. 1989;10:432-435.

84. Cianci P, Lueders H, Lee H, Shapiro R, Green B, Williams C. Hyperbaric oxygen and burn fluid requirements: Observations in 16 patients with 40-80% TBSA burns. Undersea Biomed Res. 1988;15(Suppl):14.

85. Hart GB, O'Reilly RR, Broussard ND, Cave RH, Goodman DB, Yanda RL. Treatment of burns with hyperbaric oxygen. Surg Gynecol Obstet. 1974 Nov;139(5):693-696.

86. Waisbren BA, Schutz D, Collentine G, Banaszak E. Hyperbaric oxygen in severe burns. Burns. 1982;8:176-179.

87. Merola L, Piscitelli F. Considerations on the use of HBO in the treatment of burns. Ann Med Nav. 1978;83:515.

88. Cianci P, Williams C, Lueders H, Lee H, Shapiro R, Sexton J, Sato R. Adjunctive hyperbaric oxygen in the treatment of thermal burns - an economic analysis. J Burn Care Rehabil. 1990;11:140-143.

89. Cianci P, Sato R. Adjunctive hyperbaric oxygen therapy in the treatment of thermal burns: A review. Burns. 1994 Feb;20(1):5-14.

90. Maxwell G, Meites H, Silverstein P. Cost effectiveness of hyperbaric oxygen therapy in burn care. Presented at: Winter Symposium on Baromedicine; 1991; Aspen, CO.

91. Cianci P, Sato R, Green B. Adjunctive hyperbaric oxygen reduces length of hospital stay, surgery, and the cost of care in severe burns. Undersea Biomed Research Suppl. 1991;18:108.

92. Hammarlund C, Svedman C, Svedman P. Hyperbaric oxygen treatment of healthy volunteers with UV-irradiated blister wounds. Bums. 1991;17:296-301.

93. Niezgoda JA, Cianci P, Folden BW, Ortega RL, Slade JB, Storrow AB. The effect of hyperbaric oxygen therapy on a burn wound model in human volunteers. Plast Reconstr Surg. 1997;99(6):1620-1625.

94. Brannen AL, Still J, Haynes M, Orlet H, Rosemblum F, Law E, Thompson WO. A randomized prospective trial of hyperbaric oxygen in a referral burn center population. Am Surg. 1997;63:205-208.

95. Sutherland AM, Clarke HA, Katz J, Katznelson R. Hyperbaric Oxygen Therapy: A New Treatment for Chronic Pain? Pain Practice. 2015;2(1):1-9.

96. Ramussen VM, Borgen AE, Jansen EC, Rotboll Nielsen PH, Werner MU. Hyperbaric Oxygen Therapy Attenuates Central Sensitization Induced by a Thermal Injury in Humans. Acta Anaesthesiologica Scandinavica. 2015;59:749-762.

97. Chong SJ, Kan EM, Song C, Soh CR, Lu J. Work in Progress – Characterization of Early Thermal Burns and the Effects of Hyperbaric Oxygen Treatment: A Pilot Study. Diving and Hyperbaric Medicine. 2013;43(3):157-161.

98. Jones LM, Rubadue C, Brown NV, Khandelwal S, Coffey RA. Evaluation of TCOM/HBOT Practice Guideline for the Treatment of Foot Burns Occurring in Diabetic Patients. Burns. 2015;41:536-541.

99. Zhang Q, Chang Q, Cox RA, Gong X, Gould LJ. Hyperbaric Oxygen Attenuates Apoptosis and Decreases Inflammation in an Ischemic Wound Model. J Invest Dermatol. 2008;128(8):2102-2112.

100. Fosen KM, Thom SR. Hyperbaric Oxygen, Vasculogenic Stem Cells, and Wound Healing. Antioxidants & Redox Signaling. 2014;21(11):1634-1646.

101. Thom SR, Bhopale VM, Velazquez OC, Goldstein LJ, Thom LH, Buerk DG. Stem Cell Mobilization by Hyperbaric Oxygen. Am J Physiol Heart Circ. Physiol. 2006;290:H1378-H1386.

102. Thom SR, Milovanova TN, Yang M, Bhopale VM, Sorokina EM, Uzun G, Malay DS, Troiano MA, Hardy KR, Lambert DW, Logue CJ, Margolis DJ. Vasculogenic Stem Cell Mobilization and Wound Recruitment in Diabetic Patients: Increased Cell Number and Intracellular Protein Content Associated with Hyperbaric Oxygen Therapy. Wound Rep Reg. 2011;19:149-161.

103. Stewart RJ, Yamaguchi KT, Cianci PE, Knost PM, Samadani S. Mason SW, Roshdieh B. Effects of Hyperbaric Oxygen on Adenosine Triphosphate in Thermally Injured Skin. Surg Forum. 1988;39:87.

104. Stewart RJ, Yamaguchi KT, Cianci PE, Mason WW, Roshdieh BB, Dabbassi N. Burn wound Levels of ATP after Exposure to Elevated Levels of Oxygen. Proceedings of the American Burn Association, New Orleans. 1989:67.

105. Sureda A, Batle JM, Martorell M, Capo X, Tejada S, Tur JA, Pons A. "Antioxidant Response of Chronic Wounds to Hyperbaric Oxygen Therapy." PLoS One 2016;11(9):e0163371.

106. Shirani K, Pruitt B, Mason A. The influence of inhalation injury and pneumonia on burn mortality. Ann Surg. 1986;205:82-87.

107. Balkissoon R, Shusterman DJ. Occupational upper airway disorders. Semin Respir Crit Care Med. 1999;20:569-580.

108. Rabinowitz, PM, Siegel MD. Acute inhalation injury. Clin Chest Med. 2002;23(4):707.

109. Grim PS, Nahum A, Gottlieb L, Wilbert C, Hawe E, Sznajder J. Lack of measurable oxidative stress during HBO therapy in burn patients. Undersea Biomed Res. 1989;16(Suppl):22.

110. Ray CS, Green G, Cianci P. Hyperbaric oxygen therapy in burn patients: Cost effective adjuvant therapy (abstract). Undersea Biomed Res. 1991;18(Suppl):77.
111. Villanueva E, Bennett MH, Wasiak J, Lehm JP. Hyperbaric oxygen therapy for thermal burns (Review). Cochrane Database Syst Rev. 2004;(3):CD004727.
112. Hunt JL, Sato RM, Baxter CR. Early Tangential Excision and Immediate Mesh Auto-grafting of Deep Dermal Hand Burns. Annals Surg. 1979;189(2):147-151. (Orig paper)
113. Sato RM, Beesinger DE, Hunt JL, Baxter CR. Early Excision and Closure of the Burn Wound. Current Topics in Burn Care. TL Wachtel et al.(eds) Rockville, Aspen Publication;1983. Pp.65-76.(Orig paper)
114. Sato RM, Baxter CT. Tangential Excision of the Burn Wound. Recent Advances in Emergency and Definitive Burn Wound Care. Proceedings of a Symposium Sponsored by Valley Medical Center (Fresno, CA). March 1977:16-24. CV2.
115. Sato R, Beesinger D, Hunt J, Baxter C. Early Excision and Closure of the Burn Wound. Critical Care Quarterly. 1978;1(3):51-62. CV4.
116. Hunt JL, Sato RM. Acute Electrical Burns. Uncommon Problems in Emergency Medicine. Miahcel I. Greenberg (ed). Philadelphia, F. A. Davis Company; 1982. Pp:183-195. CV11.
117. Hunt JL, Sato RM. Early Excision of Full Thickness Hand and Digit Burns: Factors Affecting Morbidity. J Trauma. 1982;22(5):414-419. CV12.
118. Kowalczyk L. Catastrophic costs: hospitals, insurers, some R.I. fire victims face huge medical bills. The Boston Globe. 2003 Feb 28.
119. Hunt JL, Sato RM, Baxter CR. Early tangential excision and immediate mesh auto-grafting of deep dermal hand burns. Annals Surg. 1979;189(2):147-151.
120. Sato RM, Beesinger DE, Hunt JL, Baxter CR. Early excision and closure of the burn wound. In: Wachtel TL et al., editors. Current topics in burn care. Rockville, MD: Aspen Publications; 1983. Pp. 65-76.
121. Nichter LS, Morwood DT, Williams GS, Spence RJ. Expanding the limits of composite grafting: A case report of successful nose replantation assisted by hyperbaric oxygen therapy. Plast Reconstr Surg. 1991;87:337-340.
122. Kindwall EP. The use of drugs under pressure. In: Kindwall EP, Whelan HT, editors. Hyperbaric medicine practice. 2nd ed. Flagstaff, AZ: Best Publishing Co.; 1999. P. 326.
123. Personal experience of the authors in a regional burn center.
124. Grube BJ, Marvin JA, Heimbach DM. Therapeutic hyperbaric oxygen: Help or hindrance in burn patients with carbon monoxide poisoning? J Burn Care Rehabil. 1988;9.
125. Cost statistics (1997-98) from hospital patient accounts, home facility of the authors.
126. Ong YS, Samual M, Song C. Meta-analysis of early excision of burns. Burns. 2006;32(2):145-150.
127. Engrav LH, Heimbach DM, Rivara FP et al. Harborview burns 1974-2009. PlosOne. 2012;7(7):1-23.
128. Blaisdell LL, Chace R, Hallagan LD, Clark DE. A half century of burn epidemiology and burn care in a rural state. J Burn Care Res. 2012 May-Jun;33(3):347-353.
129. Rowan MP, Cancio LC, Elster EA, Burmeister DM, Rose LF, Natesan S, Chan RK, Christy RJ, Chung KK. Burn Wound Healing and Treatment: Review and Advancements. Critical Care. 2015;DOI 10.1186/s13054-01509861-2.
130. Boykin JV Jr. Letter to the Editor, Undersea Hyperb Med. 2013Mar-Apr;40(2):212.

of afferent fibers without a real sensory injury.[54-55] In rats, Thompson and colleagues demonstrated that HBO_2 can reduce pain and mechanical hypersensitivity.[56] Repetitive and long-term HBO_2 exposure has led to transient inhibition of thermal hyperalgesia and thermal/mechanical hypersensitivity, respectively.[57] Zhao et al. explored the likely relationship between HBO_2 and antinociceptive reaction in animal model. They demonstrated that one HBO_2 exposure could produce a short-term antinociceptive effect and inhibition of mechanical and thermal hyperalgesia. Several HBO_2 exposures resulted in inhibition of astrocyte activation with a consequent worsening of neuropathic pain.[41] HBO_2 significantly decreased both prostaglandin E_2 and IL-1β production.[58] However, this concept is still debated in the scientific literature. Indeed, other studies showed that HBO_2 relieved neuropathic pain by reducing TNF-α production but not IL-1β.[59] We suggest that these different mechanisms might be simultaneously operative, since we are aware of the underlying regulation processes of TNF-α and IL-1 in causing neuropathic pain.[57] Moreover, specific inhibition of NO production led to a vanishing short-term antinociceptive action of HBO_2. Thus, it has been proposed that NO synthesis induced by HBO_2 is relevant in lightening hyperalgesia.[60] A recent study confirmed that this may be the main HBO_2 mechanism of action regarding antinociceptive effect.[61]

Osteogenic Process Promotion

Several clinical studies support the benefits of HBO_2 in patients afflicted with aseptic hip osteonecrosis and aseptic condylar knee necrosis.[62-64] Camporesi, et al. demonstrated with a seven-year follow up the reversal of femoral head necrosis in a small group of patients treated with a series of HBO_2 treatments at 2 ATA (202.6 kPa).[62] However, the underlying mechanisms of action are still unclear. Recent data demonstrate that intermittent supplementation of O_2 to hypoxic bone provides osteoblast stimulation and bone tissue regeneration in a study examining the effect of HBO_2, pressure, and hyperoxia on RANKL-induced (receptor activator of nuclear factor-kappa B-induced) osteoclast formation in RAW 264.7 cells and human peripheral blood monocytes (PBMC).[65] A recent study, in which magnetic resonance imaging (MRI) was obtained at T_0 and about one year from the end of HBO_2 treatments to follow lesion size, also investigated HBO_2 upregulation on serum osteoprotegerin (OPG) and/or inhibition of osteoclast activation.[66] The same group showed that HBO_2 results in an anti-inflammatory action in patients with avascular necrosis of the femoral head (AVNFH). HBO_2 results in a decreased amount of circulating TNF-α and IL-6. HBO_2 acting on TNF-α and IL-6, key bone-resorbing cytokines and their synergistic effects, which could conceivably be responsible for beneficial clinical effects.[29] In conclusion, multiple mechanism of the beneficial action of HBO_2 exposure continue to be discussed and elucidated.

References

1. Yarbrough O, Behnke A. The treatment of compressed air illness. J Ind Hyg Toxicol. 1939;21:213–8.
2. Churchill-Davidson I, Sanger C, Thomlinson R. High-pressure oxygen and radiotherapy. Lancet (London, England). 1955 May 28;268(6874):1091–5.
3. Boerema I, Huiskes J, Kroll J, Kroon B, Lokin E, Meyne N. High atmospheric pressure as an aid to cardiac surgery. Arch Chir Neerl. 1956;8(3):193–211.
4. Brummelkamp WH, Hogendijk J, Boerema I. Treatment of anaerobic infections (clostridial myositis) by drenching the tissues with oxygen under high atmospheric pressure. Surgery. 1961 Mar 1;49(3):299–302.
5. Smith G, Ledingham IM, Sharp GR, Norman JN, Bates EH. Treatment of coal-gas poisoning with oxygen at 2 atmospheres pressure. Lancet. 1962 Apr 21 [cited 2019 Feb 22];279(7234):816–9.
6. Muth CM, Shank ES. Gas Embolism. N Engl J Med [Internet]. 2000 Feb 17;342(7):476–82.
7. Thom SR. Oxidative stress is fundamental to hyperbaric oxygen therapy. J Appl Physiol. 2009 Mar;106(3):988–95.
8. Vorosmarti J. Hyperbaric oxygen therapy. Am Fam Physician. 1981 Jan;23(1):169–73.
9. Clark J, Whelan HT. Hyperbaric medicine practice. In: Kindwall & H.T. Whelan, editor. Best Publishing Company; 1994.
10. Davis JC. Hyperbaric oxygen therapy. J Intensive Care Med. 1989 Mar 30;4(2):55–7.
11. Camporesi EM, Bosco G. Mechanisms of action of hyperbaric oxygen therapy. Undersea Hyperb Med. 2014;41(3):247–52.
12. Thom SR. Hyperbaric oxygen: its mechanisms and efficacy. Plast Reconstr Surg. 2011 Jan;127:131S–141S.
13. Falanga V. Wound healing and its impairment in the diabetic foot. Lancet. 2005 Nov 12;366(9498):1736–43.
14. Marx RE. Osteoradionecrosis: a new concept of its pathophysiology. J Oral Maxillofac Surg. 1983 May;41(5):283–8.
15. Hunt TK, Aslam RS, Beckert S, Wagner S, Ghani QP, Hussain MZ, et al. Aerobically derived lactate stimulates revascularization and tissue repair via redox mechanisms. Antioxid Redox Signal. 2007 Aug;9(8):1115–24.
16. Milovanova TN, Bhopale VM, Sorokina EM, Moore JS, Hunt TK, Hauer-Jensen M, et al. Lactate stimulates vasculogenic stem cells via the thioredoxin system and engages an autocrine activation loop involving hypoxia-inducible factor 1. Mol Cell Biol. 2008 Oct 15;28(20):6248–61.
17. Bosco G, Yang Z, Nandi J, Wang J, Chen C, Camporesi EM. Effects of hyperbaric oxygen on glucose, lactate, glycerol and anti-oxidant enzymes in the skeletal muscle of rats during ischaemia and reperfusion. Clin Exp Pharmacol Physiol. 2007 Jan;34(1–2):70–6.
18. Sharifi M, Fares W, Abdel-Karim I, Petrea D, Koch JM, Adler D, et al. Inhibition of restenosis by hyperbaric oxygen: a novel indication for an old modality. Cardiovasc Radiat Med. 2002;3(3–4):124–6.
19. Sharifi M, Fares W, Abdel-Karim I, Koch JM, Sopko J, Adler D, et al. Usefulness of hyperbaric oxygen therapy to inhibit restenosis after percutaneous coronary intervention for acute myocardial infarction or unstable angina pectoris. Am J Cardiol. 2004 Jun 15;93(12):1533–5.
20. Yang ZJ, Bosco G, Montante A, Ou XI, Camporesi EM. Hyperbaric O2 reduces intestinal ischemia-reperfusion-induced TNF-alpha production and lung neutrophil sequestration. Eur J Appl Physiol.2001 Jul 5;85(1–2):96–103.
21. Yang Z, Nandi J, Wang J, Bosco G, Gregory M, Chung C, et al. Hyperbaric oxygenation ameliorates indomethacin-induced enteropathy in rats by modulating TNF-α and IL-1β production. Dig Dis Sci. 2006 Aug 13;51(8):1426–33.
22. Baynosa RC, Naig AL, Murphy PS, Fang XH, Stephenson LL, Khiabani KT, et al. The effect of hyperbaric oxygen on nitric oxide synthase activity and expression in ischemia-reperfusion injury. J Surg Res. 2013 Jul;183(1):355–61.
23. Hampson NB, Piantadosi CA, Thom SR, Weaver LK. Practice recommendations in the diagnosis, management, and prevention of carbon monoxide poisoning. Am J Respir Crit Care Med. 2012 Dec 1;186(11):1095–101.
24. Vann RD, Butler FK, Mitchell SJ, Moon RE. Decompression illness. In: The Lancet. Elsevier; 2011. Pp: 153–64.
25. Moon RE. Hyperbaric oxygen treatment for air or gas embolism. Undersea Hyperb Med. 2014;41(2):159–66.
26. Thom SR, Bhopale VM, Mancini DJ, Milovanova TN. Actin S-nitrosylation inhibits neutrophil beta2 integrin function. J Biol Chem. 2008 Apr 18;283(16):10822–34.
27. Mori H, Shinohara H, Arakawa Y, Kanemura H, Ikemoto T, Imura S, et al. Beneficial effects of hyperbaric oxygen pretreatment on massive hepatectomy model in rats. Transplantation [Internet]. 2007 Dec 27 [cited 2019 Feb 22];84(12):1656–61.
28. Yang ZJ, Xie Y, Bosco GM, Chen C, Camporesi EM. Hyperbaric oxygenation alleviates MCAO-induced brain injury and reduces hydroxyl radical formation and glutamate release. Eur J Appl Physiol. 2010 Feb 23;108(3):513–22.
29. Bosco G, Vezzani G, Mrakic Sposta S, Rizzato A, Enten G, Abou-Samra A, et al. Hyperbaric oxygen therapy ameliorates osteonecrosis in patients by modulating inflammation and oxidative stress. J Enzyme Inhib Med Chem. 2018 Dec;33(1):1501–5.
30. Gorbach SL, Bartlett JG. Anaerobic Infections. N Engl J Med. 1974 May 23;290(21):1177–84.

31. Zanon V, Rossi L, Castellani E, Camporesi EM, Palù G, Bosco G. Oxybiotest project: microorganisms under pressure. Hyperbaric oxygen (HBO) and simple pressure interaction on selected bacteria. Med Gas Res. 2012 Sep 11;2(1):24.

32. Mader JT, Brown GL, Guckian JC, Wells CH, Reinarz JA. A mechanism for the amelioration by hyperbaric oxygen of experimental staphylococcal osteomyelitis in rabbits. J Infect Dis. 1980 Dec;142(6):915–22.

33. Almzaiel AJ, Billington R, Smerdon G, Moody AJ. Effects of hyperbaric oxygen treatment on antimicrobial function and apoptosis of differentiated HL-60 (neutrophil-like) cells. Life Sci. 2013 Jul 30;93(2–3):125–31.

34. Wu Y, Klapper I, Stewart PS. Hypoxia arising from concerted oxygen consumption by neutrophils and microorganisms in biofilms. Pathog Dis. 2018 Jun 1;76(4).

35. Kolpen M, Lerche CJ, Kragh KN, Sams T, Koren K, Jensen AS, et al. Hyperbaric oxygen sensitizes anoxic pseudomonas aeruginosa biofilm to ciprofloxacin. Antimicrob Agents Chemother. 2017 Nov;61(11).

36. Lerche CJ, Christophersen LJ, Kolpen M, Nielsen PR, Trøstrup H, Thomsen K, et al. Hyperbaric oxygen therapy augments tobramycin efficacy in experimental Staphylococcus aureus endocarditis. Int J Antimicrob Agents. 2017 Sep;50(3):406–12.

37. Sanford NE, Wilkinson JE, Nguyen H, Diaz G, Wolcott R. Efficacy of hyperbaric oxygen therapy in bacterial biofilm eradication. J Wound Care. 2018 Jan 1;27(Sup1):S20–8.

38. Ishii Y, Miyanaga Y, Shimojo H, Ushida T, Tateishi T. Effects of hyperbaric oxygen on procollagen messenger RNA levels and collagen synthesis in the healing of rat tendon laceration. Tissue Eng. 1999 Jun;5(3):279–86.

39. Weisz G, Lavy A, Adir Y, Melamed Y, Rubin D, Eidelman S, et al. Modification of in vivo and in vitro TNF-alpha, IL-1, and IL-6 secretion by circulating monocytes during hyperbaric oxygen treatment in patients with perianal Crohn's disease. J Clin Immunol. 1997 Mar;17(2):154–9.

40. Tsai H-M, Gao C-J, Li W-X, Lin M-T, Niu K-C. Resuscitation from experimental heatstroke by hyperbaric oxygen therapy. Crit Care Med. 2005 Apr;33(4):813–8.

41. Zhao LL, Davidson JD, Wee SC, Roth SI, Mustoe TA. Effect of hyperbaric oxygen and growth factors on rabbit ear ischemic ulcers. Arch Surg. 1994 Oct 1;129(10):1043.

42. Gleadle JM, Ratcliffe PJ. Hypoxia and the regulation of gene expression. Mol Med Today. 1998 Mar 1;4(3):122–9.

43. Haroon ZA, Raleigh JA, Greenberg CS, Dewhirst MW. Early wound healing exhibits cytokine surge without evidence of hypoxia. Ann Surg. 2000 Jan;231(1):137–47.

44. Thom SR, Bhopale V, Fisher D, Manevich Y, Huang PL, Buerk DG. Stimulation of nitric oxide synthase in cerebral cortex due to elevated partial pressures of oxygen: an oxidative stress response. J Neurobiol. 2002 May;51(2):85–100.

45. Thom SR, Fisher D, Zhang J, Bhopale VM, Ohnishi ST, Kotake Y, et al. Stimulation of perivascular nitric oxide synthesis by oxygen. Am J Physiol Circ Physiol. 2003 Apr;284(4):H1230–9.

46. Boykin J V, Baylis C. Hyperbaric oxygen therapy mediates increased nitric oxide production associated with wound healing: a preliminary study. Adv Skin Wound Care. 2007 Jul;20(7):382–8.

47. Kendall AC, Whatmore JL, Harries LW, Winyard PG, Smerdon GR, Eggleton P. Changes in inflammatory gene expression induced by hyperbaric oxygen treatment in human endothelial cells under chronic wound conditions. Exp Cell Res. 2012 Feb 1;318(3):207–16.

48. Oter S, Korkmaz A, Topal T, Ozcan O, Sadir S, Ozler M, et al. Correlation between hyperbaric oxygen exposure pressures and oxidative parameters in rat lung, brain, and erythrocytes. Clin Biochem. 2005 Aug;38(8):706–11.

49. Palzur E, Zaaroor M, Vlodavsky E, Milman F, Soustiel JF. Neuroprotective effect of hyperbaric oxygen therapy in brain injury is mediated by preservation of mitochondrial membrane properties. Brain Res. 2008 Jul 24;1221:126–33.

50. Brentnall M, Rodriguez-Menocal L, De Guevara R, Cepero E, Boise LH. Caspase-9, caspase-3 and caspase-7 have distinct roles during intrinsic apoptosis. BMC Cell Biol. 2013 Jul 9;14(1):32.

51. Hink J, Jansen E. Are superoxide and/or hydrogen peroxide responsible for some of the beneficial effects of hyperbaric oxygen therapy? Med Hypotheses. 2001 Dec;57(6):764–9.

52. Vlodavsky E, Palzur E, Soustiel JF. Hyperbaric oxygen therapy reduces neuroinflammation and expression of matrix metalloproteinase-9 in the rat model of traumatic brain injury. Neuropathol Appl Neurobiol. 2006 Feb;32(1):40–50.

53. Tracey DJ, Walker JS. Pain due to nerve damage: are inflammatory mediators involved? Inflamm Res. 1995 Oct;44(10):407–11.

54. Zhang J-M, An J. Cytokines, inflammation, and pain. Int Anesthesiol Clin. 2007;45(2):27–37.

55. Ren K, Torres R. Role of interleukin-1beta during pain and inflammation. Brain Res Rev. 2009 Apr;60(1):57–64.

56. Thompson CD, Uhelski ML, Wilson JR, Fuchs PN. Hyperbaric oxygen treatment decreases pain in two nerve injury models. Neurosci Res. 2010 Mar;66(3):279–83.

57. Gu N, Niu J-Y, Liu W-T, Sun Y-Y, Liu S, Lv Y, et al. Hyperbaric oxygen therapy attenuates neuropathic hyperalgesia in rats and idiopathic trigeminal neuralgia in patients. Eur J Pain. 2012 Sep;16(8):1094–105.

58. Inamoto Y, Okuno F, Saito K, Tanaka Y, Watanabe K, Morimoto I, et al. Effect of hyperbaric oxygenation on macrophage function in mice. Biochem Biophys Res Commun. 1991 Sep 16;179(2):886–91.

59. Li F, Fang L, Huang S, Yang Z, Nandi J, Thomas S, et al. Hyperbaric oxygenation therapy alleviates chronic constrictive injury-induced neuropathic pain and reduces tumor necrosis factor-alpha production. Anesth Analg. 2011 Sep;113(3):626–33.

60. Ohgami Y, Zylstra CC, Quock LP, Chung E, Shirachi DY, Quock RM. Nitric oxide in hyperbaric oxygen-induced acute antinociception in mice. Neuroreport. 2009 Oct 7;20(15):1325–9.

61. Zelinski LM, Ohgami Y, Chung E, Shirachi DY, Quock RM. A prolonged nitric oxide-dependent, opioid-mediated antinociceptive effect of hyperbaric oxygen in mice. J Pain. 2009 Feb;10(2):167–72.

62. Camporesi EM, Vezzani G, Bosco G, Mangar D, Bernasek TL. Hyperbaric oxygen therapy in femoral head necrosis. J Arthroplasty. 2010 Sep 1;25(6):118–23.

63. Bosco G, Vezzani G, Enten G, Manelli D, Rao N, Camporesi EM. Femoral condylar necrosis: treatment with hyperbaric oxygen therapy. Arthroplast today. 2018 Dec;4(4):510–5.

64. Camporesi EM, Vezzani G, Zanon V, Manelli D, Enten G, Quartesan S, et al. Review on hyperbaric oxygen treatment in femoral head necrosis. Undersea Hyperb Med. 2017;44(6):497–508.

65. Hadi H Al, Smerdon GR, Fox SW. Hyperbaric oxygen therapy suppresses osteoclast formation and bone resorption. J Orthop Res. 2013 Jul;31(11).

66. Vezzani G, Quartesan S, Cancellara P, Camporesi EM, Mangar D, Bernasek T, et al. Hyperbaric oxygen therapy modulates serum OPG/RANKL in femoral head necrosis patients. J Enzyme Inhib Med Chem. 2017;32(1):707–11.

CHAPTER 16

Side Effects of Hyperbaric Oxygen Therapy

Matteo Paganini MD, Enrico M. Camporesi MD

Abstract

Several complications of hyperbaric oxygen therapy have been described in the literature, with varying degrees of seriousness. Middle ear barotrauma and sinus squeeze are the two most frequent and benign side effects, noted in up to 2% of treated patients. Another frequent complaint is claustrophobia, occurring in both multiplace and monoplace hyperbaric chambers. Other more rare but more severe side effects are related to oxygen toxicity, typically after multiple exposures required for chronic treatments. Progressive myopia, usually transient and reversible after stopping the treatments, or pulmonary symptoms, such as cough and inspiratory pain, are the most common oxygen toxicity clinical manifestations, while the more serious oxygen-induced seizures happen rarely, at higher O_2 pressures, and often during acute treatments in acidotic patients (e.g. carbon monoxide poisoning). For these reasons, a thorough medical history and physical examination should precede every hyperbaric oxygen treatment, in order to identify subjects at risk of complications and to choose the right treatment protocol tailored to that patient.

General Considerations

Oxygen is among the world's most used drugs in the health care practice. But like any drug, it should be used along with clinical acumen, seeking a balance between its unquestioned beneficial effects and its subtle intrinsic harming potential.[1] This assumption is certainly true with hyperbaric oxygen (HBO_2) therapy, in which the great therapeutic effects demonstrated in the last decades must outweigh the risks of the treatment.[2]

While the previous chapters focused on therapeutic indications, in this part we'll provide the reader with the necessary knowledge regarding complications of HBO_2 in order to counterbalance treatment decisions and avoid potentially dangerous consequences for the patients. More important, this information should be shared with patients in order to obtain their written informed consent prior to treatment.

Otorhinolaryngology

Several anatomical structures in the head are within bony structures and air-filled, which makes them susceptible to HBO_2-related injuries.

Middle ear barotrauma (MEB) is the most common side effect of HBO_2,[3-4] accounting for approximately 2% of patients in a review of 1,446 subjects treated with 31,599 sessions. The inability to adequately perform compensation maneuvers results in middle ear pressure variations beyond physiological limits, thus damaging especially the eardrum and the surrounding structures. MEB can be prevented in most patients by teaching auto-inflation techniques or in selected cases, with the application of tympanostomy tubes (e.g. for intubated or uncooperative patients). Pseudoephedrine was effective in preventing MEB in a randomized clinical trial in divers,[5] while topical nasal oxymetazoline hydrochloride proved to be ineffective.[6]

MEB patients with a history of Eustachian tube dysfunction are predisposed to the development of serous otitis media during treatments.[7] It has also been demonstrated that HBO_2 is capable of causing a reversible derangement in the middle ear chemoreceptor reflex arc that may impair middle ear aeration.[8] These two mechanisms can facilitate the development of this complication, which can lead to infection, which often requires the interruption of HBO_2 and referral to an otolaryngologist.

Sinus squeeze is the second most common HBO_2 complication[3] and usually occurs in patients with concomitant upper respiratory tract infections or allergic rhinitis. Therapy with decongestant nasal spray, antihistamines, and/ or steroid nasal spray may allow the patient to continue hyperbaric therapy.[6]

Ophthalmology

Pathogenesis of ocular complications during HBO_2 is probably related to the increase of reactive oxygen and nitrogen species and the relative lack of antioxidant protective mechanisms of the eye, a structure naturally exposed to the dangerous interaction between light radiation and cells.[9] A baseline ophthalmology pre-examination and frequent monitoring are suggested to establish pre-existing and detect early sign of ophthalmic pathology, especially in patients at risk (e.g., those over 50 years of age and those with diabetes mellitus, irradiation therapy of the head and neck, and systemic steroid therapy).

Progressive myopia (PM) is the most common ocular complication,[9] observed in patients undergoing prolonged periods of daily HBO_2.[10-13] Usually it reverses completely within a few days to several weeks after the last HBO_2 session.[10,12] Since the literature offers contradictory findings, the underlying mechanisms of PM development remain obscure, but the most accepted theory is that the change in refraction is due to an increased refractive index of the crystalline lens during prolonged HBO_2.[11-12] In the sample studied by Lyme in 1978, half of the patients developed PM after HBO_2 (4-52 weeks of daily exposures at 2.5 atmospheres absolute [ATA] [253.32 kPa]) without showing ocular pressure and fundus oculi changes or variations in the lens (no opacities or worsening of previously present opacities).[12] On the other hand, Palmquist in 1984 studied patients receiving an extremely prolonged HBO_2 course (150-850 daily exposures at 2-2.5 ATA [202.65-253.32 kPa]), and all patients except one developed PM (many with cataracts).[13] More recent literature found a greater incidence of PM in higher pressure protocols of HBO_2 (greater at 2.4 ATA [243.18 kPa] than at 2.0 ATA [202.65 kPa]),[14-15] or when a hood was used instead of an oronasal mask,[16] suggesting the role of trans-corneal oxygen diffusion in the pathogenesis of PM.

Paired with PM, cataract development may be associated with prolonged HBO_2. Oxygen plays a fundamental role in this pathology because, even though the crystalline lens is an avascular tissue, high levels of available oxygen lead to an increase in oxidative stress and protein denaturation. The above-published reports,[10-13] as well as extensive clinical experience in major hyperbaric centers, indicate that new cataracts do not develop within 20-50 sessions. However, extension of HBO_2 beyond 100 sessions may be associated with increased risk of irreversible cataract development.[13] Of note, only one instance of early cataract development has been reported in a 49-year-old woman who had only 48 HBO_2 treatments over a period of 11 weeks, with persistence of the disease at follow-up. Although HBO_2 treatment is a possible cause, the pathogenesis in this case may have been related to other factors.[17]

It has been hypothesized that reactive oxygen species may be involved in the pathophysiology of both keratoconus and retinal injury,[9] and indeed acute exposure to PO_2 exceeding 3 ATA can induce reversible visual field changes (see below). However, to date we are unaware of any direct link between clinical HBO_2 treatment and development of either keratoconus or retinal injury.

The contraction of peripheral vision[18-19] and the reduction in the electrical response of retinal glial cells to light[20] are other reversible effects of HBO_2 on visual function. These effects are only described in oxygen pressure-duration combinations that greatly exceed common applications of HBO_2. Exceptions to this general rule include a single case of reversible vision loss during a relatively brief oxygen exposure in an individual with a previous history of retrobulbar neuritis.[21]

Pulmonology

Pulmonary manifestations of oxygen poisoning are often cited as major concerns. Oxygen tolerance limits that avoid these manifestations are well defined for continuous exposures in healthy human volunteers.[22-23] Pulmonary symptoms are not produced by usual HBO_2 protocols, such as daily exposures to oxygen at 2.0 or 2.4 ATA (202.65 or 243.18 kPa) for 120 or 90 minutes, respectively, but become apparent after about six hours at 2.0 ATA.[24] Pathogenesis seems to be related to damage from reactive oxygen species.[25] Main symptoms associated with pulmonary oxygen toxicity starts with a burning sensation with inspiration, progressing to a nonproductive cough. If oxygen administration is continued, symptoms can progress to dyspnea on exertion, as an early manifestation of ARDS. Of note, the rate of onset of these symptoms can be relatively slowed by intermittent air-breathing periods ("air breaks"). Most of the symptoms diminish promptly after the interruption of the treatment, while the burning sensation can take one to three days to disappear.[26]

Pulmonary mechanical and gas exchange functions seem early impaired during prolonged daily HBO_2 sessions, and the patterns of manifestations vary on protocols used and on subjects' baseline pulmonary status. The scarcely available literature detected small decrements in lung volumes and flow rates (both in expiratory and inspiratory flows), carbon monoxide diffusing capacity and alveolar-arterial gradient,[27] whose clinical significance is questionable, but more research is needed in this field to compare the benefits and risks of prolonged HBO_2 in subjects affected by restrictive and obstructive pulmonary diseases. Of note, no differences in gas exchanges were found comparing healthy volunteers and patients with pulmonary dysfunction.[28-29]

Although rare, pulmonary barotrauma during decompression has been reported in patients with lung disease, including airway obstruction.[30-32] Overdistension and rupture of alveoli due to gas trapping can result in pneumothorax, pneumomediastinum or even arterial gas embolism. Significant air trapping (as in obstructive pulmonary diseases) and a history of spontaneous pneumothorax are concerning and should be carefully assessed in the pre-hyperbaric treatment evaluation.

Central Nervous System

Typical manifestations of oxygen toxicity in the central nervous system include the following: nausea; vomiting; numbness; twitching; dizziness; olfactory, acoustic, or gustatory sensations; and in its most severe form, nonfocal tonic-clonic seizures.[33-34]

Generally, the higher the time and oxygen pressure for the treatment, the greater the incidence of seizures. One study reported that all 36 divers breathing 100% oxygen at 3.7 ATA (374,90 kPa) experienced symptoms.[33-34] Early estimates reported an incidence of HBO_2-related seizures of around 0.01% per treatment (1.0 per 10,000 sessions at 2.0-3.0 ATA [202.65-303.98 kPa]),[3-4,35] while more recent studies suggest a higher incidence of 0.024% in 5,193 patients from 8 different facilities[36] (2.4 per 10,000 sessions at 2.4 ATA [243.18 kPa]). The higher incidence in the latter group could be related to the use of a head tent for HBO_2, while in earlier studies this aspect is not clearly specified and possibly due to unrecognized air leaks allowed by a poorly fitting face mask causing some reduction in inspired PO_2. The incidence of seizures in patients treated for carbon monoxide intoxication is higher (1.8%),[37] presumably due to intrinsic neuronal toxicity of carbon monoxide and possibly associated metabolic changes, which may contribute to lowering of the epileptic threshold.

Treatment of hyperoxic seizures consists of immediate reduction of inspired PO_2 by switching the breathing gas to room air. Evidence regarding the need for subsequent anticonvulsant treatment is scarce and anecdotal and is usually based on personal preference of the responsible physician. Decompression is contraindicated during active convulsions because of seizure-related glottis closure and the consequent potential development of lung barotrauma. Hyperoxic seizure recurrence is uncommon, and neither occurrence of a hyperoxia-related seizure or a past history of seizures preclude HBO_2.

Pediatric Considerations

The critically ill pediatric patient can safely receive HBO_2 in a multiplace chamber when personnel with appropriate experience are available. Complications included hypotension (63%), bronchospasm (34%), hemotympanum (13%) and progressive hypoxemia (6%). Of note, one child was accidentally extubated during transport.[37]

The development of retrolental fibroplasia (RF) is frequently seen after the exposure of the premature retina to relatively low levels of hyperoxia.[38] In the incompletely developed vascularization of the retina, hyperoxia starts a vicious cycle of vasoconstriction, depletion of growth factors, arrest of retinal neovascularization, hypoperfusion and ischemia. The result is an exaggerated rebound production of growth factors leading to disorganized angiogenesis and fibrosis.[2,39] RF could be concerning also in the unborn, but no cases are reported in literature even in the offspring of pregnant women treated with HBO_2 for conditions such as carbon monoxide poisoning, usually with a single session. However, pregnant women should only be treated with HBO_2 for emergency indications, when the risks of withholding the treatment outweigh those of harming the fetus.

Long-Term Evaluation of Side Effects

Currently, little is known about possible long-term effects of HBO_2. Davis and colleagues studied this issue in 1998 at the United States Air Force School of Aerospace Medicine. Their analysis included 563 patients that received more than 20 daily, 90 minutes long, hyperbaric oxygen treatments at 2.4 ATA (243.18 kPa). The follow-up period was six months to eight years and no chronic or late effects potentially related to HBO_2 were recorded, except for the development of cataracts in only two predisposed patients (a poorly controlled diabetic and a 67-year-old man taking high doses of corticosteroids).[3]

Monoplace Chambers Considerations

Monoplace hyperbaric chambers (MoHCs) are extensively used in the United States but rarely in other countries. A review by Lind describes the pros and cons regarding the choice of a MoHC in several clinical contexts.[40] Even if the use of multiplace hyperbaric chambers seems to be economically and logistically challenging, these may be better suited for the critical unstable patient who needs special equipment and advanced support during the treatment. Moreover, multiplace hyperbaric chambers can be used to treat several casualties at the same time (e.g. multiple carbon monoxide intoxications). On the other hand, MoHCs are cost-effective, versatile, and require less staffing (no inside attendant for adults), but the capacity to adequately monitor the critical patient can be limited. Of note, the reported incidence of complications during use of a MoHCs remains low (Table 1).[41]

Table 1. Adverse Events during Hyperbaric Oxygen Treatment in Monoplace Chambers

	Total events in 2 year	Adverse events per 10,000 sessions
Number of treatments	463,293	---
Complications	1870	40
Ear pain	928	20
Confinement anxiety	407	8
Hypoglycemic event	244	5
Shortness of breath	112	2
Seizure	88	2
Sinus pain	66	1
Chest pain	25	1

Other Considerations

Claustrophobia appears to be present in about 2% of the general population and may cause some degree of confinement anxiety, even in a multiplace chamber. Beyond reassurance, relaxation techniques and coaching, mild sedation is occasionally required for such individuals to continue the therapy.[3]

Dental barotrauma can happen during HBO_2 especially during decompression but has been mostly reported in divers.[42] Infections are a major predisposing factor, but the pathogenesis is not clear. Gas trapped under a root can cause pain, dental stress and in extreme reported cases odontocrexis (dental explosion).

Conflict of Interest

The authors have declared that no conflict of interest exists with this submission.

References

1. Cousins JL, Wark PA, Mcdonald VM. Acute oxygen therapy: a review of prescribing and delivery practices. Int J Chron Obstruct Pulmon Dis. 2016;11:1067-75.
2. Heyboer M, Sharma D, Santiago W, Mcculloch N. Hyperbaric oxygen therapy: side effects defined and quantified. Adv Wound Care (New Rochelle). 2017;6(6):210-224.
3. Davis JC, Dunn JM, Heimbach RD. Hyperbaric medicine: patient selection, treatment procedures, and side effects. In: Davis JC, Hunt TK, eds. Problem wounds: the role of oxygen. New York: Elsevier; 1988. Pp:225-235.
4. Davis JC. Hyperbaric oxygen therapy. J Intensive Care Med 1989;4:55-57.
5. Brown M, Jones J, Krohmer J. Pseudoephedrine for the prevention of barotitis media: a controlled clinical trial in underwater divers. Ann Emerg Med. 1992;21:849-852.
6. Carlson S, Jones J, Brown M, Hess C. Prevention of hyperbaric-associated middle ear barotrauma. Ann Emerg Med. 1992;21:1468-1471.
7. Fernau JL, Hirsch BE, Derkay C, Ramasastry S, Schaefer SE. Hyperbaric oxygen therapy: effect on middle ear and eustachian tube function. Laryngoscope. 1992;102:48-52.
8. Shupak A, Atias J, Aviv J, Melamed Y. Oxygen diving-induced middle ear under-aeration. Acta Otolaryngol Stockh. 1995;115:422-426.
9. McMonnies CW. Hyperbaric oxygen therapy and the possibility of ocular complications or contraindications. Clin Exp Optom. 2015;98(2):122-5.
10. Anderson B Jr, Farmer JC Jr. Hyperoxic myopia. Trans Am Ophthalmol Soc 1978;76:116-124.
11. Anderson B Jr, Shelton DL. Axial length in hyperoxic myopia. In: Bove AA, Bachrach AJ, Greenbaum LJ Jr, eds. Underwater and hyperbaric physiology IX. Proceedings of the ninth international symposium on underwater and hyperbaric physiology. Bethesda, MD: Undersea and Hyperbaric Medical Society; 1987. Pp:607-611.
12. Lyne AJ. Ocular effects of hyperbaric oxygen. Trans Ophthalmol Soc. 1978; 98:66-68.
13. Palmquist BM, Philipson B, Barr PO. Nuclear cataract and myopia during hyperbaric oxygen therapy. Br J Ophthalmol.1984;68:113-117.
14. Churchill S, Hopkins RO, Weaver LK. Incidence and duration of myopia while receiving hyperbaric oxygen (HBO$_2$) therapy. Undersea Hyperbaric Med 1997;24 (Suppl):36.
15. Dedi D, Prager T, Jacob R, Chan A, Fife C. Visual acuity changes in patients undergoing hyperbaric oxygen therapy. Undersea Hyperbaric Med 1998;25(Suppl):34.
16. Evanger K, Haugen OH, Irgens A, Aanderud L, Thorsen E. Ocular refractive changes in patients receiving hyperbaric oxygen administered by oronasal mask or hood. Acta Ophthalmol. 2004;82:449-453.
17. Gesell LB, Adams BS, Kob DG. De novo cataract development following a standard course of hyperbaric oxygen therapy. Undersea Hyperbaric Med 2000;27 (Suppl): 56-57.
18. Behnke AR, Forbes HS, Motley EP. Circulatory and visual effects of oxygen at 3 atmospheres pressure. Am J Physiol. 1936;114:436-442.
19. Lambertsen CJ, Clark JM, Gelfand R, Pisarello J, Cobbs WH, Bevilacqua JE, Schwartz DM, Montabana DJ, Leach CS, Johnson PC, Fletcher DE. Definition of tolerance to continuous hyperoxia in man. An abstract report of predictive studies V. In: Bove AA, Bachrach AJ, Greenbaum LJ Jr, eds. Underwater and hyperbaric physiology IX. Proceedings of the ninth international symposium on underwater and hyperbaric physiology. Bethesda, MD: Undersea and Hyperbaric Medical Society; 1987. Pp:717-735.
20. Clark JM, Lambertsen CJ, Montabana DJ, Gelfand R, Cobbs WH. Comparison of visual function effects in man during continuous oxygen exposures at 3.0 and 2.0 ATA for 3.4 and 9.0 hours. Undersea Biomed Res. 1988;15(suppl):32.
21. Nichols CW, Lambertsen CJ, Clark JM. Transient unilateral loss of vision associated with oxygen at high pressure. Arch Ophthalmol. 1969;81:548-552.
22. Clark JM, Thom SR. Oxygen under pressure. In: Brubakk AO, Neuman TS, eds. Bennett and Elliott's physiology and medicine of diving, 5th ed. Philadelphia: W.B. Saunders; 2003. Pp:358-418.
23. Lambertsen CJ. Effects of hyperoxia on organs and their tissues. In: Robin E, ed. Extrapulmonary manifestation of respiratory disease. New York: Marcel Dekker; 1978. Pp:239-303.
24. Kindwall EP. Working under increased barometric pressure. In: Francis TJR, ed. Encyclopedia of Occupational Health and Safety. Geneva: International Labor Organization; 2011.
25. Tsan MF Superoxide dismutase and pulmonary oxygen toxicity: lessons from transgenic and knockout mice (Review). Int J Mol Med. 2001 Jan;7(1):13-9.
26. Clark JM, Lambertsen CJ. Rate of development of pulmonary O$_2$ toxicity in man during O$_2$ breathing at 2.0 ATA. J Appl Physiol. 1971;30:739–752.

27. Thorsen E, Aanderud L, Aasen TB. Effects of a standard hyperbaric oxygen treatment protocol on pulmonary function. Eur Respir J. 1998;12:1442-1445.

28. Weaver LK, Howe S. Normobaric measurement of O_2 tension of blood in subjects exposed to hyperbaric oxygen. Chest. 1992;102:1175-1181.

29. Weaver LK, Howe S. Arterial oxygen tension of patients with abnormal lungs treated with hyperbaric oxygen is greater than predicted. Chest. 1994;106:1134-1139.

30. Bond GF. Arterial gas embolism. In: Davis JC, Hunt TK, eds. Hyperbaric oxygen therapy. Bethesda, MD: Undersea Medical Society;1977. Pp:141-152.

31. Wolf HK, Moon RE, Mitchell PR, Burger PC. Barotrauma and air embolism in hyperbaric oxygen therapy. Am J Forensic Med Pathol. 1990;11:149-153.

32. Sloan EP, Murphy DG, Hart R, Cooper MA, Turnbull T, Barreca RS, Ellerson B. Complication and protocol considerations in carbon monoxide-poisoned patients who require hyperbaric oxygen therapy: report from a ten-year experience. Ann Emerg Med. 1989;18:629-634.

33. K.W. Donald: Oxygen poisoning in man. I. Br Med J.1:667-672. 1947.

34. K.W. Donald: Oxygen poisoning in man. II. Br Med J.1:712-717. 1947.

35. Hart GB, Strauss MB. Central nervous system oxygen toxicity in a clinical setting. In: Bove AA, Bachrach AJ, Greenbaum LJ, eds. Undersea and hyperbaric physiology IX. Proceedings of the ninth international symposium on underwater and hyperbaric physiology. Bethesda, MD: Undersea and Hyperbaric Medical Society; 1987. Pp:695-699.

36. Sherlock S, Way M, Tabah A. Audit of practice in Australasian hyperbaric units on the incidence of central nervous system oxygen toxicity. Diving Hyperb Med. 2018;48(2):73-78.

37. Keenan HT, Bratton SL, Norkool DM, Brogan TV, Hampson NB. Delivery of hyperbaric oxygen therapy to critically ill, mechanically ventilated children. J Crit Care. 1998;13:7-12.

38. Patz A. Effect of oxygen on immature retinal vessels. Invest Ophthalmol. 1965;4:988-999.

39. Sola A, Chow L, Rogido M. [Retinopathy of prematurity and oxygen therapy: a changing relationship]. An Pediatr (Barc). 2005;62(1):48-63.

40. Lind F. A pro/con review comparing the use of mono- and multiplace hyperbaric chambers for critical care. Diving Hyperb Med. 2015;45(1):56-60.

41. Beard T, Watson B, Barry R, Stewart D, Warriner R: Analysis of adverse events occurring in patients undergoing adjunctive hyperbaric oxygen treatment: 2009-2010 (Abstract) UHM Vol. 38-5 - section G, p. 455. 2011.

42. Zadik Y, Drucker S. Diving dentistry: a review of the dental implications of scuba diving. Australian Dent J. 2011;56:265–271.

CHAPTER 17

Oxygen Pretreatment and Preconditioning

Enrico M. Camporesi MD, Matteo Paganini MD, Gerardo Bosco MD, PhD

Abstract

Pretreatment with hyperbaric oxygen results in preconditioning, that is the induction of physiological and pathophysiological protective changes (e.g. genetic or enzymatic modifications) against predictable, extreme, environment-induced and disease-related damages. This therapy is nowadays emerging as a useful adjunct in diving medicine, as well as in the treatment of acute and chronic diseases.

Oxygen pretreatment before diving has been extensively documented in recreational, technical, commercial and military diving. Its use for tissue denitrogenation has an important role in the prevention of decompression sickness, resulting in a lesser post-diving micronuclei load. Hyperbaric oxygen pretreatment has also been used in patients before exposure to several clinical situations with beneficial effects. Preconditioning with hyperbaric oxygen increases the antioxidant resiliency of the body, especially against the consequences of ischemia-reperfusion injury. The mechanisms of action are only partially understood, but this therapy has been successfully applied before coronary artery bypass grafting and is a promising technique in several other systems or procedures. Future efforts in research should be undertaken to better understand the basic knowledge about preconditioning and, most important, to help in the translation of current discoveries towards the clinical context.

Rationale

As previously defined by Murry in 1986, the term "pretreatment" describes the act of exposing a patient to a controlled stimulus before a crucial and similar event affects that subject. This pretreatment is intended to cause in the patient "preconditioning," that is the induction of physiological and pathophysiological protective changes (e.g. genetic or enzymatic modifications) against predictable, extreme, environment-induced and disease-related damages.[1] In the last decade, a number of researchers reported several experiences of oxygen (O_2) preconditioning after breathing normobaric (NBO_2) or hyperbaric oxygen (HBO_2). The duration and modality of O_2 pretreatment can influence the modality of preconditioning and, therefore, cause different expression patterns of these changes at a biomolecular level, as well as macroscopically.

In the most practical form, a short pretreatment period with inhaled 100% NBO_2 has been historically used to increase the body's O_2 reserves. For example, several techniques of preoxygenation are recommended before the induction of general anesthesia, as a safety maneuver to prevent dangerous tissue deoxygenation in patients with a difficult airway and at risk of prolonged laryngoscopy time (such as pregnant women, small children and the obese).[2] Moreover, a short O_2 pretreatment has also been used in extreme environments such as breath-hold diving to prolong useful apnea time.[3]

Oxygen causes peculiar physiological and pathophysiological responses during and after an extended exposure. In fact, a prolonged (one hour at sea level) O_2 inhalation at rest can result in a significant heart rate and cardiac output decrease, in parallel with a peripheral vascular resistance increase.[4] These effects are probably the consequence exerted by hyperoxia on the autonomic nervous system, resulting in a reduction of sympathetic and an increase of parasympathetic tone that can persist for more than one hour after restoring normal environmental air conditions.[5] Therefore, the effects of the prolonged O_2 administration could be useful to counterbalance potentially dangerous responses to non-physiological selected environmental or clinical circumstances.

Apart from the prolonged and repetitive use of O_2 in mountain climbing, aviation and space medicine,[6] this chapter will describe the effects of prolonged NBO_2 and prolonged HBO_2 pretreatment and will show currently known biomolecular and macroscopical changes in diving medicine and in selected clinical situations.

Diving Medicine Applications

O_2 pretreatment can be successfully utilized for recreational, technical, commercial[7] and military diving[6] for the prevention of potential complications connected with underwater activities.

In the case of decompression sickness (DCS), an immediate treatment with normobaric O_2 is fundamental. Its use on the scene of a diving accident and during the prompt evacuation to definitive treatment in the hyperbaric chamber positively affects the outcome of these patients and can be life-saving, as discussed in Chapter 7: Decompression Sickness.[8] However, it is important to remember that the development of DCS relies on two main features: the rapid decrease in hydrostatic pressure and the expansion of gas micronuclei into bubbles.[9]

As suggested by an early study, micronuclei of inert nitrogen (N_2) gas exist within living tissue under normal conditions.[10] With this assumption, a number of researchers have recently confirmed that pretreatment with NBO_2 or HBO_2 can significantly remove N_2, reduce micronuclei and therefore prevent bubble formation after decompression.[9,11-12] In fact, O_2 may replace N_2 inside micronuclei by diffusion and then is consumed, thus progressively reducing the size and removing micronuclei from tissues.[6,12-15] Moreover, tissue exposure to hyperoxia causes denitrogenation, that is the elimination of inert N_2 normally present in tissues by diffusion into the bloodstream, thus reducing the likelihood of bubble formation.[16] Oxygen also seems to enhance the metabolism of lymphatic vessels, thus promoting the removal of proteins coated by micronuclei,[17] although the exact mechanisms remain still poorly understood. Of note, it has been proposed that exercise can increase the preventive effects of O_2 pretreatment through an increase of ventilation, tissue perfusion and gas diffusion,[18] and thus allow a shorter time of O_2 pretreatment.

After such pretreatments, the delay for the regeneration of micronuclei population can range from a few hours up to 100 hours.[19] Specifically, Castagna and colleagues showed that 30 minutes of NBO_2 pretreatment before repetitive open-water air dives provides a significant reduction in decompression-induced bubble production (assessed with a Doppler ultrasound and bubble formation score).[6] Surprisingly, this protective effect was also extended to a subsequent dive, even though repetitive diving is known to increase bubble production[20] and therefore the risk of DCS.[21]

Researchers have recently shown that compared to NBO_2 pretreatment, HBO_2 pretreatment may have an enhanced protective effect against DCS development in humans. For example, pretreatment with O_2 at 1.6 atmospheres absolute (ATA) (162.12 kPa) for 25 minutes significantly reduced bubble score detected with Doppler ultrasound compared to NBO_2 pretreatment, suggesting more efficient denitrogenation and denucleation.[12] Subsequent studies in open-water divers demonstrated that underwater O_2 breathing at a depth of 6 or 12 msw led to lower bubble scores than O_2 pretreatment at the surface.[9]

Questions have been raised about a possible contribution of activated platelets in the pathogenesis of DCS,[22] and indeed O_2 pretreatment may attenuate platelet activation. Recent work has demonstrated reduced platelet activation after HBO_2,[12] or NBO_2 and underwater HBO_2 pretreatment, [9, 23] thus opening the way to further research in this new application of O_2 pretreatment against DCS.

Hyperbaric Medicine Applications

HBO_2 preconditioning has been used in patients before exposure to potentially dangerous clinical situations with beneficial effects, but the mechanisms of action have not yet been clearly ascertained or completely translated into clinical practice.

Ischemia-reperfusion (I/R) is a pathologic phenomenon during which reperfusion of ischemic tissue by oxygenated blood increases numbers and activities of oxidants generated in tissues, causing injury. In particular, reperfusion increases the hazardous effects of early ischemic injury mainly by enhancing inflammation in two ways: first by the release of cytokines and reactive O_2 species such as hydroxyl radical ($\bullet OH$), superoxide radical (O_2-), and hydrogen peroxide (H_2O_2), and second by activation of the complement system.[24]

All tissues can be involved in I/R. Basic science research in the field has focused on animal models demonstrating the tolerance and vulnerability of different tissues and organs such as kidney, liver, lung, testis, brain, heart muscle, skeletal muscle, and intestine.[25-31] Some important enzymatic pathways involved in the ischemic response have been shown to be influenced by HBO_2 therapy, such as the increased expression of HIF-1α,[32] but in recent years there has been an increasing amount of clinical research in this area. This has resulted in increased understanding of the mechanisms of I/R and its causes, which may be natural (e.g. atherosclerotic occlusive disease, arterial thrombosis or embolism, and vascular trauma) or iatrogenic (such as organ transplantation or when a prolonged bloodless surgical field is needed during a surgical procedure[26,33]). In this context, the pretreatment with O_2 is intended to activate endogenous protective mechanisms to potentially reduce the morphologic and functional sequelae of a prolonged ischemic insult.

Cardiac Surgery

Despite constant improvement in surgical techniques and anesthetic management, I/R injury remains an inevitable effect of cardiac surgery. I/R can be a consequence of aortic clamping during cardiopulmonary bypass (CPB) and is a cause of perioperative complications and mortality in coronary artery bypass grafting (CABG).[34] Among the most frequent complications, I/R is responsible for reperfusion-induced arrhythmias, myocardial stunning, microvascular obstruction and reperfusion injury, as a result of apoptosis and several other changes occurring in myocardiocytes that manifests clinically as low cardiac output in the acute or as heart failure in the chronic setting.[35-36]

Oxygen preconditioning of the heart was firstly described in a canine myocardium I/R injury model.[37] Since then, intense research on possible applications of preconditioning before cardiac surgery has been undertaken, including the use of volatile anesthetic gases[34] and artificially induced peripheral limb ischemia.[38-40] In particular, the latter technique has shown an interesting twofold timing of increased protection: an early "first window" developing within minutes from the pretreatment lasting a few hours, and a "second window" occurring from about 12-24 hours to three to four days after delivering the ischemic stimulus. This finding has also been applied to the prevention of high-altitude illness.[41] More recently, several studies have linked HBO_2 preconditioning with better outcomes after CABG [Table 1]. Positive effects of HBO_2 preconditioning on the heart were prominent in terms of better cardiovascular hemodynamic parameters, length of stay in intensive care unit, hospital length of stay, perioperative complications, and cardiac injury.[42-43] More important, HBO_2 pretreatment seems useful for on-pump but not for off-pump CABG surgery patients, thus confirming the role of CPB in the pathogenesis of I/R injury.[43] Moreover, trials in this field showed not only a better cardiac function in patients pretreated with HBO$_2$ but also reduced systemic inflammatory response and neuropsychometric dysfunction,[44] less cerebral inflammation and increased cerebral protection.[43]

Table 1. Evidence of HBO$_2$ Preconditioning Usefulness in Patients Undergoing CABG

	Design	HBO$_2$ protocol	Outcome measured	Main results
Alex, 2005[44]	Randomized, double-blind trial	3 sessions at 2.4 ATA (243.18 kPa)	inflammatory response; neuropsychometric dysfunction. HBO$_2$ vs. control	HBO$_2$ resulted in: ↓ inflammatory response and neuropsychometric dysfunction
Yogaratnam, 2010[42]	Randomized controlled clinical trial	1 session at 2.5 ATA (253.32 kPa) for 90 min	Cardiovascular hemodynamic parameters; LOS in ICU; perioperative complications. HBO$_2$ vs. control	HBO$_2$ resulted in: ↓ PVR, troponin T, LOS in ICU, perioperative complications, blood loss; ↑ SV and LVSW
Li 2011[43]	Randomized controlled clinical trial	1 session/day for 5 days at 2.0 ATA (202.65 kPa) for 70 min each	Cardiovascular hemodynamic and vital parameters; cerebral inflammatory markers and S100B protein; HBO$_2$ vs. control, and in-pump vs. on-pump	HBO$_2$ resulted in: ↓ troponin I, inotrope use, ventilator hours, LOS in ICU and hospital; ↑ hemodynamic parameters, serum CAT activity. ↓ S100B and NSE in on-pump + HBO$_2$ pretreated.
Jeysen 2011[45]	Randomized controlled clinical trial	At 2.4 ATA (243.18 kPa) 30 + 30 minutes	eNOS and HSP72 on right atrium biopsies	No significant changes in eNOS and HSP72

HBO$_2$: hyperbaric oxygen; CABG: coronary artery bypass grafting; SV: stroke volume; LVSW: left ventricle stroke work; PVR: pulmonary vascular resistance; eNOS: nitric oxide synthase; HSP72: heat shock protein 72.

Central Nervous System

The brain and the spinal cord have a unique sensitivity to ischemia due to their high metabolism, dependence on constant glucose delivery and peculiar features of neurons. Despite excellent results in the treatment of several affections of the central nervous system and a high interest in the topic, most of the existing literature is restricted to animal models.[36] Reports have indicated that HBO$_2$ preconditioning in pre-clinical trials cause controlled oxidative stress and subsequent transcription of various antioxidative enzymes in the central nervous system including not only catalase (CAT), superoxide dismutase, peroxidases, and heme oxygenase-1 but also heat-shock proteins, Nrf-2 and eNOS/nNOS enzymes.[46-49] However, clinical trials designed to assess the utility of HBO$_2$ pretreatment on neurological outcomes have failed thus far to show benefit, although the results of these trials could have been biased because the populations studied consisted mostly of elderly people with comorbidities and polytherapy.[36]

Neurological impairment has been frequently reported after cardiac surgery. Sequelae can be mild (such as postoperative cognitive dysfunction and postoperative delirium) or be as severe as stroke.[50] The etiology of cardiac surgery-related cerebral injuries is probably multifactorial, arising from an interaction among cerebral microemboli, global cerebral hypoperfusion, inflammation, cerebral temperature modulation and genetic susceptibility.[51] In this field, trials of HBO$_2$ therapy preconditioning have shown reduced postoperative cognitive dysfunction.[44,52]

Other Systems and Perspectives of Future Research

Studies have demonstrated that NBO_2 and HBO_2 preconditioning may have a beneficial effect on other organ systems, for example induction of heme oxygenase 1 and its protective role in liver I/R injury.[53] HBO_2 preconditioning has been shown to reduce the incidence of pulmonary infections in oncologic patients undergoing a pancreaticoduodenectomy (Whipple procedure).[54] Studies on the effects of HBO_2 preconditioning on surgical outcomes are short-term and scarce. Future studies should assess both short and long-term outcomes.

HBO_2 pretreatment administered underwater has been shown to have two effects on peripheral blood lymphocytes. First, compared with HBO_2 administered in the dry, CAT enzyme activity in circulating lymphocytes, as well as superoxide dismutase and glutathione peroxidase mRNA genes expression patterns, were higher in underwater. Second, no intracellular calcium increase was found in lymphocytes, suggesting a preserved calcium homeostasis. Both these results were interpreted as an enhanced antioxidant defense but these mechanisms need further assessments.[23]

Only one study addressed the usefulness of HBO_2 in patients admitted for unstable angina or acute myocardial infarction and undergoing percutaneous transluminal coronary intervention. However, results of this study are questionable because of a restricted sample size and to a non-rigorous methodology (among patients allocated in the HBO_2 arm, some received pretreatment while the other part received HBO_2 *after* the procedure).[55]

Skin flap grafting is a widely used technique in plastic surgery, affected by I/R injury which significantly impacts the survival of the graft. Basic science studies in rats suggest an association of HBO_2 pretreatment with antioxidative effects, better vascularization of the flap, decreased expression of adhesive molecules on T-cells (reducing rejection) and resistance to I/R injury.[56] The clinical usefulness of these observations will need confirmation in human studies.

The interaction of HBO_2 therapy with drugs could be a future interesting research field. For example, Yang and colleagues suggested a protective effect of HBO_2 therapy against indomethacin-induced enteropathy.[57] Future investigations will also have to take into account confounding effects exerted by various diseases and medications on NO synthesis, apoptosis, autophagy, and gene transcription.[36] We therefore suggest a multidisciplinary approach for the translation of the above-mentioned experiments in the clinical context, and the subsequent integration of NBO_2 and HBO_2 into consensus-based international guidelines.

Conflict of Interest

The authors have declared that no conflict of interest exists with this submission.

References

1. Murry CE, Jennings RB, Reimer KA. Preconditioning with ischemia: a delay of lethal cell injury in ischemic myocardium. Circulation. 1986;74(5):1124-36.
2. Bouroche G, Bourgain JL. Preoxygenation and general anesthesia: a review. Minerva Anestesiol. 2015;81(8):910-20.
3. Otis AB, Rahn H, Fenn WO. Alveolar gas changes during breath holding. Am J Physiol. 1948;152(3):674-86.
4. Waring WS, Thomson AJ, Adwani SH, Rosseel AJ, Potter JF, Webb DJ, Maxwell SR. Cardiovascular effects of acute oxygen administration in healthy adults. J Cardiovasc Pharmacol. 2003;42:245-250.
5. Thomson AJ, Drummond GB, Waring WS, Webb DJ, Maxwell SR. Effects of short-term isocapnic hyperoxia and hypoxia on cardiovascular function. J Appl Physiol. 2006;101:809-816.
6. Castagna O, Gempp E, Blatteau JE. Pre-dive normobaric oxygen reduces bubble formation in scuba divers. Eur J Appl Physiol. 2009;106:167-172.
7. Piepho T, Ehrmann U, Werner C, Muth CM. Oxygen therapy in diving accidents. Anaesthesist. 2007;56:44-52.
8. Vann RD, Denoble PJ, Howle LE, Weber PW, Freiberger JJ, Pieper CF. Resolution and severity in decompression illness. Aviat Space Environ Med. 2009;80:466-471.
9. Bosco G, Yang ZJ, Di Tano G, Camporesi EM, Faralli F, Savini F, Landolfi A, Doria C, Fano G. Effect of in-water oxygen prebreathing at different depths on decompression-induced bubble formation and platelet activation. J Appl Physiol. 2010;108:1077-1083.
10. Evans A, Walder DN. Significance of gas micronuclei in the aetiology of decompression sickness. Nature. 1969;222(5190):251-2.
11. Arieli R, Boaron E, Arieli Y, Abramovich A, Katsenelson K. Oxygen pretreatment as protection against decompression sickness in rats: pressure and time necessary for hypothesized denucleation and renucleation. Eur J Appl Physiol. 2011;111:997-1005.
12. Landolfi A, Yang Z, Savini F, Camporesi E, Faralli F, Bosco G. Pre-treatment with hyperbaric oxygenation reduces bubble formation and platelet activation. Sport Sciences for Health. 2006;1:122-128.
13. Arieli Y, Arieli R, Marx A. Hyperbaric oxygen may reduce gas bubbles in decompressed prawns by eliminating gas nuclei. J Appl Physiol. 2002;92:2596-2599.
14. Butler BD, Little T, Cogan V, Powell M. Hyperbaric oxygen pre-breathe modifies the outcome of decompression sickness. Undersea Hyperb Med. 2006;33:407-417.
15. Katsenelson K, Arieli Y, Abramovich A, Feinsod M, Arieli R. Hyperbaric oxygen pretreatment reduces the incidence of decompression sickness in rats. Eur J Appl Physiol. 2007;101:571-576.
16. Behnke AR. The isobaric (oxygen window) principle of decompression. In: The new thrust seaward. Transactions of the third annual conference of marine technology society. San Diego, CA: Marine Technology Society; 1967.
17. Balestra C, Germonpre P, Snoeck T, Ezquer M, Leduc O, Leduc A, Willeput F, Marroni A, Cali Corleo R, Vann R. Normobaric oxygen can enhance protein captation by the lymphatic system in healthy humans. Undersea Hyperb Med. 2004;31:59-62.
18. Webb JT, Pilmanis AA. Preoxygenation time versus decompression sickness incidence. SAFE J. 1999;29:75-78.
19. Younth DE. On the evolution, generation, and regeneration of gas cavitation nuclei. J Acoust Soc Am. 1982;71:1473-1481.
20. Dunford RG, Vann RD, Gerth WA, Pieper CF, Huggins K, Wacholtz C, Bennett PB. The incidence of venous gas emboli in recreational diving. Undersea Hyperb Med. 2002;29:247-259.
21. Hamilton RW, Thalmann ED. Decompression practice. In: Brubakk AO, Neuman TS, editors. Bennett & Elliott's Physiology and Medicine of Diving. 5th ed. New York, NY: Elsevier Science; 2003. Pp. 455-500.
22. Pontier JM, Gempp E, Ignatescu M. Blood platelet-derived microparticles release and bubble formation after an open-sea air dive. Appl Physiol Nutr Metab. 2012;37(5):888-92.
23. Morabito C, Bosco G, Pilla R, Corona C, Mancinelli R, Yang Z, Camporesi EM, Fano G, Mariggio MA. Effect of pre-breathing oxygen at different depth on oxidative status and calcium concentration in lymphocytes of scuba divers. Acta Physiol (Oxf). 2011;202:69-78.
24. Gorsuch WB, Chrysanthou E, Schwaeble WJ, Stahl GL. The complement system in ischemia-reperfusion injuries. Immunobiology. 2012;217(11):1026-33.
25. Yu SY, Chiu JH, Yang SD, Yu HY, Hsieh CC, Chen PJ, Lui WY, Wu CW. Preconditioned hyperbaric oxygenation protects the liver against ischemia-reperfusion injury in rats. J Surg Res. 2005;128:28-36.
26. Grisotto PC, dos Santos AC, Coutinho-Netto J, Cherri J, Piccinato CE. Indicators of oxidative injury and alterations of the cell membrane in the skeletal muscle of rats submitted to ischemia and reperfusion. J Surg Res. 2000;92:1-6.

The controversy is illustrated by the fascinating RCT published in 2013 by Efrati et al, concerning the treatment of a different chronic neurological condition: post-ischemic stroke from six to 36 months after the event.[32] In this unblinded trial (with no attempt to provide a sham therapy), patients improved in functional and quality-of-life scores after 40 sessions of HBO_2 for 90 minutes at 2 ATA over two months. The cross group, who continued their standard rehabilitation, showed no such improvement for two months, after which they, too, received HBO_2 therapy, and showed similar improvements. The authors concluded they had shown "convincing results demonstrating that HBO_2 therapy, can induce significant neurological improvement in poststroke patients." They attribute these changes to the activation of neuroplasticity in the brain by HBO_2 therapy.

These authors maintain a true sham therapy for HBO_2 cannot be devised because confinement in the chamber and breathing air or oxygen, even at trivial pressures, constitutes an active comparator. Perhaps serendipitously, the magnitude of any treatment effect happens to be similar at all oxygen, nitrogen and pressure doses used to date. Those who prosecute this view suggest the best we can do in this situation is to use the continuation of standard treatment alone. This position means we can never hope to conduct a sham-controlled, blinded study in hyperbaric therapy. If true, the implications for generating robust evidence to support hyperbaric practice that would convince both colleagues in other fields to use it, and funding authorities to pay for it, are grave.

An alternative view is that once again these authors have shown that a series of exposures in the hyperbaric chamber lead to a powerful placebo or participation effect. Which view prevails will be the subject of another fascinating chapter in the evolution of hyperbaric practice and will involve the use of more rigorous trial design with the parallel administration of both real and sham HBO_2 therapy, and blinding of patients, researchers and outcome assessors alike. For a more complete discussion of the issues and implications, see Mitchell 2014 and Bennett 2014.[33-34] This controversy has further to run and can only be resolved with a mutually acceptable form of sham exposure.

The second area of controversy is the treatment of problem diabetic wounds. Two recent sham-controlled RCTs have both suggested HBO_2 therapy is not effective in this condition, despite a strongly held consensus view among hyperbaric physicians that this is one of the best supported indications.[35-36] Fedorko 2016 enrolled 107 diabetic patients with Wagner Grades 2 to 4 foot lesions and reported the primary outcome of "failure to meet amputation criteria."[35] Although described as a study of chronic diabetic wounds, the minimum period of ulceration was only four weeks (the mean was about 10 months). The outcome was short-term at 12 weeks after starting treatment—the first six weeks of which the patients received the randomized intervention. The sample size was modest and despite interrogating the references, it is not clear how the sought-after difference of 28% in the incidence of major amputation was obtained. There was no discussion of the minimum clinically important difference the authors wished to exclude. Assessment of the outcome has become contentious. While the protocol indicated assessment of amputation criteria was to be done at consultation with a vascular surgeon, most assessments were done remotely using clinical notes and wound photographs. The authors reported criteria for major amputation (metatarsal or above) were similar in the two groups (odds ratio 0.91 [95% CI 0.37, 2.28], P = 0.846). Interestingly, there was only one actual amputation (a toe in the sham group) performed during the study period.

Santema 2018 enrolled 120 diabetic patients with ischemic wounds and found a statistically non-significant 10% improvement in limb salvage at one year with the addition of HBO_2 therapy to standard care (RD 10% [95% CI –4 to 23]) and a similarly non-significant in amputation free survival benefit with HBO_2 therapy (RD 13% [95% CI –2 to 28]).[36] The latter achieved statistical significance on a per protocol analysis including only those who completed the course of HBO_2 therapy. They rather starkly concluded that in patients with lower limb ischemia and diabetes, additional HBO_2 therapy didn't improve wound healing and limb salvage significantly. This conclusion seems a little definitive given the authors were unable to achieve their planned sample size to detect a limb salvage improvement of 12% (close to their measured estimate) and failure to discuss what might be a reasonable threshold for clinical significance (the minimum clinically important difference that should be excluded before rejecting a therapy). If their estimate is close to the truth, many would argue that an NNT of 10 for limb salvage at one year is well worth confirming. A further factor confounding the clear interpretation of this trial was that 35% of those allocated to HBO_2 therapy were unable to complete the course of treatment, further reducing power in this study. Intervening medical factors played a part, but the authors specifically mention the burden of daily travel over long distances to receive treatment—a reminder of the "tyranny of distance" that operates in many parts of the world in relation to HBO_2 therapy facilities.

The treatment of selected problem wounds will remain an area of debate for some time yet.

These two areas of controversy both speak to the importance of thoroughly planning RCTs and the great practical difficulty in achieving high-quality results with a low risk of bias. This seems a cross the field is required to bear given the historical difficulty of obtaining funding. For Santema 2018 the problem was limited funding mandating a 30-month maximum recruitment window that constrained power and for Fedorko 2016 it appears changes to the protocol after ethics review may have fundamentally altered the estimation of amputation rates, while the study seems both underpowered to exclude important differences and the primary outcome too short-term to be meaningful. The high potential for bias in the open design of Efrati 2013 is problematic and any attempt at sham controlling and blinding is currently, and conveniently, unacceptable to some.

The Cochrane Collaboration

It is generally accepted that results from well-designed double-blind prospective RCTs are the gold standard for directing clinical decision-making. As discussed above, one of the problems with hyperbaric literature has been that many RCTs were not designed with sufficient power or applicability to provide definitive clinical guidance. In many cases, small trials produced results at odds with each other, making interpretation problematic. The Cochrane Collaboration is an international non-profit and independent organization, dedicated to making up-to-date, accurate information about the effects of health care readily available worldwide. The aim is to assist health care workers and their patients to make decisions about health care. The Collaboration produces and disseminates systematic reviews of health care interventions and promotes the search for evidence in the form of clinical trials and other studies of interventions.

While not the first to synthesize data from many small trials to produce a single measure of effect size and confidence, the Cochrane Collaboration has been collating evidence since the opening of the first Cochrane Centre in 1992 under the auspices of the British National Health Service. The by-then-independent Cochrane Collaboration was formally declared in October 1993 and rapidly expanded to become a global entity. In June 2018, the Database of Systematic Reviews (CDSR) has more than 7,000 systematic reviews of the randomized evidence through many areas of clinical medicine (http://www.cochranelibrary.com/cochrane-database-of-systematic-reviews/). A total of 32 such reviews examine the therapeutic use of hyperbaric oxygenation and are included in Appendix 1. Combined with economic data, such reviews of efficacy can be used to estimate the cost-effectiveness of HBO_2 therapy for common indications. Some of these have been in a published doctoral thesis.[37] Publication in the CDSR does not guarantee that a review is free of errors and biases. Cochrane reviews must be read with the same critical eye as any other research report. While the aim of reviews is to produce an unbiased summary of the highest level of evidence, those with the motivation and expertise to perform reviews often have strong opinions in the area they are reviewing. Supporters of the collaboration suggest that these problems are likely to be of greater magnitude in non-explicit reviews of the same material, and there is some evidence that this is true.[38]

Conclusion

While not the only research methodology of value in assisting clinicians with making decisions, RCTs have a unique role because of the low propensity for bias and the ability to assume causality. Hyperbaric medicine has been widely criticized for lacking a decent evidence basis. There are, in fact, many relevant RCTs, but these can be difficult to locate, scattered as these reports are through the literature of dozens of medical and surgical specialties. Recently, these RCTs have become easier to find with the development of specialist electronic search engines and dedicated diving and hyperbaric RCT databases.

Clinicians need to develop some skills in both critical appraisal and the basic interpretation of medical statistics in order to get the most out of the literature. Using a checklist while reading core research reports is one useful approach.

Good clinical research is time-consuming, costly and difficult. This article has touched only briefly upon a few issues pertinent to the conduct of a rigorous RCT. The interested individual is encouraged to read further regarding design of RCTs.[4-17]

References

1. Medicare Services Advisory Committee. Review of interim funded service: Hyperbaric oxygen therapy for the treatment of chronic non-diabetic wounds and non-neurological soft tissue radiation injuries. MSAC Application 1054.1 Assessment Report, Commonwealth Government of Australia. ISBN 978-1-74241-605-2, 18 July 2016. http://www.msac.gov.au/internet/msac/publishing.nsf/Content/1054.1-public.
2. Health Quality Ontario. Hyperbaric oxygen therapy for the treatment of diabetic foot ulcers: a health technology assessment. Ontario health technology assessment series. 2017;17(5):1.
3. Health Technology Assessment Program, Washington State Health Care Authority. Hyperbaric oxygen therapy (HBOT) for tissue damage, including wound care and treatment of central nervous system (CNS) conditions. Final Evidence Report. 15 February 2013. https://www.hca.wa.gov/assets/program/021513_hbot_final_report[1].pdf
4. Wittes J, ed. (Special Design Issue). Controlled clinical trials. 1998;19(4):313-418.
5. Frieden TR. Evidence for health decision making—beyond randomized, controlled trials. New England Journal of Medicine. 2017 Aug 3;377(5):465-75.
6. Moher D, Hopewell S, Schulz KF, et al. CONSORT 2010 Explanation and elaboration: updated guidelines for reporting parallel group randomised trials. BMJ 2010;340:c869.
7. Machin D, Campbell MJ, Fayers PM, Pinol APY. Sample size tables for clinical studies, 2nd ed. Blackwell Science Ltd. Malden, MA. 1997.
8. Phillips B, Ball C, Sackett D, et al. Oxford Centre for Evidence-based Medicine http://www.cebm.net/ (last accessed January 2013).
9. Ho PM, Peterson PN, Masoudi FA. Key issues in outcomes research Evaluating the evidence. Is there a rigid hierarchy? Circulation. 2008;118:1675-1684.
10. Hopewell S, Dutton S, Yu LM, Chan AW, Altman DG. The quality of reports of randomised trials in 2000 and 2006: comparative study of articles indexed in PubMed. BMJ 340: c723.
11. Treweek S, Zwarenstein M. What kind of randomised trials do patients and clinicians need? Evidence Based Medicine 2009;14:101-103.
12. Zwarenstein M, Treweek S, Gagnier JJ, et al. Improving the reporting of pragmatic trials: an extension of the CONSORT statement.BMJ 2008;337:a2390.
13. Foëx BA. The ethics of clinical trials. Anaesthesia & Intensive Care Medicine. 2009 Feb 1;10(2):98-101.
14. Freedman B. Equipoise and the ethics of clinical research. N Engl J Med. 1987;317:141-145.
15. Veatch R. The irrelevance of equipoise. Journal of Medical Philosophy 2007;32:167-183.
16. Ubel PA, Silbergleit R. Behavioral equipoise: A way to resolve ethical stalemates in clinical research. The American Journal of Bioethics. 2008;11:1-8.
17. Kahneman D, Tversky A. The psychology of preferences. Scientific American. 1982;246:160–173.
18. Truzzi M. On the extraordinary: an attempt at clarification. Zetetic Scholar. 1978;1:11.
19. Sackett DL, Straus SE, Richardson WS, Rosenberg W, Haynes RB (2000). Evidence-based medicine: How to practice and teach EBM (2nd ed.). Edinburgh: Churchill Livingstone, 2000:1.
20. Evidence-Based Medicine Working Group. Evidence-based medicine. A new approach to teaching the practice of medicine. JAMA 1992; 268:2420-2425.
21. Sackett DL, Straus SE, Richardson WS, Rosenberg W, Haynes RB. Teaching methods relevant to the clinical application of the results of critical appraisals to individual patients. In: Evidence-based medicine. How to practice and teach EBM (2nd Ed). Churchill Livingstone; London. 2000.
22. Bennett MH, Connor D, Lehm JP. The database of randomized controlled trials in hyperbaric medicine (DORCTHIM). http://hboevidence.unsw.wikispaces.net/.
23. Morris AH. Randomized clinical trials (Editorial). Trans Am Soc Artif Intern Organs 1991;27:41-42.
22. The Oxford Centre for Evidence-based Medicine. http://www.cebm.net/ (Accessed January 2013).
24. Turner JA, Deyo RA, Loeser JD, Korff MV, Fordyce WE. The importance of placebo effects in pain treatment and research. JAMA 1994;271:1609-1614.
25. UK Parliamentary Committee Science and Technology Committee. Evidence Check 2: Homeopathy 2010. February 2010:10-12. Evidence Check 2: Homoepathy 2010 (accessed January 2013).
26. McCarney R, Warner J, Iliffe S, van Haselen R, Griffin P, Fisher P. The Hawthorne effect: a randomised, controlled trial. BMC Medical Research Methodology. 2007;7:30.
27. Clarke RE, Catalina Tenorio LM, Hussey JR, Toklu AS, Cone DL, Hinojosa JG, et al. Hyperbaric oxygen treatment of chronic refractory radiation proctitis: a randomised and controlled double-blind crossover trial with long-term follow-up. International Journal of Radiation Oncology, Biology, Physics. 2008;72:134-143.

28. Weaver LK, Hopkins RO, Churchill S, Haberstock D. Double-blinding is possible in hyperbaric oxygen (HBO$_2$) randomized clinical trials (RCT) using a minimal chamber pressurization as control (abstract). Undersea and Hyperbaric Med. 1997;24(Suppl):36.

29. Weaver LK, Churchill SK, Bell J, Deru K, Snow GL. A blinded trial to investigate whether 'pressure familiar' individuals can determine chamber pressure. Undersea and Hyperbaric Medicine. 2012;39:801-5.

30. Jansen T, Mortensen CR, Tvede MF. It is possible to perform a double-blind hyperbaric session: a double-blinded randomized trial performed on healthy volunteers. Undersea Hyperb Med. 2009 Sep-Oct;36(5):347-51.

31. Wolf G, Cifu D, Baugh L, Carne W, Profenna L. The effect of hyperbaric oxygen on symptoms after mild traumatic brain injury. Journal of Neurotrauma. 2012. Pp:2606-2612.

32. Efrati S, Fishlev G, Bechor Y, Volkov O, Bergan J, et al. Hyperbaric oxygen induces late neuroplasticity in post stroke patients – randomized prospective trial. PLoS ONE 2013;8(1):e53716.

33. Mitchell SJ, Bennett MH. Unestablished indications for hyperbaric oxygen therapy. Diving Hyperb Med. 2014 Dec 1;44(4):228-34.

34. Bennett MH. Hyperbaric medicine and the placebo effect. Diving Hyperb Med. 2014 Dec 1;44:235-40.

35. Fedorko L, Bowen JM, Jones W, Oreopoulos G, Goeree R, Hopkins RB, O'Reilly DJ. Hyperbaric oxygen therapy does not reduce indications for amputation in patients with diabetes with nonhealing ulcers of the lower limb: a prospective, double-blind, randomized controlled clinical trial. Diabetes Care. 2016 Mar 1;39(3):392-9.

36. Santema KT, Stoekenbroek RM, Koelemay MJ, Reekers JA, van Dortmont LM, Oomen A, Smeets L, Wever JJ, Legemate DA, Ubbink DT. Hyperbaric Oxygen Therapy in the Treatment of Ischemic Lower-Extremity Ulcers in Patients With Diabetes: Results of the DAMO2CLES Multicenter Randomized Clinical Trial. Diabetes care. 2018 Jan 1;41(1):112-9.

37. Bennett MH. The evidence basis of diving and hyperbaric medicine - a synthesis of the high level clinical evidence with meta-analysis. http://trove.nla.gov.au/.

38. Jørgensen AW, Hilden J, Gøtzsche PC. Cochrane reviews compared with industry supported meta-analyses and other meta-analyses of the same drugs: systematic review. BMJ 2006;333:782.

Appendix 1: Randomized Clinical Trials in Hyperbaric Medicine

This list includes abstracts when there has been no more complete report.

Acute Thermal Burns

1. Hart GB, O'Reily RR, Broussard N, Cave RH, Goodman DB, Yanda RL. Treatment of burns with hyperbaric oxygen. Surg Gynecol Obstet. 1974;139:693-696.
2. Hammarlund C, Svedman C, Svedman P. Hyperbaric oxygen treatment of healthy volunteers with U.V.-irradiated blister wounds. Burns. 1991;17(4):296-301.
3. Brannen AL, Still J, Haynes M, Orlet H, Rosenblum F, Law E, Thompson WO. A randomized prospective trial of hyperbaric oxygen in a referral burn center population. Am Surgeon. 1997;63(3):205-208.
4. Niezgoda JA, Cianci P, Folden BW, Ortega RL, Slade JB, Storrow AB. The effect of hyperbaric oxygen therapy on a burn wound model in human volunteers. Plastic and Reconstructive Surgery. 1997;99:1620-1625.
5. Xu N, Li Z, Luo X. [Effects of hyperbaric oxygen therapy on the changes in serum sIL-2R and Fn in severe burn patients]. Zhonghua Zheng Xing Shao Shang Wai Ke Za Zhi. 1999; 15(3):220-223.
6. Villanueva E, Bennett MH, Wasiak J, Lehm JP. Hyperbaric oxygen therapy for thermal burns (Cochrane Review). In: The Cochrane Library (Issue 3, 2004). Chichester, UK: John Wiley & Sons, Ltd.
7. Ma L, Li P, Shi Z, Hou T, Chen X, Du J. A prospective, randomized, controlled study of hyperbaric oxygen therapy: effects on healing and oxidative stress of ulcer tissue in patients with a diabetic foot ulcer. Ostomy Wound Manage. 2013 Mar 1;59(3):18-24.
8. Rasmussen VM, Borgen AE, Jansen EC, Rotbøll Nielsen PH, Werner MU. Hyperbaric oxygen therapy attenuates central sensitization induced by a thermal injury in humans. Acta Anaesthesiologica Scandinavica. 2015 Jul 1;59(6):749-62.

Acute Myocardial Ischemia and Cardiac Surgery

9. Cameron AJV, Gibb BH, Ledingham IMcA. A controlled clinical trial of hyperbaric oxygen in the treatment of acute myocardial infarction. Proceedings of the Second International Congress. London: ES Livingston; 1965. P:277.
10. Thurston JGB, Greenwood TW, Bending MR, Connor H, Curwen MP. A controlled investigation into the effects of hyperbaric oxygen on mortality following acute myocardial infarction. Q J Med, New Series, XLII. 1973;168:751-770.
11. Swift PC, Turner JH, Oxer HF, O'Shea JP, Lane GK. Myocardial hibernation identified by hyperbaric oxygen treatment and echocardiography in postinfarction. Am Heart J. 1992;124:1151-1158.
12. Dekleva MN, Ostojic M, Vujnovic D. Hyperbaric oxygen and thrombolysis in acute myocardial infarction: a preliminary report. In: Sitinen SA, Leinio M, eds. Proceedings of the Twenty-first Annual Meeting of the European Underwater and Baromedical Society (EUBS), Helsinki, Finland; 1995. Pp:9-13.
13. Shandling AH, Ellestad MH, Hart GB, Crump R, Marlow D, Van Natta B, Messenger JC, Strauss M, Stavitsky Y. Hyperbaric oxygen and thrombolysis in myocardial infarction: The "Hot MI" Study. Am Heart J. 1997;143(3):544-550.
14. Stavitsky Y, Shandling AH, Ellestad MH, Hart GB, Van Natta B, Messenger JC, Strauss M, Dekleva MN, Alexander JM, Mattice M, Clarke D. Hyperbaric oxygen and thrombolysis in myocardial infarction: the 'HOT MI' randomised multicenter study. Cardiology. 1998; 90:131-136.
15. Vlahovic A, Neskovic AN, Dekleva M, Putnikovic B, Popovic ZB, Otasevic P, Ostojic M. Hyperbaric oxygen treatment does not affect left ventricular chamber stiffness after myocardial infarction treated with thrombolysis. American Heart Journal. 2004;148:J1-J7.
16. Sharifi M, Fares W, Abdel-Karim I, Koch MJ, Sopdo J, Adler D. Usefulness of hyperbaric oxygen therapy to inhibit restenosis after percutaneous coronary intervention for acute myocardial infarction or unstable angina pectoris. Am J Cardiol. 2004;93:1533-1535.
17. Dekleva M, Neskovic A, Vlahovic A, Putnikovic B, Beleslin B, Ostojic M. Adjunctive effect of hyperbaric oxygen treatment after thrombolysis on left ventricular function in patients with acute myocardial infarction. Am Heart J. 2004 Oct;148(4).

18. Alex J, Laden G, Cale A, Bennett S, Flowers K, Madden L, Gardiner E, McCollum T, Griffin S. Pretreatment with hyperbaric oxygen and its effect on neuropsychometric dysfunction and systemic inflammatory response after cardiopulmonary bypass: A prospective randomised double-blind trial. Journal of Thoracic and Cardiovascular Surgery. 2005;130(6):1623-30.

19. Yogaratnam JZ, Laden G, Madden LA, Guvendik L, Cowen M, Greenman M, Seymour AM, Cale A, Griffin S. Hyperbaric oxygen preconditioning promotes cardioprotection following ischemic reperfusion injury by improving myocardial function, limiting necrosis and enhancing the induction of Hsp72. Undersea and Hyperbaric Medicine. 2007;34(4):301-302.

20. Li Y, Dong H, Chen M, Liu J, Yang L, Chen S, Xiong L. Preconditioning with repeated hyperbaric oxygen induces myocardial and cerebral protection in patients undergoing coronary artery bypass graft surgery: a prospective, randomized, controlled clinical trial. J Cardiothorac Vasc Anesth. 2011 Dec;25(6):908-16. doi:10.1053/j.jvca.2011.06.017. Epub 2011 Aug 25.

21. Jeysen ZY, Gerard L, Levant G, Cowen M, Cale A, Griffin S. Research report: the effects of hyperbaric oxygen preconditioning on myocardial biomarkers of cardioprotection in patients having coronary artery bypass graftsurgery. Undersea Hyperb Med. 2011 May-Jun;38(3):175-85.

22. Bennett MH, Lehm JP, Jepson N. Hyperbaric oxygen therapy for acute coronary syndrome. Cochrane Database of Systematic Reviews 2015, Issue 7. Art. No.: CD004818. DOI: 10.1002/14651858.CD004818.pub4.

Altitude Sickness

23. Kasic J, Yaron M, Nicholas R, Lickteig J, Roach R. Treatment of acute mountain sickness: hyperbaric versus oxygen therapy. Annals of Emergency Medicine. 1991;20:1109-1112.

24. Bartsch P, Merki B, Hofstetter D, Maggiorini M, Kayser B, Oelz O. Treatment of acute mountain sickness by simulated descent: a randomised controlled trial. British Medical Journal. 1993;306:1098-1101.

25. Kayser B, Jean D, Herry JP. Pressurization and acute mountain sickness. Aviation Space and Environmental Medicine.1993;64(10):928-37.

Audiovestibular

26. Goto F, Fujita T, Kitoni Y, Kanno M, Kamei T, Ishii H. Hyperbaric oxygen and stellate ganglion blocks for idiopathic sudden hearing loss. Acta Otolaryngol. 1979;88:335-342.

27. Pilgramm M, Schumann K. Hyperbaric oxygen therapy for acute acoustic trauma. Archives of Otolaryngology.1985;241:247-254.

28. Pilgramm M. Clinical and animal experiment studies to optimise the therapy for acute acoustic trauma. Scandinavian Audiology (Suppl).1991;34:103-122.

29. Carlson S, Jones J, Brown M, Hess C. Prevention of hyperbaric-associated middle ear barotrauma. Annals of Emergency Medicine.1992;21:1468-1471.

30. Hoffman G, Bohmer D, Desloovere C. Hyperbaric oxygenation as a treatment of chronic forms of inner ear hearing loss and tinnitus. In: Wen-ren Li, pres. Proceedings of the Eleventh 30. International Congress on Hyperbaric Medicine (Fuzhou, China). Flagstaff, Arizona: Best Publishing Co.;1993. Pp.146-152.

31. Hoffman G, Bohmer D, Desloovere C. Hyperbaric oxygenation as a treatment of chronic forms of inner ear hearing loss and tinnitus (abstract). In: Wen-ren Li, pres. Proceedings of the Eleventh International Congress on Hyperbaric Medicine (Fuzhou, China). Flagstaff, Arizona: Best Publishing Co.; 1993. Pp:26-27.

32. Hoffman G, Bohmer D, Desloovere C. Hyperbaric oxygenation as a treatment for sudden deafness and acute tinnitus. In: Wen-ren Li, pres. Proceedings of the Eleventh International Congress on Hyperbaric Medicine (Fuzhou, China). Flagstaff, Arizona: Best Publishing Co.; 1993. Pp:141-145.

33. Dauman, R, Poisot D, Cros AM, Zennaro O, Bertrand B, Duclos JY, Esteben D, Milacic M, Boudey, Bebear JP. (Sudden deafness: A randomized comparative study of 2 administration modalities of hyperbaric oxygen therapy combined with naftidrufuryl). Rev Laryngol Otoal Rhino. 1993;114(1):53-58.

34. Cavallazzi G, Pignataro L, Capaccio P. Italian experience in hyperbaric oxygen therapy for idiopathic sudden sensorineural hearing loss. In Proceedings of the International Joint Meeting on Hyperbaric and Underwater Medicine. Marroni A, Oriani G, Wattel F, eds. Grafica Victoria, Bologna; 1996. Pp:647-649.

35. Schwab B, Flunkert C, Heermann R, Lenarz T. HBO in the therapy of cochlear dysfunctions - first results of a randomized study. Collected manuscripts of XXIV Annual Scientific Meeting of the European Underwater and Baromedical Society, M Gennser, ed. Stockholm; 1998. Pp:40-42.

36. Mutzbauer T, Mueller P, Tetzlaff K, et al. Is eustachian tube ventilatory function (ETVF) impairment after oxygen diving mediated by free radicals? Undersea and Hyperbaric Medicine 2000; 27(suppl):16.

37.	Fattori B. Sudden hypoacusis treated with hyperbaric oxygen therapy: a controlled study. Ear, Nose and Throat Journal 2001;80(9):655-660.

38.	Topuz E., Yigit O, Cinar U, Seven H. Should hyperbaric oxygen be added to treatment in idiopathic sudden sensorineural hearing loss. Eur Arch Otorhinolaryngol. 2004;261:393-396.

39.	Phillips JS, Jones SEM. Hyperbaric oxygen as an adjuvant treatment for malignant otitis externa. Cochrane Database of Systematic Reviews 2005, Issue 2. Art. No.: CD004617.

40.	Stiegler P, Matzi V, Lipp C, Kontaxis A, Klemen H, Walch C, Smolle-Jüttner F. Hyperbaric oxygen (HBO2) in tinnitus: influence of psychological factors ontreatment results? Undersea Hyperb Med. 2006 Nov-Dec;33(6):429-37.

41.	Cekin E, Cincik H, Ulubil SA, Gungor A. Effectiveness of hyperbaric oxygen therapy in management of sudden hearing loss. J Laryngol Otol. 2009 Jun;123(6):609-12.

42.	Cvorovic L, Jovanovic MB, Milutinovic Z, Arsovic N, Djeric D. Randomized prospective trial of hyperbaric oxygen therapy and intratympanic steroid injection as salvage treatment of sudden sensorineural hearing loss. Otology & Neurotology. 2013 Aug 1;34(6):1021-6.

43.	Ng AW, Muller R, Orton J. Incidence of middle ear barotrauma in staged versus linear chamber compression during hyperbaric oxygen therapy: a double blinded, randomized controlled trial. Undersea & Hyperbaric Medicine: Journal of the Undersea and Hyperbaric Medical Society, Inc. 2017;44(2):101-7.

44.	Bennett MH, Weibel S, Wasiak J, Schnabel A, French C, Kranke P. Hyperbaric oxygen therapy for acute ischaemic stroke. Cochrane Database of Systematic Reviews 2014, Issue 11. Art. No.: CD004954. DOI: 10.1002/14651858.CD004954.pub3.

Avascular Necrosis

45.	Vezzani G, Caberti L, Cantadori L, Mordacci M, Nicolopolou A, Pizzola A, Valesi M. Hyperbaric oxygen therapy (HBO$_2$) for idiopathic avascular femoral head necrosis (IAFHN): a prospective double-blind randomized trial. Undersea and Hyperbaric Medicine 2005; 32(4):272-273.

46.	Hsu SL, Wang CJ, Lee MS, Chan YS, Huang CC, Yang KD. Cocktail therapy for femoral head necrosis of the hip. Arch Orthop Trauma Surg. 2010 Jan;130(1):23-9. doi: 10.1007/s00402-009-0918-5.

47.	Camporesi EM, Vezzani G, Bosco G, Mangar D, Bernasek TL. Hyperbaric oxygen therapy in femoral head necrosis. J Arthroplasty. 2010 Sep;25(6 Suppl):118-23.

Carbon Monoxide Poisoning

48.	Raphael JC, Elkharrat D, Jars-Guincestre MC, Chastang C, Chasles V, Verken JB, Gajdos P. Trial of normobaric and hyperbaric oxygen for acute carbon monoxide intoxication. Lancet. 1989;2(8660):414-419.

49.	Ducasse JL, Izard PH, Celsis P, Leclercq Ch, Marc-Vergnes JP, Cathala B. Moderate carbon monoxide poisoning: Hyperbaric or normobaric oxygenation? In: Bakker DJ, Schmutz J, eds. Hyperbaric Medicine Proceedings, 2nd Swiss Symposium on Hyperbaric Medicine. Basel, Switzerland: Foundation for Hyperbaric Medicine; 1990. Pp:289-297.

50.	Ducasse JL, Celsis P, Marc-Vergnes JP. Non-comatose patients with acute carbon monoxide poisoning: Hyperbaric or normobaric oxygenation? Undersea Hyperbaric Med. l995;22(1):9-15.

51.	Thom SR, Taber RL, Mendiguren II, Clark JM, Hardy KR, Fisher AB. Delayed neuropsychologic sequelae after carbon monoxide poisoning: Prevention by treatment with hyperbaric oxygen. Ann Emerg Med. l995;25(4):474-480.

52.	Jay GD, Tetz DJ, Hartigan CF, Lane LL, Aghababian RV. Portable hyperbaric oxygen therapy in the emergency department with the modified Gamow bag. Annals of Emergency Medicine. 1995;26:707-711.

53.	Mathieu D, Wattel F, Mathieu-Nolf M, Durak C, Tempe JP, Bouachour G, Sainty JM. Randomized prospective study comparing the effect of HBO versus 12 hours NBO in non-comatose CO poisoned patients: results of the interim analysis. In: Proceedings of the International Joint Meeting on Hyperbaric and Underwater Medicine, Marroni A, Oriani G, Wattel F eds. Grafica Victoria, Bolognia; 1996. P:331.

54.	Scheinkestel CD, Bailey M, Myles PS, Jones K, Cooper DJ, Millar IL, Tuxen DV. Hyperbaric or normobaric oxygen for acute carbon monoxide poisoning: a randomised controlled clinical trial. Medical Journal of Australia. 1999;170:203-210.

55.	Weaver LK, Hopkins RO, Chan KJ, et al. Hyperbaric oxygen for acute carbon monoxide poisoning. New England Journal of Medicine. 2002;1347(14):1057-1066.

56.	Hampson NB, Dunford RG, Ross DE, Wreford-Brown CE. A prospective, randomized clinical trial comparing two hyperbaric treatment protocols for carbon monoxide poisoning. Undersea and Hyperbaric Medicine. 2006;33(1):27-32.

57. Hopkins RO, Weaver LK, Valentine KJ, Mower C, Churchill S, Carlquist J. Apolipoprotein E genotype and response of carbon monoxide poisoning to hyperbaric oxygen treatment. Am J Respir Crit Care Med. 2007 Nov 15;176(10):1001-6.

58. Annane D, Chadda K, Gajdos P, Jars-Guincestre M-C, Chevret S, Raphael J-C. Hyperbaric oxygen therapy for acute domestic carbon monoxide poisoning: two randomised controlled trials. Intensive Care Medicine. 2011;8658:414-419.

59. Buckley NA, Stanbrook MB, McGuigan MA, Bennett M, Lavonas E. Hyperbaric oxygen for carbon monoxide poisoning. Cochrane Database Syst Rev. 2011;(1):CD002041.

Cerebral Palsy and Autism

60. Collet J-P, Vannasse M, Marois P, et al. Hyperbaric oxygen for children with cerebral palsy: a randomised multicentre trial. Lancet. 2001;357:582-586.

61. Hardy P, Collet JP, Goldberg J, Ducruet T, Vanasse M, Lambert J, Marois P, et al. Neuropsychological effects of hyperbaric oxygen therapy in cerebral palsy. Developmental Medicine and Child Neurology. 2002;44:436-446.

62. Mathai SS, Bansali P, Singh Gill B, Nagpal S, John MJ, Aggarwal H, Bhatt V. Effects of hyperbaric oxygen therapy in children with cerebral palsy. Proceedings of the International Conference on Diving and Hyperbaric Medicine, Barcelona 7-10 September 2005:193-197.

63. Packard M. The Cornell Study. http://www.netnet.net/mums//.

64. Rossignol, DA, et al. Hyperbaric treatment for children with autism: a multicenter, randomised, double blind, controlled trial. BMC Paediatrics. 2009;9:21.

65. Granpeesheh D, Tarbox J, Dixon D, Wilke A, Allen M, Bradstreet J. Randomized trial of hyperbaric oxygen therapy for children. Research in Autism Spectrum Disorders. 2010;4:268-275.

66. Sampanthavivat M, Singkhwa W, Chaiyakul T, Karoonyawanich S, Ajpru H. Hyperbaric oxygen in the treatment of childhood autism: a randomised controlled trial. Diving Hyperb Med. 2012 Sep;42(3):128-33.

67. Xiong T, Chen H, Luo R, Mu D. Hyperbaric oxygen therapy for people with autism spectrum disorder (ASD). Cochrane Database of Systematic Reviews 2016, Issue 10. Art. No.: CD010922. DOI: 10.1002/14651858.CD010922.pub2

Cognitive Performance and Psychology

68. Boyle E, Aparico A, Canosa F, Owen D, Dash HH. Hyperbaric oxygen and acetazolamide in the treatment of senile cognitive functions. In: Trapp WG, Bannister EW, Davison AJ, Trapp PA, eds. Proceedings of the Fifth International Hyperbaric Conference. Burnaby, Canada: Simon Fraser University; 1974. Pp:432-438.

69. Raskin A, Gershon S, Crook T, Sathananthan G, Ferris S. The effects of hyperbaric and normobaric oxygen on cognitive impairment in the elderly. Archives of General Psychiatry 1978;35:50-56.

70. Allen KD, Danforth JS, Drabman RS. Videotaped modeling and film distraction for fear reduction in adults undergoing hyperbaric oxygen therapy. Journal of Consulting and Clinical Psychology. 1989;57:554-558.

71. Xiao Y, Wang J, Jiang S, Luo H. Hyperbaric oxygen therapy for vascular dementia. Cochrane Database of Systematic Reviews 2012, Issue 7. Art. No.: CD009425.

72. Vadas D, Kalichman L, Hadanny A, Efrati S. Hyperbaric Oxygen Environment Can Enhance Brain Activity and Multitasking Performance. Frontiers in integrative neuroscience. 2017 Sep 27;11:25.

73. Feng JJ, Li YH. Effects of hyperbaric oxygen therapy on depression and anxiety in the patients with incomplete spinal cord injury (a STROBE-compliant article). Medicine. 2017 Jul;96(29).

Crush Injury

74. Bouachour G, Cronier P, Gouello JP, Toulemonde JL, Talha A, Alquier PH. Hyperbaric oxygen therapy in the management of crush injuries: A randomized double-blind placebo-controlled clinical trial. J Trauma. 1996;41(2):333-339.

75. Cronier P, Bouachour G, Talha A, Gouello JP, Toulemonde JL, Merienne JF, Alquier P. The effectiveness of hyperbaric oxygen in post-traumatic skin lesions. Journal of Bone and Joint Surgery – British Volume. 1997;79(Suppl 1):56.

76. Lindstrom T, Gullichsen K, Lertola K, Niinikoski J. Effects of hyperbaric oxygen therapy on perfusion parameters and transcutaneous oxygen measurements in patients with intramedullary nailed tibial shaft fractures. Undersea and Hyperbaric Medicine. 1998;25:87-91.

77. Millar IL, Williamson OD, Cameron PA. Hyperbaric oxygen in lower limb trauma (HOLLT): Designing a randomised controlled multi-centre study. Undersea and Hyperbaric Medicine. 2007;34(4):299.

78. Bennett MH, Stanford RE, Turner R. Hyperbaric oxygen therapy for promoting fracture healing and treating fracture non-union. Cochrane Database of Systematic Reviews 2012, Issue 11. Art. No.: CD004712.

Enhancement of Radiotherapy

79. Cade IS, McEwen JB. Megavoltage radiotherapy in hyperbaric oxygen: A controlled trial. Cancer. 1967;20:817-821.
80. Brenk Van den HAS. Hyperbaric oxygen in radiation therapy: Investigations of dose-effect relationships in tumour response and tissue damage. Am J Roentgenology. 1968;102:8-26.
81. Van Den Brenk HA. Hyperbaric oxygen in radiation therapy. An investigation of dose-effect relationships in tumour response and tissue damage. American Journal of Roetgenology. 1968;102:8-26.
82. Faust DS, Brady LW, Kazem B, Germon PA. Hybaroxia and radiation therapy in carcinoma of the cervix (Stage III and IV): A clinical trial. In: Wada J, Takashi I, eds. Proceedings of the Fourth International Congress on Hyperbaric Medicine (Sapporo, Japan). Baltimore: Williams & Wilkins; 1970. Pp:410-414.
83. Henk JM. Hyperbaric oxygen in radiotherapy of head and neck carcinoma. Clin Radiol. 1970;21:223-231.
84. Tobin DA, Vermund H. A randomised study of hyperbaric oxygen as an adjunct to regularly fractionated radiation therapy for clinical treatment of advanced neoplastic disease. Am J Roentgenol Radium Ther Nucl Med. 1971;3:613-621.
85. Plenk HP. Hyperbaric radiation therapy. Preliminary results of a randomized study of cancer of the urinary bladder and review of the "oxygen experience." Am J Roentgenol Radium Ther Nucl Med. 1972;114(1):152-157.
86. Shigematsu Y, Fuchihata, Makino T, Inoue T. Radiotherapy with reduced fraction in head and neck cancer, with special reference to hyperbaric oxygen radiotherapy in maxillary sinus carcinoma (a controlled study). In: Sugahara T, Scott OCA, eds. Fraction Size in Radiobiology and Radiotherapy. Tokyo: Igako Shoin; 1973. Pp:180-187.
87. Dische S. The hyperbaric oxygen chamber in the radiotherapy of carcinoma of the uterine cervix. Br J Radiol. 1974. Pp:99-107.
88. Glassburn JR, Damsker JI, Brady LW, Faust DS, Antoniades J, Prasavinichai S, Lewis GC, Torpie RJ, Asbell SO. Hyperbaric oxygen and radiation treatment of advanced cervical cancer. Proceedings of the Fifth International Hyperbaric Congress. Simon Fraser University; 1974. Pp:813-819.
89. Chang CH, Conley JJ, Herbert C. Radiotherapy of advanced carcinoma of the oropharyngeal region under hyperbaric oxygenation. Am J Roentgenol Radium Ther Nucl Med. 1975;117(3):509-516.
90. Fletcher GH, Lindberg RD, Carderao JB, Wharton JT. Hyperbaric oxygen as a radiotherapeutic adjuvant in advanced cancer of the uterine cervix: Preliminary results of a randomized trial. Cancer. 1977;39(2):617-23.
91. Henk JM, Smith CW. Radiotherapy and hyperbaric oxygen in head and neck cancer. Interim report of second clinical trial. Lancet. 1977;8029(2):104-105.
92. Henk JM, Kunkler PB, Smith CW. Radiotherapy and hyperbaric oxygen in head and neck cancer: Final report of first controlled clinical trial. Lancet. 1977;8029(2):101-103.
93. Perrins D, Wiernik G. The medical research council's working party on radiotherapy and hyperbaric oxygen. Controlled trials in carcinoma of the bladder. Br J Radiol. 1978;51(611):876-878.
94. Watson ER, Halnan KE. Hyperbaric oxygen and radiotherapy: A medical research council trial in carcinoma of the cervix. Br J Radiol. 1978;51:879-887.
95. Cade IS, Dische S, Watson ER, Wiernik G, Sutherland I. Hyperbaric oxygen and radiotherapy: a medical research council trial in carcinoma of the bladder. Br J Radiol. 1978; 51:876-878.
96. Cade IS, McEwen JB, Dische S, Saunders MI, Watson ER, Halnan KE, Wiernik G, Perrins DJD, Sutherland I. Hyperbaric oxygen and radiotherapy: A medical research council trial in carcinoma of the bladder. Br J Radiol. 1978;51(611):876-878.
97. Cade IS, McEwen JB. Clinical trails of radiotherapy in hyperbaric oxygen at Portsmouth (1964-1976). 1978;29:333-338.
98. Ward AJ, Dixon B. Carcinoma of the cervix: Results of a hyperbaric oxygen trial associated with the use of the cathetron. Clin Radiology. 1979;30(4):383-387.
99. Berry GH, Dixon B, Ward AJ. The leeds results of radiotherapy in HBO for carcinoma of the head and neck. Clin Radiol. 1979;30:591-592.
100. Sause WT, Plenk HP. Radiation therapy of head and neck tumours: a randomised study of treatment in air vs. treatment in hyperbaric oxygen. International Journal of Radiation Oncology, Biology and Physics. 1979;5:1833-1836.
101. Brady Lw, Plenk HP, Hanley JA, Glassburn JR, Kramer S, Parker RG. Hyperbaric oxygen for carcinoma of the cervix - stages IIB, IIIB and IVA: Results of a randomized study by the radiation therapy oncology group. Int J Radiation Oncology Biol Phys 1981;7(8):991-998.

102. Henk JM. Late results of a trial of hyperbaric oxygen and radiotherapy in head and neck cancer: A rationale for hypoxic cell sensitizers? Int J Radiat Oncol Biol Phys. 1986;12(8):1339-1341.

103. Sealy R, Cridland S, Barry L. Irradiation with misonidazole and hyperbaric oxygen: Final report on arandomized trial in advanced head and neck cancer. Int J Radiat Oncol Biol Phys. 1986;12(8):1343-1346.

104. Dische S, Saunders M, Sealy R, Werner I, Verma N, Foy C, Bentzen S. Carcinoma of the cervix and the use of hyperbaric oxygen with radiotherapy: a report of a randomised controlled trial. Radiotherapy and Oncology. 1999;53:93-98.

105. Haffty BG, Peters LJ. Radiation therapy with hyperbaric oxygen at 4 atmospheres pressure in the management of squamous cell carcinoma of the head and neck: results of a randomized clinical trial. The Cancer Journal from Scientific American, 1999;5:341-347.

106. Bennett MH, Feldmeier J, Smee R, Milross C. Hyperbaric oxygenation for tumour sensitisation to radiotherapy. Cochrane Database of Systematic Reviews 2018, Issue 4. Art. No.: CD005007. DOI: 10.1002/14651858.CD005007.pub4.

Headache

107. Fife CE, Meyer JS, Berry JM. Hyperbaric oxygen and acute migraine pain: Preliminary results of a randomized blinded trial. Undersea Biomed Res. 1992;19(5):106-107.

108. Hill RK. A blinded, cross-over controlled study on the use of hyperbaric oxygen in the treatment of migraine headache. Undersea Biomed Res. 1992;19(5):106.

109. Myers DE, Myers RAM. A preliminary report on hyperbaric oxygen in the relief of migraine headache. Headache. 1995;35:197-199.

110. Wilson JR, Foresman BH, Gamber RG, Wright T. Hyperbaric oxygen in the treatment of migraine with aura. Headache. 1998;38:112-115.

111. Nilsson Remahl AIM, Ansjon R, Lind F, Waldenlind E. Hyperbaric oxygen treatment of active cluster headache: a double-blind placebo-controlled cross-over study. Cephalalgia. 2002; 22:730-739.

112. Eftedal OS, Lydersen S, Helde G, White L, Brubakk AO, Stovner LJ. A randomised, double-blind study of the prophylactic effect of hyperbaric oxygen therapy on migraine. Cephalalgia. 2004; 24:639-644.

113. Bennett MH, French C, Schnabel A, Wasiak J, Kranke P, Weibel S. Normobaric and hyperbaric oxygen therapy for the treatment and prevention of migraine and cluster headache. Cochrane Database of Systematic Reviews 2015, Issue 12. Art. No.: CD005219. DOI: 10.1002/14651858.CD005219.pub3.

Inflammatory and Autoimmune Clinical Conditions

114. Racic G, Denoble PJ, Sprem N, Bojic L, Bota B. Hyperbaric oxygen as a therapy of Bell's palsy. Undersea and Hyperbaric Medicine. 1997;24:35-38.

115. Van Hoof E, Coomans D, De Becker P, Meeusen R, Cluydts R, De Meirleir K. Hyperbaric therapy in chronic fatigue syndrome. Journal of the Chronic Fatigue Syndrome. 2003;11(3):37-49.

116. Yildiz S, Kiralp MZ, Akin A, Keskin, I, Ay H, Dursun H, Cimsit M. A new treatment modality for fibromyalgia syndrome: hyperbaric oxygen therapy. Journal of International Medical Research. 2004;32: 263-267.

117. van Ophoven A, Rossbach G, Pajonk F, Hertle L. Safety and efficacy of hyperbaric oxygen therapy for the treatment of interstitial cystitis a randomised, sham controlled, double blind trial. Journal of Urology. 2006;176:1442-1446.

118. Holland NJ, Bernstein JM, Hamilton JW. Hyperbaric oxygen therapy for Bell's palsy. Cochrane Database of Systematic Reviews 2012, Issue 2. Art. No.: CD007288.

119. Pagoldh M, Hultgren E, Arnell P, Eriksson A. Hyperbaric oxygen therapy does not improve the effects of standardized treatment in a severe attack of ulcerative colitis: a prospective randomized study. Scandinavian journal of gastroenterology. 2013 Sep 1;48(9):1033-40.

120. Gallego-Vilar D, García-Fadrique G, Povo-Martin I, Salvador-Marin M, Gallego-Gomez J. Maintenance of the response to dimethyl sulfoxide treatment using hyperbaric oxygen in interstitial cystitis/painful bladder syndrome: a prospective, randomized, comparative study. Urologia internationalis. 2013;90(4):411-6.

121. Efrati S, Golan H, Bechor Y, Faran Y, Daphna-Tekoah S, Sekler G, Fishlev G, Ablin JN, Bergan J, Volkov O, Friedman M. Hyperbaric oxygen therapy can diminish fibromyalgia syndrome–prospective clinical trial. PloS one. 2015 May 26;10(5):e0127012.

Miscellaneous

122. Hutchinson JH, Kerr MM, Inall JA, Shanks RA. Controlled trials of hyperbaric oxygen and tracheal intubation in asphyxia neonatorum. Lancet. 1966;7444:935-939.

123. Allen KD, Danforth JS, Drabman RS. Videotaped modeling and film distraction for fear reduction in adults undergoing hyperbaric oxygen therapy. Journal of Consulting and Clinical Psychology. 1989;57:554-558.

124. Verrazo G, Coppola L, Luongo C, Sammartino A, Giunta R, Grassia A, Ragone R, Tirelli A. Hyperbaric oxygen, oxygen-ozone therapy, and rheological parameters of blood in patients with peripheral occlusive arterial disease. Undersea and Hyperbaric Medicine. 1995; 22:17-22.

125. Kiralp MZ, Yildiz S, Vural D, Keskin I, Ay H, Dursun H. Effectiveness of hyperbaric oxygen therapy in the treatment of complex regional pain syndrome. The Journal of International Medical Research. 2004; 32:258-262.

126. Risberg J, Englund M, Aanderud L, Eftedal O, Flook V, Thorsen E. Venous gas embolism in chamber attendants after hyperbaric exposure. Undersea Hyperb Med. 2004 Winter;31(4):417-29.

127. Levett D, Bennett MH, Millar I. Adjunctive hyperbaric oxygen for necrotizing fasciitis (Protocol). Cochrane Database of Systematic Reviews 2009, Issue 3. Art. No.: CD007937.

128. Nogueira-Filho GR, Rosa BT, David-Neto JR. Effects of hyperbaric oxygen therapy on the treatment of severe cases of periodontitis. Undersea Hyperb Med. 2010 Mar-Apr;37(2):107-14.

129. Xiong T, Li H, Zhao J, Dong W, Qu Y, Wu T, Mu D. Hyperbaric oxygen for term newborns with hypoxic ischemic encephalopathy (Protocol). Cochrane Database of Systematic Reviews 2011, Issue 8. Art. No.: CD009248.

130. Wu Z, Cai J, Chen J, Huang L, Wu W, Luo F, Wu C, Liao L, Tan J. Autologous bone marrow mononuclear cell infusion and hyperbaric oxygen therapy in type 2 diabetes mellitus: an open-label, randomized controlled clinical trial. Cytotherapy. 2014 Feb 1;16(2):258-65.

Multiple Sclerosis

131. Fischer BH, Marks M, Reigh T. Hyperbaric oxygen treatment of multiple sclerosis: A randomized, placebo controlled, double-blind study. New Engl J Med. 1983;308:181-186.

132. Wood J, Stell R, Unsworth I, Lance J, Skuse N. A double-blind trial of hyperbaric oxygen in the treatment of multiple sclerosis. Medical Journal of Australia. 1985;143:238-241.

133. Erwin CW, Massey EW, Brendle AC. Hyperbaric oxygen influences on the visual evoked potentials in multiple sclerosis patients. Neurology. 1985;35(suppl 1):104.

134. Barnes MP, Cartlidge NEF, Bates D, French JM, Shaw DA. Hyperbaric oxygen and multiple sclerosis: Short-term results of a placebo-controlled, double-blind trial. Lancet. 1985;1:297-300.

135. Murthy KN, Maurice PB, Wilmeth JB. Double-blind randomized study of hyperbaric oxygen (HBO) versus placebo in multiple sclerosis (MS). Neurology. 1985;35(Suppl):104.

136. Nieman J, Nilsson B, Barr P, Perrins D. Hyperbaric oxygen in chronic progressive multiple sclerosis: visual evoked potentials and clinical effects. Journal of Neurology, Neurosurgery and Psychiatry. 1985;48:497-500.

137. Slater GE, Anderson DA, Sherman R, Ettinger MG, Haglin J, Hitchcock C. Hyperbaric oxygen and multiple sclerosis: a double-blind, controlled study. Neurology. 1985;35(Suppl 1):315.

138. Wiles CM, Clarke CRA, Irwin HP, Edgar EF, Swan AV. Hyperbaric oxygen in multiple sclerosis: A double blind trial. Br Med J. 1986;292(6517):367-371.

139. Confavreux C, Mathieu C, Chacornac R, Aimard G, Devic M. Hyperbaric oxygen in multiple sclerosis. A double-blind randomised placebo-controlled study. La Presse Medicale. 1986;15:1319-1322.

140. L'Hermitte F, Roullet E, Lyon-Caen O, et al. Hyperbaric oxygen treatment of chronic multiple sclerosis. Results of a placebo-controlled, double-blind study in 49 patients. Revue de Neurologie. 1986;142:201-206.

141. Harpur GD, Suke R, Bass BH. Hyperbaric oxygen therapy in chronic stable multiple sclerosis: double-blind study. Neurology. 1986;36:988-991.

142. Barnes MP, Bates D, Cartlidge NEF, French JM, Shaw DA. Hyperbaric oxygen and multiple sclerosis: Final results of a placebo-controlled, double-blind trial. J Neurol Neurosurg Psychiatry. 1987;50:1402-1406.

143. Worthington JA, DeSouza LH, Forti A. A double-blind controlled cross-over trial investigating the efficacy of hyperbaric oxygen in patients with multiple sclerosis. In: Rose FS, Jones R, eds. Multiple Sclerosis: Immunological, Diagnostic and Therapeutic Aspects. London: John Libbey Publications;1987.

144. Hart G, Rowe MJ, Myers LW. A controlled study of hyperbaric oxygen treatment in multiple sclerosis. J Hyperbaric Med. 1987;2(1):1-5.

145. Massey EW, Shelton DL, Greenberg J, Wewin W, Saltzman H, Bennett PB. Hyperbaric oxygen in multiple sclerosis: Double blind crossover study of 18 patients. Neurology. 1985;35(Suppl. 1):104. (Also in: Bove AA, Bachrach AJ, Greenbaum LJ, Jr., eds. 9th International Symposium on Underwater and Hyperbaric Physiology. Bethesda, Maryland: Undersea and Hyperbaric Medical Society;1987. Pp:859-857.)

146. Oriani G, Barbieri S, Cislaghi G. Long-term hyperbaric oxygen in multiple sclerosis: A placebo-controlled, double-blind trial with evoked potentials studies. J Hyperbaric Med. 1990;5(4):237-245.

147. Oriani G, Magni R, Musini A, Meazza D, Brancato R. A new electrophysiological test to assess ophthalmological benefits of hyperbaric therapy. Proceedings of the 10th International Congress on Hyperbaric Medicine, Amsterdam. Best Publishing, Flagstaff, Arizona; 1992.Pp:104-109.
148. Bennett MH, Heard R. Hyperbaric oxygen therapy for multiple sclerosis. Cochrane Database of Systematic Reviews 2004, Issue 1. Art. No.: CD003057.

Ophthalmology

149. Bojic L, Kovacevic H, Gosavic S, Denoble P. The effect of hyperbaric oxygen on glaucoma: A prospective study. In: Bakker DJ, Schmutz J, eds. Hyperbaric Medicine Proceedings, 2nd Swiss Symposium on Hyperbaric Medicine. Basel, Switzerland: Foundation for Hyperbaric Medicine;1990. Pp:273-275.
150. Oriani G, Magni R, Musini A, Meazza D, Brancato R. A new electrophysiological test to assess ophthalmological benefits of hyperbaric therapy. In: Bakker DJ, Cramer FS, Kley AJvd, van Merkesteyn JPR, eds. Proceedings of the Tenth International Congress on Hyperbaric Medicine (Amsterdam, Netherlands), Flagstaff, Arizona: Best Publishing Co.;1990. Pp:104-109.
151. Recupero SM, Cruciani F, Picardo V, Sposato PA, Tamanti N, Abdolrahimzadeh S. Hyperbaric oxygen therapy in the treatment of secondary keratoendotheliosis. Ann Ophthalmol. l992;24(12):448-452.
152. Bojic L, Kovacevic H, Andric d, Romanovic D, Petri NM. Hyperbaric oxygen dose of choice in the treatment of glaucoma. Arh Hig Rada Toksikol .1993;44(3):239-247.
153. Bojic L, Racic G, Gosovic S. The effect of hyperbaric oxygen breathing on the visual field in glaucoma. Acta Ophthalmol. 1993;71:315-319.
154. Vingolo E, Pelaia, Forte R. Rocco M, Giusti C, Rispole E. Does hyperbaric oxygen (HBO) delivery rescue retinal photoreceptors in retinitis pigmentosa? Documenta Opthalmologica; 1999;97:33-39.
155. Jalabi MW, Abidia A, Kuhan G. The safety and effect of hyperbaric oxygen therapy in patients with diabetic retinopathy - a double-blind randomised-controlled trial. Undersea and Hyperbaric Medicine. 2001;28(suppl):57.
156. Rozenek R, Brennan FF, Banks JC, Russo AC, Lacourse MG, Strauss MB. Does hyperbaric oxygen exposure affect high-intensity, short-duration exercise performance? Journal of Strength and Conditioning Research. 2007;21(4):1037-1041.

Physiology and Pharmacology

157. Merritt GJ, Slade JB. Influence of hyperbaric oxygen on the pharmacokinetics of single-dose gentamicin in healthy volunteers. Pharmacotherapy. 1993;13(4):382-385.
158. Peliai P, Rocco M, De Blasi R, Spadetta G, Alampi D, Araimo F, Nicolucci S. Assessment of lipid peroxidation in hyperbaric oxygen therapy: protective role of N-acetylcysteine. Minerva Anestesiologia. 1995;61:133-139.
159. Shupak A, Abramovich A, Adir Y, Goldenberg I, Ramon Y, Halpern P, Ariel A. Effects on pulmonary function of daily exposure to dry or humidified hyperbaric oxygen. Respiratory Physiology.1997;108:241-246.
160. Stephens M, Frey M, Mohler H. Effect of caffeine consumption on tissue oxygen levels during hyperbaric oxygen treatment. Undersea and Hyperbaric Medicine. 1999;26:93-97.
161. Thomas PS, Hakim TS, Trang LQ, Hosain SI, Camporesi EM. The synergistic effect of sympathectomy and hyperbaric oxygen exposure on transcutaneous PO2 in healthy volunteers. Anesthesia and Analgesia. 1999;88:67-71.
162. Ueno S, Tanabe G, Kihara K, Aoki D, Arikawa K, Dogomori H, Aikou T. Early postoperative hyperbaric oxygen therapy modifies neutrophile activation. Hepato-Gastroenterology. 1999;46:1798-1799.
163. Granowitz EV, Skulsky EJ, Benson RM, Wright J, Garb JL, Cohen ER, Smithline EC, Brown RB. Exposure to increased pressure or hyperbaric oxygen suppresses interferon-gamma secretion in whole blood cultures of healthy humans. Undersea and Hyperbaric Medicine. 2002;29(3):216-225.
164. Muth CM, Glenz Y, Klaus M, Radermacher P, Speit G, Leverve X. Influence of an orally effective SOD on hyperbaric oxygen-related cell damage. Free Radic Res. 2004 Sep;38(9):927-32.
165. Bader N, Bosy-Westphal A, Koch A, Mueller MJ. Influence of vitamin C and E supplementation on oxidative stress induced by hyperbaric oxygen in healthy men. Ann Nutr Metab. 2006;50(3):173-6.
166. Fagher K, Katzman P, Löndahl M. Hyperbaric oxygen therapy reduces the risk of QTc interval prolongation in patients with diabetes and hard-to-heal foot ulcers. Journal of Diabetes and its Complications. 2015 Nov 1;29(8):1198-202.
167. Mutzbauer TS, Schneider M, Neubauer B, Weiss M, Tetzlaff K. Antioxidants may Attenuate Plasma Erythropoietin Decline after Hyperbaric Oxygen Diving. International journal of sports medicine. 2015 Nov;36(13):1035-40.

Preconditioning, Postoperative Care and Transplantation

168. Williamson OD, Millar I, Venturoni C. Hyperbaric oxygen and the management of open tibial fractures. Journal of Bone and Joint Surgery – British Volume, Orthopaedic proceedings 2005;88-B(Suppl II):323.

169. Tang X, Yin X, Zhang T, Peng H. The effect of hyperbaric oxygen therapy on clinical outcomes of patients after resection of meningiomas with conspicuous peritumoral brain edema. Undersea and Hyperbaric Medicine. 2011;38(2):109-115.

170. Yuan JB, Yang LY, Wang YH, Ding T, Chen TD, Lu Q. Hyperbaric oxygen therapy for recovery of erectile function after posteriorurethral reconstruction. Int Urol Nephrol. 2011 Sep;43(3):755-61.

171. Ueno S, Sakoda M, Kurahara H, Iino S, Minami K, Ando K, Mataki Y, Maemura K,Ishigami S, Shinchi H, Natsugoe S. Safety and efficacy of early postoperative hyperbaric oxygen therapy with restriction of transfusions in patients with HCC who have undergone partial hepatectomy. Langenbecks Arch Surg. 2011 Jan;396(1):99-106.

172. Eskes A, Vermeulen H, Lucas C, Ubbink DT. Hyperbaric oxygen therapy for treating acute surgical and traumatic wounds. Cochrane Database of Systematic Reviews 2013, Issue 12. Art. No.: CD008059. DOI: 10.1002/14651858.CD008059.pub3.

173. Bosco G, Casarotto A, Nasole E, Camporesi E, Salvia R, Giovinazzo F, Zanini S, Malleo G, Di Tano A, Rubini A, Zanon V. Preconditioning with hyperbaric oxygen in pancreaticoduodenectomy: a randomized double-blind pilot study. Anticancer research. 2014 Jun 1;34(6):2899-906.

174. Ravaioli M, Baldassare M, Vasuri F, Pasquinelli G, Laggetta M, Valente S, De VP, Neri F, Siniscalchi A, Zanfi C, Bertuzzo VR. Strategies to Restore Adenosine Triphosphate (ATP) Level After More than 20 Hours of Cold Ischemia Time in Human Marginal Kidney Grafts. Annals of transplantation. 2018 Jan;23:34-44.

Sham and Blinding

175. Weaver LK, Hopkins RO, Churchill S, Haberstock D. Double-blinding is possible in hyperbaric oxygen (HBO$_2$) randomized clinical trials (RCT) using a minimal chamber pressurization as control (abstract). Undersea and Hyperbaric Med. 1997;24(Suppl):36.

176. Abidia A, Kuhan G, Laden G. The placebo effect of hyperbaric oxygen therapy- fact or fiction? Undersea and Hyperbaric Medicine. 2001;28(suppl):57-58.

177. Jansen T, Mortensen CR, Tvede MF. It is possible to perform a double-blind hyperbaric session: a double-blinded randomized trial performed on healthy volunteers. Undersea Hyperb Med. 2009 Sep-Oct;36(5):347-51.

178. Weaver LK, Churchill SK, Bell J, Deru K, Snow GL. A blinded trial to investigate whether 'pressure-familiar' individuals can determine chamber pressure. Undersea Hyperb Med. 2012 Jul-Aug;39(4):801-5.

Sports and Athletic Performance

179. Cabric M, Medved R, Denoble P, Zivkovic M, Kovacevic H. Effect of hyperbaric oxygenation on maximal aerobic performance in a normobaric environment. Journal of Sports Medicine and Physical Fitness. 1991;31:362-366.

180. Soolsma SJ, Clement DB, Connell DC, McKenzie DC, Taunton JB, Staples JR, Logan MA, Davidson RD. The effect of intermittent hyperbaric oxygen on short term recovery from grade II medial collateral injuries. Allan McGavin Sports Medicine Centre, Vancouver BC, Canada. 1995.

181. Borromeo CN, Ryan JL, Marchetto PA, Peterson R, Bove AA. Hyperbaric oxygen therapy for acute ankle sprains. American Journal of Sports Medicine. 1997;25:619-625.

182. Borer RC, Rozenek R, Russo AC, Strauss MB. Delayed onset of muscle soreness, neutrophil inflammatory response and hyperbaric oxygen therapy. Undersea and Hyperbaric Medicine. 1999 (Suppl); 26:12.

183. Staples JR, Clement DB, Taunton JE, McKenzie DC. Effects of hyperbaric oxygen on a human model of injury. Am Journal of Sports Medicine. 1999;27:600-605.

184. McGavock J, Lecomte J, Delaney J. Effect of hyperbaric oxygen on aerobic performance in a normobaric environment. Undersea and Hyperbaric Medicine. 1999; 26(4):219-224.

185. Mekjavic IB, Exner J, Tesch PA, Eiken O. Hyperbaric oxygen therapy does not affect recovery from delayed onset muscle soreness. Medicine and Science in Sports and Exercise. 2000;32:558-563.

186. Harrison BC, Robinson D, Davison BJ, Foley B, Seda E, Byrnes WC. Treatment of exercise-induced muscle injury via hyperbaric oxygen therapy. Medicine and Science in Sports and Exercise. 2001;33(1):36-42.

187. Webster AL, Syrotuik DG, Bell GJ, Jones RL, Hanstock CC. Effects of hyperbaric oxygen on recovery from exercise-induced muscle damage in humans. Clinical Journal of Sport Medicine. 2002;12:139-150.

188. Babul S, Rhodes EC, Taunton J, Lepawsky M. Effects of intermittent exposure to hyperbaric oxygen for the treatment of acute soft tissue injury. Clinical Journal of Sports Medicine. 2003;13:138-147.

189. Germain G, Delaney J, Moore G, Lee P, Lacroix V, Montgomery D. Effect of hyperbaric oxygen therapy on exercise-induced muscle soreness. Undersea and Hyperbaric Medicine. 2003;30(2):135-145.

190. Bennett MH, Best TM, Babul-Wellar S, Taunton JE. Hyperbaric oxygen therapy for delayed onset muscle soreness and closed soft tissue injury. Cochrane Database of Systematic Reviews 2005, Issue 4. Art. No.: CD004713.

191. Shimoda M, Enomoto M, Horie M, Miyakawa S, Yagishita K. Effects of hyperbaric oxygen on muscle fatigue after maximal intermittent plantar flexion exercise. The Journal of Strength & Conditioning Research. 2015 Jun 1;29(6):1648-56.

192. Branco BH, Fukuda DH, Andreato LV, da Silva Santos JF, Esteves JV, Franchini E. The effects of hyperbaric oxygen therapy on post-training recovery in jiu-jitsu athletes. PloS one. 2016 Mar 9;11(3):e0150517.

Stroke

193. Sarno MT, Sarno JE, Diller L. The effect of hyperbaric oxygen on communication function in adults with aphasia secondary to stroke. Journal of Speech and Hearing Research. 1972;15:42-48.

194. Anderson DC, Bottini AG, Jagiella WM, Westphal B, Ford S, Rockswold GL, Leowenson RB. A pilot study of hyperbaric oxygen in the treatment of human stroke. Stroke 1991;22(9):1137-1142.

195. Nighoghossian N, Trouillas P, Adeleine P, Salord F. Hyperbaric oxygen in the treatment of acute ischemic stroke. A double-blind pilot study. Stroke. l995;26(8):1369-1372.

196. Sansone A, Gulotta G, Sparacia B, Alongi A, Savoia G, Sparacia GV. Effect of hyperbaric oxygen therapy on neurologic recovery after focal cerebral ischaemia. British Journal of Anaesthesia. 1997;78(Suppl 1):73-4.

197. Rusyniak DE, Kirk MA, May JD, et al. Hyperbaric oxygen therapy in acute ischemic stroke. Results of the hyperbaric oxygen in acute ischaemic stroke trial pilot study. Stroke. 2003;34:571-574.

198. Imai K, Mori T, Izumoto H, Takabatake N, Kuneida T, Watanabe M. Hyperbaric oxygen combined with intravenous edaravone for treatment of acute embolic stroke: a pilot clinical trial. Neurological Medicine and Surgery (Tokyo). 2006;46:373-378.

199. Tang X-P, et al. Effects of early hyperbaric oxygen therapy on clinical outcome in postoperative patients with intracranial aneurysm. UHM. 2011;38(6):493-501.

200. Efrati S, Fishlev G, Bechor Y, Volkov O, Bergan J, et al. Hyperbaric oxygen induces late neuroplasticity in post stroke patients – randomized prospective trial. PLoS ONE. 2013;8(1):e53716.

201. Bennett MH, Weibel S, Wasiak J, Schnabel A, French C, Kranke P. Hyperbaric oxygen therapy for acute ischaemic stroke. Cochrane Database of Systematic Reviews 2014, Issue 11. Art. No.: CD004954. DOI: 10.1002/14651858.CD004954.pub3.

202. Xu Q, Fan SB, Wan YL, Liu XL, Wang L. The potential long-term neurological improvement of early hyperbaric oxygen therapy on hemorrhagic stroke in the diabetics. Diabetes research and clinical practice. 2018 Apr 1;138:75-80.

Tissue Injury and Chemotherapy

203. Xin PJ, Miao GC, Zong WC, Rong WS, Min LJ, Yingying C, An ZS, Song LT. The influence of hyperbaric oxygenation on chemotherapy effect in patients with malignant lymphoma. In: Wen-ren Li, pres. Proceedings of the Eleventh International Congress on Hyperbaric Medicine (Fuzhou, China). Flagstaff, Arizona: Best Publishing Co.;1993. Pp:44-47.

204. Heys SD, Smith IC, Ross JA, Gilbert FJ, Brooks J, Semple S, Miller ID, Hutcheon A, Sarker T, Eremin O. A pilot study with long term follow up of hyperbaric oxygen pretreatment in patients with locally advanced breast cancer undergoing neo-adjuvant chemotherapy. Undersea and Hyperbaric Medicine. 2006;33(1):33-43.

Tissue Injury Due to Radiation and Bisphosphonates

205. Tobey RE, Kelly JF. Osteoradionecrosis of the jaws. Otolaryngol Clin North Am. 1979;12(1):183-186.

206. Marx RE. Prevention of osteoradionecrosis: A randomized prospective clinical trial of hyperbaric oxygen versus penicillin. J Am Dent Assoc. 1985;(III):49-54.

207. Marx RE. Radiation injury to tissue. In: Kindwall EP, ed. Hyperbaric Medicine Practice. Flagstaff, Arizona: Best Publishing Co.;1994. Pp:447-503.

208. Hulshof M, Stark N, Van der Kleij A, Sminia P, Smeding M, Gonzalez D. Hyperbaric oxygen therapy for cognitive disorders after irradiation of the brain. Strahlentherapie und Onkol. 2001;177:192-8.

209. Pritchard J, Anand P, Broome J, Davis C, Gothard L, Hall E, Maher J, McKinna F, Millington J, Misra VP, Pitkin A, Yarnold JR. Double-blind randomized phase II study of hyperbaric oxygen in patients with radiation-induced brachial plexopathy. Radiother Oncol 2001. Mar;58(3):279-86.

210. Denton AS, Andreyev JJ, Forbes A, Maher J. Non surgical interventions for late radiation proctitis in patients who have received radical radiotherapy to the pelvis. Cochrane Database of Systematic Reviews 2002, Issue 1. Art. No.: CD003455.

211. Denton AS, Maher J. Interventions for the physical aspects of sexual dysfunction in women following pelvic radiotherapy. Cochrane Database of Systematic Reviews 2003, Issue 1. Art. No.: CD003750.

212. Annane D, Depondt J, Aubert P, Villart M, Gehanno P, Gajdos P, Chevret S. Hyperbaric oxygen therapy for radionecrosis of the jaw: a randomised, placebo-controlled, double-blind trial from the ORN96 study group. Journal of Clinical Oncology. 2004;22(24):1-8.

213. Lewis AL, Hardy KR, Huang ET, Bolotin T, Clark JM, Thom SR. Hyperbaric oxygen therapy decreases gross haematuria and improves quality of life in patients with radiation cystitis. Undersea and Hyperbaric Medicine. 2005;32(4):236.

214. Gesell LB, Warnick RE, Brenerman JC, Vogt CJ, Lindsell CJ. A randomized, controlled trial of hyperbaric oxygen therapy for brain radionecrosis. Undersea and Hyperbaric Medicine; 2005;32(4): 235-236.

215. Sidik S, Hardjodisastro D, Setiabudy R, Gondowiardjo S. Does hyperbaric oxygen administration decrease side effect and improve quality of life after pelvic radiation? Acta Med Indones. 2007;39(4):169-173.

216. Schoen PJ, Raghoebar GM, Bouma J, Reintsema H, Vissink A, Sterk W, Roodenburg JL. Rehabilitation of oral function in head and neck cancer patients after radiotherapy with implant-retained dentures: effects of hyperbaric oxygen therapy. Oral Oncol. 2007 Apr;43(4):379-88.

217. Clarke RE, Catalina Tenorio LM, Hussey JR, Toklu AS, Cone DL, Hinojosa JG, et al. Hyperbaric oxygen treatment of chronic refractory radiation proctitis: a randomised and controlled doubleblind crossover trial with long-term follow-up.International Journal of Radiation Oncology, Biology, Physics. 2008;72:134-143.

218. Esposito M, Grusovin MG, Patel S, Worthington HV, Coulthard P. Interventions for replacing missing teeth: hyperbaric oxygen therapy for irradiated patients who require dental implants. Cochrane Database of Systematic Reviews 2008, Issue 1. Art. No.: CD003603.

219. Teguh DN, Levendag PC, Noever I, Voet P, van der Est H, van Rooij P, Dumans AG, de Boer MF, van der Huls MP, Sterk W, Schmitz PI. Early hyperbaric oxygen therapy for reducing radiotherapy side effects: early results of a randomized trial in oropharyngeal and nasopharyngeal cancer. Int J Radiat Oncol Biol Phys. 2009 Nov 1;75(3):711-6.

220. Gothard J, Haviland J, Bryson P. Randomised phase II trial of hyperbaric oxygen therapy in patients with chronic arm lymphoedema after radiotherapy for cancer. Radiotherapy and Oncology. 2010;97:101-107.

221. Shao Y, Lu GL, Shen ZJ. Comparison of intravesical hyaluronic acid instillation and hyperbaric oxygen in the treatment of radiation-induced hemorrhagic cystitis. BJU Int. 2012 Mar;109(5):691-4.

222. Freiberger JJ, Padilla-Burgos R, McGraw T, Suliman HB, Kraft KH, Stolp BW, Moon RE, Piantadosi C. What is the role of hyperbaric oxygen in the management of bisphosphonate-related osteonecrosis of the jaw: a randomized controlled trial of hyperbaric oxygen as an adjunct to surgery and antibiotics. J Oral Maxillofac Surg. 2012 Jul;70(7):1573-83.

223. Esposito M, Worthington HV. Interventions for replacing missing teeth: hyperbaric oxygen therapy for irradiated patients who require dental implants. Cochrane Database of Systematic Reviews 2013, Issue 9. Art. No.: CD003603. DOI: 10.1002/14651858.CD003603.pub3.

224. Svalestad J, Hellem S, Thorsen E, Johannessen AC. Effect of hyperbaric oxygen treatment on irradiated oral mucosa: microvessel density. International journal of oral and maxillofacial surgery. 2015 Mar 1;44(3):301-7.

225. Glover M, Smerdon GR, Andreyev HJ, Benton BE, Bothma P, Firth O, Gothard L, Harrison J, Ignatescu M, Laden G, Martin S. Hyperbaric oxygen for patients with chronic bowel dysfunction after pelvic radiotherapy (HOT$_2$): a randomised, double-blind, sham-controlled phase 3 trial. The Lancet Oncology. 2016 Feb 1;17(2):224-33.

226. Rollason V, Laverrière A, MacDonald LCI, Walsh T, Tramèr MR, Vogt-Ferrier NB. Interventions for treating bisphosphonate-related osteonecrosis of the jaw (BRONJ). Cochrane Database of Systematic Reviews 2016, Issue 2. Art. No.: CD008455. DOI: 10.1002/14651858.CD008455.pub2.

227. Bennett MH, Feldmeier J, Hampson NB, Smee R, Milross C. Hyperbaric oxygen therapy for late radiation tissue injury. Cochrane Database of Systematic Reviews 2016, Issue 4. Art. No.: CD005005. DOI: 10.1002/14651858.CD005005.pub4.

Traumatic Brain Injury

228. Holbach KH, Wassman H, Kolberg T. Improved reversibility of the traumatic mid-brain syndrome following the use of hyperbaric oxygen. Acta Neurochirurgica. 1974;30:247-256.

229. Artru F, Chacornac R, Deleuze R. Hyperbaric oxygenation for severe head injuries. Preliminary results of a controlled study. European Neurology. 1976;14:310-318.

CHAPTER 19

Hyperbaric Oxygen for Symptoms Following Mild Traumatic Brain Injury

Lindell K. Weaver MD

Abstract

Hyperbaric oxygen for chronic problems after brain injury is considered investigational. The United States military has sponsored four randomized, double-blind clinical trials of hyperbaric oxygen for persistent post-concussive symptoms after mild traumatic brain injury. One of these trials found no within-group changes in post-concussive symptoms, but post-traumatic stress symptoms improved with hyperbaric oxygen at 2.0 atmospheres absolute (ATA). Two of these trials reported symptom improvement in both the hyperbaric oxygen sham groups. The fourth trial found improvement in post-concussive symptoms with hyperbaric oxygen but not sham, more dramatically in those with post-traumatic stress disorder, but improvement at six months in eye tracking in both groups. Symptom improvements were not significant at 12 months. Another study (open-label, crossover design) from the University of Tel Aviv in civilians with mild traumatic brain injury reported improved symptoms, cognitive function, and brain SPECT scans after hyperbaric oxygen. Further research is indicated regarding optimal pressure and frequency of hyperbaric oxygen and patient selection to ultimately lead to a phase III efficacy trial.

Rationale

Introduction and Definitions

Disability from brain injury, particularly traumatic brain injury (TBI), affects millions in the United States (US).[1] While some have advocated for hyperbaric oxygen (HBO$_2$) to improve functional outcome and long-standing symptoms after brain injury, HBO$_2$ is considered investigational for chronic brain injury problems. Results from several clinical trials of HBO$_2$ for persistent post-concussive symptoms after mild TBI are available, as are meta-analyses and summaries provided by the Samueli Institute[2] and the Veterans Health Administration,[3] though these reviews do not include the most recent clinical trial.[4]

Evidence-Based Review

Because of the number of US military combat personnel TBI,[5] anecdotal information that hyperbaric oxygen may improve outcome,[6-7] (Table 1) and interest from Congress, the US Department of Defense sponsored four, phase II, blinded, sham-controlled randomized trials of US service members with chronic symptoms after mild TBI. The US military-sponsored trials of HBO$_2$ for post-concussive symptoms were relatively small[8] and only one had long-term follow-up with high rates.[4] In addition, a randomized, non-blinded, crossover study in civilians with mild TBI is available from the University of Tel Aviv.[9] These five studies are summarized in Table 1 and Table 2.

Table 1. Literature Review

Study Type	Year	Investigators	N (TBI)	Patient Population	Timing of HBO₂	HBO₂ Protocol	Adverse Events	Results/Conclusions
Prospective, no control group	1985	Neubauer[18]	17	TBI, prolonged coma, randomly selected. Age 4 to 63. Excluded patients with excessive ventricular enlargement by CT.	1.5 to 23 mos.	1.5 – 2.0 ATA/60 min, 40-120 tx	None reported	16 of 17 had improved Glasgow Coma Score after course of HBO₂
Case Report	1991	Eltorai and Monroy[19]	1	58 y/o M, TBI with anoxic insult.	48 dys.	2.0 ATA/90 min, 24 tx	None reported	Recovered consciousness during first tx. Residual cognitive deficits.
Case Report	1992	Neubauer and Gottlieb[20]	2	Long-term closed head injuries	Not described	1.5 ATA/60 min, 18 and 134 tx	None reported	Improved blood flow by SPECT, "substantial clinical improvement"
Not specified	1994	Harch, et al.[21]	12	12 patients had TBI, 6 had other brain injury.	Average 3.7 yrs. post-insult (0.2- 15.2 yrs)	1.5 – 1.75 ATA/90 min, 40-80 tx	Two patients stopped at 40 and 60 sessions for "personal reasons and sinusitis"	All patients had improved SPECT scans. All patients had motor, behavioral, personality, or cognitive gains.
Case Report	1994	Neubauer, et al.[7]	1	40 y/o male, MVA, TBI with anoxic insult, total life support	7 mos.	1.5 – 1.75 ATA/60 min, 161 tx	None reported	Improved SPECT scan and cognitive function, ambulatory, communicative, and independent.
Case Report	1996	Harch, et al.[22]	1	23 y/o female, MVA with partial recovery, left with mutism, motor problems, affective problems	5.5 yrs.	1.5 ATA/90 min, 80 tx	None reported	Improved SPECT scan, behavior, mood swings, balance, and gait.
Prospective, no control group	1997	Keim, et al.[23]	4	10 patients reported, 4 with closed head injury.	Up to 11 yrs.	1.5 ATA/90 min, up to 120 tx	None reported	All had clinical improvement. Computed quantitative SPECT improved +205% for TBI patients.
Retrospective, selected cases, no control group	2002	Golden, et al.[24]	13	25 adults, 25 children, selected from 300 case files. 26% had TBI, 74% had other neurological disorders.	Average 5 yrs. post-insult	1.25 – 2.5 ATA/60 min, 2 to 12 times per week. Duration of course not specified.	None reported	Improved SPECT after HBO₂. Three children had declines in cerebral blood flow.

Table 1. Literature Review (continued)

Study Type	Year	Investigators	N (TBI)	Patient Population	Timing of HBO$_2$	HBO$_2$ Protocol	Adverse Events	Results/Conclusions
Case Report	2002	Neubauer and Gerstenbrand [25]	3	Of 5 cases presented, 3 patients with TBI: 1) 24 y/o male, coma for 4 months, sem-comatose 6 months 2) 89 y/o female, coma for 1 month, nursing home for 9 months, G-tube, spastic paralysis, aphasia 3) 21 y/o male, MVA, semi-ambulatory, poor motor skills, cognitive deficits	1) 1 yr. 2) 1.5 yrs. 3) 2 yrs.	1) 1.5 – 1.75 ATA/60 min, 600 tx 2) 1.1 ATA/60 min, 38 tx 3) 1.5 – 1.75 ATA/60 min, 64 tx	None reported	1) Returned to self-sufficiency, some residual motor disability and a mild speech impediment 2) Became much more alert, spasticity and speech improved 3) Improved SPECT scan, more alert and oriented, some cognitive deficits
Case Report	2002	Harch [26]	3	Of 450 patients with brain injury, plus all phone and email consultations, presents 37 patients who developed "untoward signs and symptoms during HBO$_2$." Four were treated for TBI. 1) 60 y/o male, stroke with TBI (fall) 2.5 years later. 2) 2 y/o "shaken baby" 3) 19 y/o female with TBI from MVA 4) 21 y/o male TBI complicated by cerebral edema, developed seizure disorder and frontal lobe abscess.	1) 3 mos. 2) 22 mos. 3) 5 mos. 4) 6 yrs.	1) 1.5 ATA/90 min, 70 tx 2) 1.75 ATA/60 min, 78 tx 3) 2.0 ATA/90 min, 10 tx, then 1.5 ATA/60 min, 40 tx 4) 1.5 – 1.75 ATA/60 min, 39 tx, then 1.25 ATA/60 min	1) "Oxygen toxicity." Peak improvement at 65 tx, rapid deterioration at 70 tx. Returned to peak level after 8-10 weeks of no HBO$_2$ 2) "Oxygen toxicity." At 38 tx, seizure frequency and medication requirement decreased. At 78 tx, seizure activity much worse than baseline. 3) "Oxygen toxicity" at 2.0 atm abs. No improvement with after 10 tx, SPECT after this course interpreted as "seizures." After second round of 40 tx, improvement in functions, SPECT showed resolution of toxicity. 4) No improvement at 1.5 atm abs, deterioration at 1.75 atm abs. Tx at 1.25 atm abs had some improvement, total number of sessions not provided.	Oxygen toxicity can occur at 1.5 and 1.75 atm abs in patients with chronic TBI.

Table 1. Literature Review (continued)

Study Type	Year	Investigators	N (TBI)	Patient Population	Timing of HBO₂	HBO₂ Protocol	Adverse Events	Results/Conclusions
Prospective pilot study, matched normal controls and matched head-injured controls	2004	Barrett, et al.[27-28]	5	3 males, 2 females. 4 subjects had closed head injuries, 1 had gunshot wound to head with bifrontal lobectomy	> 3 yrs. post-injury	1.5 ATA/60 min, 120 tx	"Oxygen toxicity." One patient had clinical improvement at 80 tx. At 110 tx, patient experienced bizarre uncontrollable behavior. SPECT imaging one year later showed deterioration in blood flow below baseline.	HBO₂ did not produce any clinical change, statistical analysis of SPECT showed no improvement in cerebral blood flow with HBO₂, SPECT scan after one HBO₂ did not predict outcome. Earlier abstract of this work reported that the results suggested "HBO₂ at 1.5 ATA is a promising therapy."
Case Report	2004	Harch and Neubauer[29]	1	Female infant with battered child syndrome and anoxic injury, cardiac arrest. Left paraplegic, with rectal prolapse, dependent on feeding tube, 5-8 seizures per day	4 mos.	1.5 ATA/60 min, 80 tx	None reported	Improved SPECT imaging, resolved rectal prolapse, removal of feeding tube. More social and interactive, no seizure activity.
Prospective, normal and head-injured controls	2006	Golden, et al.[30]	11	21 adults and 21 children, 26% with traumatic brain injury	Not reported	Not reported. Mean 28 to 35 tx.	Not reported	HBO₂ group had greater improvements than either control group.
Prospective, no controls	2006	Shi, et al.[31]	310	Ages 12-78 years, mean 45 years, all with traumatic brain injury and persistent symptoms.	Most (212) had HBO₂ within 1-6 mos. of TBI, 19 had HBO₂ > 12 mos. from TBI.	0.1 Mpa, 96% oxygen/90 min, daily sessions for 20 days, 2 courses.	None reported	SPECT imaging: 252 abnormal pre-HBO₂, 92 abnormal post-HBO₂. Similar improvements in clinical symptoms. 7 patients with previously abnormal CT had normal CT post HBO₂
Case Report	2007	Hardy, et al.[32]	1	54 y/o male with TBI from MVA	11 mos.	2.0 ATA/60 min plus 20 min compression/ decompression, 20+60 tx	None reported	HBO₂ produced electrophysiological and sensorimotor improvements after 20 sessions, which had all but disappeared one year later. Beneficial effects were restored with additional HBO₂ sessions, including improved cognitive function.

Table 1. Literature Review (continued)

Study Type	Year	Investigators	N (TBI)	Patient Population	Timing of HBO₂	HBO₂ Protocol	Adverse Events	Results/Conclusions
Prospective series, matched head-injured controls	2008	Lin, et al.[33]	22	Age ≥16 years, moderate to severe TBI, not ventilator-dependent, GCS 3 to 12	Target 1 month, actual 27.5±5.8 days from TBI	2.0 ATA/90 min plus 15-minute compression and 15 minute decompression, 20 tx	Two subjects with seizures during first week. Two subjects with ear barotraumas, received tympanostomy.	Significant short-term improvement in Glasgow Coma Scale (GCS) in HBO₂ group. No difference between groups in Glasgow Outcome Scale (GOS) at 6 months. Authors suggest this is due to the insensitivity of the GOS tool.
Case Report	2009	Harch, et al.[34]	1	25 y/o male with mild-to-moderate blast-induced TBI and PTSD. Complaints of headaches, tinnitus, sleep disruption, blurred vision, irritability, depression, fatigue, decreased hearing, imbalance, cognitive problems, PTSD.	3 yrs post-injury	1.5 ATA/60 min, 39 tx in 26 calendar days (BID)	None reported	Headaches resolved after first session. After 12 sessions, resolution of sleep disruption and depression. By end of course, improvement in fatigue, imbalance, cognitive problems. Complete resolution of PTSD. No improvement in tinnitus or blurred vision. Improved blood flow by SPECT scan.
Case Report	2009	Wright, et al.[35]	2	2 airmen injured in IED blast. Complaints of headaches, sleep disruption, irritability. Cognitive dysfunction compared to pre-morbid testing.	8 mos post-injury	1.5 ATA/60 min, 1 subject 40 sessions, 1 subject 80 sessions	None reported	Headaches resolved in first 2 weeks of HBO₂. Both returned to pre-injury function by ANAM and symptoms.
Pilot study, no controls	2010	Harch, et al.[36]	15	15 veterans with blast-induced mTBI. Neuropsychological testing, symptom questionnaires, and SPECT scanning before and after intervention (interval 35 days).	1-5 yrs post-injury, mean 2.6 years	1.5 ATA/60 min, 40 sessions (BID)	None reported	Improvement in cognitive testing and symptom reports. Improvement in SPECT scans.

Table 1. Literature Review (continued)

Study Type	Year	Investigators	N (TBI)	Patient Population	Timing of HBO₂	HBO₂ Protocol	Adverse Events	Results/Conclusions
Pilot study, controlled, blinded	2012	Wolf, et al.[10,37-40]	50	50 active duty military personnel with TBI. Participants completed cognitive testing before and after intervention. Biomarkers were also collected	3-71 months post-injury	Active: 2.5 ATA/90 min, 100% O₂, 30 sessions Sham control: 1.3 ATA/90 min, room air, 30 sessions	Difficulty with pressure equalization in ears/sinuses (52 incidents), generally resolved in-chamber. Pressure-related events were more common in the HBO₂ group than in the sham group. There were 2 sinus squeeze events and 4 confinement anxiety events. Seven participants reported worsening headaches and 3 reported nausea. No pneumothorax, seizure, claustrophobia, or fire.	Both HBO₂ and sham arms had improvement in IMPACT symptoms and cognitive performance and PTSD symptoms. Subgroup with PTSD had better response with HBO₂ on PCL-M. No significant differences on IMPACT. In a subset of 28 participants who had measurement of circulating stem cells, HBO₂ was associated with stem cell mobilization and improved cognitive function.
Prospective feasibility study, no controls	2013	Churchill, et al.[41]	28	63 adults with brain injury (stroke, anoxia, trauma) who could participate in outcome assessments. Neuropsychological, neurological, and physical therapy outcomes assessed pre-HBO₂, post-HBO₂, and 6 months post-HBO₂. Some participants also had speech and neuroimaging.	1-30 yrs post-injury, mean 7 years	1.5 ATA/60 min, 60 sessions	HBO₂-related adverse events included: myopia (3), tympanostomy tubes (3), and otitis externa (1). Other protocol-related adverse events included test anxiety (1) and fatigue (1). No pneumothorax, seizure, claustrophobia, or fire.	Conducting a definitive clinical trial in the study population is feasible. HBO₂-related adverse events and most participants tolerated study participation. Participants generally reported symptom improvement. There was little objective effect on neuropsychological or speech outcomes. Favorable changes were noted on neuroimaging, but the relationship to clinical improvement is unknown.

Table 1. Literature Review (continued)

Study Type	Year	Investigators	N (TBI)	Patient Population	Timing of HBO₂	HBO₂ Protocol	Adverse Events	Results/Conclusions
Prospective, unblinded cross-over study	2013	Boussi-Gross, et al.[9]	56	56 adults with mild TBI. Evaluated at baseline, 2 months, and 4 months.	1-5 years post-injury	HBO₂ group (n=32) (1.5 ATA, 100% O₂) Crossover group (n=24) (1.5 ATA, 100% O₂, after a 2-month control period) 40 chamber sessions, 60 min door-to-door	Not reported.	Improvement in cognitive performance and quality of life compared to control period. SPECT imaging showed increased brain activity with HBO₂.
Prospective, controlled, blinded	2014	Cifu, et al.[11,42-44]	61	61 active duty military personnel with mild TBI. Symptoms, cognitive testing, and eye tracking tested before, after, and 3 months after chamber sessions.	3-39 months post-injury, mean 8.5 months	HBO₂ 2.0 equivalent (2.0 ATA, >99% O₂) HBO₂ 1.5 equivalent (2.0 ATA, 75% O₂) Sham (2.0 ATA, 10.5% O₂) 40 chamber sessions, 60 min door-to-door	Not reported.	No significant within-group changes on RPQ, cognitive function, or balance. No clinical improvements with eye tracking. Significant improvement on PCL-M with HBO₂ 2.0 ATA.
Prospective, controlled, blinded	2015	Miller, et al.[12,45]	72	72 active duty military personnel with mild TBI. Symptom and cognitive testing before chamber sessions, after 20 chamber sessions, and after 40 chamber sessions (13 weeks post-randomization).	At least 4 months after most recent mild TBI, mean 23 months	HBO₂ (1.5 ATA, >99% O₂) Sham (1.2 ATA, air) Local care (no intervention) 40 chamber sessions 60 min door-to-door	Two participants withdrew from chamber sessions due to claustrophobia and worsening of headaches.	Worsening or no change on measures in local care group. Sham and HBO₂ groups had significant within-group improvements but no between-group differences.
Retrospective	2015	Tal, et al.[46]	10	10 patients, 4 with mild TBI. Cognitive testing and MRI before and after HBO₂.	6 months to 27 years after injury	1.5 ATA, >99% O₂ 50-70 chamber sessions 60 min door to door	Not reported	Improved whole brain perfusion and cognitive performance with HBO₂.

Table 1. Literature Review (continued)

Study Type	Year	Investigators	N (TBI)	Patient Population	Timing of HBO₂	HBO₂ Protocol	Adverse Events	Results/Conclusions
Prospective, case-controlled study	2017	Harch, et al.[47]	30	30 active duty and veteran military personnel. Assessed at baseline, immediately after HBO₂ and at 6 months (symptoms, cognitive testing, SPECT imaging).	At least 1 year after injury, mean 3 years	HBO₂ (1.5 ATA, >99% O₂) 40 chamber sessions Administered twice per day 60 min duration	One participant withdrew due to middle ear barotrauma and bronchospasm. Other adverse events were mild ear barotrauma, transient deterioration in symptoms, and anxiety unrelated to claustrophobia.	Significant improvements in neurological exam, symptoms, cognitive testing, and SPECT imaging.
Retrospective	2017	Tal, et al.[48]	15	15 patients, 8 with mild TBI. MRI and cognitive testing before and after HBO₂.	6 months to 27 years after injury	2.0 ATA, >99% O₂ 60 sessions 90 min at pressure	Not reported.	HBO₂ improved cognitive function, diffusion tensor imaging, and cerebral perfusion.
Prospective, controlled, blinded	2018	Weaver, et al.[4]	71	71 active duty and veteran military personnel. Comprehensive assessments at baseline, 13 weeks (post-chamber sessions), and 6 months, with telephone questionnaires at 12 months.	3-60 months from injury, mean 25 months	HBO₂ (1.5 ATA, >99% O₂) Sham (1.2 ATA, air) 40 chamber sessions 60 min door-to-door	Some minor, non-limiting barotrauma during 43 chamber sessions, more frequent in the HBO₂ group. No chamber-related serious adverse events.	Improvements in post-concussive and PTSD symptoms, sleeps, and anger control with HBO₂, not sham. Greatest at 13 weeks and in the subset with PTSD. Few changes in other outcomes.
Retrospective	2018	Hadanny, et al.[49]	154	154 adult TBI patients, of which 69 had mild TBI. Participants underwent cognitive and brain SPECT before and after HBO₂ course.	3 months to 33 years from injury, mean 4.6 years	40-70 daily HBO₂ sessions 60-90 min at pressure, 1.5-2.0 ATA	12% of patients reported adverse events, which included mild ear barotrauma and palpitations/dyspnea.	Improvement in global cognitive scores, memory, and attention with HBO₂. Changes to SPECT imaging in the prefrontal and temporal areas.

NOTE: ATA means atmospheres absolute.

Table 2. Randomized Trials of HBO$_2$ for Persistent Post-Concussive Symptoms after Mild TBI (adapted)[4]

	U.S. Air Force[10,37-39]	U.S. Navy/VCU[11,14,42-44]	U.S. Army: HOPPS[12,14,45]	U.S. Army: BIMA[4]	University of Tel Aviv[9]
Study arms	HBO$_2$ (n=25) (2.4 ATA, >99% O$_2$) Sham (n=25) (1.3 to 1.2 ATA, air)	HBO$_2$ 2.0 equivalent (n=21) (2.0 ATA, >99% O$_2$) HBO$_2$ 1.5 equivalent (n=21) (2.0 ATA, 75% O$_2$) Sham (n=18) (2.0 ATA, 10.5% O$_2$)	HBO$_2$ (n=24) (1.5 ATA, >99% O$_2$) Sham (n=25) (1.2 ATA, air) Local care (n=23) (no intervention)	HBO$_2$ (n=36) (1.5 ATA, >99% O$_2$) Sham (n=35) (1.2 ATA, air)	HBO$_2$ group (n=32) (1.5 ATA, 100% O$_2$) Crossover group (n=24) (1.5 ATA, 100% O$_2$, after a 2-month control period)
Sessions	30 sessions 90 minutes at pressure	40 sessions 60 minutes door to door	40 sessions 60 minutes door to door	40 sessions 60 minutes door to door	40 sessions 60 minutes door to door
Sites	Brooks City-Base, Texas Recruited from Camp Lejeune, North Carolina, 29 Palms, California, and other military installations	Naval Air Station, Pensacola, Florida Recruited from Camp Lejeune, North Carolina, and Quantico, Virginia	Fort Carson, Colorado Camp Lejeune, North Carolina Camp Pendleton, California Fort Gordon, Georgia	Fort Carson, Colorado Camp Lejeune, North Carolina Joint Base Lewis-McChord, Washington	Assaf-Harofeh Medical Center, Israel
Participants	Mean age 28 years 48 males Mean education 12 years Mean 3.4 prior concussions 33 blast 8 blunt force 9 blast and blunt force PTSD rate 50%	Mean age 23 years 60 males Education not reported 25% had >1 concussion All had at least 1 blast injury	Median age 31 years 69 males 66% had some college or more Mean 3 lifetime concussions 51 had blast injury as their most recent injury PTSD rate 66%	Mean age 33 years 70 males 82% had some college or more Mean 3.6 prior concussions 23 blast 14 blunt force 34 blast and blunt force PTSD rate 49%	Mean age 44 years 24 males Mead education level 15.2 years All blunt force injury PTSD not assessed
Qualifying injury	Neurologist-confirmed TBI diagnosis >3 months from injury 3 participants had >mild TBI	TBI-specialist confirmed diagnosis >3 months from injury	Structured interview >4 months from injury	Structured interview >3 months from injury	Diagnosis method not reported 1-6 years from injury
Head injuries during participation	Not reported	Not reported	2 participants had an additional mild TBI (over 13 weeks)	5 participants had an additional mild TBI (over 12 months)	Not reported
Outcome assessments	IMPACT, PCL-M before, weekly, and after chamber sessions	RPQ, PCL-M, eye tracking, cognitive, and balance measures before and after chamber sessions and 3 months later.	Post-concussive symptoms, quality of life, neuropsychological testing before and after chamber sessions.	Comprehensive outcome assessments at baseline, 13 weeks, and 6 months. Questionnaires at 12 months.	Neuropsychological testing, quality of life, gamma camera SPECT
Travel requirement	2-month relocation for chamber sessions and testing	2-month relocation for chamber sessions	None	Travel to Colorado Springs, Colorado at baseline, 13 weeks, and 6 months for assessments.	Not reported

Table 2. Randomized Trials of HBO₂ for Persistent Post-Concussive Symptoms After Mild TBI (adapted)[4] (continued)

	U.S. Air Force[10,37-39]	U.S. Navy/ VCU[11,14,42-44]	U.S. Army: HOPPS[12,14,45]	U.S. Army: BIMA[4]	University of Tel Aviv[9]
Compliance	Not reported	All received intervention as assigned.	24/49 (49%) assigned to chamber sessions received 40 sessions. 34/49 (69%) received ≥30 sessions. 3 sham participants received no chamber sessions.	59/71 (83%) completed 40 sessions (see Figure 2).	4 dropped out during chamber period

Protocol adherence not reported |
| **Analysis** | Not reported | Per protocol. 60/61 included in primary analysis. 10 participants excluded from cognitive performance analysis due to failed validity testing. | Intent-to-treat | Intent-to-treat | Per protocol. 6 excluded for problems on cognitive tests, 4 for inconsistent medication use. |
| **Key results** | Both HBO₂ and sham arms had improvement in IMPACT symptoms and cognitive performance and PTSD symptoms.

Subgroup with PTSD had better response with HBO₂ on PCL-M. No significant differences on IMPACT. | No significant within-group changes on RPQ, cognitive function, or balance. No clinical improvements with eye tracking.

Significant improvement on PCL-M with HBO₂ 2.0 ATA. | Worsening or no change on measures in local care group.

Sham and HBO₂ groups had significant within-group improvements but no between-group differences. | Improvements in post-concussive and PTSD symptoms, sleeps, and anger control with HBO₂, not sham. Greatest at 13 weeks and in the subset with PTSD.

Few changes in other outcomes. | Improvement in cognitive performance and quality of life compared to control period.

SPECT imaging showed increased brain activity with HBO₂. |

Briefly, the US Air Force study (n=50) showed improvement in both the sham and HBO₂ (2.4 ATA) groups in post-concussive symptoms, cognitive performance, and post-traumatic stress disorder (PTSD) symptoms. In the subgroup of participants with PTSD, the HBO₂ group had improved PTSD symptoms.[10] In the US Navy/VCU study (n=60), all participants were exposed to 2.0 ATA but each of the three arms breathed different concentrations of oxygen (10.5%, 75%, 100%).[11] PTSD symptoms improved significantly in the HBO₂ 2.0 ATA group, but other within-group changes were not significant.

The first of the trials sponsored by the US Army, HOPPS, randomized participants to receive no-intervention local care, sham, or HBO₂ (1.5 ATA). Over 13 weeks, the local care group reported worsened symptoms. Participants who went in the chamber, regardless of allocation to sham or HBO₂, had improved post-concussive symptoms, but there was no significant difference symptom severity between those two groups at 13 weeks.[12]

In the second US Army trial, BIMA, symptom severity was significantly lower in the HBO₂ (1.5 ATA) group compared to sham after 40 sessions (13 weeks). The favorable difference seen at 13 weeks was greatest in the subset with PTSD. By six and 12 months, most differences between groups were no longer significant.[4] Interestingly, the eye tracking outcomes were strikingly abnormal at baseline in both groups, but at 13 weeks and six months both groups had significant improvement, without difference between HBO₂ and sham.[13]

The study done by investigators at the University of Tel Aviv enrolled 56 civilians with post-concussive symptoms that were one to six years after mild TBI. The study was a prospective crossover design, randomized but not blinded. There was no sham comparator. After HBO_2, cognitive function, quality of life, and SPECT imaging were improved.[9]

Only BIMA incorporated long-term outcomes beyond six months. While an effort was made to obtain long-term outcomes from the US Navy/VCU and HOPPS studies, the number of respondents was low, limiting conclusions.[14]

Interpreting the synthesized results of these five studies is challenging. While all the studies tested HBO_2 for persistent post-concussive symptoms, the studies examined different populations and utilized different chamber pressures, sham designs, and outcome measures. The most similar studies, the two US Army studies, used the same sham and HBO_2 interventions and post-concussive symptom outcomes. However, in HOPPS, participants improved with both interventions, while in BIMA only those who received HBO_2 improved. The reason for this different result is not known. BIMA participants were older, had more education, and were less likely to have PTSD (49% compared to 64% in HOPPS) and more likely to complete 40 sessions (83% vs. 49% in HOPPS). The intervention group size was approximately 50% larger in BIMA. Some of the study sites were different, and fewer screened participants enrolled in BIMA (17% vs. 27% in HOPPS), possibly because of the travel requirements and extensive evaluations required.

In the University of Tel Aviv, U.S. Air Force, and HOPPS studies, participants who went into chambers reported improvement in post-concussive symptoms regardless of receiving HBO_2 or sham, while the non-chamber control groups (local care in HOPPS, crossover period in the University of Tel Aviv study) did not improve during that interval. Some attributed this improvement to placebo or Hawthorne effects,[15] while others suggested that a low-pressure air sham offers advantage to the damaged brain.[16] The military studies utilized sham controls to minimize bias. Blinding of study participants in HBO_2 studies is challenging because the participant might discover their allocation if they do not experience a change in pressure.[17] Three of the military studies utilized a minimal pressure sham (e.g., 1.2 ATA, breathing room air), while the US Navy/VCU study compressed all participants to 2 ATA and provided 10.5% oxygen to sham participants, which exposed participants to increased partial pressures of nitrogen. None of these studies were designed to determine whether a low-pressure air exposure is therapeutic for post-concussive symptoms. BIMA results did not support a therapeutic sham effect (except for eye tracking measures), or a placebo/participation effect, but the improvements in the sham arms in the other studies suggest that further investigation of a "therapeutic sham" should be considered.

All these studies were exploratory, phase II clinical trials, and conclusions about efficacy cannot be made. However, given the heterogeneity of these brain-injured participants (age, injury type and number, time from injury to intervention, rates of PTSD, extensive pharmacotherapy, etc.), that any intervention would demonstrate improvement with such small sample sizes deserves attention. Given the prevalence and importance of brain injury, further studies should be done.

Acknowledgments

Col Brian F. McCrary DO (USAF), LCDR Kevin Marrs PhD (USN), Col R. Scott Miller MD, Cheryl Dicks, Kayla Deru, Nicole Close PhD, and Col Marla DeJong PhD (USAF) contributed to the earlier editions of this review.

References

1. Zaloshnja E, Miller T, Langlois JA, Selassie AW. Prevalence of long-term disability from traumatic brain injury in the civilian population of the United States, 2005. J Head Trauma Rehabil. 2008 Nov-Dec;23(6):394-400.
2. Crawford C, Teo L, Yang E, Isbister C, Berry K. Is hyperbaric oxygen therapy effective for traumatic brain injury? A rapid evidence assessment of the literature and recommendations for the field. J Head Trauma Rehabil. 2017 May/Jun;32(3):E27-E37.
3. Peterson K, Bourne D, Anderson J, Boundy E, Helfand M. Evidence brief: hyperbaric oxygen therapy (HBOT) for traumatic brain injury and/or post-traumatic stress disorder. Portland, OR: Evidence-Based Synthesis Program (ESP), Portland VA Health Care System; 2018.
4. Weaver LK, Wilson SH, Lindblad AS, et al. Hyperbaric oxygen for post-concussive symptoms in United States military service members: a randomized clinical trial. Undersea Hyperb Med. 2018;45(2):129-156.
5. Terrio H, Brenner LA, Ivins BJ, et al. Traumatic brain injury screening: preliminary findings in a US Army Brigade Combat Team. J Head Trauma Rehabil. 2009 Jan-Feb;24(1):14-23.
6. Harch PG. The dosage of hyperbaric oxygen in chronic brain injury. In: Joiner JT, editor. The proceedings of the 2nd international symposium on hyperbaric oxygenation for cerebral palsy and the brain-injured child. Flagstaff, AZ: Best Publishing; 2002. Pp. 31-56.
7. Neubauer RA, Gottlieb SF, Pevsner NH. Hyperbaric oxygen for treatment of closed head injury. South Med J. 1994 Sep;87(9):933-936.
8. Weaver LK, Cifu D, Hart B, Wolf G, Miller S. Hyperbaric oxygen for post-concussion syndrome: design of Department of Defense clinical trials. Undersea Hyperb Med. 2012 Jul-Aug;39(4):807-814.
9. Boussi-Gross R, Golan H, Fishlev G, et al. Hyperbaric oxygen therapy can improve post concussion syndrome years after mild traumatic brain injury - randomized prospective trial. PLoS One. 2013;8(11):e79995.
10. Wolf G, Cifu D, Baugh L, Carne W, Profenna L. The effect of hyperbaric oxygen on symptoms after mild traumatic brain injury. J Neurotrauma. 2012 Nov 20;29(17):2606-2612.
11. Cifu DX, Hart BB, West SL, Walker W, Carne W. The effect of hyperbaric oxygen on persistent postconcussion symptoms. J Head Trauma Rehabil. 2014 Jan-Feb;29(1):11-20.
12. Miller RS, Weaver LK, Bahraini N, et al. Effects of hyperbaric oxygen on symptoms and quality of life among service members with persistent postconcussion symptoms: a randomized clinical trial. JAMA Intern Med. 2015 Jan;175(1):43-52.
13. Lindblad AS, Weaver LK, Wetzel PA, et al. Eyetracker outcomes in a randomized trial of hyperbaric oxygen or sham in participants with persistent post-concussive symptoms. Undersea Hyperb Med. 2017;44(5):441-442.
14. Skipper LD, Churchill S, Wilson SH, Deru K, Labutta RJ, Hart BB. Hyperbaric oxygen for persistent post-concussive symptoms: long-term follow-up. Undersea Hyperb Med. 2016;43(5):601-613.
15. Hoge CW, Jonas WB. The ritual of hyperbaric oxygen and lessons for the treatment of persistent postconcussion symptoms in military personnel. JAMA Intern Med. 2015 Jan;175(1):53-54.
16. Harch PG. Hyperbaric oxygen therapy for post-concussion syndrome: contradictory conclusions from a study mischaracterized as sham-controlled. J Neurotrauma. 2013 Dec 01;30(23):1995-1999.
17. Weaver LK, Churchill SK, Bell J, Deru K, Snow GL. A blinded trial to investigate whether 'pressure-familiar' individuals can determine chamber pressure. Undersea Hyperb Med. 2012 Jul-Aug;39(4):801-805.
18. Neubauer R. The effect of hyperbaric oxygen in prolonged coma. Possible identification of marginally functioning brain zones. Medicina Subacquea ed Iperbarica. 1985;5(3):75-79.
19. Eltorai I, Monroy R. Hyperbaric oxygen therapy leading to recovery of a 6-week comatose patient afflicted by anoxic encephalopathy posttraumatic edema. Journal of Hyperbaric Medicine. 1991;6(3):189-198.
20. Neubauer R, Gottlieb SF. Amelioration of long term head injuries with hyperbaric oxygen-documentation via SPECT brain imaging (abs). Undersea Biomed Res. 1992;19(Suppl):66-67.
21. Harch P, Gottlieb SF, Van Meter K, Staab P. HMPAO SPECT brain imaging and low pressure HBOT in the diagnosis and treatment of chronic traumatic, ischemic, hypoxic and anoxic encephalopathies (abs). Undersea Hyperb Med. 1994;21 (Suppl):30.
22. Harch P, Van Meter K, Neubauer R, Gottlieb SF. Use of HMPAO SPECT for assessment of response to HBO in ischemic/hypoxic encephalopathies. In: Jain K, editor. Textbook of hyperbaric medicine. 1996. Pp. 480-491.
23. Keim L, Aita J, Hankins J, Spethman T, Shalberg P. Quantitative SPECT scanning in the assessment of patients with ischemic/traumatic brain injury treated with HBO (abs). Chest. 1997 112(3 (suppl)):918.
24. Golden ZL, Neubauer R, Golden CJ, Greene L, Marsh J, Mleko A, editors. Improvement in cerebral metabolism in chronic brain injury after hyperbaric oxygen therapy. 2nd International Symposium on Hyperbaric Oxygenation for Cerebral Palsy and the Brain-injured Child. Flagstaff, AZ: Best Publishing Company; 2002.

25. Neubauer R, Gerstenbrand F, editors. Hyperbaric oxygen facilitates neurorehabilitation. 3rd World Congress in Neurological Rehabilitation; 2002 April 3-6, 2002; Venice, Italy: Medimond Inc.

26. Harch P, editor. The dosage of hyperbaric oxygen in chronic brain injury. 2nd International Symposium on Hyperbaric Oxygenation for Cerebral Palsy and the Brain-injured Child.Flagstaff, AZ: Best Publishing Company; 2002.

27. Barrett K, Harch P, Masel B, Patterson J, Corson K, Mader J. Cognitive and cerebral blood flow improvements in chronic stable traumatic brain injury induced by 1.5 ATA hyperbaric oxygen (abs). Undersea Hyperb Med. 1998;25(Suppl):9.

28. Barrett K, Masel B, Patterson J, Scheibel R, Corson K, Mader J. Regional CBF in chronic stable TBI treated with hyperbaric oxygen. Undersea Hyperb Med. 2004 Winter;31(4):395-406. Epub 2005/02/03. eng.

29. Harch PG, Neubauer R. HBO therapy in global cerebral ischemia/anoxia and coma. In: Jain K, editor. Textbook of hyperbaric medicine. 4th ed. Cambridge, MA: Hogrefe & Huber Publishers; 2004. Pp. 223-261.

30. Golden Z, Golden CJ, Neubauer RA. Improving neuropsychological function after chronic brain injury with hyperbaric oxygen. Disabil Rehabil. 2006 Nov 30;28(22):1379-1386.

31. Shi XY, Tang ZQ, Sun D, He XJ. Evaluation of hyperbaric oxygen treatment of neuropsychiatric disorders following traumatic brain injury. Chin Med J (Engl). 2006 Dec 5;119(23):1978-1982. Epub 2007/01/04. eng.

32. Hardy P, Johnston KM, De Beaumont L, et al. Pilot case study of the therapeutic potential of hyperbaric oxygen therapy on chronic brain injury. J Neurol Sci. 2007 Feb 15;253(1-2):94-105. Epub 2007/01/20. eng.

33. Lin JW, Tsai JT, Lee LM, et al. Effect of hyperbaric oxygen on patients with traumatic brain injury. Acta Neurochir Suppl. 2008;101:145-149. Epub 2008/07/23. eng.

34. Harch PG, Fogarty EF, Staab PK, Van Meter K. Low pressure hyperbaric oxygen therapy and SPECT brain imaging in the treatment of blast-induced chronic traumatic brain injury (post-concussion syndrome) and post traumatic stress disorder: a case report. Cases J. 2009;2:6538.

35. Wright JK, Zant E, Groom K, Schlegel RE, Gilliland K. Case report: Treatment of mild traumatic brain injury with hyperbaric oxygen. Undersea Hyperb Med. 2009 Nov-Dec;36(6):391-399.

36. Harch P, Andrews S, Fogarty E, et al. Hyperbaric oxygen therapy treatment of chronic mild-moderate blast-induced traumatic brain injury/post concussion syndrome with post traumatic stress disorder: pilot trial (abs). Eight World Congress on Brain Injury; March 10-14, 2010; Washington DC2010.

37. Wolf EG, Prye J, Michaelson R, Brower G, Profenna L, Boneta O. Hyperbaric side effects in a traumatic brain injury randomized clinical trial. Undersea Hyperb Med. 2012 Nov-Dec;39(6):1075-1082.

38. Scorza KA, McCarthy W, Miller RS, Carne W, Wolf EG. Hyperbaric oxygen effects on PTSD and mTBI symptoms: a subset analysis. Undersea Hyperb Med. 2013;40(6):548.

39. Wolf EG, Baugh LM, Kabban CM, Richards MF, Prye J. Cognitive function in a traumatic brain injury hyperbaric oxygen randomized trial. Undersea Hyperb Med. 2015 Jul-Aug;42(4):313-332.

40. Shandley S, Wolf EG, Schubert-Kabban C, et al. Increased circulating stem cells and better cognitive performance in traumatic brain injury subjects following hyperbaric oxygen therapy. Undersea Hyperb Med. 2017;44(3):257-269.

41. Churchill S, Weaver LK, Deru K, et al. A prospective trial of hyperbaric oxygen for chronic sequelae after brain injury (HYBOBI). Undersea Hyperb Med. 2013 Mar-Apr;40(2):165-193.

42. Cifu DX, Walker WC, West SL, et al. Hyperbaric oxygen for blast-related postconcussion syndrome: three-month outcomes. Ann Neurol. 2014 Feb;75(2):277-286.

43. Walker WC, Franke LM, Cifu DX, Hart BB. Randomized, sham-controlled, feasibility trial of hyperbaric oxygen for service members with postconcussion syndrome: cognitive and psychomotor outcomes 1 week postintervention. Neurorehabil Neural Repair. 2014;28(5):420-432.

44. Cifu DX, Hoke KW, Wetzel PA, Wares JR, Gitchel G, Carne W. Effects of hyperbaric oxygen on eye tracking abnormalities in males after mild traumatic brain injury. J Rehabil Res Dev. 2014;51(7):1047-1056.

45. Churchill S, Miller RS, Deru K, Wilson SH, Weaver LK. Simple and procedural reaction time for mild traumatic brain injury in a hyperbaric oxygen clinical trial. Mil Med. 2016 May;181(5 Suppl):40-44.

46. Tal S, Hadanny A, Berkovitz N, Sasson E, Ben-Jacob E, Efrati S. Hyperbaric oxygen may induce angiogenesis in patients suffering from prolonged post-concussion syndrome due to traumatic brain injury. Restor Neurol Neurosci. 2015;33(6):943-951.

47. Harch PG, Andrews SR, Fogarty EF, Lucarini J, Van Meter KW. Case control study: hyperbaric oxygen treatment of mild traumatic brain injury persistent post-concussion syndrome and post-traumatic stress disorder. Med Gas Res. 2017 Jul-Sep;7(3):156-174.

48. Tal S, Hadanny A, Sasson E, Suzin G, Efrati S. Hyperbaric oxygen therapy can induce angiogenesis and regeneration of nerve fibers in traumatic brain injury patients. Front Hum Neurosci. 2017;11:508.

49. Hadanny A, Abbott S, Suzin G, Bechor Y, Efrati S. Effect of hyperbaric oxygen therapy on chronic neurocognitive deficits of post-traumatic brain injury patients: retrospective analysis. BMJ Open. 2018 Sep 28;8(9):e023387.

APPENDIX A.

Approved Indications for HBO₂ Therapy

Disorder	HBO$_2$ Mechanism	Typical Dose	Utilization Review	Level of Evidence[1]	Class of Recommendation[1]
Air or gas embolism	Bubble reduction Inert gas washout Modulation of ischemia-reperfusion injury and inflammation Treatment of ischemia	U.S. Navy Treatment Table 6 or equivalent 1 to clinical plateau	10	C-LD	I
Carbon monoxide poisoning, acute	CO washout Treatment of ischemia Modulation of ischemia-reperfusion injury and inflammation	Up to 3 ATA (303.98 kPa) 1–3 sessions or to clinical plateau	3	A	IIa
Clostridial myositis Clostridial myonecrosis	Inhibition of toxins Suppresses organism growth Treatment of ischemia	2.4–3 ATA (243.18 kPa –303.98 kPa) 3 times in first 24 hours Twice daily for the next 2–5 days	10	B-NR	I
Crush injury Compartment syndrome Acute traumatic ischemia	Treats ischemia Limits edema Modulation of ischemia-reperfusion injury and inflammation	2–2.4 ATA (202.65–243.18 kPa) 2 times per day 2–7 days	14	B-R	I
Decompression sickness	Bubble reduction Inert gas washout Modulation of ischemia-reperfusion injury and inflammation Treatment of ischemia	U.S. Navy Treatment Table 6 or equivalent 1 to clinical plateau	10	C-LD	I
Central retinal artery occlusion	Treatment of ischemia Modulation of ischemia-reperfusion injury	2–2.8 ATA (202.65–283.71 kPa) or Table 6 or equivalent Twice daily to clinical plateau (typically less than 1 week) plus 3 days	3 days after clinical plateau	C-LD	IIb
Diabetic foot ulcer	Treat ischemia Modulation of inflammation Inhibition of infection Upregulation of growth factors, growth factor receptors, and circulating stem cells Angiogenesis	2–2.5 ATA (202.65–253.32 kPa) Daily for 3–4 weeks, based on healing response	30	A	I

cytokines, 32, 35, 53-54, 58, 164-165, 205, 311, 328-331, 333, 345

    TGF-beta, 165

D

deafness, 212, 220, 224-229, 365

debridement, 32, 37-39, 42, 47, 49-50, 52, 54, 56-57, 59, 78, 109-110, 136, 139, 167-170, 172, 176, 233, 239, 243-244, 247-251, 253, 255-256, 259, 262-265, 267-270, 272-286, 288, 304, 313-314, 321

decompression, iii, x, xiii, xviii, xxi, 1, 3-4, 8-10, 12, 90, 102, 153-158, 160-162, 170, 312, 318, 327, 329, 332, 337-339, 343-344, 348, 356, 382-383, 394

decompression illness (DCI). *See also* decompression sickness, xiii, 4, 9-10, 12, 19, 90, 153-158, 160-162, 332, 348, 356

decompression-induced bubble formation, 348

decompression sickness (DCS), iii, x, xiii, xviii, 1-2, 4, 8-10, 75, 102, 153-162, 170, 312, 327, 329, 343-345, 348, 394

    symptoms of DCS, 154

    treatment for altitude-induced, 154

delayed radiation injury, 163-166, 171, 181, 200-201

dermal elements, 305-307, 311, 317

dermal ischemia, 243, 301, 303, 308, 319-320

diabetes, xiii, 36-37, 47-48, 50, 52, 55, 57, 72-76, 88, 101, 204, 225, 242, 252, 262, 267, 292, 328, 336, 359, 363, 370-371, 373, 376-377

diabetic foot ulcers (DFUs), 34, 36-37, 41, 43, 72, 74-76, 268, 275, 282, 291-292, 362, 376-377

diabetic gangrene, 74

diagnostic imaging, 2

diffuse axonal injury (DAI), xiii, 78

diving, iii, v, ix, xvii, xviii, xxi, xxiii, xxiv, 1, 3-4, 6, 9-10, 12, 30, 76, 79, 115, 131, 149, 153-156, 160-162, 226, 229, 298, 322, 340-341, 343-344, 348, 351, 354, 361, 363, 365, 367, 371, 376

double-blinding, 356, 363, 372

E

efficacy of HBO, xi, 34, 44, 64, 117, 119, 128, 154, 312, 317

endothelial cells, 2, 8-9, 32, 73, 77, 97, 106, 124, 150, 225, 255, 262, 305, 328, 330, 333

Environmental Protection Agency (EPA), 82, 94

enzyme activity, 98, 347

epidural abscess, 233, 235, 237, 288

epidural empyema. *See also* intracranial abscess, 231

equation, 64, 293

eustachian tube dysfunction, 336

evidence-based medicine (EBM), xiii, 110, 115, 118, 125, 351-354, 362

explanatory trial, 352

eye, 13, 15, 19-21, 25, 28-30, 62, 184-185, 253, 336, 360, 375, 379, 385, 387-389, 391

    anatomy of the eye, 15

    See also central retinal artery occlusion (CRAO), optic neuritis, and myopia

F

fetal distress, 87

fibroatrophic effect, 164

fibroblasts, 32-33, 73, 128

fire, x, xv, 82, 102-103, 301, 323, 384

fixation hardware, 263, 265, 268, 270, 285-286

flaps. *See also* compromised flaps, iii, 117-136, 138-142, 145, 147, 163, 168, 170-171, 175-176, 181, 198, 258, 277, 280, 284, 291, 315, 319, 396

fluorescein angiogram, xiv, 17, 19, 22, 26

Food and Drug Administration (FDA), xiii, 260, 294

Fournier's gangrene, 241-242, 248-249, 251, 257, 259, 261

free radicals, 107, 205, 320, 329, 365

free radical scavengers, 165

frostbite, 135

G

gas embolism, iii, x, xiii, xvi, xviii, 1-3, 5-13, 153, 160-162, 327, 329, 332, 337, 341, 370, 394

    arterial, x, xiii, xviii, 1-3, 5-12, 153, 161-162, 327, 337, 341

    venous xvi, 1-2, 5-6, 8, 160, 370

gas gangrene. *See also* clostridial myonecrosis, iii, 105-115, 239, 247, 249, 261, 327

Glasgow Coma Scale (GCS), xiv, 375, 383

grafts. *See also* compromised grafts, iii, 39, 117-120, 125-134, 139, 142, 147, 265, 287, 314-315, 319, 350, 372, 376, 396

normobaric hyperoxia, 375

normobaric oxygen (NBO$_2$), xv, 17-19, 34-35, 81, 84, 88, 102, 154, 207, 294-295, 298, 343-345, 347-348, 366-367

NSAIDs, 4, 158, 242, 260

O

obliterative endarteritis, 164

omphalitis, 242-243, 247, 260-261

ophthalmic artery, 15-16, 21

ophthalmology, xviii, xix, xx, 17, 22, 28-30, 201, 336, 371

optic neuritis, 184-185

optic neuropathy, 185, 201

osteoclasts, 264, 395

osteogenesis, 264, 287, 291

osteomyelitis. *See also* refractory osteomyelitis, iii, 61, 126, 129, 135, 138, 142, 145, 151, 167, 177, 232-233, 237, 263-292, 321, 329, 333, 395

    chronic, 129, 263-265, 284, 287-292

    cranial, 268, 280

    long bone, 272, 275-277

    mandibular, 167, 278-279, 290-291

    spinal, 233, 276, 279-280, 290, 292

    sternal, 268, 274, 281-282, 284, 292

osteoradionecrosis (ORN), xv, 129, 163, 166-167, 176, 186, 190, 192, 197-199, 201, 289, 291, 332, 373-374, 395

Oxford Centre for Evidence-Based Medicine (CEBM), xiii, 118, 125, 351-352, 362

oxidant(s), 96, 98, 303, 345, 350

oxidative stress, 35, 68, 73, 75, 84-85, 95, 97-98, 187, 308, 312, 322, 328-330, 332-333, 336, 346, 349, 364, 371, 376

oxygen debt, 293-294, 296, 298

oxygen radicals, 124, 137-138

oxyhemoglobin dissociation curve, 85, 95

P

partial pressure of oxygen (PO$_2$), xv, 32-35, 61, 71, 89, 97, 108, 127, 155, 169, 203, 207, 232, 263-264, 270, 327-328, 336-338, 371

patent foramen ovale, 8

peripheral arterial occlusive disease (PAOD), xv, 77

pharmacology, xi, 371

physiology, ix, xxi, 9, 17, 28, 31-32, 35, 47, 133, 150, 160-161, 266-267, 305, 340-341, 348, 352, 370-371

pilot studies, 355

platelet activation, 344, 348

platelet derived growth factor (PDGF), xv, 36-37, 73, 330

platelet thromboemboli, 303

pneumonia, 6, 11, 105, 252, 254, 301-302, 322

pneumothorax, 3, 153, 249-250, 274, 337, 384

polymorphonuclear leukocytes (PMNs), xv, 32, 89, 106, 239, 254, 329

position paper, xii

post-antibiotic effect, 240

post-concussion syndrome (PCS), xv, 375, 390-391

pragmatic trials, 352, 362

preconditioning, iii, xxiv, 99, 306, 343, 345-350, 365, 372

preoxygenation, 343, 348

pressure ulcers, 275

problem wounds. *See also* diabetic foot ulcers (DFUs), iii, 31, 34, 48, 57, 64, 74, 114, 142, 288, 292, 340, 360, 395

progressive bacterial gangrene, 251

progressive myopia. *See also* myopia, xv, 335-336

pulmonary barotrauma, 1-3, 6, 8, 10-11, 153, 337

pulmonary oxygen toxicity, xxiv, 283, 337, 340

pyogenic infection, 231

R

radiation cystitis, 177-178, 200, 374

radiation injury, 72, 163-166, 169, 171, 174, 179-181, 183, 186, 188-189, 197, 200-201, 357, 373

    chronic. See also mandibular radiation necrosis, 166

    delayed, 163-166, 171, 181, 200-201

radiation-induced brain necrosis, 183

radiation-induced enteritis, 179

radiation-induced myelitis, 183, 185

radiation-induced proctitis, 179-180

radiation-induced sacral plexopathy, 185

radiotherapy, 197-200, 202, 280, 327, 332, 368-369, 374

randomized controlled trials (RCTs), iii, 26, 37, 41, 102, 111, 171, 206-207, 214, 216-219, 257, 282, 351-362, 397

    ethics of conducting, 353

randomized trials, 46, 86, 89-90, 102, 181, 206, 351, 353, 378-379, 387-388

reactive nitrogen species (RNS), xv, 35, 328

reactive oxygen species (ROS), xv, 32, 35, 85, 137-138, 188, 306, 328, 330, 336-337

recompression, xiv, 3, 9-10, 153-157, 161-162

red cell aggregation, 303

refractory osteomyelitis, iii, 142, 151, 263-265, 267, 270-278, 280, 282-292, 395

reimbursement, xi, 31, 37, 40, 64-65, 257, 310

Report of the Decompression Illness Adjunctive Therapy Committee of the Undersea and Hyperbaric Medical Society, 157

Report of the Hyperbaric Oxygen Therapy Committee, 110

respiratory distress syndrome, xiii, 8, 12, 103, 312

resuscitation, 4, 6, 12, 102, 154-155, 157, 296, 298, 315, 333

resuscitative weight gain, 309

retinal artery occlusion, iii, xiii, xix, xxii, 15-16, 25, 28-30, 62, 79, 394

retinal detachment, 17, 62, 79

revascularization, 38-39, 44, 50-51, 76, 118, 141, 147, 265, 320, 332

rhinocerebral mucormycosis, 232, 237, 253, 262

rhinocerebral zygomycosis, 252

Rhizopus species, 254-255

S

sample size, 48, 86, 245, 311, 347, 355-356, 359-360, 362, 378

secondary injury, 307

seizures, 1, 18, 250, 335, 337-338, 381-383
    as a side effect of HBO, 250, 335

serous otitis, 336

severe anemia, iii, 293-294, 296-297, 300, 395

shock, 81, 83, 85, 98, 105, 153, 160, 242-243, 247, 249, 260, 293, 298-299, 307, 321, 346, 376
    burn, 307
    septic, 247

shocks (electric-like), 164

silver sulfadiazine, 307-308, 316

sinus barotrauma, 283

sinus squeeze. *See also* sinus barotrauma, 335-336, 384

skeletal muscle compartment syndrome (SMCS), xv, 135-136, 140-144, 146

skin perfusion pressure (SPP), xvi, 34

smoke inhalation, 81, 92-93, 102-103, 312

soft tissue infection, 47, 126, 246, 249, 251-252, 259-261, 395

SPECT scan, 380-383

spinal osteomyelitis, 233, 276, 279-280, 290, 292

splanchnic hypoperfusion, 307-308

statistical analysis, 40, 44, 156, 351, 355-356, 382

stem cell mobilization, 34, 71-72, 197, 321-322, 384

stem, xv, 34-37, 50, 52, 71-74, 77, 164-166, 183, 197, 256, 308, 311, 317, 321-322, 328, 332, 350, 384, 391, 394-396

sternal osteomyelitis, 268, 274, 281-282, 284, 292

steroids, 23, 55-58, 120, 131, 164, 183-185, 213, 224-226, 228, 255

stroke, 8, 10-11, 17, 28, 40, 66, 76, 99, 160, 204, 220, 225, 253, 302, 320, 346, 350, 359, 363, 366, 373, 381, 384

subdural empyema. *See also* intracranial abscess, 231, 233

sudden sensorineural hearing loss (SSHL). *See also* idiopathic sudden sensorineural hearing loss, iii, xvi, 203, 220, 224-229, 366, 396

Sulfamylon, 316

supine position, 3

supplemental oxygen, 2, 16-21, 83, 86, 88, 91, 164

T

tension pneumothorax, 3

the bends. *See also* decompression sickness

thermal burns, iii, 301, 312, 322-323, 364

thromboemboli, 303

tinnitus, 81, 84, 203, 206, 208, 213, 215, 218, 220, 226-228, 365-366, 383

tissue inhibitor of metalloproteinase-1 (TIMP-1), 36

tissue oxygenation, 3, 31, 33, 39, 59, 85-86, 137, 165, 207

toxic shock syndrome, 105, 242-243, 249, 260

transcutaneous oximetry, 59, 72, 129, 376
    as a predictor of wound healing, 376

trauma, xi, xxiii, 6, 11, 17, 54-55, 77, 101-103, 108, 114-115, 117-118, 127, 135-136, 138, 141-142, 145-146, 149-151, 164, 203, 208, 220, 226, 231, 241-242, 248, 251-253, 255, 262, 264, 275, 287-290, 296, 298, 302, 319, 323, 345, 365-367, 384, 390 traumatic brain injury (TBI). *See also* mild traumatic brain injury (mTBI), iii, xv, xvi, 41, 99-101, 333, 357-358, 363, 374-375, 379-391

treatment algorithm, 249, 300

trials registration, 357

troponin I, xiii, 87, 93, 346

tympanostomy tubes, 335, 384

U

U.S. Navy treatment tables, 156, 161

Undersea and Hyperbaric Medical Society (UHMS), i-ii, v, ix-xii, xvi-xxii, xxiv, 4, 9-10, 28-30, 40, 46-47, 71, 90, 94, 102, 156-158, 161-163, 183, 201, 220, 222, 226, 272, 292, 298, 319, 327, 340-341, 354, 366, 370, 375-376

Undersea and Hyperbaric Medicine, ix, xvii, xviii, xix, xx, xxi, xxii, 31, 145, 198, 363, 365-367, 369-374, 376

Undersea Biomedical Research, ix

Undersea Medical Society, v, vi, xvi, 161-162, 287, 291, 319, 341

utilization review, iii, xii, 5, 26, 31, 48-49, 51-53, 58, 60, 62, 64, 90-91, 110, 129, 145, 157, 189, 233, 257, 283-284, 286, 296, 315-316, 394-395

V

vaginal necrosis, 181

vascular endothelial growth factor (VEGF), xvi, 36-37, 73, 99, 124, 131-132, 184, 312, 330, 376

vascular insufficiency, 29, 123, 251, 290

vascular oxidative stress, 84

venous gas embolism (VGE), xvi, 1, 3

venous stasis ulcers, 62

venous thromboembolism, 4, 157

vision loss, 15-17, 19-21, 26, 337

vitreous hemorrhage, 17

W

Wagner grading system, 38, 45

white cell adhesion, 303

World Health Organization (WHO), xvi, 46, 82, 222, 229, 357

wound bed, 33, 118, 123, 129

wound desiccation, 305

wound healing, xxiv, 31-36, 38, 40, 42, 44-45, 47-50, 58-59, 63-64, 71-76, 78, 109, 121, 126, 129, 131-132, 137, 144-145, 149, 175, 186, 188, 199, 272, 276, 302, 308, 312, 317-318, 320-323, 330, 332-333, 359, 376

wound hypoxia, 39, 71, 321

wounds, non-healing. *See also* problem wounds and diabetic foot ulcers (DFUs), 328, 376

X

xanthine oxidase, xvi, 85, 306

Z

zone of coagulation, 302

zone of stasis, 301-302, 305, 308, 317, 321

zygomycosis, 237, 252-256, 261-262
  rhinocerebral, 252

zygomycotic gangrenous cellulitis, 243, 251